Cardiovascular Imaging

Cardiovascular Imaging

Edited by Jared Peters

hayle
medical

New York

Hayle Medical,
750 Third Avenue, 9th Floor,
New York, NY 10017, USA

Visit us on the World Wide Web at:
www.haylemedical.com

ISBN: 978-1-63241-585-1

Cataloging-in-Publication Data

Cardiovascular imaging / edited by Jared Peters.
    p. cm.
Includes bibliographical references and index.
ISBN 978-1-63241-585-1
1. Cardiovascular system--Imaging. 2. Heart--Imaging.
3. Cardiovascular system--Diseases--Diagnosis. 4. Diagnostic imaging. I. Peters, Jared.
RC683.5.I42 C37 2019
616.107 54--dc23

Contents

Preface

Cardiovascular imaging is undertaken to investigate a heart condition. Various techniques are used for cardiac imaging such as coronary catheterization, intravascular ultrasound, echocardiogram, cardiac CT scan, cardiac PET scan, cardiac MRI, etc. Coronary catheterization requires blood sampling and monitoring of blood pressure by inserting a catheter into the heart to determine heart function. Intravascular ultrasound is an imaging technique that uses a long, thin, specially designed catheter that is attached to ultrasound equipment to visualize the interior wall of blood vessels and visualize the lumen. An echocardiogram is done by using ultrasonic waves for the visualization of the heart chamber and blood flow. This book explores all the important aspects of cardiovascular imaging in the present day scenario. It strives to provide a fair idea about this discipline and to help develop a better understanding of the latest advances within this field. Scientists and students actively engaged in cardiovascular imaging will find this book full of crucial and unexplored concepts.

Significant researches are present in this book. Intensive efforts have been employed by authors to make this book an outstanding discourse. This book contains the enlightening chapters which have been written on the basis of significant researches done by the experts.

Finally, I would also like to thank all the members involved in this book for being a team and meeting all the deadlines for the submission of their respective works. I would also like to thank my friends and family for being supportive in my efforts.

Editor

Evaluation of left atrial function in patients with iron-deficiency anemia by two-dimensional speckle tracking echocardiography

Jiaqi Shen, Qiao Zhou, Yue Liu, Runlan Luo, Bijun Tan and Guangsen Li[*]

Abstract

Background: Iron-deficiency anemia (IDA) is a global health problem and a common medical condition that can be seen in everyday clinical practice. And two-dimensional speckle tracking echocardiography (2D-STE) has been reported very useful in evaluating left atrial (LA) function, as well as left ventricular (LV) function. The aim of our study is to evaluate the LA function in patients with IDA by 2D-STE.

Methods: 65 patients with IDA were selected. This group of patients was then divided into two groups according to the degree of hemoglobin: group B (Hb > 90 g/L) and group C (Hb60 ~ 90 g/L). Another 30 healthy people were also selected as control group A. Conventional echocardiography parameters, such as left atrial diameter (LAD), peak E and A of mitralis (E, A), E/A, end-diastolic thickness of ventricular septum (IVST d), end-diastolic thickness of LV posterior wall (PWTd) and left ventricular end-diastolic dimension (LVDd) were obtained from these three groups. Left atrial minimum volume (LAVmin), left atrial pre-atrial contraction volume (LAVp) and left atrial maximum volume (LAVmax) were measured by Simpson's rule, whereas left atrial active ejection fraction (LAAEF) and left atrial passive ejection fraction (LAPEF) were obtained from calculation. Two-dimensional images were acquired from apical four-chamber view and two-chamber view to store images for offline analysis. The global peak atrial longitudinal strain and strain rate of systolic LV (GLSs, GLSRs) as well as early and late diastolic LV strain rate (GLSRe, GLSRa) curves of LA were acquired in each LA segment from basal segment to top segment of LA by 2D-STE.

Results: Compared with group A, there were no differences between group B and group A (all $P > 0.05$). The LAAEF and GLSRa were significantly higher in group C compared with those of group A and group B (all $P < 0.01$). The LAPEF, GLSs, GLSRs and GLSRe were significantly lower in group C compared with those of group A and group B (all $P < 0.01$).

Conclusions: 2D-STE could evaluate the LA function in patients with IDA.

Keywords: Two-dimensional speckle tracking echocardiography, Left atrial function, Iron-deficiency anemia

Abbreviations: 2D-STE, Two-dimensional speckle tracking echocardiography; E/A, Ratio of peak early and late diastolic velocities; GLSRa, The global peak longitudinal strain rate of late diastolic left ventricular; GLSRe, The global peak longitudinal strain rate of early diastolic left ventricular; GLSRs, The global peak longitudinal strain rate of systolic left ventricular; GLSs, The global peak longitudinal strain of systolic left ventricular; IDA, Iron-deficiency anemia; IVSTd, End-diastolic thickness of ventricular septum; LA, Left atrial; LAAEF, Left atrial active emptying fraction; LAD, Left atrial dimension; LAPEF, Left atrial passive emptying fraction; LAVmax, Left atrial maximum volume; LAVmin, LA minimum volume; LAVp, LA pre-atrial volume; LVDd, Left ventricular end-diastolic diameter; LVDs, Left ventricular systolic dimension; PWTd, End-diastolic thickness of LV posterior wall

* Correspondence: liguangsen09@163.com
Department of Ultrasound, The Second Affiliated Hospital of Dalian Medical University, Dalian 116027, China

Background

World Health Organization (WHO) defines Anemia as hemoglobin levels < 13 g/dL (hematocrit < 39 %) in males, < 12 g/dL (hematocrit < 36 %) in non-pregnant females, and < 11 g/dL (hematocrit <33 %) in pregnant females [1]. Iron deficiency and iron-deficiency anemia (IDA) are global health problems and common medical conditions that can be seen in everyday clinical practice [2]. WHO estimates that 42 % of pregnant women, 30 % of non-pregnant women (aged 15 to 50 years), 47 % of preschool children (aged 0 to 5 years), and 12.7 % of men older than 15 years worldwide are anemic [3]. Anemia affects one-fourth of world's population, accounted for 8.8 % of the total global burden of disease [4]. Iron deficiency is the predominant cause of anemia across countries, with women more commonly afflicted than men [4]. Although the prevalence of iron-deficiency anemia somehow has recently declined, iron deficiency continues to be the top-ranking cause of anemia worldwide. Iron deficiency may result from inadequate iron intake and absorption, increased iron requirements for growth, and excessive iron losses [5].

Based on the physiological significance of oxygen transported to myocardial tissue, anemia may be a cause of more severe cardiovascular diseases or a sign of other severe diseases that occur in the body. The physiologic response to anemia is a compensatory increase in cardiac output in order to maintain adequate oxygen delivery [6]. Patients are asymptomatic with mild anemia. Dyspnea and fatigue may occur when anemia is further aggravated. In severe cases, iron-deficiency anemia can lead to LV dysfunction and heart failure [6]. It has reported that myocardial contractility would decrease when hemoglobin was below 7 g/dL [7] and chronic anemia would result in increased LV end-diastolic pressure as well as decreased functional reserve [8]. Frequent research has been conducted on LA structural and functional remodeling, which is a cause of LV diastolic dysfunction, therefore the significance of LA has drawn much attention nowadays [9]. Increased left atrial size has been shown as an important predictor of target organ damage and multiple adverse cardiovascular events [10, 11].

2D-STE is a new technology to accurately evaluate LA function in normal subjects [12]. It has the advantage in accurate quantification of myocardial deformation and being angle independent [13, 14]. Hence the goal of the research is to evaluate the LA function in patients with IDA by 2D-STE.

Methods

Study population

Between November 2014 and April 2016, we studied 65 patients between the age of 22 and 65 with IDA, (male:

female = 1:5.5). 38 patients with IDA were caused by gynecological disease such as uterine leiomyoma, adenomyosis and increased menstrual flow. 18 patients with IDA were caused by digestive system disease such as subtotal gastrectomy. Another 9 cases with IDA were caused by unknown reasons. We rejected other causes of heart disease such as coronary heart disease, hypertension, congenital heart disease, diabetes mellitus, systemic lupus erythematosus, cardiopulmonary surgery and any grade of valvular stenosis etc. According to the degree of hemoglobin, 65 patients were classified into mild group (34 patients, 90 g/L ≤ Hb < 120 g/L, aged 25–65 years, mean age: 48.8 ± 14.1 years, male: female = 7:27, IDA duration were all between 7 months and 15 years,mean time: 6.5 ± 3.3 years) and moderate group (31 patients, 60 g/L ≤ Hb < 90 g/L aged 22–62 years, mean age: 47.6 ± 16.6 years, male: female = 6:25, IDA duration were all between 8 months and 14 years,mean time: 6.2 ± 3.6 years). In addition, we did not have enough patents with severe IDA as patients with hemoglobin below 60 g/L were very rare to find, and in most of all cases were being cured immediately, thus their duration at severe anemia stage did not last long. The control group consisted of 30 healthy volunteers (aged 23–64 years, mean age: 47.0 ± 14.5 years, male: female = 6:24). All of them had no cardiovascular diseases with all examinations results shown as normal. This study was consented by the Second Affiliated Hospital's Ethics Committee of Dalian Medical University on human research and all patients were being informed and consented to participate in this research.

Clinical and laboratory examination

All patients had completed a physical examination, From which height and weight were measured, and body mass index (BMI, kg/m^2) and body surface area (BSA, m^2) were calculated. Blood pressure and blood glucose were measured before echocardiographic examination. A 12-lead standard resting electrocardiogram (ECG) was performed among all patients.

Conventional echocardiography

An ultrasound system (Vivid E9, GE Medical Health, USA) and an M5S-D probe (1.5–4.5 MHz) were used for the study. Every subject had a conventional echocardiography examination in sinus rhythm. Every subject was connected with ECG and was in the left lateral decubitus position, eupnea. The parameters were measured by conventional echocardiography, such as left ventricular end-diastolic dimension (LVDd), end-diastolic thickness of ventricular septum (IVSTd), end-diastolic thickness of LV posterior wall (PWTd) and left atrial chamber dimension (LAD). Early (E) and late (A) diastolic mitral inflow velocities were measured by pulsed wave

Doppler, and E/A ratio was also calculated. Maximal, preatrial contraction, and minimal LA volume were acquired by the biplane modified Simpson's rule [15]. The maximum LA volume (LAVmax) was obtained before standard mitral valve opening. The precontraction LA volume (LAVp) was obtained at the precise beginning of the ECG P wave, and the minimum LA volume (LAVmin) was obtained precisely at the late diastolic left ventriculus. Then left atrial active ejection fraction (LAAEF) and left atrial passive ejection fraction (LAPEF) were calculated using the following formulas [16, 17]: passive emptying index (LAPEF) was calculated by ([LAVmax-LAVpre-a]/LAVmax), active emptying index (LAAEF) was calculated by ([LAVpre-a-LAVmin]/LAVpre-a). Standard apical four- and two-chamber views were acquired according to the guidelines of the American Society of Echocardiography (3 consecutive heart cycles). Images were stored for offline analysis.

Speckle tracking

Standard images obtained in 2D mode were analyzed using the EchoPAC software. Frame rates were controlled between 40 and 60 frames/sec. The endocardial interfaces of left atrial were demonstrated completely and they were traced manually by using a point-and-click method at the end of atrial contraction. Epicardial surface tracing were then generated automatically by the software and were changed manually based on the thickness of LA wall. The LA wall was then divided into 6 segments automatically. If some segments were unavailable due to unsatisfactory tracking quality, these images would be removed. At the end, the final results were acquired in both four and two chamber views. Longitudinal strain and strain rate curves were generated for global LA wall. Global peak LA longitudinal strain rate of early and late diastolic LV (GLSRe, GLSRa), as well as the global peak LA longitudinal strain and strain rate of systolic LV (GLSs, GLSRs) were obtained. Last but not the least, the peak longitudinal systolic strain of LV was obtained and their absolute values were compared.

Statistical analysis

The data were analyzed with SPSS 17.0 for Windows system. Numeric variables were presented as mean ± standard deviation (SD). One-way Analysis of Variance (ANOVA) was performed to test for statistically significant differences among the four groups. Continuous data were compared between differences among individual groups using the Student-Newman-Keuls post-test. All statistical tests were two sided, and $p < 0.01$ was set for statistical significance. Intra-observer analysis of global longitudinal strain and strain rate in the 4-chamber view were conducted two months after completion of the initial measurements (SJQ). For inter-observer

Table 1 Demographic and clinical characteristics of the study population

Demographic characteristics/Risk factors	Group A (n = 30)	Group B (n = 34)	Group C (n = 31)
Male: female ratio	6:24	7:27	6:25
Age, years (mean ± SD)	47.0 ± 14.5	48.8 ± 14.1	47.6 ± 16.6
Duration of IDA (years)	0	6.5 ± 3.3	6.2 ± 3.6
Heart rate(rates/min)	71 ± 12	72 ± 9	70 ± 10
Body mass index(kg/m2)	22.4 ± 2.6	23.2 ± 2.9	22.5 ± 2.7
Systolic arterial pressure(mmHg)	120 ± 11	123 ± 13	121 ± 14
Diastolic arterial pressure(mmHg)	73 ± 7	75 ± 9	73 ± 10
Blood glucose (mmol/L)	4.52 ± 0.37	4.73 ± 0.42	4.62 ± 0.28

variability, a second observer (LGS) analyzed 20 % of the initial images. Intra-observer variability and inter-observer variability were assessed using the intra-class correlation coefficient (ICC).

Results

Demographic and clinical characteristics

Demographic and clinical characteristics of the three groups are presented in Table 1. There were no significant differences among the three groups with respect to age, gender, duration of IDA, heart rates, body mass index, systolic arterial pressure, diastolic arterial pressure or blood glucose level (all P > 0.05).

Table 2 Echocardiographic characteristics of the study populations

Variables	Group A (n = 30)	Group B (n = 34)	Group C (n = 31)
LAD(mm)	32.69 ± 2.43	34.00 ± 2.80	37.49 ± 1.61*#
LVDd(mm)	43.51 ± 2.45	43.90 ± 2.36	44.35 ± 2.92
IVSTd(mm)	8.79 ± 0.67	9.10 ± 0.41	9.20 ± 0.60
PWTd(mm)	8.82 ± 0.76	9.06 ± 0.33	9.16 ± 0.53
E velocity(m/s)	0.96 ± 0.15	0.90 ± 0.18	0.72 ± 0.12*#
A velocity(m/s)	0.77 ± 0.15	0.78 ± 0.12	1.05 ± 0.16*#
E/A	1.13 ± 0.39	1.14 ± 0.34	0.70 ± 0.06*#
LAVmax(ml)	35.53 ± 2.66	37.09 ± 3.51	55.71 ± 8.72*#
LAVmin(ml)	14.19 ± 1.32	14.47 ± 1.39	22.27 ± 3.93*#
LAVp (ml)	20.66 ± 1.54	20.65 ± 1.50	36.92 ± 5.57*#
LAPEF(%)	41.87 ± 3.23	43.33 ± 2.58	33.33 ± 2.60*#
LAAEF(%)	31.42 ± 2.39	29.95 ± 3.18	40.01 ± 6.17*#

LAD left atrial dimension, *LVDd* left ventricular end-diastolic diameter, *IVSTd* end-diastolic thickness of ventricular septum, *PWTd* end-diastolic thickness of LV posterior wall, *E/A* ratio of peak early and late diastolic velocities, *LAVmax* Left atrial maximum volume, *LAVmin* LA minimum volume, *LAVp* LA pre-atrial volume, *LAPEF* left atrial passive emptying fraction, *LAAEF* left atrial active emptying fraction. *P <0.01 versus the control group. #P <0.01 versus the mild group

Table 3 Left atrial strain and strain rate

Variables	Group A (n = 30)	Group B (n = 34)	Group C (n = 31)
GLSs(%)	37.23 ± 5.26	35.33 ± 4.58	29.12 ± 4.83*#
GLSRs(s-1)	1.78 ± 0.26	1.71 ± 0.32	1.49 ± 0.11*#
GLSRe(s-1)	−2.12 ± 0.46	−2.05 ± 0.38	−1.57 ± 0.07*#
GLSRa(s-1)	−1.45 ± 0.11	−1.45 ± 0.24	−1.70 ± 0.16*#

GLSs/GLSRs the globle peak longitudinal strain rate of systolic left ventricular, GLSRa the globle peak longitudinal strain rate of late diastolic left ventricular, GLSRe the globle peak longitudinal strain rate of early diastolic left ventricular, *P <0.01 versus the control group. #P <0.01 versus the mild group

Traditional echocardiographic parameters

There were no significant differences between group B and group A (all $P > 0.05$). None of LVDd, IVSTd and PWTd were significant among the three groups. The LAD, LAVp, LAVmax, LAVmin, A and LAAEF of group C were significantly higher than those of groups A and B. E, E/A and LAPEF of group C were significantly lower than those of groups A and B (all $P < 0.01$) (Seen in Table 2).

Left atrial strain and strain rate

The group B was not significant compared with the control group (all $P > 0.05$). The GLSRa of group C were significantly higher than that of group A and B ($P < 0.01$). The GLSRe, GLSs, GLSRs of group C were significantly lower than those of group A and B (all $P < 0.01$) (Seen in Table 3). The 2D-STE strain rate curves of the three groups were shown in Fig. 1, 2 and 3.

Left ventricular longitudinal strain

Meanwhile, the LV longitudinal strain values was manifested in the study. The strain value of the moderate group was reduced, compared with both control group and the mild group (all P < 0.01) (Seen in Table 4).

The inter- and intra-observer results revealed good reproducibility and small variability by using 2D-STE in evaluation of patients with IDA (Seen in Table 5).

Discussion

Anemia has been shown to be an important factor in increasing cardiac output to maintain adequate oxygen supply to the tissues [6]. The transition from a high-output (compensated) state to a state of LV dysfunction (decompensated) begin at the hemoglobin below 7 g/dL in iron-deficient patients. The reduction of hemoglobin level is related to future increased morbidity and mortality [18]. So early diagnosis and treatment in iron deficiency can greatly improve quality of life and can promptly reduce hospitalization rate, unemployment rate and ultimately, reduce medical consumption [19]. Therefore it has a significant prognosis to allow for early and correct diagnosis.

The LA function is an important factor influencing cardiac output [20] by regulating the filling pressure of the left ventricular with its reservoir, conduit and pump functions. Although LA structural and functional remodeling is a barometer of LV diastolic dysfunction [21], there were no studies to reveal the changes of LA function in patients with IDA. Previous reports have shown that some disease (hypertension, atrial fibrillation,

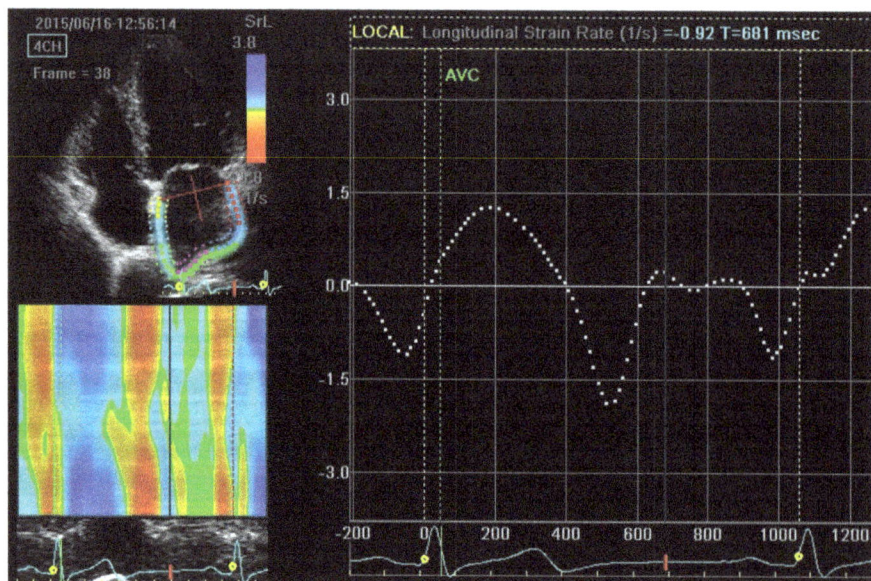

Fig. 1 Measurement of global longitudinal left atrial strain rate from an apical four-chamber view of group A

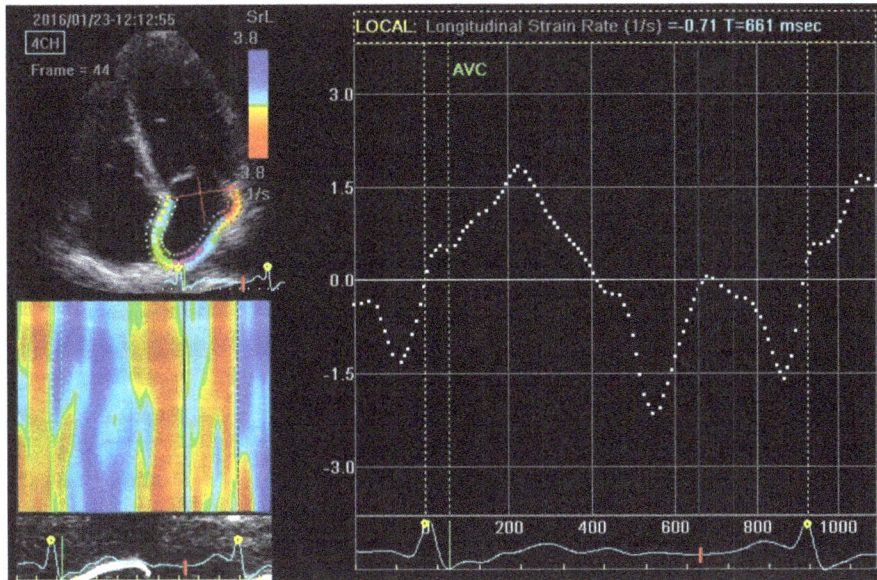

Fig. 2 Measurement of global longitudinal left atrial strain rate from an apical four-chamber view of group B

coronary artery disease, etc.) may lead to left atrial phasic dysfunction evaluated by 2D-STE [22, 23]. Additionally, the longitudinal strain and strain rate, which are inversely related to LA wall fibrosis, have been reported to be a feasible and reproducible method to assess LA myocardial function [24, 25]. So we try to evaluate the LA function in patients with IDA by 2D-STE.

In our study, there were no significant differences between group B and group A (all $P > 0.05$). None of LVDd, IVSTd and PWTd were significant among the three groups. The longitudinal strain of LV from basal to apical were decreased in the moderate group compared to the control and mild group (all $P < 0.01$). The LAD, LAVp, LAVmax, LAVmin, A and LAAEF of group C were significantly higher than those of groups A and B (all $P < 0.01$). E, E/A and LAPEF of group C were significantly lower than those of group A and B (all $P < 0.01$). We found that the conventional echocardiography parameters and strain and strain rate of LA, and

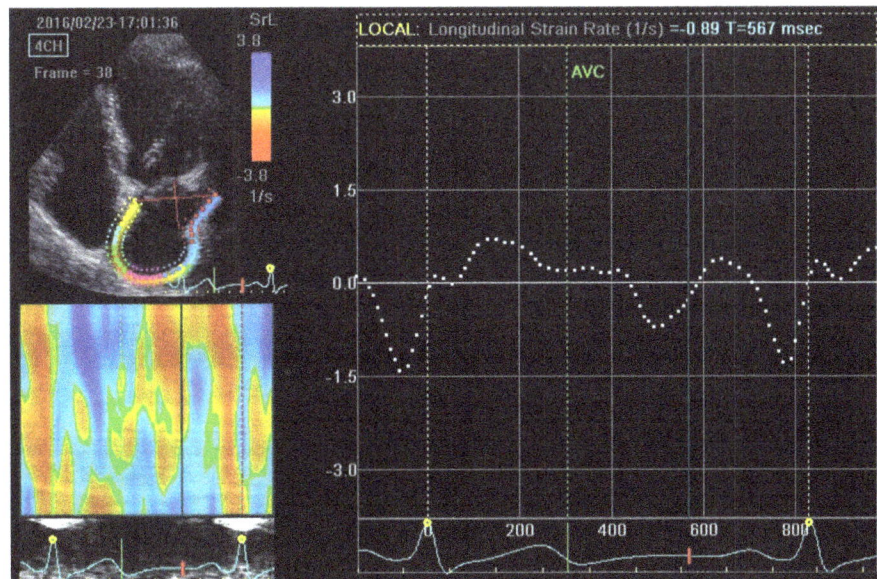

Fig. 3 Measurement of global longitudinal left atrial strain rate from an apical four-chamber view of group C

Table 4 Left ventricular peak longitudinal strain

Variables	Group A (n = 30)	Group B (n = 34)	Group C (n = 31)
Basal(%)	−20.4 ± 4.5	−20.8 ± 4.8	−16.2 ± 4.8a#
Middle(%)	−21.8 ± 4.2	−22.3 ± 5.1	−17.1 ± 5.2*#
Apical(%)	−25.4 ± 5.3	−25.8 ± 4.7	−20.4 ± 4.6*#

*P <0.01 versus the control group. #P <0.01 versus the mild group

longitudinal strain of LV were changed with the decrease in hemoglobin concentration. When Hb > 90 g/L, there were no obvious differences between the parameters of group B and group A compared with the control group. This suggested that the structure and function did not have obvious change in the mild group. When Hb 60–90 g/L, LAAEF and GLSRa of group C were higher than those of groups A and B. LAPEF, GLSs, GLSRe and GLSRs of group C were lower than group A and B. This meant that the LA longitudinal myocardial deformation had impaired in this stage.

However, LA abnormalities are associated with abnormal diastolic function of the LV [26–28]. LA conduit function is correlated with LV early diastolic function [29], LA reservoir function is correlated with LV systolic function [30, 31], and LA pump function is associated with LV late diastolic function [32, 33]. The result of our study had agreed to these above. At some degree, decreasing strain values means rising LV filling pressure. Based on the results, we found the following: the value of GLSs and GLSRs, the reservoir function which receives blood from the pulmonary veins during ventricular systole was decreased in the moderate group. GLSRe and LAPEF, the conduit function for transporting blood from the pulmonary veins to the LV were also decreased in the moderate group. They indicated that the movements of myocardial tissue had slowed down. These results were consistent with the longitudinal strain of LV and had indicated the LV diastolic dysfunction in the moderate group, which had associated with chronic myocardial ischemia and hypoxia [6]. Both ischemia and hypoxia may lead to LA remodeling. On the other hand, the increase of LV filling pressure could result in increasing of LA afterload, which then could affect transporting blood from the pulmonary veins to the LA.

GLSRa and LAAEF, the parameters for the functional evaluation of the pump phase that established the final LV end-diastolic volume were increased in the moderate group. Perhaps it was due to the strong contraction of left atrial, which was caused by increasing length of left atrial myocardial fibers and rising LA pressure according to the Frank-Starling mechanism [34]. In addition, compared to the control and mild groups, the LV global longitudinal strain decreased in the moderate group (Table 4). Studies have manifested that longitudinal strain could be sensitive to subtle LV dysfunction, which allowed investigation of earlier stages of myocardium. In the study, the investigation of strain values in the moderate group was decreased and it was a good illustration of the sensitivity of 2D-STE in detecting earlier cardiac dysfunction. Therefore LA function and LV function are interactional. Nowadays, many clinicians cognize the importance to assess the role of left atrial function in prognosis of multiple adverse cardiovascular events, including death. After the study, most of patients in the study were made aware of the important effects of anemia to their hearts. They had all actively accepted the clinical treatment, and the result may have effectively prevented further cardiac dysfunction.

Clinical implications

2D-STE is a sensitive tool for evaluating LA function in patients with IDA. The application of 2D-STE in patients with IDA may help clinicians to identify earlier changes of LA function. It greatly helps in early detection of abnormal LA function, even indicates clinical therapy. An aggressive therapeutic and preventive approach could improve the outcome of this disease.

Limitations

Our study had several limitations. First, we only analyzed a part of LA wall in apical four- and two-chamber views, but in some studies, another three segments from apical three-chamber view were also included [35]. Secondly, lack of standardization could make our result incomparable with others. Thirdly, the obesity, such as lung weight may impede image quality and the unclear endocardium may also affect the result. Lastly, only 65 patients were selected in this study, the objects in the

Table 5 Inter and intra-observer analyses for LA strain and strain rate

	Intra-observer				Inter-observer			
	R	bias(%)	LOA(%)	ICC	R	bias(%)	LOA(%)	ICC
GLSs	0.80	2.39	−5.48 ~ 6.75	0.853	0.82	2.29	−6.18 ~ 4.97	0.875
GLSRs	0.85	1.28	−4.42 ~ 2.95	0.901	0.84	1.19	−5.54 ~ 4.69	0.885
GLSRe	0.81	2.14	−6.58 ~ 5.10	0.867	0.79	2.75	−8.42 ~ 3.13	0.821
GLSRa	0.90	0.65	−1.04 ~ 2.35	0.969	0.96	0.59	−0.13 ~ 1.87	0.993

R coefficient of determination, *LOA* limit of agreement, *ICC* intra-class correlation coefficient

research were relatively small and only limited number of patients in extremely severe group could be obtained. In these situations, we would select more samples to study in the future.

Conclusions

2D-STE could significantly evaluate the left atrial function in patients with IDA. And in our study, GLSs, GLSRs, GLSRe and GLSRa, the new LA function parameters, which are measured by 2D-STE, exert better potential for the accurate assessment of LA dysfunction in patients with IDA.

Acknowledgement
Greatly appreciated for the supports from Prof. Li, who participated in the analysis, interpretation and statistics of date, as well as critical revision. Also thanks for the help of Qiao Zhou, Yue Liu, Runlan Luo and Bijun Tan, who participated in collection of cases and the final approval of the article. Those authors are all from Department of Ultrasound, the Second Affiliated Hospital of Dalian Medical University, China.

Funding
Not applicable for the section.

Authors' contributions
SJQ: Collection and design of data, analysis and interpretation of data, and drafting the article. ZQ, LY, LRL and TBJ: Collection of data and final approval of the article. LGS: Conception and analysis of data, interpretation and statistics of date, critical revision, and final approval of the article.

Competing interests
All authors declare that they have no competing interests.

References
1. Cappellini MD, Motta I. Anemia in Clinical Practice-Definition and Classification: Does Hemoglobin Change With Aging? Semin Hematol. 2015;52(4):261–9.
2. Camaschella C. Iron-deficiency anemia. N Engl J Med. 2015;372(19):1832–43.
3. McLean E, Cogswell M, Egli I, Wojdyla D, de Benoist B. Worldwide prevalence of anaemia, WHO Vitamin and Mineral Nutrition Information System, 1993–2005. Public Health Nutr. 2009;12(4):444–54.
4. Kassebaum NJ, Jasrasaria R, Naghavi M, Wulf SK, Johns N, Lozano R, Regan M, Weatherall D, Chou DP, Eisele TP, Flaxman SR, Pullan RL, Brooker SJ, Murray CJ. A systematic analysis of global anemia burden from 1990 to 2010. Blood. 2014;123(5):615–24.
5. Pasricha SR, Drakesmith H, Black J, Hipgrave D, Biggs BA. Control of iron deficiency anemia in low- and middle-income countries. Blood. 2013; 121(14):2607–17.
6. Hegde N, Rich MW, Gayomali C. The cardiomyopathy of iron deficiency. Tex Heart Inst J. 2006;33(3):340–4.
7. Georgieva Z, Georgieva M. Compensatory and adaptive changes in microcirculation and left ventricular function of patients with chronic iron-deficiency anaemia. Clin Hemorheol Microcirc. 1997;17(1):21–30.
8. Rakusan K, Cicutti N, Kolar F. Effect of anemia on cardiac function, microvascular structure, and capillary hematocrit in rat hearts. Am J Physiol Heart Circ Physiol. 2001;280(3):1407–14.
9. Blume GG, Mcleod CJ, Barnes ME, Seward JB, Pellikka PA, Bastiansen PM, Tsang TS. Left atrial function: Physiology, assessment, and clinical implications. Eur J Echocardiogr. 2011;12(6):421–30.
10. Amin MG, Tighiouart H, Weiner DE, Stark PC, Griffith JL, MacLeod B, Salem DN, Sarnak MJ. Hematocrit and left ventricular mass: the Framingham Heart study. J Am Coll Cardiol. 2004;43(7):1276–82.
11. Cameli M, Lisi M, Righini FM, Mondillo S. Novel echocardiographic techniques to assess left atrial size,anatomy and function. Cardiovasc Ultrasound. 2012;10:4.
12. Cianciulli TF, Saccheri MC, Lax JA, Bermann AM, Ferreiro DE. Two-dimensional speckle tracking echocardiography for the assessment of atrial function. World J Cardiol. 2010;2(7):163–70.
13. Cameli M, Lisi M, Mondillo S, Padeletti M, Ballo P, Tsioulpas C, Bernazzali S, Maccherini M. Left atrial longitudinal strain by speckle tracking echocardiography correlates well with left ventricular filling pressures in patients with heart failure. Cardiovasc Ultrasound. 2010;21(8):14.
14. Galderisi M, Henein MY, D'hooge J, Sicari R, Badano LP, Zamorano JL, Roelandt JR. Recommendations of the European Association of Echocardiography: How to use echo-Doppler in clinical trials: Different modalities for different purposes. Eur J Echocardiogr. 2011;12(5):339–53.
15. Yoon YE, Kim HJ, Kim SA, Kim SH, Park JH, Park KH, Choi S, Kim MK, Kim HS, Cho GY. Left atrial mechanical function and stiffness in patients with paroxysmal atrial fibrillation. Cardiovasc Ultrasound. 2012;20(3):140–5.
16. Moyssakis I, Papadopoulos DP, Kelepeshis G, Gialafos E, Votteas V, Triposkiadis F. Left atrial systolic reserve inidiopathic vs. ischaemic-dilated cardiomyopathy. Eur J ClinInvest. 2005;35(6):355–61.
17. Paraskevaidis IA, Dodouras T, Adamopoulos S, Kremastinos DT. Left atrial functional reserve in patients with nonischemic dilated cardiomyopathy: an echocardiographic dobutamine study. Chest. 2002;122(4):1340–7.
18. Komajda M, Anker SD, Charlesworth A, Okonko D, Metra M, Di Lenarda A, Remme W, Moullet C, Swedberg K, Cleland JG, Poole-Wilson PA. The impact of new onset anaemia on morbidity and mortality inchronic heart failure: results from COMET. Eur Heart J. 2006;27(12):1440–6.
19. Kaitha S, Bashir M, Ali T. Iron deficiency anemia in inflammatory bowel disease. World J Gastrointest Pathophysiol. 2015;6(3):62–72.
20. Tsang TS, Abhayaratna WP, Barnes ME, Miyasaka Y, Gersh BJ, Bailey KR, Cha SS, Seward JB. Prediction of cardiovascular outcomes with left atrial size: is volume superior to area or diameter? J Am Coll Cardiol. 2006; 47(5):1018–23.
21. Laukkanen JA, Kurl S, Eränen J, Huttunen M, Salonen JT. Left atrium size and the risk of cardiovascular death in middle-aged men. Arch Intern Med. 2005; 165(15):1788–93.
22. Hong J, Gu X, An P, Luo T, Lv Q, Kang J, He Y, Hu R, Liu X, Ma C. Left atrial functional remodeling in lone atrial fibrillation: a two-dimensional speckle tracking echocardiographic study. Echocardiography. 2013;30(9):1051–60.
23. Miyoshi H, Oishi Y, Mizuguchi Y, Iuchi A, Nagase N, Ara N, Oki T. Effect of anincrease in left ventricular pressure overload on left atrialleftventricular coupling in patients with hypertension: Atwo-dimensional speckle tracking echocardiographicstudy. Echocardiography. 2013;30(6):658–66.
24. Kim D, Shim CY, Cho IJ, Kim YD, Nam HS, Chang HJ, Hong GR, Ha JW, Heo JH, Chung N. Incremental value of left atrial global longitudinal strain for prediction of post stroke atrial fibrillation in patients with acute ischemic stroke. Cardiovasc Ultrasound. 2016;24(1):20–7.
25. Shao C, Zhu J, Chen J, Xu W. Independent prognostic value of left atrial function by two-dimensional speckle tracking imaging in patients with non -ST-segment-elevation acute myocardial infarction. BMC Cardiovasc Disord. 2015;15:145.
26. Morris DA, Gailani M, Vaz Pérez A, Blaschke F, Dietz R, Haverkamp W, Ozcelik C. Left atrial systolic and diastolic dysfunction in heart failure with normal left ventricular ejection fraction. J Am Soc Echocardiogr. 2011;24(6):651–62.
27. Santos AB, Kraigher-Krainer E, Gupta DK, Claggett B, Zile MR, Pieske B, Voors AA, Lefkowitz M, Bransford T, Shi V, Packer M, McMurray JJ, Shah AM, Solomon SD. Impaired left atrial function in heart failure with preserved ejection fraction. Eur J Heart Fail. 2014;16(10):1096–103.
28. Kocabay G, Karabay CY, Colak Y, Oduncu V, Kalayci A, Akgun T, Guler A, Kirma C. Left atrial deformation parameters in patients with non-alcoholic fatty liver disease: A 2D speckle tracking imaging study. Clin Sci (Lond). 2014;126(4):297–304.
29. Okamatsu K, Takeuchi M, Nakai H, Nishikage T, Salgo IS, Husson S, Otsuji Y, Lang RM. Effects of aging on left atrialfunction assessed by two-dimensional speckle tracking echocardiography. J Am Soc Echocardiogra. 2009;22(1):70–5.
30. Rabbat MG, Wilber D, Thomas K, Malick O, Bashir A, Agrawal A, Biswas S, Sanagala T, Syed MA. Left atrial volume assessment in atrial fibrillation using multimodalityimaging: a comparison of echocardiography, invasive three-dimensional CARTO and cardiac magnetic resonance imaging. Int J Cardiovasc Imaging. 2015;31(5):1011–8.
31. Barbier P, Solomon SB, Schiller NB, Glantz SA. Left atrial relaxation and left ventricular systolic functiondetermine left atrial reservoir function. Circulation. 1999;100(4):427–36.

2

Feasibility and relevance of compound strain imaging in non-stenotic arteries: comparison between individuals with cardiovascular diseases and healthy controls

Martijn F.H. Maessen[1], Thijs M.H. Eijsvogels[1,3], Ayla Grotens[1], Maria T.E. Hopman[1], Dick H.J. Thijssen[1,3] and Hendrik H.G. Hansen[2*]

Abstract

Background: Compound strain imaging is a novel method to noninvasively evaluate arterial wall deformation which has recently shown to enable differentiation between fibrous and (fibro-)atheromatous plaques in patients with severe stenosis. We tested the hypothesis that compound strain imaging is feasible in non-stenotic arteries and provides incremental discriminative power to traditional measures of vascular health (i.e., distensibility coefficient (DC), central pulse wave velocity [cPWV], and intima-media thickness [IMT]) for differentiating between participants with and without a history of cardiovascular diseases (CVD).

Methods: Seventy two participants (60 ± 7 years) with non-stenotic arteries (IMT < 1.1 mm) were categorized in healthy participants (CON, $n = 36$) and CVD patients ($n = 36$) based on CVD history. Participants underwent standardised ultrasound-based assessment (DC, cPWV, and IMT) and compound strain imaging (radial [RS] and circumferential [CS] strain) in left common carotid artery. Area under receiver operating characteristics (AROC)-curve was used to determine the discriminatory power between CVD and CON of the various measures.

Results: CON had a significantly ($P < 0.05$) smaller carotid IMT (0.68 [0.58 to 0.76] mm) than CVD patients (0.76 [0.68 to 0.80] mm). DC, cPWV, RS, and CS did not significantly differ between groups ($P > 0.05$). A higher CS or RS was associated with a higher DC (CS: $r = -0.32; p < 0.05$ and RS: $r = 0.24; p < 0.05$) and lower cPWV (CS: $r = 0.24; p < 0.05$ and RS: $r = -0.25; p < 0.05$). IMT could identify CVD (AROC: 0.66, 95%-CI: 0.53 to 0.79), whilst the other measurements, alone or in combination, did not significantly increase the discriminatory power compared to IMT.

Conclusions: In non-stenotic arteries, compound strain imaging is feasible, but does not seem to provide incremental discriminative power to traditional measures of vascular health for differentiation between individuals with and without a history of CVD.

Keywords: Strain imaging, Myocardial infarction, Ultrasound imaging, Cardiovascular assessment, Intima media thickness

* Correspondence: Rik.Hansen@radboudumc.nl
[2]Department of Radiology and Nuclear Medicine, Radboud university
medical center, Medical UltraSound Imaging Center (MUSIC), P.O. Box 9101
(766), 6500, HB, Nijmegen, The Netherlands
Full list of author information is available at the end of the article

Background

Atherosclerosis is a multifactorial disease, which affects the vasculature and usually develops in humans over the course of years to decades [1]. Early detection of people at risk for CVD is of paramount importance to prevent life threatening events, such as stroke or myocardial infarction. Results from large cohort studies [2, 3] indicate that several vascular markers obtained via ultrasound techniques, such as the distensibility coefficient (DC), central pulse wave velocity (cPWV), or intima-media thickness (IMT), improve cardiovascular risk stratification. Recent studies also investigated the performance of carotid artery wall strain parameters by commercially available speckle tracking techniques for CVD risk stratification [4–6]. Park et al. observed a significant correlation between circumferential strain, the amount of cardiovascular risk factors and the Framingham Risk Score [4]. Catalano et al. found that peak systolic circumferential strain adjusted for pulse pressure could differentiate between three cardiovascular risk groups, whereas for instance IMT could not [6]. Although these results are very promising, these commercial techniques were initially developed for myocardial strain estimation. All commercially available packages for myocardial strain estimation use either B-mode data or the envelope signal of the raw radiofrequency data for tracking. [7] It is known that more accurate strain estimation can be performed when using the underlying raw ultrasound radiofrequency (RF) data, because it contains the phase information of the ultrasound signal [8, 9]. Recently, several RF-based strain techniques specifically designed to evaluate arterial wall strain have been developed [10–15]. Some of these techniques have already been validated against post-endarterectomy histology and/or magnetic resonance imaging derived plaque composition [16–19]. In all of these validation studies patients with severe amounts of stenosis (>50%) were included. Whether these RF-based techniques are also feasible in non-stenotic arteries and provide information that can discriminate between healthy, asymptomatic subjects and those with a history of cardiovascular disease, needs to be explored. Despite the promising findings for speckle-tracking-based strain analysis, it is also still unclear if the information provided by RF-based strain imaging has additional value for cardiovascular risk stratification over traditional measures of conduit arteries, such as cPWV or IMT.

In this study, we tested whether compound strain imaging, an in house built and validated RF-based strain imaging technique designed for transverse imaging planes, is feasible in non-stenotic arteries and provides information that has additional value compared to traditional measures of conduit arteries (i.e., cPWV, DC or IMT) for discrimination between participants with and without a history of CVD.

Methods

Participants

A total of 72 male participants aged 46 to 77 years with non-stenotic arteries were included. Based on CVD history the participants were categorized in healthy, asymptomatic controls (CON, n = 36) and CVD patients (CVD, n = 36). CVD participants suffered from a myocardial infarction in the past and used cardiovascular medication (anticoagulants, antihypertensive, or lipid lowering agents). Smokers and diabetics were excluded from the study. The Local Committee on Research Involving Human Subjects of the region Arnhem and Nijmegen approved the study. All participants gave their written informed consent.

Study Design

During this cross-sectional study, participants underwent comprehensive vascular assessment including traditional measures (DC, cPWV, and IMT) and compound strain imaging.

Vascular Measurements

All measurements were performed in supine position, in a temperature-controlled room, and following a ≥ 6 h fast, ≥18 h abstinence from caffeine, alcohol and vitamin supplements, and at least 24 h after strenuous physical activity by the participant. Measurements began after a resting period in the supine position for at least 15 min [20].

Traditional vascular measurement: distensibility coefficient, central pulse wave velocity, and IMT
Distensibility coefficient
DC was assessed with a 9 MHz (L5–13) linear transducer connected to an Accuvix V10 ultrasound system (Samsung Medison, Seoul South Korea) in a transverse plane. Blood pressure was obtained in the right arm [21] and measured twice using a sphygmomanometer. Distensibility was measured twice in the left common carotid artery 1.5 and 2.0 cm upstream of the bulbous in the transverse plane.

Central pulse wave velocity
cPWV was measured using a three-lead electrocardiogram and an Echo-Doppler ultrasound machine (Waki Doppler, Atys Medical, Soucieu en Jarrest, France) at the left carotid artery and right common femoral artery [2]. The distances were measured between sternal notch and site of measurement for the carotid artery and common femoral artery via the umbilicus [2]. To estimate the travel distance between the carotid and femoral site, we subtracted the distance between the carotid location to the suprasternal notch from the distance between the suprasternal notch and the femoral site [22]. At least 10 cardiac cycles were recorded for the analysis.

Intima-media thickness

IMT of the left common carotid was recorded using a T3000 ultrasound system (Terason Teratech Corporation, Boston, United States) equipped with an 8.5 MHz 12 L5 linear transducer. To normalize vascular tonus the participants received 400 µg of sublingual glyceryl trinitrate (nitric oxide donor) before the IMT measurement [23]. Therefore, the IMT measurement took place after DC and compound strain imaging. Image sequences of ≥10 s were recorded 1.5 to 2.0 cm distally of the bifurcation of the common carotid, while having the vessel in a longitudinal imaging plane. Wall thickness were collected from two distinct angles and the mean value is presented.

Compound strain imaging

Vascular radial strain was assessed with a 9 MHz (L5–13) linear transducer connected to an Accuvix V10 ultrasound system (Samsung Medison, Seoul South Korea) equipped with a dedicated multi-angle acquisition mode for compound strain imaging and with an interface providing ultrasound RF data. The subject was lying in supine position, with no pillow beneath the head. Blood pressure was manually measured using a sphygmomanometer in the right arm before each recording. Cumulative radial (RS) and circumferential (CS) strains from peak systole to end diastole were determined in the left common carotid. The end-diastolic phase was based on the carotid distention (pressure) waveform and defined as the time at which minimal lumen diameter was measured. The probe was placed at the location where the IMT was the thickest in the left common carotid artery. Whenever there was no location with a thicker IMT, the probe was placed between 1.5 and 2.0 cm upstream of the bulbous. Radiofrequency datasets of the carotid artery in a transverse plane were recorded twice for 3 seconds.

Data Analysis

Traditional vascular measurement: distensibility coefficient, cPWV, and IMT

DC was calculated from M-mode (Eq. 1) [2] and derived from a diameter curve that was obtained by manually indicating the lumen-intima interfaces for the near and far wall at peak systole, after which the software automatically traced the interfaces from systole to systole. DC values of measurement 1 and 2 were averaged per artery.

$$\frac{\text{diameter systole}^2 - \text{diameter diastole}^2}{\text{diameter diastole}^2 \times PP}$$

$$((1)\text{distensibility})$$

$$PP = \text{Systolic Blood Pressure} - \text{Diastolic Blood Pressure}$$

$$((2)\text{PulsePressure})$$

cPWV was calculated in Matlab (MATLAB and Statistics Toolbox Release R2014, The MathWorks, Inc., Natick, United States) and was based on the interval between the R-wave on the electrocardiogram and onset of the Doppler waveform. The onset of the Doppler waveform was semi-automatically detected by the software and only major deviations were operator corrected.

Intima-media thickness of the left common carotid artery was examined using custom-designed off-line edge-detection and wall-tracking software written in LabVIEW (LabVIEW 6.02, National Instruments, Austin, TX, USA). This DICOM-based software is largely independent of investigator bias and has been previously described in detail [24, 25]. Briefly, each recording was converted to a DICOM file at a frame rate of 30 Hz. Detection of the far wall media-adventitia interface was performed on every frame selected. The mean intima-media thickness was calculated via: (1/3 × systolic wall thickness) + (2/3 × diastolic wall thickness) [26]. All files were analyzed blinded by an independent researcher.

Compound strain imaging

Strain parameters (RS and CS) were calculated from the radiofrequency data using custom made software written in Matlab R2014 (The MathWorks Inc., USA) [10, 19]. First ultrasonic frames were identified that corresponded to the systolic and diastolic phases (maximum and minimum lumen diameter, respectively) in an M-mode view of the image line that crossed the vessel lumen center. For each systolic frame a region-of-interest corresponding to the upper half segment of the vessel wall was manually selected for which strains were to be computed, tracked and accumulated from systole to diastole. Strain calculation was performed using a 2D cross-correlation based coarse-to-fine strain estimation strategy followed by displacement compounding, tracking, rotation and 2D least squares strain estimation, see Table 1 for detailed settings of the compound strain estimation [8, 10, 27, 28]. The algorithm provided strain values for every 62.5 µm (vertically) by 200 µm (horizontally) of tissue. Of all strain values in the region-of-interest, the 90th percentile of the maximal strain was defined as the final result of the strain analysis. Strain was normalized with respect to a reference pulse pressure of 40 mmHg. Strain values of measurement 1 and 2 were averaged.

Statistical Analysis

This study was exploratory by design, since we had no information about RF-based strain in patients with cardiovascular diseases in non-stenotic arteries. Participants' characteristics as well as vascular characteristics (DC, cPWV, IMT, RS, and CS) of the left common carotid of the participants were summarized with means and standard deviations or median and interquartile

Table 1 Settings of the strain estimation algorithm

	Iteration 1	Iteration 2	Iteration 3	Iteration 4[y]	Strain Estimation
Data input	Envelope	RF data	RF data	RF data	Radial displacements
Pre-kernel size (mm x mm)	1.3×0.6^a	0.6×0.6^a	0.3×0.6^a	0.3×0.6^a	-
Post-kernel size (mm x mm)	1.9×1.8^a	0.9×1.8^a	0.5×1.8^a	0.5×1.8^a	-
Axial kernel overlap (%)	80	80	80	80	-
Lateral kernel overlap (%)	67	67	67	67	-
Median filter size (mm x mm)	2.2×1.8^a	1.1×1.8^a	0.6×1.8^a	0.9×0.6^{az} 0.6×0.6^{az}	$21° \times 0.5$ mm^x
2D least squares strain estimator size (° x mm)	-	-	-	-	$9° \times 0.5$ mm^x

[a]Axial x lateral direction; y with sub-sample aligning (24); z-filter settings after compounding (15) for the cumulated horizontal and vertical displacements, respectively; x-filter sizes defined in circumferential x radial direction, because of conversion to polar grid with a spacing of 1° circumferentially and 100 μm radially (22)

range (IQR). Parameters were checked for normality using a *Shapiro-Wilk* test and Q-Q plots. An independent Student's *t* in case of normal distribution or *Mann-Whitney U* test for all other cases was used to analyse differences in participant characteristics and differences in compound strain imaging of non-stenotic carotid arteries between CVD and CON. To determine the coherence between traditional vascular measurements (DC, cPWV, IMT, RS, and CS) and compound strain imaging, correlation coefficients were calculated via *Spearman's Rank* test for the total group and subgroups (CVD and CON). The Holm-Bonferoni method was used to correct for multiple pairwise testing [29]. Area under receiver operating characteristics (AROC)-curve was used to determine the discriminatory power of DC, cPWV, IMT, RS and CS. The different vascular measurements were combined to determine whether this increased the discriminatory power to detect CVD. All statistical analyses were performed using SPSS 22.0 software (IBM Corp. Released 2013. IBM SPSS Statistics for Windows, Version 22.0. Armonk, NY: IBM Corp.). Statistical significance was assumed at $p < 0.05$ (two-sided).

Results

Characteristics Participants
Age, weight, and body mass index did not significantly differ between CVD and CON (Table 2). CON were

Table 2 Participant characteristics of total and according to presence cardiovascular diseases

	Total group n = 72	Controls n = 36	CVD patients n = 36	p value
Characteristics				
Age (years)	60 ± 7	59 ± 7	61 ± 6	0.41
Body height (cm)	178 ± 7	180 ± 7	176 ± 6	0.011
Body mass (kg)	81 ± 11	81 ± 11	81 ± 12	0.98
Body Mass Index (kg/m^2)[a]	25.3 [23.6 to 27.0]	24.9 [23.3 to 26.9]	25.6 [24.2 to 27.9]	0.20
Mean arterial pressure (mmHg)[a]	97 [91 to 105]	100 [93 to 106]	94 [90 to 100]	0.035
Diastolic blood pressure (mmHg)[a]	79 [75 to 88]	83 [77 to 91]	77 [73 to 82]	0.011
Systolic blood pressure (mmHg)	131 [123 to 142]	136 [124 to 142]	128 [120 to 139]	0.19
Cardiovascular medication use				
Anticoagulant (n)		-	35 (97%)	
Antihypertensive agents (n)		-	29 (81%)	
Lipid lowering agents (n)		-	32 (89%)	
Vascular measurements				
Radial strain (%)[a]	4.2 [3.2 to 6.5]	4.2 [3.2 to 6.4]	4.8 [3.6 to 6.5]	0.50
Circumferential strain (%)[a]	−10.0 [−13.6 to −6.5]	−10.2 [−14.9 to −7.0]	−8.8 [−13.2 to −6.2]	0.29
Distensibility[a]	0.27 [0.19 to 0.37]	0.27 [0.20 to 0.35]	0.29 [0.18 to 0.40]	0.77
Central pulse wave velocity[a]	8.0 [6.8 to 10.1]	7.8 [6.5 to 10.0]	8.0 [7.2 to 10.2]	0.22
Intima to media thickness (mm)[a]	0.72 [0.61 to 0.78]	0.68 [0.58 to 0.76]	0.76 [0.68 to 0.80]	0.023

P-value refers to an independent *Student's t* or *Mann-Whitney U* test (two-sided) between controls and CVD patients. Data is presented as mean and standard deviation (normal distribution) or median and interquartile range (non-normal distribution)
[a]*Mann-Whitney U* test

taller compared to CVD (CON: 180 ± 7 cm vs. CVD: 176 ± 6 cm; $P = 0.011$) and had a higher mean arterial pressure (CON: 100 mmHg [IQR: 93–106] vs. CVD: 94 mmHg [IQR: 90–100] mmHg; $P = 0.035$) (Table 2). Within the CVD group, anticoagulant ($n = 35$ [97%]) medications were used most frequently, followed by lipid lowering ($n = 32$ [89%]) and antihypertensive agents ($n = 29$ [81%]), whereas the control group did not use medications (Table 2).

Vascular Measures
The participants did not show visible atherosclerotic plaques during the vascular measurements. All compound strain measures took place approximately 1.5 to 2.0 cm below the bifurcation of the carotid artery. DC and cPWV did not significantly differ between CON and CVD (Table 2). CON demonstrated a smaller intima-media thickness of carotid artery compared to CVD (Table 2). RS and CS not significantly differ between CON and CVD, respectively (Table 2).

Pairwise comparison: traditional measures vs. Compound strain imaging
Spearman rank analysis revealed that a higher CS or RS was associated with a higher DC and lower cPWV in the total group (Table 3). A higher DC was associated with a lower cPWV. IMT did not correlate with DC, cPWV, CS, and RS (Table 3).

Area Under Receiver Operating Characteristic Curve
DC, cPWV, RS, and could not discriminate between CVD or CON (Table 4). The IMT was able to identify CVD with a best cut-off for the carotid IMT of 0.70 mm (sensitivity: 74%, specificity: 58%). Although combinations of IMT and RS, CS, DC, or cPWV increased the

Table 3 Spearman rank correlations between vascular measurements

	RS	CS	DC	cPWV	IMT	
RS		**-0.72****	0.28	−0.34*	-0.05	CON
		-0.75**	0.23	−0.26	-0.15	CVD
CS	**-0.73****		−0.34*	0.42*	0.07	CON
			-0.24	0.04	0.24	CVD
DC	0.27*	**−0.32****		-0.26	0.14	CON
				-0.30	−0.17	CVD
cPWV	−0.25*	0.24*	−0.28*		0.28	CON
					-0.38*	CVD
IMT	-0.08	0.19	0.01	0.01		

RS radial strain, CS circumferential strain, DC distensibility coefficient,
CON controls, CVD patients with history of cardiovascular disease
*P < 0.05 **P < 0.01; numbers in bold remain statistical significant after correcting for multiple testing with the Holm-Bonferroni method [9]

Table 4 Area under the Receiver Operator Curve to determine the discriminatory power to detect patients with cardiovascular diseases for Radial Strain (RS), Circumferential Strain (CS), Distensibility Coefficient (DC), central Pulse Wave Velocity (cPWV), Intima-Media Thickness (IMT)

Parameter	AUC (95% CI)	P value
RS	0.57 (0.44 to 0.71)	0.28
CS	0.55 (0.41 to 0.68)	0.50
DC	0.48 (0.34 to 0.62)	0.76
cPWV	0.58 (0.45 to 0.72)	0.22
IMT	0.66 (0.53 to 0.79)	0.023
Combinations		
IMT + RS	0.64 (0.51 to 0.78)	0.04
IMT + CS	0.66 (0.53 to 0.79)	0.02
IMT + DC	0.65 (0.52 to 0.78)	0.03
IMT + cPWV	0.66 (0.53 to 0.79)	0.02
IMT + RS + CS	0.71 (0.59 to 0.84)	0.002
IMT + RS + CS + DC	0.71 (0.59 to 0.84)	0.002
IMT + RS + CS + DC + pPWV	0.71 (0.59 to 0.84)	0.003

RS radial strain, CS circumferential strain, DC distensibility coefficient, IMT intima-media thickness

AUC, this was not statistically different from IMT only (Table 4).

Discussion
The present study revealed that compound strain imaging is coherent to traditional measures of vascular stiffness (DC and cPWV). Compound strain imaging seems a feasible technique to measure carotid wall deformation, which are indirectly related to wall stiffness. However, compound strain imaging does not provide an incremental discriminative value to traditional measures of vascular health to discriminate between CVD and asymptomatic controls with non-stenotic arteries.

Measuring Vascular Strain In Non-Stenotic Arteries
Strain estimation in the arterial wall is challenging because of the small structure of the arterial wall. Compound strain imaging was validated in severely stenotic arteries (>70% stenosis) [30] and demonstrated good correlation with local plaque composition. A larger area to calculate strain was present in these stenotic plaques than in the present study where none of the participants had severely stenotic arteries (IMT$_{total group}$: 0.73 [0.61–0.78] mm), making a correct estimation of strain more challenging and probably more susceptible for errors. We can speculate that strain could provide additional information on changes of arterial elastic properties. The cPWV (carotid-fermoral) is considered the gold standard measurement to determine arterial stiffness [2]. Our results indicate that strain, DC, and cPWV are related

measurements, since we observed a statistically significant correlation. Compound strain imaging seems technically feasible to measure in non-stenotic arteries. It is however questionable what additional information strain provides next to DC or cPWV when there is no or hardly any plaque present. Given the fact that compound strain imaging requires complex and intensive calculations, whereas DC and cPWV are relatively straightforward to determine and calculate, we would recommend using the DC or cPWV instead of strain to obtain an (indirect) measure for arterial stiffness in non-stenotic arteries.

Vascular stiffness vs. Vascular structure

Elastic and structural properties of the arteries are influenced by different (lifestyle) factors [31–36]. In general, elasticity parameters seem to adjust in week-months by changing lifestyle (i.e., physical activity) [35, 36] or medication usage [32]. Possibly, the reason why strain and distensibility could not discriminate between CVD or CON relates to the use of antihypertensive agents within the CVD group (Table 2). Antihypertensive agents are known to improve vascular compliance [31, 32], which may have reduced the arterial stiffness of the participants with CVD.

In the present study IMT was significantly larger among CVD patients compared to controls, despite that participants with CVD used (lipid lowering) medication. These results align with other studies, which demonstrated participants with prevalent CVD have an increased IMT compared to disease-free controls [37–40]. Lifestyle interventions (e.g., diet, physical activity) and usage of lipid lowering agents following myocardial infarction reduces the progression of the IMT [33, 34]. IMT is therefore considered a more chronic stable index for the evaluation of vascular health. Care should be taken when evaluating vascular health in patients with CVD, since (lifestyle) interventions may reduce vascular stiffness, whereas structural measures may be better to evaluate long-term arterial properties and discriminate between chronically diseased and control participants.

Limitations

A few methodological considerations should be taken into account to the present study. This study was cross-sectional by design and is subject to the inherent limitations of that approach. During this study, we could not evaluate the predictive value of compound strain imaging, since our CVD patient group already had the disease. Secondly, the offline analysis of the strain data is semi-automatic. The arterial wall was not always detected by the program and had to be retraced by the researcher. However, each measurement was evaluated by two researchers to determine whether the arterial wall was correctly traced. After consensus was met, the measurement was included

in the statistical analysis. Third, DC was calculated using the pulse pressure of the right brachial artery instead of the local pulse pressure of the carotid artery. Due to pressure amplification [41] it is possible that we overestimated the pulse pressure in the carotid artery, since the amplitude of a pressure wave is higher in peripheral arteries than central arteries. However, with natural ageing the difference in arterial stiffness between central and peripheral arteries declines [41], which causes a fall in pressure amplification. Fourth, in the present study, we used a Doppler device to measure the cPWV. However, applanation tonometry is generally recognized as a more reliable technique to measure cPWV [42]. Fifth, in the past, we have gone through extensive efforts to improve the analysis [24, 25] and procedures to examine carotid IMT [23]. Nonetheless, we understand this approach may be slightly different compared to typically adopted protocols in the literature (including large cohort studies). We emphasize that, due to our protocol, generalizability against larger epidemiologic studies is inappropriate. Finally, all the participants of the study were men, which limits the generalizability of the present study.

Conclusion

In non-stenotic arteries, compound strain imaging is a feasible technique to determine arterial wall deformation, but did not shown an incremental discriminative value next to DC, cPWV, or IMT in this study. This suggests that, in patients with non-stenotic arteries, compound strain imaging provides limited additional insight next to traditional measures of vascular health (DC, cPWV, or IMT) when differentiating between CVD patients and asymptomatic controls.

Abbreviations
AROC: Area under Receiver operating characteristics; CON: Asymptomatic controls; CVD: Cardiovascular diseases; IMT: Intima-media thickness; IQR: Interquartile range

Funding
TMHE is financially supported by a European Commission Horizon 2020 grant [Marie Sklodowska-Curie Fellowship 655,502]. DHJT is financially supported by the Netherlands Heart Foundation (2009 T064).

Authors' contributions
Conception and design of data: MH, HH; Acquisition of data: MM, DT; Data analysis: MM, AG; Interpretation of data: MM, TE, DT, HH; Drafting the manuscript: MM, HH; Critical revision and final approval of the manuscript: TE, AG, MH, DT.

Competing interests
The authors declare that they have no competing interests.

Author details
[1]Department of Physiology, Radboud university medical center, Nijmegen, The Netherlands. [2]Department of Radiology and Nuclear Medicine, Radboud university medical center, Medical UltraSound Imaging Center (MUSIC), P.O. Box 9101 (766), 6500, HB, Nijmegen, The Netherlands. [3]Research Institute for Sports and Exercise Sciences, Liverpool John Moores University, Liverpool, UK.

References
1. Falk E. Pathogenesis of atherosclerosis. J Am Coll Cardiol. 2006;47(8 Suppl):C7–12.
2. Laurent S, Cockcroft J, Van Bortel L, Boutouyrie P, Giannattasio C, Hayoz D, Pannier B, Vlachopoulos C, Wilkinson I, Struijker-Boudier H, et al. Expert consensus document on arterial stiffness: methodological issues and clinical applications. Eur Heart J. 2006;27(21):2588–605.
3. Polak JF, Pencina MJ, Pencina KM, O'Donnell CJ, Wolf PA, D'Agostino RB Sr. Carotid-wall intima-media thickness and cardiovascular events. N Engl J Med. 2011;365(3):213–21.
4. Park HE, Cho GY, Kim HK, Kim YJ, Sohn DW. Validation of circumferential carotid artery strain as a screening tool for subclinical atherosclerosis. J Atheroscler Thromb. 2012;19(4):349–56.
5. Bjallmark A, Lind B, Peolsson M, Shahgaldi K, Brodin LA, Nowak J. Ultrasonographic strain imaging is superior to conventional non-invasive measures of vascular stiffness in the detection of age-dependent differences in the mechanical properties of the common carotid artery. Eur J Echocardiogr. 2010;11(7):630–6.
6. Catalano M, Lamberti-Castronuovo A, Catalano A, Filocamo D, Zimbalatti C. Two-dimensional speckle-tracking strain imaging in the assessment of mechanical properties of carotid arteries: feasibility and comparison with conventional markers of subclinical atherosclerosis. Eur J Echocardiogr. 2011;12(7):528–35.
7. Leung KY, Bosch JG. Automated border detection in three-dimensional echocardiography: principles and promises. Eur J Echocardiogr. 2010;11(2): 97–108.
8. Lopata RG, Nillesen MM, Hansen HH, Gerrits IH, Thijssen JM, de Korte CL. Performance evaluation of methods for two-dimensional displacement and strain estimation using ultrasound radio frequency data. Ultrasound Med Biol. 2009;35(5):796–812.
9. Ma C, Varghese T. Comparison of cardiac displacement and strain imaging using ultrasound radiofrequency and envelope signals. Ultrasonics. 2013;53(3):782–92.
10. Hansen HH, Lopata RG, Idzenga T, de Korte CL. Full 2D displacement vector and strain tensor estimation for superficial tissue using beam-steered ultrasound imaging. Phys Med Biol. 2010;55(11):3201–18.
11. McCormick M, Varghese T, Wang X, Mitchell C, Kliewer MA, Dempsey RJ. Methods for robust in vivo strain estimation in the carotid artery. Phys Med Biol. 2012;57(22):7329–53.
12. Korukonda S, Nayak R, Carson N, Schifitto G, Dogra V, Doyley MM. Noninvasive vascular elastography using plane-wave and sparse-array imaging. IEEE Trans Ultrason Ferroelectr Freq Control. 2013;60(2):332–42.
13. Poree J, Garcia D, Chayer B, Ohayon J, Cloutier G. Noninvasive Vascular Elastography With Plane Strain Incompressibility Assumption Using Ultrafast Coherent Compound Plane Wave Imaging. IEEE Trans Med Imaging. 2015;34(12):2618–31.
14. Hasegawa H, Kanai H. Phase-sensitive lateral motion estimator for measurement of artery-wall displacement–phantom study. IEEE Trans Ultrason Ferroelectr Freq Control. 2009;56(11):2450–62.
15. Maurice RL, Ohayon J, Fretigny Y, Bertrand M, Soulez G, Cloutier G. Noninvasive vascular elastography: theoretical framework. IEEE Trans Med Imaging. 2004;23(2):164–80.
16. Naim C, Cloutier G, Mercure E, Destrempes F, Qin Z, El-Abyad W, Lanthier S, Giroux MF, Soulez G. Characterisation of carotid plaques with ultrasound elastography: feasibility and correlation with high-resolution magnetic resonance imaging. Eur Radiol. 2013;23(7):2030–41.
17. Liu F, Yong Q, Zhang Q, Liu P, Yang Y. Real-time tissue elastography for the detection of vulnerable carotid plaques in patients undergoing endarterectomy: a pilot study. Ultrasound Med Biol. 2015;41(3):705–12.
18. Huang C, Pan X, He Q, Huang M, Huang L, Zhao X, Yuan C, Bai J, Luo J. Ultrasound-Based Carotid Elastography for Detection of Vulnerable Atherosclerotic Plaques Validated by Magnetic Resonance Imaging. Ultrasound Med Biol. 2016;42(2):365–77.
19. Hansen HH, de Borst GJ, Bots ML, Moll FL, Pasterkamp G, de Korte CL. Validation of Noninvasive In Vivo Compound Ultrasound Strain Imaging Using Histologic Plaque Vulnerability Features. Stroke. 2016;47(11):2770–5.
20. Thijssen DH, Black MA, Pyke KE, Padilla J, Atkinson G, Harris RA, Parker B, Widlansky ME, Tschakovsky ME, Green DJ. Assessment of flow-mediated dilation in humans: a methodological and physiological guideline. Am J Phys Heart Circ Phys. 2011;300(1):H2–12.
21. Godia EC, Madhok R, Pittman J, Trocio S, Ramas R, Cabral D, Sacco RL, Rundek T. Carotid artery distensibility: a reliability study. J Ultrasound Med. 2007;26(9):1157–65.
22. Weber T, Ammer M, Rammer M, Adji A, O'Rourke MF, Wassertheurer S, Rosenkranz S, Eber B. Noninvasive determination of carotid-femoral pulse wave velocity depends critically on assessment of travel distance: a comparison with invasive measurement. J Hypertens. 2009;27(8):1624–30.
23. Thijssen DH, Scholten RR, van den Munckhof IC, Benda N, Green DJ, Hopman MT. Acute change in vascular tone alters intima-media thickness. Hypertension. 2011;58(2):240–6.
24. Potter K, Green DJ, Reed CJ, Woodman RJ, Watts GF, McQuillan BM, Burke V, Hankey GJ, Arnolda LF. Carotid intima-medial thickness measured on multiple ultrasound frames: evaluation of a DICOM-based software system. Cardiovasc Ultrasound. 2007;5:29.
25. Potter K, Reed CJ, Green DJ, Hankey GJ, Arnolda LF. Ultrasound settings significantly alter arterial lumen and wall thickness measurements. Cardiovasc Ultrasound. 2008;6:6.
26. Thijssen DH, De Groot PC, van den Bogerd A, Veltmeijer M, Cable NT, Green DJ, Hopman MT. Time course of arterial remodelling in diameter and wall thickness above and below the lesion after a spinal cord injury. Eur J Appl Physiol. 2012;112(12):4103–9.
27. Lopata RG, Hansen HH, Nillesen MM, Thijssen JM, De Korte CL. Comparison of one-dimensional and two-dimensional least-squares strain estimators for phased array displacement data. Ultrason Imaging. 2009;31(1):1–16.
28. Hansen HH, Lopata RG, Idzenga T, de Korte CL. An angular compounding technique using displacement projection for noninvasive ultrasound strain imaging of vessel cross-sections. Ultrasound Med Biol. 2010;36(11):1947–56.
29. Goeman JJ, Solari A. Multiple hypothesis testing in genomics. Stat Med. 2014;33(11):1946–78.
30. Hansen HHG, De Borst GJ, Bots ML, Moll F, Pasterkamp G, De Korte CL. Noninvasive compound ultrasound elastography for vulnerable plaque detection: in vivo validation. Eur Heart J. 2013;34(suppl 1):28.
31. Dudenbostel T, Glasser SP. Effects of antihypertensive drugs on arterial stiffness. Cardiol Rev. 2012;20(5):259–63.
32. Ong KT, Delerme S, Pannier B, Safar ME, Benetos A, Laurent S, Boutouyrie P, investigators. Aortic stiffness is reduced beyond blood pressure lowering by short-term and long-term antihypertensive treatment: a meta-analysis of individual data in 294 patients. J Hypertens. 2011;29(6):1034–42.
33. Crouse JR, Furberg CD, Espeland MA, Riley WA. B-Mode Ultrasound: A Noninvasive Method for Assessing Atherosclerosis. In: Willerson JT, HJJ W, Cohn JN, Holmes DR, editors. Cardiovascular Medicine. London: Springer London; 2007. p. 1783–96.
34. Thijssen DH, Cable NT, Green DJ. Impact of exercise training on arterial wall thickness in humans. Clin Sci. 2012;122(7):311–22.
35. Tanaka H, Dinenno FA, Monahan KD, Clevenger CM, DeSouza CA, Seals DR. Aging, habitual exercise, and dynamic arterial compliance. Circulation. 2000;102(11):1270–5.
36. Ashor AW, Lara J, Siervo M, Celis-Morales C, Oggioni C, Jakovljevic DG, Mathers JC. Exercise modalities and endothelial function: a systematic review and dose-response meta-analysis of randomized controlled trials. Sports Med. 2015;45(2):279–96.
37. Burke GL, Evans GW, Riley WA, Sharrett AR, Howard G, Barnes RW, Rosamond W, Crow RS, Rautaharju PM, Heiss G. Arterial wall thickness is associated with prevalent cardiovascular disease in middle-aged adults. The Atherosclerosis Risk in Communities (ARIC) Study. Stroke. 1995;26(3):386–91.
38. Linhart A, Dostalova G, Belohlavek J, Vitek L, Karetova D, Ingrischova M, Bojanovska K, Polacek P, Votavova R, Cifkova R. Carotid intima-media thickness in young survivors of acute myocardial infarction. Exp Clin Cardiol. 2012;17(4):215–20.
39. Polak JF, Pencina MJ, Meisner A, Pencina KM, Brown LS, Wolf PA, D'Agostino RB Sr. Associations of carotid artery intima-media thickness (IMT) with risk factors and prevalent cardiovascular disease: comparison of mean common carotid artery IMT with maximum internal carotid artery IMT. J Ultrasound Med. 2010;29(12):1759–68.

3

Stress echo 2020: the international stress echo study in ischemic and non-ischemic heart disease

Eugenio Picano[1*], Quirino Ciampi[2], Rodolfo Citro[3], Antonello D'Andrea[4], Maria Chiara Scali[5], Lauro Cortigiani[6], Iacopo Olivotto[7], Fabio Mori[7], Maurizio Galderisi[8], Marco Fabio Costantino[9], Lorenza Pratali[1], Giovanni Di Salvo[10], Eduardo Bossone[3], Francesco Ferrara[3], Luna Gargani[1], Fausto Rigo[11], Nicola Gaibazzi[12], Giuseppe Limongelli[13], Giuseppe Pacileo[4], Maria Grazia Andreassi[1], Bruno Pinamonti[14], Laura Massa[14], Marco A. R. Torres[15], Marcelo H. Miglioranza[16], Clarissa Borguezan Daros[17], José Luis de Castro e Silva Pretto[18], Branko Beleslin[19], Ana Djordjevic-Dikic[19], Albert Varga[20], Attila Palinkas[21], Gergely Agoston[20], Dario Gregori[22], Paolo Trambaiolo[23], Sergio Severino[24], Ayana Arystan[25], Marco Paterni[1], Clara Carpeggiani[1] and Paolo Colonna[26]

Abstract

Background: Stress echocardiography (SE) has an established role in evidence-based guidelines, but recently its breadth and variety of applications have extended well beyond coronary artery disease (CAD). We lack a prospective research study of SE applications, in and beyond CAD, also considering a variety of signs in addition to regional wall motion abnormalities.

Methods: In a prospective, multicenter, international, observational study design, > 100 certified high-volume SE labs (initially from Italy, Brazil, Hungary, and Serbia) will be networked with an organized system of clinical, laboratory and imaging data collection at the time of physical or pharmacological SE, with structured follow-up information. The study is endorsed by the Italian Society of Cardiovascular Echography and organized in 10 subprojects focusing on: contractile reserve for prediction of cardiac resynchronization or medical therapy response; stress B-lines in heart failure; hypertrophic cardiomyopathy; heart failure with preserved ejection fraction; mitral regurgitation after either transcatheter or surgical aortic valve replacement; outdoor SE in extreme physiology; right ventricular contractile reserve in repaired Tetralogy of Fallot; suspected or initial pulmonary arterial hypertension; coronary flow velocity, left ventricular elastance reserve and B-lines in known or suspected CAD; identification of subclinical familial disease in genotype-positive, phenotype- negative healthy relatives of inherited disease (such as hypertrophic cardiomyopathy).

Results: We expect to recruit about 10,000 patients over a 5-year period (2016-2020), with sample sizes ranging from 5,000 for coronary flow velocity/ left ventricular elastance/ B-lines in CAD to around 250 for hypertrophic cardiomyopathy or repaired Tetralogy of Fallot. This data-base will allow to investigate technical questions such as feasibility and reproducibility of various SE parameters and to assess their prognostic value in different clinical scenarios.

(Continued on next page)

* Correspondence: picano@ifc.cnr.it
[1]Institute of Clinical Physiology, National Research Council, Pisa, Italy
Full list of author information is available at the end of the article

(Continued from previous page)

Conclusions: The study will create the cultural, informatic and scientific infrastructure connecting high-volume, accredited SE labs, sharing common criteria of indication, execution, reporting and image storage of SE to obtain original safety, feasibility, and outcome data in evidence-poor diagnostic fields, also outside the established core application of SE in CAD based on regional wall motion abnormalities. The study will standardize procedures, validate emerging signs, and integrate the new information with established knowledge, helping to build a next-generation SE lab without inner walls.

Keywords: Effectiveness, Imaging, Prognosis, Stress echocardiography

Background

For a long time, the scope of stress echo (SE) remained focused on coronary artery disease (CAD) [1, 2]. In the last ten years, SE has exploded in its breadth and variety of applications [3, 4]. From a one-fits-all approach (wall motion by 2D-echo in the patient with known or suspected CAD), the field has progressed to an omnivorous, next-generation laboratory employing a variety of technologies (from M-Mode to 2D, from pulsed, continuous, color and tissue Doppler to lung ultrasound) on patients covering the entire spectrum of severity (from elite athletes to patients with end-stage heart failure) and ages (from children with congenital heart disease to the elderly with aortic stenosis) [4] (Fig. 1). As a consequence of this rapid growth, the clinical use of SE often lacks the necessary supportive evidence and is slowed by unavoidable confusion on methodological issues in a rapidly evolving field. This situation represents a challenge and an opportunity for the SE community. It is a challenge, because in other fields of cardiology we currently lack the level of evidence collected in the last 30 years that led SE based on the detection of regional wall motion abnormalities to play a central role in CAD and heart failure management, as acknowledged in specialty [5, 6] and general cardiology guidelines [7–10]. It is also an opportunity, because today SE has the unprecedented advantages of economic sustainability, lack of radiation, portability and versatility making it especially attractive in the current era of increasing societal concerns about cardiac imaging costs and long-term risks due to ionizing radiation [11].

"Stress echo 2020" (SE2020) is a prospective, multicenter, international, observational study, involving > 100 SE laboratories, with short-term, mid-term, and long-term aims: 1) In the short term (12 months), to create the cultural, digital and scientific infrastructure connecting high volume, accredited SE labs, sharing common criteria of indication, performance, reporting and image storage of SE; 2) In the mid-term (2 to 3 years), to obtain original safety, feasibility, and outcome data in evidence-poor diagnostic fields, also outside the established core application of SE in CAD [12]: contractile reserve for prediction of cardiac resynchronization or medical therapy response; stress B-lines in heart failure; hypertrophic cardiomyopathy; heart failure with preserved ejection fraction; mitral and aortic valve function after transcatheter or surgical aortic valve implantation; outdoor SE in extreme physiology; right ventricular contractile reserve in repaired Tetralogy of Fallot; exercise-induced pulmonary artery pressure rise in predicting outcome in at risk, borderline or early established pulmonary arterial hypertension; added value of new, second- and third-generation parameters (coronary flow velocity reserve, left ventricular elastance reserve and B-lines) for refining prognosis based on regional wall motion abnormalities, within and outside CAD; identification of subclinical familial disease in genotype-positive and phenotype–negative healthy relatives at risk for hypertrophic cardiomyopathy or familial dilated cardiomyopathy or pulmonary hypertension; 3) In the long-term (at the end of the 5-year project), to establish an up and running platform for future prospective, randomized, outcome studies with selective interventions on specific diseases based on SE results.

Methods

In a prospective, multicenter, international, observational study design, > 100 SE labs will be networked with systematic clinical, laboratory and imaging data collection at the time of SE and with structured follow-up information.

The study theater is the international network of cardiology SE laboratories, and the study is endorsed and promoted by the Italian Society of Cardiovascular Echography. The main documents (from protocols to case report form to software and website platform) will be in English, so that selected highly motivated and experienced centers may join specific subprojects, setting the stage for an international upscaling of the project in the coming years. The starting point of the recruitment phase was a recent electronic survey by the Italian Society of Cardiovascular Echography, in 2015 censoring 134 laboratories with moderate- (>100/year) to high- (>400/year) volume SE activities [13], which were precisely interrogated for interest in participation to SE2020. Laboratories from Brazil, Serbia, and Hungary have already joined the project. The recruitment plan forecasts 500 patients by the end of 2016, with doubling of the rate of enrollment in subsequent years, in parallel with the

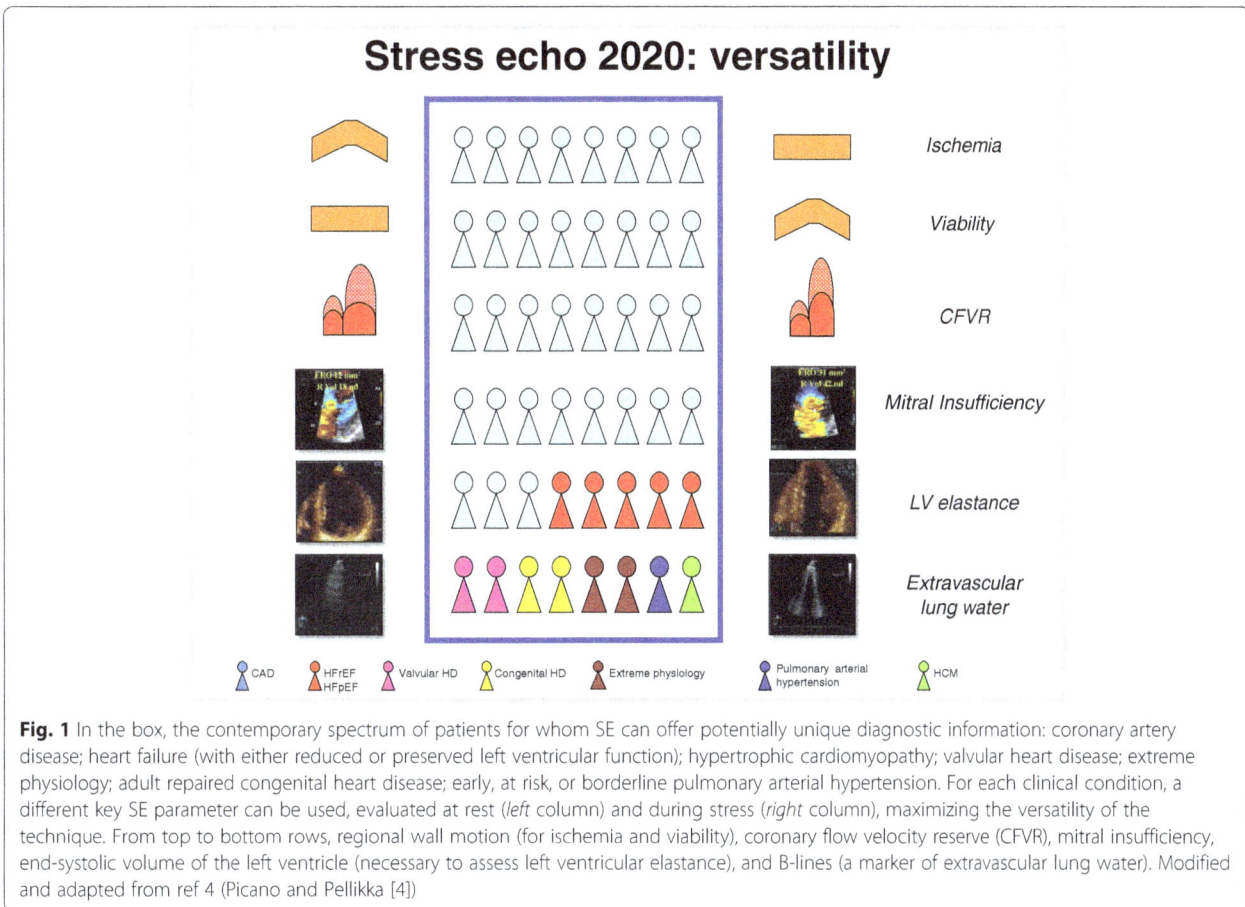

Fig. 1 In the box, the contemporary spectrum of patients for whom SE can offer potentially unique diagnostic information: coronary artery disease; heart failure (with either reduced or preserved left ventricular function); hypertrophic cardiomyopathy; valvular heart disease; extreme physiology; adult repaired congenital heart disease; early, at risk, or borderline pulmonary arterial hypertension. For each clinical condition, a different key SE parameter can be used, evaluated at rest (*left* column) and during stress (*right* column), maximizing the versatility of the technique. From top to bottom rows, regional wall motion (for ischemia and viability), coronary flow velocity reserve (CFVR), mitral insufficiency, end-systolic volume of the left ventricle (necessary to assess left ventricular elastance), and B-lines (a marker of extravascular lung water). Modified and adapted from ref 4 (Picano and Pellikka [4])

increasing number of recruiting labs fulfilling quality control criteria, reaching the target number of 100 at the end of the 5-year schedule.

Data collection

As recommended by guidelines, we will adopt a 17-segment model of the left ventricle, with 1-to-4 segmental scoring system [5, 6]. Stress protocols are harmonized according to recent European and North-American scientific societies' guidelines, with semi-supine exercise recommended and pharmacological stress dosages up to 40 mcg/kg/min for dobutamine, up to 0.84 mg/kg in 6 min for dipyridamole, and up to a 4-min step of 200 microg/kg/min for adenosine [5, 6]. With dobutamine, atropine (up to 1 mg) can be administered in patients with suspected CAD (protocol 9), and it is associated with a higher rate of complications in those with a history of neuropsychiatric symptoms, reduced left ventricular function, or small body habitus. The maximal allowed dobutamine dose is 20 mcg/kg/min in patients with aortic stenosis, in whom higher doses are less safe and probably unnecessary [13]. All laboratories will share a standardized case report form coded in a database format to facilitate retrieval and communication. For

applications outside CAD and for CAD testing with vasodilator stress, no atropine is given on top of pharmacological stress.

Although data collection with a dedicated project-specific case report form is allowed, we encourage implementing a dedicated, free ad-hoc system for data storage and reporting developed at the National Research Council, Institute of Clinical Physiology. The software provides a suitable informatics infrastructure for the SE 2020 Italian multicenter study, with an intuitive graphic interface, eye-catching graphic format and convenient reporting option. It could represent the trade-off between the comprehensive information required by scientific standards and the smooth workflow priority of busy, high-volume, clinically-driven activities [14]. As an illustrative example, the report page for regional wall motion abnormalities and Wall Motion Score Index is shown in Fig. 2. The software was developed and tested in Italian and the translation of the last release in other languages (English, Portuguese and Serbian) is currently in progress.

Data analysis

Data will be expressed as mean ± standard deviation (normally distributed data, such as wall motion score

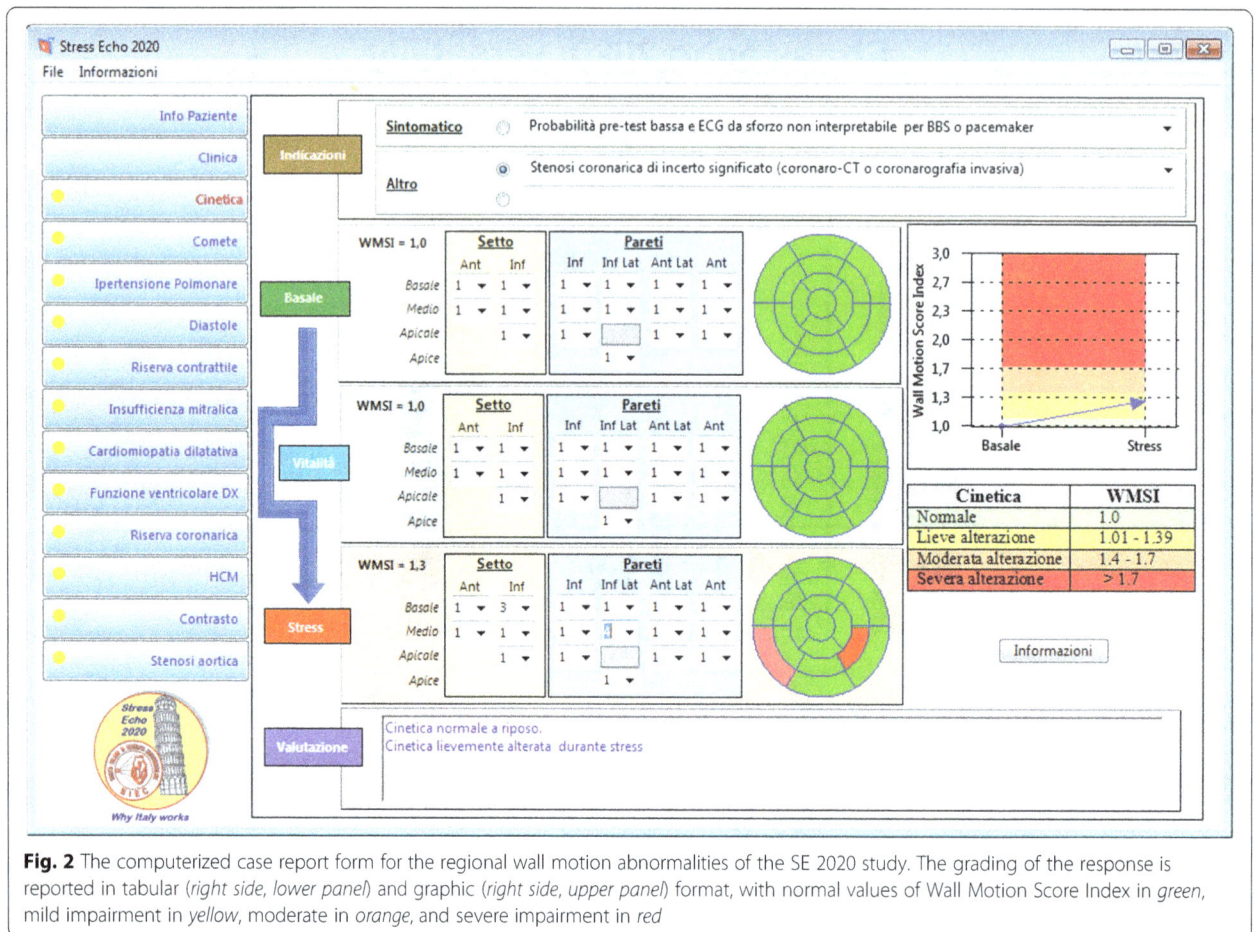

Fig. 2 The computerized case report form for the regional wall motion abnormalities of the SE 2020 study. The grading of the response is reported in tabular (*right side, lower panel*) and graphic (*right side, upper panel*) format, with normal values of Wall Motion Score Index in *green*, mild impairment in *yellow*, moderate in *orange*, and severe impairment in *red*

index), median and inter-quartile (25th, 75th) range (non-normally distributed data, such as B-lines) or per cent frequency (categorical data, such as presence or absence of severe mitral regurgitation), with absolute numbers. In patients with coronary angiographic information, diagnostic sensitivity, specificity, positive and negative predictive value will be assessed for any combination of the wall motion score index, coronary flow velocity reserve, left ventricular contractile reserve and B-lines.

One-sample comparisons will be performed using Wilcoxon test, and the chi-squared test without Fisher's correction for categorical data. Event rates will be estimated with Kaplan–Meier curves and compared by the log-rank test. Univariable analyses by Cox proportional hazards models will be performed to assess the association between each candidate variable and outcome. All variables with $P < 0.20$ by univariable analysis will be considered as candidate variables for the multivariable analyses. Goodness of fit of the models will be based on C-statistics and its variants, adjusting for optimism using bootstrap replications (at least 1000). A receiver operating characteristic analysis will be used to obtain the best prognostic

predictor for the individual SE variables. We will also analyze the data according to a clinically guided stepwise procedure, where the variables will be included in the model in the same order in which they are actually considered by the cardiologist. Statistical significance will be set at $p < 0.05$.

Quality control

It is well-known that the diagnostic performance of SE is closely related to the level of expertise of the cardiologist-echocardiographer performing the test, since the evaluation of regional wall motion is subjective and qualitative, with considerable variability even among experienced centers of undisputed reputation [15]. The reproducibility and accuracy of wall motion reading can be substantially increased with limited training [16] and through development of conservative, pre-specified reading criteria [17]. Therefore, quality control of the diagnostic performance in the various laboratories is a must in order to enter meaningful information in the data bank. The burden of quality control is on the hub center of the principal investigator of each subproject, where various spoke centers may converge. For the general project, the hub center for regional wall motion analysis is Pisa-CNR, in coordination with the principal investigator. There are five different levels of quality control, with increasing levels of complexity:

1. Level 1, pre-requisite: a volume activity of the lab of at least 100 SE tests per year, which is the requirement for credentialing of SE activity by scientific societies [18].
2. Level 2, spoke centers read hub SE images, consisting in 20 selected studies for regional wall motion analysis. The concordance requires identification of test negativity/positivity and, in positive tests, the correct localization of the ischemic zone. For each test, a multiple choice 6-answer test is given. The criterion of ≥ 90% concordance (at least 18 out of 20 studies) is required, as previously described for first-generation SE multicenter studies [19, 20].
3. Level 3, hub centers read spoke centers studies, consisting in 20 any-quality consecutive studies recorded by the spoke center. The criterion of ≥ 80% concordance (at least 16 out of 20 studies) is required, as previously described for first-generation SE multicenter studies [19].
4. Level 4, core lab reading. All centers should grant full access to images of SE studies entered in the data bank for audit or reading by core lab laboratory, which is the standard for specific subprojects such as number 10 for genetic SE, when every effort needs to be made to minimize variability and a single reader will analyze all studies acquired by different centers, as required by recommendations for small-to-medium sample studies, when resources allow [20].
5. Level 5, specific protocols quality control. Although the SE quality control has proved to work well for regional wall motion analysis, novel SE applications involve different parameters, methodology of acquisition and reading criteria. Therefore, for each subproject, a web-based training session and quality control is organized by the specific hub center and principal investigator to assure consistency of data [21]. The principal investigator of each subproject will prepare a set of 20 studies with rest-stress images. For each test, a multiple choice 6-answers test is given (only 1 correct). The criterion of ≥90% concordance (at least 18 out of 20 studies) is required. The specific signs tested for certification are: end-diastolic and end-systolic volume changes (protocol 1); B-lines (protocol 2, 4, 6 and 9); left ventricular outflow tract gradient (protocol 3 and 10); E/e' (protocol 4); mitral regurgitation quantitative assessment (protocol 5); aortic stenosis quantitative assessment (protocol 5); right ventricular function (protocol 7); pulmonary arterial systolic pressure

measurements during stress (protocol 8); coronary flow velocity reserve (protocol 9); left ventricular elastance (protocol 9); global longitudinal strain (protocol 4 and 10).

This study is also intended as a special level of voluntary accreditation and expertise in the specific field of interest, well above the volume activity criteria requested by guidelines. The accreditation process is run and certified by the Italian scientific society of echocardiography strictly following criteria and procedures of the European association of cardiovascular imaging to ensure standardization and independence of the process. When not otherwise specified, resting and SE measurements are performed according to the latest joint recommendations of European and North-American societies [22]. A simplified view of each lab's road to SE2020 is shown in Fig. 3: the essential pre-requisite is the high-volume activity of the lab, with readers' certification of competence from national or international societies and written declaration of interest in SE2020. After adoption of dedicated SE computerized software by the lab (allowing direct entry of the information in a format compatible with the data bank) and voluntary certification for project-specific SE reading, the center can start recruiting.

Overall study design

We will collect the experience of Italian, Brazilian, Hungarian and Serbian SE labs over the 5-year period from 2016 to 2020. In this broader framework, 10 sub-projects will address specific patients' subsets. The target population ranges from 250-patient samples for protocols focused on specific diseases (such as protocol 7 in repaired tetralogy of Fallot) to 2,500 for protocols on heart failure (number 2) to 5,000 to all-comers with known or suspected CAD tested with novel indices (number 9) (Table 1).

Different study projects will cover the entire spectrum of disease, age and clinical status of current patients. The recruited participants are "the wellest of the well" (super-fit athletes entering project 6), the "worried well" (young first-degree relatives of patients with hypertrophic cardiomyopathy or familiar forms of dilated cardiomyopathy or pulmonary arterial hypertension, in project 10), the "suspected sick" (for instance patients with suspected diastolic heart failure or CAD as in projects 4 and 9), up to the "sickest of the sick" (for instance, patients with advanced heart failure or valvular heart disease entering projects 1, 2 and 5). Some degree of overlap is unavoidably present for some projects, for instance with subjects eligible for project 2 who are also recruitable for project 1 (if they undergo cardiac resynchronization therapy) or for project 5 (if they have heart failure with preserved ejection fraction). Over time, patients may move from one project to another: for

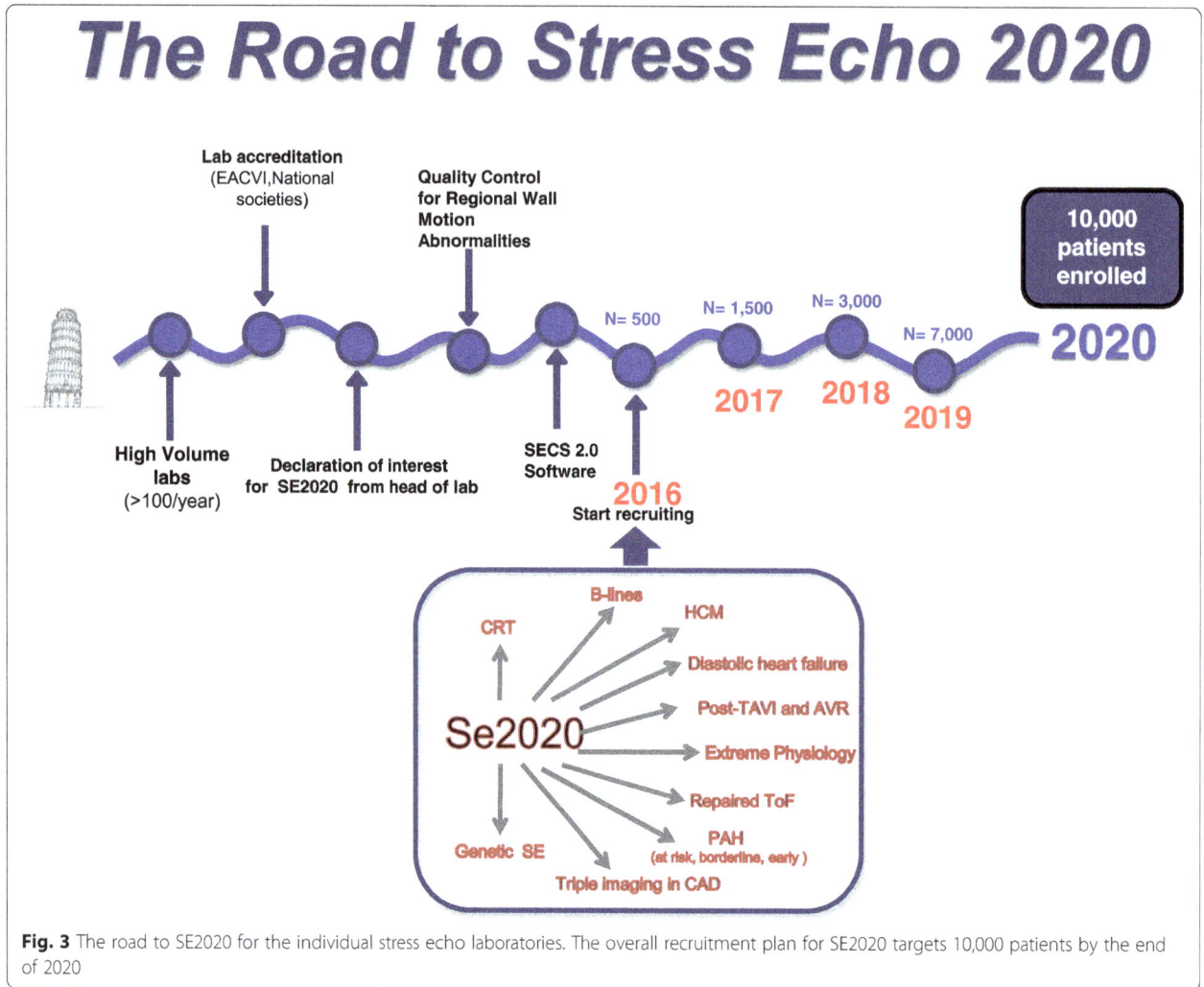

Fig. 3 The road to SE2020 for the individual stress echo laboratories. The overall recruitment plan for SE2020 targets 10,000 patients by the end of 2020

Table 1 The 10 subprojects

Number	Acronym	Patients	Main parameter	Sample size
1-Cardiac Resynchronization Therapy forecast	CHEF	Prior to cardiac resynchronization therapy	Wall Motion Score Index	500
2-B-lines in heart failure	BHEF	Heart failure	Left ventricular Contractile Rererve	2,500
3-SE in Hypertrophic cardiomyopathy	SEHCA	Hypertrophic cardiomyopathy	Left ventricular outflow tract gradient	250
4- SE in diastolic heart failure	SEDIA	Heart failure preserved ejection fraction	E/e'	250
5-SE in Transvalvular or surgical aortic valve replacement	SETA	After aortic valve replacement	Mitral insufficiency	250
6-SE outdoor	SEO	Extreme exercise	B-lines	250
7-SE in repaired tetralogy of Fallot	SETOF	Repaired Fallot	Tricuspid annular plane systolic excursion	250
8-Doppler SE in pulmonary arterial hypertension	DOPSAH	Pulmonary arterial hypertension (early, borderline, at risk)	Systolic pulmonary arterial pressure	250
9-Diagnosis of CAD by triple imaging SE	DITSE	Known or suspected CAD	Coronary Flow velocity reserve	5,000
10-Genetic SE	GENES	Preclinical dilated or hypertrophic cardiomyopathy	Left ventricular outflow tract gradient	250

instance, first-degree relatives of hypertrophic cardiomyopathy patients with negative phenotype enrolled in project 10 may subsequently develop overt forms of disease and be enrolled in project 3. All these potential grayzone situations will be readily identified in individual SE reports. The investigator is allowed to enter the patient in only one subproject at a given time.

Although the setting will be mainly the Italian cardiological community, all essential documents will be written in English and we plan to extend the project to other communities with long-standing history of cooperation and experience in multicenter trials. Brazilian, Hungarian and Serbian centers are already recruiting and additional laboratories from other countries are now entering the process of accreditation. The project is curiosity-driven, independent from sponsors, and clinically oriented. However, after the planning and start-up phase, support from public or private funding agencies or industries is possible – provided that it is unrestricted and does not interfere in any way with data collection and analysis.

There is no bonus payment for subject recruitment and subject referral. Enrolled patients are referred to the SE lab for clinically-driven indications. Each patient signs an informed consent form allowing scientific utilization of data, respectful of privacy rights, at the time of testing. The study project was submitted by the coordinating center of the principal investigator on

January 31, 2016 and approved in its revised form by the Rome-1 ethical committee on July 20, 2016 (protocol number 1487/Lazio1). Ethics committee approval will be sought by each participating center, as needed.

Inclusion criteria shared by all projects are: 1- age < 85 years and > 18 years (except for project 7 regarding repaired Tetralogy of Fallot and project 10 regarding healthy relatives of patients with familial disease, in which children > 10 years can enter the study after parental consent); 2- technically acceptable acoustic window at rest (with at least 14 segments well visualized in at least one projection).

Exclusion criteria shared by all projects are: 1- presence of prognosis-limiting comorbidities, such as advanced cancer, reducing life expectancy to < 1 year; 2- pregnancy/lactation; 3- unwillingness to give informed consent and to enter a regular follow-up program.

SE data will be available to the referring physician.

A brief synopsis of each project is presented for each sub-study, which places emphasis on different parameters tailored on the specific diagnostic question (Fig. 4).

CHEF
Cardiac resynchronization tHErapy Forecast.

Background
Cardiac resynchronization therapy is increasingly used in patients with heart failure, but the identification of

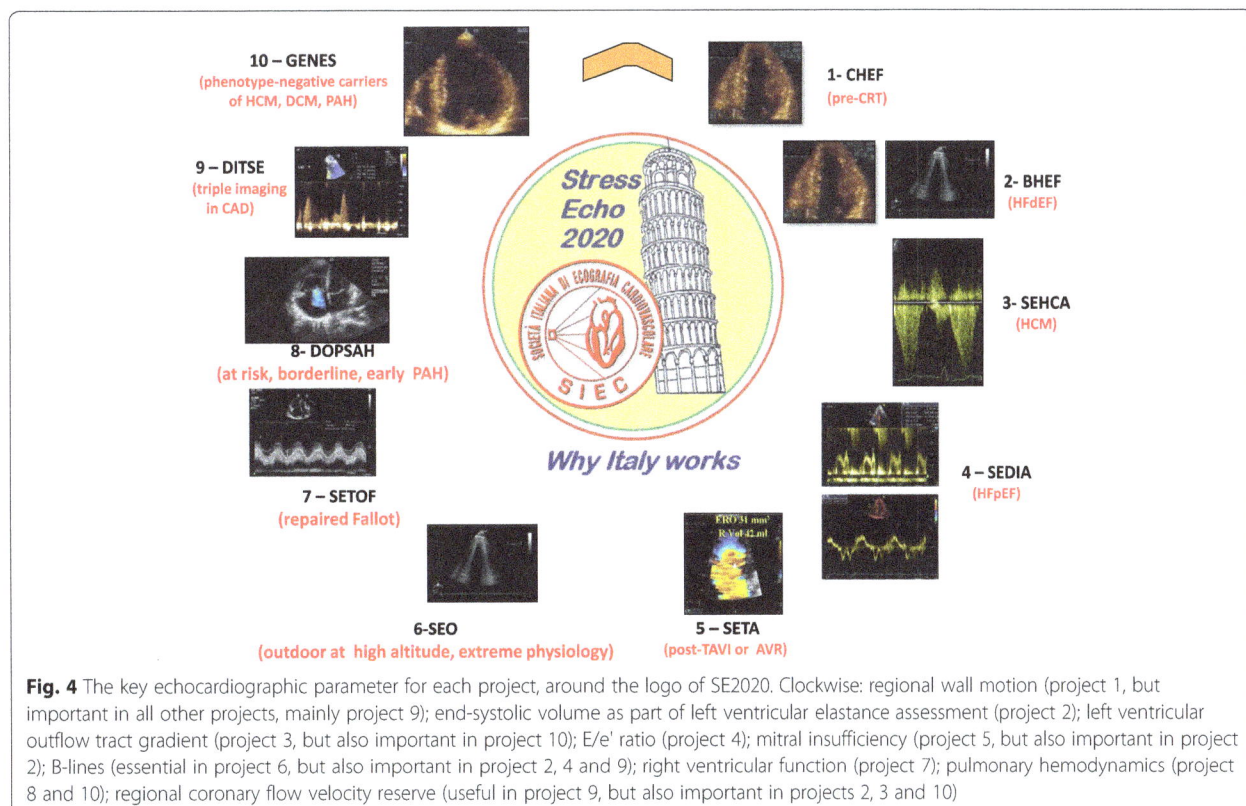

Fig. 4 The key echocardiographic parameter for each project, around the logo of SE2020. Clockwise: regional wall motion (project 1, but important in all other projects, mainly project 9); end-systolic volume as part of left ventricular elastance assessment (project 2); left ventricular outflow tract gradient (project 3, but also important in project 10); E/e' ratio (project 4); mitral insufficiency (project 5, but also important in project 2); B-lines (essential in project 6, but also important in project 2, 4 and 9); right ventricular function (project 7); pulmonary hemodynamics (project 8 and 10); regional coronary flow velocity reserve (useful in project 9, but also important in projects 2, 3 and 10)

"responders" remains challenging, since up to 1 in 3 patients do not show symptomatic improvement with this costly and demanding electrical therapy [10]. QRS width remains the single established criterion to assess intraventricular dyssynchrony according to guidelines; however, there is no accepted consensus on which imaging parameter is best to predict cardiac resynchronization therapy response. Inconsistent results have been obtained with several echocardiographic indices of left ventricular dyssynchrony [23]. The presence of myocardial contractile reserve assessed during SE predicted the response to cardiac resynchronization therapy: the use of SE had obvious potential for a better selection of cardiac resynchronization therapy candidates, in whom a preserved contractility is related to a higher percentage of clinical and echocardiographic responders to cardiac resynchronization therapy [24–27].

Aims

The primary aim is to evaluate the feasibility of several indices of SE (including the well- established, such as wall motion score index, and more innovative ones such as left ventricular elastance) in the evaluation of patient candidates for cardiac resynchronization therapy. The secondary aim is to assess the value of each of these parameters (alone or in combination) in predicting the symptomatic and functional improvement in the short-term (1 week to 1 month) after electrical or medical therapy. The tertiary aim is to assess the prognostic value of SE indices for prognostic stratification in the medium-long term.

Methods

Patients evaluated prior to cardiac resynchronization therapy, with class I, IIa or IIb for cardiac resynchronization therapy according to ESC 2016 guidelines [10], and therefore with ejection fraction ≤ 35% (by 2-D Simpson method, or real time 3D echocardiography) and QRS duration ≥ 130 ms. Contractile reserve will be assessed during stress (exercise or dobutamine or vasodilators) through variations in Wall Motion Score Index and with more advanced parameters such as left ventricular elastance reserve, as the peak stress/baseline ratio of end-systolic pressure/ end-systolic volume [28]. All other echocardiographic parameters of interest (left ventricular ejection fraction, E/e', mitral regurgitation, tricuspid annular plane systolic excursion, septal flash, apical rocking, left anterior descending artery coronary flow velocity whenever possible) will also be assessed at baseline and peak stress. All patients will be followed-up within 6-months to 1 year also with resting echocardiographic examination to assess left ventricular remodelling and recovery of function. Any patient excluded from cardiac resynchronization therapy and kept on optimal medical therapy will be included in the follow-up, since the presence of contractile reserve may predict the functional improvement in these patients as well [13].

Sample size calculation

If we assume a 60% response rate to cardiac resynchronization therapy, with doubling of likelihood of improvement in presence of a pre-test contractile reserve by SE, with a power of 80% and an alpha error of 5%, a sample size of 277 patients is required. About the same number is required to predict the response to medical therapy in patients eventually not undergoing cardiac resynchronization therapy.

Study hypothesis

The presence of contractile reserve is associated with a better prognosis and greater chance of functional recovery with cardiac resynchronization therapy.

BHEF

Evaluation of B-lines in HEart Failure patients with depressed ejection fraction.

Background

B- lines are a semiquantitative sign of extravascular lung water present in 1 out of 3 heart failure patients at rest and in 1 out of 2 during stress, and potentially useful for refining prognostic stratification and titrating diuretic therapy in these patients. Their prognostic power is higher during stress than at rest, and integrates the powerful stratification provided by dynamic assessment of other established predictors such as mitral regurgitation, E/e' as a surrogate of left ventricular filling pressure, ejection fraction and tricuspid annular plane systolic excursion [29, 30].

Aims

The primary aim is to assess the feasibility of several indices of SE (including the well- established such as left ventricular ejection fraction and more innovative ones such as B-lines or left anterior descending coronary flow reserve) in evaluating patients with known or suspected heart failure with reduced ejection fraction. The secondary aim is to assess the value of each of these parameters in predicting the functional impairment, indicated by New York Heart Association class, cardiac natriuretic peptides concentration, peak VO2 and other indices. The tertiary aim is to assess the prognostic value of SE indices for prognostic stratification in the medium-long -term.

Methods

We will enrol patients referred to SE (with exercise, dobutamine or dipyridamole) with known or suspected heart failure, with reduced (<40%) ejection fraction. B-lines will be scored with the 28-regions antero-lateral chest assessment as previously described at baseline and immediately after stopping exercise [31]. A simplified 8-region or 4-region scan is also allowed in order to save time without loss of critical information. All other echocardiographic parameters of interest (left ventricular ejection fraction, E/e', mitral regurgitation, tricuspid annular plane systolic excursion, left anterior descending artery coronary flow velocity whenever possible) will also be assessed at baseline and peak stress [32]. All patients will be followed-up for at least 1 year.

Sample size calculation

If we conservatively assume a 30% yearly incidence of composite end-points (death, myocardial infarction, new hospital readmission, heart transplant, ventricular assist device implantation, aborted sudden death) and a 5% incidence of death, with doubling of likelihood of events in presence of a positive SE (for B-lines increase during stress or lack of contractile reserve or severe mitral insufficiency), with a power of 95% and an alpha error of 5%, with an attrition rate of 15%, a sample size of about 2500 patients is required if the effect on mortality is evaluated.

Study hypothesis

The integrated assessment of 5 major echocardiographic variables during stress adds power to the prognostic stratification operated by isolated echocardiographic predictors in heart failure patients. The prognostically meaningful signs explore 5 key links in the patho-physiologic chain behind cardiovascular response in heart failure: left ventricular systolic function – left ventricular diastolic function - mitral valve regurgitation - lung water accumulation - right ventricular function.

SEHCA
Stress Echo in Hypertrophic Cardiomyopathy.

Background

The impact of SE in hypertrophic cardiomyopathy is limited by lack of standardization and outcome data. Current guidelines recommend SE solely for evaluation of left ventricular outflow tract obstruction [33]. However, large-scale registry data show that SE positivity for ischemic criteria (such as new wall motion abnormalities and coronary flow velocity reserve) rather than inducible gradients predict adverse outcome in hypertrophic cardiomyopathy [34]. Thus, important prognostic as well as functional information may be derived from SE, although their clinical impact remains limited due lack of standardized data collection and uniform protocols. Currently there are virtually no two centers performing SE in the same way in hypertrophic cardiomyopathy

patients, and the test remains grossly underutilized due to (unjustified) concerns with safety. Prospective, standardized, multicenter data collection is necessary to achieve comprehensive evaluation of SE potential in this disease. Of note, exercise limitation and breathlessness may be due to a number of different causes, including left ventricular outflow tract obstruction (which may increase, remain stable or decrease during exercise), functional mitral regurgitation, restrictive physiology, amplified mechanical dyssynchrony, coronary microvascular disease or – less frequently – ischemia associated with prognostically unfavorable stress-induced wall motion abnormalities. Despite similar clinical manifestations, management may differ substantially based on the mechanisms [35]. SE is the only test with the potential to discriminate the various components, allowing a targeted treatment driven by pathophysiology, but prospective data are required to substantiate this hypothesis. Of note, general consensus exists regarding the advisability of preferring physiological provocation with exercise over pharmacological stressors (particularly dobutamine due to substantial prevalence of false positives with regard to inducible obstruction).

Aims

The primary aim is to evaluate the feasibility of several indices of SE (from the well- established such as left ventricular outflow tract gradient to more innovative features such as B-lines or left anterior descending coronary flow reserve) in the evaluation of hypertrophic cardiomyopathy patients. The secondary aim is to assess the value of each of these parameters in predicting functional impairment, indicated by New York Heart Association class, European Society of Cardiology sudden cardiac death risk score and other indices. The tertiary aim is to assess the prognostic value of SE indices for prognostic stratification in the medium-long-term.

Methods

Diagnosis of hypertrophic cardiomyopathy will be based on existing guidelines [33]. Phenocopies such as infiltrative/ storage disease (eg, Fabry) will be excluded. Low-to-intermediate risk symptomatic or asymptomatic hypertrophic cardiomyopathy patients will undergo exercise SE with assessment at each stage and during recovery of wall motion, mitral insufficiency, left ventricular outflow tract gradient (in orthostatic position) and E/e'. If feasible, coronary flow velocity reserve on left anterior descending and lung ultrasound B-lines will also be assessed. Only when patients are unable to exercise, or for the specific aim of assessing coronary flow velocity reserve, will a vasodilator stress (high dose dipyridamole or adenosine without atropine) be performed. All patients will be followed-up and the prognostic value of different rest and SE parameters (also compared to standard prognostic indices) will be assessed.

Sample size calculation

The composite end-point of the study comprises death (cardiovascular and all-cause), new hospital admission for acute heart failure, newly onset atrial fibrillation, aborted sudden death, heart transplant or ventricular assist device implantation. A pilot study showed an incidence of events around 8% per year [34]. If we assume a positivity rate to SE (by composite criteria) of 40%, with doubling of likelihood of events in presence of SE positivity (by any criteria), with a power of 80%, an alpha error of 5%, and an attrition rate of 10%, a sample size of about 250 patients is required.

Study hypothesis

Hypertrophic cardiomyopathy patients with inducible wall motion abnormalities and reduced coronary flow velocity reserve (or lung ultrasound B-lines) are at substantially higher risk for subsequent unfavorable events than patients with normal wall motion and preserved coronary flow velocity reserve. Exercise capacity predicts outcome in hypertrophic cardiomyopathy patients independent of the presence and magnitude of resting or provocable obstruction.

SEDIA

Stress Echo in Diastolic Heart failure.

Background

Diastolic SE should be considered in the breathless patient with normal left ventricular ejection fraction, high cardiac natriuretic peptides and low exercise tolerance, especially in presence of cardiovascular risk factors (advanced age, arterial systemic hypertension, diabetes mellitus, obesity and sedentary lifestyle) after ruling out other common cardiac (heart valve disease, coronary artery disease) and non-cardiac causes of dyspnea (mainly anemia and chronic obstructive pulmonary disease). « Red flag » indicators of possible diastolic dysfunction include left ventricular hypertrophy, enlarged left atrium and pulmonary hypertension. During SE, findings which may account for unexplained dyspnea beyond diastolic dysfunction are left ventricular outflow tract obstruction, dynamic mitral regurgitation, and new onset regional wall motion abnormalities [36]. The diagnostic SE criteria of heart failure with preserved ejection fraction are reduced stroke volume and cardiac output reserve, high left ventricular filling pressures (average E/e' ratio > 14) and pulmonary hypertension, which also identify patients with more severe prognosis [37, 38]. In patients with heart failure and either preserved (>50%) or mid-range (40-49%) ejection fraction, SE may allow the identification of diastolic dysfunction in patients with parameters inconclusive at rest [10]. According to the latest 2016 recommendations on the evaluation of left ventricular diastolic function by echocardiography [36], diastolic stress testing would not be indicated in patients with either completely normal diastolic function at rest (in whom a severe diastolic dysfunction is unlikely to develop during stress) and in patients with ≥ grade 2 diastolic dysfunction at rest (with elevated filling pressures at rest which will likely increase further during exercise). However, testing of these patients can be valuable to assess the incremental value, if any, of newer candidate indices such as left ventricular end-diastolic volume reserve and B-lines. In addition, also patients with normal left ventricular diastolic function at rest can indeed develop increase in left ventricular filling pressures with dyspnea when exercising.

Aims

The primary aim is to evaluate the feasibility of several indices of SE (including more established such as E/e' ratio and more innovative ones such as B-lines or left ventricular diastolic volume reserve) in the evaluation of patients with known or suspected heart failure with preserved or mid-range ejection fraction. The secondary aim is to assess the value of each of these parameters in predicting the functional impairment, indicated by New York Heart Association class, cardiac natriuretic peptides concentration, peak VO2 and other indices. The tertiary aim is to assess the prognostic value of SE indices for prognostic stratification of heart failure with preserved ejection fraction in the medium-long-term.

Methods

Patients with known or suspected heart failure with preserved ejection fraction by 2016 ESC criteria will be enrolled and studied with cycle-ergometer in semi-supine SE (or treadmill). The test is especially indicated in patients with dyspnea and grade 1 diastolic dysfunction at rest, identified as mitral E/A ratio ≤ 0.8, average E/e' ratio < 10, peak tricuspid regurgitant jet velocity <2.8 m/s and left atrium volume index normal (<34 mL/m^2) or increased [36]. In patients unable to exercise, pharmacological test of choice (dobutamine or vasodilator) is allowed, but not recommended. The diastolic assessment should be included into all exercise SE tests by measuring standard Doppler-derived mitral inflow velocity, pulsed Tissue Doppler of mitral annulus, and retrograde tricuspid gradient of tricuspid regurgitation. These measurements can be performed at intermediate load of exercise and/or 1- 2 min after the end of the exercise, after obtaining wall motion acquisitions, when the heart rate decreases and mitral inflow E and A velocities appear to be well separated. As a part of the "diastolic package", we will also assess, at baseline, intermediate load (50 watts) and peak-post stress [36]: diastolic left ventricular volume index (to evaluate left ventricular diastolic volume reserve, impaired in stiff hearts, which are less dilated for any given filling pressure); systolic left ventricular volume index (for assessment of left ventricular elastance, which may unmask occult systolic dysfunction with normal ejection fraction increase); ejection fraction and both stroke volume and cardiac output (to assess conventional contractile reserve); mitral regurgitation and left ventricular outflow tract obstruction; pulmonary artery systolic pressure (from velocity of tricuspid regurgitation); B-lines during stress (to provide a direct imaging of extra-vascular lung water accumulation as a direct cause of dyspnea), since they can be present at rest in diastolic heart failure [32]. Global longitudinal strain could be optionally determined as the average of the regional longitudinal strain measured in 17-segments model from the apical long-axis, 4-chamber and 2-chamber view. Despite not being independent on preload and afterload, global longitudinal strain could be considered as an appropriate, alternative parameter of left ventricular contractile reserve [22, 39]. On the basis of currently accepted criteria, the test is considered positive for diastolic dysfunction when all of the following three conditions are met during exercise: average E/e' > 14 or septal E/e' ratio > 15, peak tricuspid regurgitant jet velocity >2.8 m/s and septal e' velocity < 7 cm/s at baseline [36].

Sample size calculation

The composite end-point of the study comprises death (cardiovascular and all-cause), new hospital admission for acute heart failure, aborted sudden death, heart transplant or ventricular assist device implantation. The expected incidence of events is around 20% per year [10]. We assume a positivity rate to SE (by composite criteria: increase in E/e' and/or increase in pulmonary artery systolic pressure and/ or decrease in septal e' velocity and/or increase in B-lines) of 30%, with doubling of likelihood of events in presence of SE positivity (by any criteria). With a power of 80%, an alpha error of 5%, and an attrition rate of 10% (for exams non-feasible and/ or for exclusion criteria during the screening phase due to previously unrecognized dynamic severe mitral regurgitation or left ventricular outflow obstruction), a sample size of about 250 patients is required.

Study hypothesis

In patients with known or suspected heart failure with reduced ejection fraction, higher left ventricular filling pressures, more B- lines and lower increases in end-diastolic volumes during stress are associated with worse prognosis.

SETA

Stress Echo in Transcatheter or surgical Aortic Valve Implantation.

Background

Transcatheter Aortic Valve Implantation is an extraordinarily effective but still a relatively novel technology, and short and long term morbidity and mortality after Transcatheter Aortic Valve Implantation remains significant. There is substantial interest in the identification and modification of factors influencing prognosis before and after the procedure. The severity of concomitant mitral regurgitation improves after the procedure in 2 out of 3 patients, but baseline moderate-severe mitral regurgitation and significant residual mitral regurgitation are associated with an increase in mortality after Transcatheter Aortic Valve Implantation and represent an important group to target with medical or transcatheter therapies in the future [40]. Stress echo plays a pivotal role in valvular heart disease [41], but its role after either Transcatheter Aortic Valve Implantation or surgical replacement is still unsettled, although it has potential to identify the presence and severity of mitral regurgitation and aortic stenosis after intervention, so as to refine the prognostic strategy and better tailor treatment.

Aims

The primary aim is to evaluate the feasibility of SE focused on mitral and aortic reserve after aortic valve replacement (with Transcatheter or surgical aortic valve implantation). The secondary aim is to assess the presence and entity of changes in valvular and ventricular function and their correlation with indices of functional severity (New York Heart Association Class, cardiac natriuretic peptides, peak VO$_2$, etc.).. The tertiary aim is to assess the prognostic value of SE indices for prognostic stratification in the medium-long-term.

Methods

Patients with previous (from 6 months to 10 years) surgical or Transcatheter Aortic Valve Implantation capable of exercising and with absent-to-moderate mitral insufficiency will be enrolled and studied with semisupine SE. The full quantitative evaluation of mitral regurgitation and aortic stenosis will be performed according to recommendations of the European Society of Cardiology. In addition, assessment of B- lines (as in protocol 2), right ventricular function (as in protocol 7), left ventricular elastance (as in protocol 1) will be performed at baseline and peak stress. Exercise will be started at 15 watts, with 5-min steps and 15-watt increments per step [13]. In patients unable to exercise, a pharmacological test of choice (dobutamine or vasodilator) is allowed, but not recommended.

Sample size calculation

The expected incidence of SE positivity (by composite criteria: increase in mean transaortic gradient > 20 mmHg and/or increase in mitral insufficiency > 1 grade and/or increase in B-lines and/or increase in systolic pulmonary artery pressure) is around 30% post- Transcatheter Aortic Valve Implantation or aortic valve surgical replacement [10]. With a power of 80%, an alpha error of 5%, and an attrition rate of 10%, a sample size of about 100 patients is required to detect a significant stress-induced increase in mitral regurgitation severity. For the prognostic analysis (tertiary end-point). If we conservatively assume a 20% yearly incidence of composite end-points (death, myocardial infarction, new hospital readmission, heart transplant, ventricular assist device implantation, aborted sudden death), with doubling of likelihood of events in presence of a positive SE (for severe mitral insufficiency and/or abnormally increased transaortic gradient and/ or B-lines and/ or abnormal pulmonary artery systolic pressure), with a power of 80% and an alpha error of 5%, a sample size of about 250 patients is required with a 3 -year follow-up.

Study hypothesis

In patients with absent-to moderate mitral regurgitation in resting transthoracic echocardiography after either surgical or Transcatheter Aortic Valve Implantation, those with lower transaortic gradient and less mitral regurgitation during stress will have a more favourable outcome than patients with higher gradients and more severe residual mitral regurgitation during stress.

SEO

Stress Echo Outdoor in Extreme conditions.

Background

SE with B-lines can also be performed outdoors, with pocket size or portable instruments, in a setting of ecological stress entirely different from standard indoor testing [4]. The diagnostic target is the diagnosis, or early subclinical identification, of life-threatening disease at high altitudes or any kind of environmental pulmonary edema. In this challenging but fascinating context, lung ultrasound detects B-lines in 20 to 40% of normal and/or super-fit subjects in extreme physiology settings, such as high altitude [42, 43], deep underwater apnea diving [44] or endurance exercise [45].

Aims

The primary aim is to evaluate the feasibility of outdoor SE focused on B-lines in the logistic setting of extreme physiology. The secondary aim is to assess the presence and amount of B-lines increase at peak stress vs baseline conditions (pre-exercise; pre-apnea; pre-ascent) and to correlate lung ultrasound findings with symptoms (such as dyspnea, cough, fatigue). The tertiary aim is to assess the prognostic value of SE indices for predicting spontaneously occurring pulmonary edema.

Methods

Subjects involved in extreme sporting events (competitive triathlon, marathon, apnea diving etc.) or ordinary exercise in extreme environments (trekking at high altitude) will undergo lung ultrasound scan for B-lines before, soon after (within 10 min) and (when positive soon after) later after (6 to 24 h) the acute extreme exercise. Additional clinical information will be collected in addition to standard case report form (including Acute Mountain Sickness scores in subjects evaluated at high altitude), and will include details on type and duration of exercise (apnea diving vs ascent trekking vs strenuous exercise at sea level etc.) [43]; environmental conditions (temperature, humidity, setting, wind etc.); location and timing of scanning, with possibility of limited scanning (8 regions instead of the standard 28) in more hostile environments.

Sample size calculation

The expected incidence of SE positivity (increase in B-lines >5 compared to rest) is around 30% [43]. With a power of 80%, an alpha error of 5%, and an attrition rate of 10%, a sample size of about 80 patients is required to detect a significant stress-induced increase in B-lines in each of the three major study subgroups: high altitude trekkers (n = 100); marathon and ultra marathon runners (n = 80) and apnea divers (n = 70).

Study hypothesis

Asymptomatic subjects with evidence of B- lines are more likely to develop clinically overt forms of environmental pulmonary edema with persistence of exposure or in the future when re-challenged under similar conditions.

SETOF

Stress Echo in operated Tetralogy of Fallot.

Background

Tetralogy of Fallot is the most common cyanotic congenital heart lesion, and since treatments became available over 70 years ago, there are now a large number of patients with repaired Tetralogy of Fallot [46]. After Tetralogy of Fallot repair, children often have residual lesions (the most common being pulmonary regurgitation) which can be treated with surgical or catheter-based pulmonary valve replacement decreasing right ventricular size but not yet correlated with improved outcome [46]. Pulmonary regurgitation can cause progressive right ventricular dilatation and dysfunction. In Tetralogy of Fallot patients morbidity and mortality are strongly related to right ventricular dysfunction. For this reason, the early detection of right ventricular dysfunction before it reaches an irreversible stage remains crucial [47]. Unfortunately, resting parameters have shown a limited ability to detect early impairment of right ventricular function. Recently, a few studies have suggested that physical or pharmacological stress may unmask abnormalities of right ventricular function in patients with repaired Tetralogy of Fallot, with normal right ventricular function under resting conditions [48–50]. Physical exercise SE allows the simultaneous assessment of right and left ventricular global and regional function and Doppler parameters [51].

Aims

The primary aim is to evaluate the feasibility of right ventricular SE in patients with repaired tetralogy of Fallot. The secondary aim is to assess the presence and amount of right ventricular contractile reserve and its correlation with indices of functional severity (NYHA class, cardiac natriuretic peptides, peak VO_2, 6-min walking test, etc.). The tertiary aim is to assess the prognostic value of SE indices for prognostic stratification in the medium and long-term.

Methods

Patients with repaired Tetralogy of Fallot or Fallot-like pathology (double-outlet right ventricle Fallot type, tetralogy of Fallot with pulmonary atresia), evaluated at least 1 year after the last surgical or percutaneous procedure, will be recruited by regional reference centers for congenital heart disease. Additional inclusion criteria are age > 10 years, height > 140 cm, New York Heart Association class I or II. Right ventricular function will be assessed at baseline and peak stress with variations (rest and peak stress) of tricuspid annular plane systolic excursion, an index of right ventricular longitudinal function, and right ventricular fractional area change (a load-dependent index of right ventricular inlet function). Due to the influence of load on these measures, they tend to reflect right ventricular arterial coupling rather than measures of right ventricular contractility per se. To distinguish between genuine right ventricular dysfunction and/or pathological increases in pulmonary vascular load, whenever possible we will combine systolic pulmonary artery pressure and right ventricular end-systolic area using echocardiography to calculate right ventricular end-systolic pressure-area relation as a surrogate of right ventricular contractility [52].

Peak systolic tricuspid annulus velocity and conventional indices of left ventricular systolic and diastolic function will also be measured at baseline and peak stress. Left ventricular function will also be assessed through measurement of ejection fraction, wall motion score index and E/e' at baseline and peak stress.

Sample size calculation

The expected incidence of SE positivity (by increase in tricuspid annular plane systolic excursion < 5 mm) is around 30% as shown by previous pilot studies [10]. With a power of 80%, an alpha error of 5%, and an attrition rate of 10%, a sample size of about 250 patients is required to detect a significant stress-induced increase in tricuspid annular plane systolic excursion. For the exploratory prognostic analysis (tertiary end-point), we conservatively assume a 20% yearly incidence of the predetermined end-point (death, myocardial infarction, new hospital readmission, heart transplant, ventricular assist device implantation, aborted sudden death), with doubling of likelihood of events in presence of a positive SE (reduced right ventricular contractile reserve). With a power of 80% and an alpha error of 5%, a sample size of about 250 patients is required with a 3 -year follow-up.

Study hypothesis

Repaired tetralogy of Fallot patients with better right (and possibly left) ventricular reserve will have less chance of developing adverse events in their natural history.

DOSPAH

Doppler Stress echo in Pulmonary Arterial Hypertension.

Background

Patients at risk of pulmonary arterial hypertension at rest may show abnormal flow-adjusted increase in pulmonary pressures during exercise and are more likely to develop subsequent resting pulmonary hypertension [53, 54]. In patients with established or borderline pulmonary arterial hypertension capable of exercising, the level of exercise-induced increase in systolic pulmonary artery pressure and a reduced right ventricular contractile reserve are associated with a poorer prognosis [55]. The potential value of exercise-stress echo can be diagnostic in patients at risk of pulmonary arterial hypertension, and prognostic in patients with early established or borderline pulmonary arterial hypertension (Group 1 of European Society of Cardiology guidelines 2015) [56].

Aims

The primary aim is to evaluate the feasibility of SE focused on pulmonary hemodynamics and right ventricular function in patients at risk, borderline or early established pulmonary arterial hypertension. The secondary aim is to assess the presence and amount of right ventricular contractile reserve and its correlation with indices of functional severity (New York Heart Association Class, cardiac natriuretic peptides, peak VO_2, etc.). The tertiary aim is to assess the prognostic value of SE for predicting increase of resting systolic pulmonary artery pressure in the medium-term (2-years follow-up).

Methods

Patients at risk, borderline, or early established pulmonary hypertension capable of exercising will be recruited by regional reference centers for pulmonary hypertension. A physical stress with exercise will be performed. A thorough non-invasive hemodynamic assessment will be performed, including evaluation of rest and peak stress of: 1) Systolic pulmonary artery pressure from maximal velocity of tricuspid Doppler regurgitant jet adding the value of the right atrial pressure estimated on the basis of diameter and inspiratory collapse index of the inferior vena cava [57]; 2) mean pulmonary artery pressure as 0.6 x systolic pulmonary artery pressure +2 [58]; 3) cardiac output from the time-velocity integral of the left ventricular outflow tract [59]. SE positivity criteria will be the absolute increase in systolic pulmonary artery pressure >50 mmHg or the delta mean pulmonary arterial pressure/cardiac output > 3 mmHg/L/min. When a good-quality tricuspid jet signal cannot be sampled, the mean pulmonary artery pressure will be estimated based on pulsed-Doppler measurement of the acceleration time of pulmonary flow, sampled at the right ventricular outflow tract as mean pulmonary arterial pressure =79 - (0.6 x Acceleration time) [60]. Right ventricular contractile reserve will be measured as described above in project 7.

Sample size calculation

The expected incidence of SE positivity is around 30% as shown by previous pilot studies [10]. With a power of 80%, an alpha error of 5%, and an attrition rate of 10%, a sample size of about 250 patients is required to detect a significant stress-induced hemodynamic changes. For the prognostic analysis (tertiary end-point), if we conservatively assume a 15% yearly incidence of the pre-determined end-point (increase in resting systolic pulmonary artery pressure > 35 mmHg), with doubling of likelihood of events in presence of a positive SE, with a power of 80% and an alpha error of 5%, a sample size of about 250 patients is required with a 3 -year follow-up.

Study hypothesis

In subjects at risk of pulmonary arterial hypertension, those with higher pulmonary artery systolic pressure and lower decrease in pulmonary vascular resistance (as delta mean pulmonary arterial pressure/cardiac output >3 mmHg/L/min) during exercise will have more chance of developing resting pulmonary hypertension in their natural history [59, 60]. In patients with established early or borderline pulmonary arterial hypertension, those with lower decrease in pulmonary vascular resistances and worse right ventricular contractile reserve during exercise will have more chances of developing adverse events in their natural history.

DITSE

Diagnosis of CAD by Triple imaging Stress Echo (wall motion, coronary flow reserve and left ventricular elastance) plus B-lines.

Background

The cornerstone of diagnosis with SE is the finding of reversible regional wall motion abnormalities. However, the potentially valuable, diagnostic and prognostic, information provided by SE extends well beyond regional wall motion. In vasodilator and also during exercise stress, a clear step-up in diagnostic sensitivity (with a modest loss in specificity) and risk stratification capability is obtained with assessment of coronary flow velocity reserve in the left anterior descending coronary artery [61–63]. In exercise and dobutamine, and also with vasodilator stress, critical gains in sensitivity can be achieved by non invasive assessment of left ventricular contractile reserve through changes in left ventricular elastance, a load-independent index of left ventricular contractility more diagnostically and prognostically valuable than changes in ejection fraction [64, 65]. Normal values of coronary flow velocity reserve are >2.0 for all stresses, while the contractile reserve normal values are >2.0 for exercise and dobutamine but >1.0 for vasodilator stress. Furthermore, evaluation of B-lines can introduce a variable of additional prognostic value indicating acute accumulation of extra-vascular lung water [30, 31].

Aims

The *primary* aim is to evaluate the feasibility (with different stresses and protocol, with or without contrast) of rest and stress-induced integrated approach during SE with the "quadruple imaging" approach: regional wall motion abnormalities (standard, *single imaging* approach), coronary flow velocity reserve on left anterior descending (advanced, *dual imaging* approach); left ventricular elastance (derived from simple raw measures of cuff sphygmomanometer systolic arterial pressures/end-systolic volume, *triple imaging* approach); extra-vascular lung water (derived from B-lines from lung sonography, *quadruple* imaging approach). The *secondary* aim is to assess the diagnostic value of each of these parameters (alone and in combination) in predicting underlying coronary anatomy independently assessed by cardiac computed tomography and/or invasive coronary angiography (required when cardiac computed tomography is positive). The *tertiary* aim is to assess the prognostic value of the integrated SE in predicting events in the medium-term follow-up (up to 2 years)

Methods

All patients ("*allcomers*") referred to the SE lab with suspected CAD (history of chest pain or asymptomatic with previous positivity of any stress test, different from SE) will be evaluated with standard regional wall motion analysis and also – whenever feasible - with left ventricular coronary flow reserve (at least on the left anterior descending coronary artery) and left ventricular elastance reserve (whatever the stress: exercise, vasodilator or dobutamine). B-lines can be assessed at baseline and soon after stress. For each stress, all the four indices (regional wall motion, coronary flow velocity reserve, left ventricular elastance reserve and B-lines) can be obtained, if possible. For coronary flow velocity reserve assessment on left anterior descending, both the maximum diastolic flow velocity and, when possible, the whole envelope to extrapolate the new parameter labelled coronary functional reserve will be measured. Also patients with known CAD referred to SE for prognostic stratification will be included and evaluated for prognostic outcome, including (when feasible) resting transthoracic echocardiography evaluation of regional and global left ventricular function to assess progression to left ventricular dilation and dysfunction (ejection fraction decrease of > 15% and below 35%).

Centers can recruit with any combination of dual imaging (regional wall motion plus at least one of the three more innovative parameters: coronary flow velocity reserve, left ventricular contractile reserve and B-lines) as dictated by the locally available technology and expertise. According to preliminary experience, the feasibility rate is expected to be highest for left ventricular contractile reserve and B-lines, and lower for more demanding coronary flow velocity reserve.

Sample size calculation

The expected incidence of SE positivity (by composite criteria: regional wall motion abnormalities in 10%; reduction in coronary flow reserve velocity in 30%, blunted left ventricular contractile reserve in 20%; B-line increase >5) is around 35% [10]. A subset of 500 patients with coronary angiography verification (by invasive angiography or coronary CT) is required for reliable estimates of feasibility, imaging time and analysis time of each parameter. For prognostic tertiary end-point, if we conservatively assume a 5% yearly incidence of composite end-points (death, myocardial infarction, new hospital readmission, heart transplant, ventricular assist device implantation, aborted sudden death), with doubling of likelihood of events in presence of a positive SE (for composite criteria), with a power of 90% and an alpha error of 5%, a sample size of about 2500 patients is required with a 3-year follow-up. If only mortality is considered, a sample size of about 5,000 patients will be required.

Study hypothesis

Quadruple imaging combining coronary flow velocity reserve on left anterior descending artery, left ventricular contractility reserve evaluation with elastance assessment and B-lines in addition to conventional regional wall motion analysis is feasible with reasonable success rate, and diagnostically useful in all patients with all stresses. Even in the absence of inducible regional wall motion abnormalities, a lower coronary flow velocity reserve on left anterior descending coronary artery and/or a reduced left ventricular contractile reserve and/or an increase in B-lines will identify patients with worse outcome. When feasible, the combination of the quadruple imaging (regional wall motion, coronary flow reserve, left ventricular elastance reserve and B-lines) yields more prognostic information than any of the four parameters considered alone.

GENES

Genetic Stress echocardiography.

Background

The identification of phenotype-negative and genotype positive carriers of pathologic mutations is an important, yet still elusive, target for clinical cardiologists, although encouraging preliminary results have been reported with SE allowing identification of dynamic gradients in hypertrophic cardiomyopathy mutation carriers prior to development of hypertrophy [66], increased pulmonary resistance in mutation carriers of familial pulmonary hypertension with normal pulmonary pressure at rest [67], and higher resting end-diastolic volumes and possibly reduced contractile reserve during stress in familial dilated cardiomyopathy mutation carriers with normal left ventricular function at rest [68].

Aims

The primary aim is to evaluate the feasibility of SE in genetically characterized (on the basis of existing recommendations) first-degree relatives of patients with genetically transmitted cardiac diseases (such as hypertrophic cardiomyopathy, familial pulmonary arterial hypertension, and familial dilated cardiomyopathy). The secondary aim is to assess the value of disease-specific sentinel-parameters during SE in predicting the carrier and non-carrier status of healthy asymptomatic relatives, with the carrier status predicted by increased left ventricular outflow tract gradient in hypertrophic cardiomyopathy, exaggerated rise in systolic pulmonary arterial pressure in familial pulmonary arterial hypertension, and by blunted left ventricular contractile reserve in familial dilated cardiomyopathy. The tertiary, exploratory aim is to assess the value of SE indices for predicting the phenotypic expression of the disease in the medium-long term.

Methods

We will initially select 75 patients (25 for each disease) with documented disease and mutant gene identified by next-generation sequencing platform using targeted disease gene panels in tertiary care centers of genetic cardiology (in Florence-Careggi, Naples-Monaldi, Pisa-CNR or Cattinara-Trieste); they will undergo standardized SE testing. Furthermore, we will enroll around 250 first-degree relatives of the initially considered probands, with similar number for each disease, all with good-quality echocardiographic imaging, normal findings at rest and age range preferentially between 10 and 21 years (since a pathological phenotype is more likely to develop in the following 5 years when a diseased genotype is present). The relatives will undergo both genetic testing for the gene identified in the proband and SE testing with centralized core lab reading by observers blinded to genetic testing results. Each SE testing will be tailored on the specific question: hypertrophic cardiomyopathy as in protocol 3 (primary endpoint: orthostatic exercise induced change in left ventricular outflow tract gradient); pulmonary hypertension as in protocol 8 (primary endpoint: rest-exercise, flow-adjusted, variation in pulmonary vascular resistances); dilated cardiomyopathy as in protocol 1 (primary endpoint: left ventricular elastance change following exercise). All enrolled subjects (both genotype-positive and genotype-negative) will undergo yearly clinical and resting transthoracic echocardiography follow-up. The criteria for disease detection in these individuals include minimal phenotypes with low cut-off values (a wall thickness > 13 mm in the anterior septum and/or posterior left ventricular wall for hypertrophic cardiomyopathy; resting pulmonary artery systolic pressure > 40 mmHg verified by cath lab for primary pulmonary hypertension; a dilated left ventricular end-diastolic volume index > 74 mL/m^2 for men or 61 mL/m^2 for women and/or ejection fraction < 45% for dilated cardiomyopathy) [22]. In all subjects, coronary flow reserve during exercise will be evaluated, since a coronary microvascular abnormality has been reported as a very early finding in both dilated and hypertrophic cardiomyopathy, and this technique, albeit demanding, is feasible with last generation technology also during exercise [63].

Sample size calculation

We conservatively assume a significant increase in left ventricular outflow tract gradient > 50 mmHg during exercise in 50% of mutation carriers (as shown in a pilot study, 66) versus 5% of non-carriers. A significant difference in prevalence of left ventricular outflow tract

gradient will be observed, with a power of 80% and an alpha error of 5% with an attrition rate of 10%, with a sample size of about 80 patients for the hypertrophic cardiomyopathy study. A similar sample size estimation is applied to the other two subprojects of familial dilated cardiomyopathy (primary SE endpoint: increase in left ventricular contractile reserve <2.0) and familial pulmonary hypertension (primary SE endpoint: increase in systolic pulmonary artery pressure > 50 mmHg), with a total sample size of about 250 subjects for the whole subproject.

Study hypothesis

SE abnormalities predict carrier status in families with genetic cardiomyopathies. In genetic carriers, SE abnormalities may predict development of overt disease at mid-term follow-up.

Discussion

The overarching aim of SE2020 is to provide data directly relevant to patient care by filling the existing evidence gap in several areas of SE. Due to health care rationing and shortage of resources for independent, patient-oriented research, the SE community should face the challenge to optimize the use of infrastructural resources to provide the evidence base necessary for tailoring the right SE to the right patient with the right technology, used by the right (properly trained and certified) cardiologist.

There are several possible kinds of added values in this project.

Clinical

Only multicenter trials can provide the necessary information for validation of any diagnostic procedure in a reasonable amount of time; otherwise, tests that are hazardous or unfeasible, or both, may become accepted before inadequacies are recognized. SE is widely validated and has stood the test of time, but this is true mainly (if not only) for CAD and heart failure applications based on regional wall motion abnormalities. New applications are conceptually innovative, based on various parameters, applied to different patients, and we cannot skip the chain of validation required to transform a promising innovation into an established procedure [3, 4].

Scientific

Enrollment of patients in 10 different studies of special interest will provide a considerable amount of unique information in a relatively short time in several areas of critical scientific interest. In particular, in all of these fields available prognostic data are absent or, when existent, suffer from relatively small sample size and include soft and heterogeneous end-points to document prognostic power. The study will also generate an intellectual and professional network which is the ideal platform for future randomized, outcome intervention trials to assess the value of SE-based interventions, which is the highest level of evidence required by guidelines to change current clinical practice and yet lacking to date for several new applications of cardiac imaging [3, 4].

Educational

With a coordinated effort endorsed by the Italian Society of Cardiovascular Echography, the stress echo community will develop, test in the field and disseminate a structured software for collecting medical history, demographic information, clinical, SE, other imaging techniques, and outcome data for patients entering the standardized Italian and international "SE lab without walls". The participants to this SE lab will voluntarily agree to share a common language of indications, execution, reporting, image storage and archiving SE information performed in accredited centers, which previously underwent quality control of reading for specific SE skills. This will help to advance the field of SE, minimizing the greatest weakness of the technique, i.e., inter-laboratory variability in reading criteria, reporting heterogeneity and lack of permanent quality control standards [16, 17].

Economic

Today SE enjoys the advantages of economic sustainability and lack of radiation, making it potentially dominant in the current era of health care rationing [69]. However, to be cost-effective the indication must be appropriate, the exam must be performed by trained personnel, and with robust evidence supporting its specific clinical use. Otherwise, SE becomes just another tree in the cardiac imaging forest of inappropriate and redundant testing [70].

Comparison with previous studies

The same conceptual and operative template of SE2020 was put in place almost 30 years ago, at the beginning of the SE era, when the Italian first-generation multicenter studies provided unique evidences for the use of pharmacological testing with dipyridamole (EPIC; Echo-Persantine International Cooperative) study and dobutamine (EDIC, Echo-Dobutamine International Cooperative) study for the diagnosis of coronary artery disease. They addressed key aspects of stress testing such as safety and prognostic value in specific patient subsets [71–74]. From 1992 to 2012, over 30 articles from this multicenter trial network were published in top peer-reviewed journals and more importantly, these results rapidly shaped clinical practice and scientific guidelines [5, 6], since practice is easier to change when based on evidence that someone contributed to building in his/her own laboratory. In the footsteps of this template, the same paradigm will be followed today with SE2020 (Table 2). At that time, the main focus was on CAD; today,

Table 2 Stress echo multicenter trials

Years	1990-2010	2016-2030
Study acronym	EPIC and EDIC	SE 2020
Main focus	CAD	CAD and beyond
Enrolling centers criteria	Selective	Inclusive
Stress	Dip and Dob	Exercise, dip (ado) and dob
Key parameters	RWMA	CFVR, B-lines, E/e', etc.
Participating centers	10+	100+
Scientific societies role	Absent	Proactive

CAD coronary artery disease, CFVR coronary flow velocity reserve, EDIC echo-dobutamine international cooperative study, EPIC, echo-persantine international cooperative study, RWMA regional wall motion abnormalities

on conditions beyond CAD. Yesterday, the key sign was wall motion with 2-D, today an array of disease-specific diagnostic markers (from B-lines with lung ultrasound to coronary flow reserve with pulsed Doppler). At that time, early adopters were interested mainly for scientific reasons; today, virtually every lab can play a role, and is motivated by clinical interest to share experiences and standardize languages in a widely deregulated field. Yesterday, the driving force and core team of investigators came from a research institute (Italian National Research Council) with a top-down approach, from a research vision; today, from a scientific society (Italian Society of Echocardiography) networking all interested clinical cardiologists with an inclusive approach generating a bottom-up strategy, where all different expertise is added in a common intellectual architecture. The rationale of first- and second-generation studies is the same. As scientists and as clinicians, we need to act on the basis of effectiveness, real-world data populated by real patients, real doctors and real problems rather than on published efficacy data collected in ideal conditions but not always representative of true life. The seed of efficacy should not be mistaken for the fruit of effectiveness, which is the value of the technique when deployed in the field. We need the fruit of effectiveness, not the seed of efficacy, to feed our patients. We also learned from the decades of experience with first-generation multicenter trials that simple protocols without economic induction can change guidelines, and cardiologists interested in SE are generous with their time and willing to do things that help them to work better and offer a contribution to clinically meaningful, patient-oriented research [19].

One generation later, in a totally different economic and scientific healthcare scenario, once again Italian and international cardiology creates a network to build up the missing evidence. At least in principle, SE2020 fully shares the four cornerstones of the landmark mega-trial GISSI, Gruppo Italiano Studio Streptochinasi nell' Infarto, which can be summarized as follows [75]: 1) sponsorship by a respected, independent, not-for profit national society: it was the national Association of Hospital Cardiologists for

GISSI, and now it is the Italian Society of Echocardiography for SE2020; 2) scientific coordination by a professional, public research institute: it was the Mario Negri of Milan for GISSI, it is now the National Research Council of Pisa for SE2020; 3) inclusivity, with the involvement of nearly all the interested professionals in the nation: it was over 300 coronary care units in GISSI, it is now > 100 echocardiography labs in SE2020; and 4) emphasis on clinically relevant topic and outcomes that directly impact every day patient care: it was thrombolytic therapy for GISSI, it is now be cardiac imaging in and outside CAD for SE2020. Hopefully, the results will help improve the practice standards for the Italian cardiology and echocardiographic community across the nation and the available practice-changing scientific evidence worldwide. In a rapidly evolving SE field, SE 2020 addresses the need for standardization clearly identified by the American Society of Echocardiography roadmap to 2020 in its research and technology recommendations [76]. The development of research registries is identified as a potentially important tool for assessing and improving the quality of care and a valuable platform for clinical research. Such registry data would be accessible to the research community, facilitating a broad range of clinical research on the effectiveness of echocardiography (in this case, of SE) for the improvement of patient management and outcome [76].

Conclusion

The study officially starts in the very same days when American poet and singer Bob Dylan is awarded the Nobel prize for literature in December 2016 – and perhaps also for SE "*the times they're in a-changin'* ". SE2020 will coordinate and channel the efforts of the echocardiographic community to keep SE where it stands now – at center stage in guidelines of CAD and heart failure – and to move on beyond CAD and above regional wall motion abnormalities, filling in the gaps in a currently evidence-poor field: "*The line it is drawn, the curse it is cast. The slow one now will later be fast, as the present now will later be past, the order is rapidly fadin'. And the first one now will later be last, for the times they are a changin*".

Abbreviations
CAD: Coronary artery disease; EDIC: Echo-dobutamine international cooperative study; EPIC: Echo-persantine international cooperative study; GISSI: Gruppo italiano studio streptochinasi nell' infarto; SE: Stress echo; SIEC: Società italiana di ecocardiografia

Authors' contributions
QC is the principal investigator responsible for coordinating all organizational, administrative and scientific aspects with the assistance of RC (deputy chief of scientific activities of the Italian Society of Echocardiography). The Italian Society of Echocardiography is a professional and scientific society recruiting members among hospital, extra-hospital and academic cardiologists, and PC is responsible for recruiting centers, governing the accreditation process and disseminating activities of SE 2020 within the society. LC is responsible for case report form harmonization of main core project and each of the 10 sub-projects; CC for data archiving and data quality control (with a technician, PL)

and data analysis (with a statistician, DG from Padua); PT for website construction and web-based learning (with web administrator computer scientist MDN); SS and AA for permanent quality control and accreditation process (with computer scientist MP); EP and QC for software development for data archiving and reporting with a computer scientist (MP). The study steering committee includes the liaison with scientific societies, such as European Association of Cardiovascular Imaging (MG), Brazilian Society of Echocardiography (MAT), Serbian Society of Cardiology (BB), Hungarian Society of Cardiology (AV). Each subproject has specific responsible investigators (appointed for a renewable 1-year term): AD'A for project 1; MCS and MM for project 2; IO (with FM as accredited reader) for project 3; MG for project 4; MFC for project 5; LP for project 6; GdiS for project 7; EB and LG (with FF as accredited reader) for project 8; FR and NG for project 9; GL, MGA (geneticist) and BP (with LM as accredited reader) for project 10. All the subproject leaders are also part of the steering committee. EP is the project chairman, responsible for overall study design, scientific coordination and final approval of all scientific, editorial and dissemination activities. All authors read and approve the final manuscript.

Competing interests
The authors declare that they have no competing interest.

Author details
[1]Institute of Clinical Physiology, National Research Council, Pisa, Italy. [2]Cardiology Division, Fatebenefratelli Hospital, Benevento, Italy. [3]Heart Department, University Hospital "San Giovanni di Dio e Ruggi d'Aragona", Salerno, Italy. [4]Division of Cardiology, Monaldi Hospital, Second University of Naples, Naples, Italy. [5]Cardiology Department, Pisa University and Nottola (Siena) Hospital, Pisa, Italy. [6]Cardiology Department, San Luca Hospital, Lucca, Italy. [7]Cardiology Department, Careggi Hospital, Florence, Italy. [8]Department of Advanced Biomedical Sciences, Federico II University Hospital, Naples, Italy. [9]Cardiology Department, San Carlo Hospital, Potenza, Italy. [10]Pediatric Cardiology Department, Brompton Hospital, London, UK. [11]Division of Cardiology, Ospedale dell'Angelo Mestre-Venice, Mestre, Italy. [12]Cardiology Department, Parma University Hospital, Parma, Italy. [13]Pediatric Cardiology Department, Monaldi Hospital Clinics, Naples, Italy. [14]Cardiology Department, University Hospital "Ospedale Riuniti", Trieste, Italy. [15]Hospital de Clinicas de Porto Alegre, Universidade Federal do Rio Grande do Sul, Porto Alegre, Brazil. [16]Cardiology Institute of Rio Grande do Sul, Porto Alegre, Brazil. [17]Cardiology Division, Hospital San José, Criciuma, Brazil. [18]Hospital Sao Vicente de Paulo, Hospital de Cidade, Passo Fundo, Brazil. [19]Cardiology Clinic, Clinical Center of Serbia, Medical School, University of Belgrade, Belgrade, Serbia. [20]Institute of Family Medicine, University of Szeged, Szeged, Hungary. [21]Department of Internal Medicine, Elisabeth Hospital, Hodmezovasarhely, Hungary. [22]Department of Biostatistics, University of Padua, Padua, Italy. [23]Department of Cardiology, Sandro Pertini Hospital, Rome, Italy. [24]Cardiology Department, Monaldi Hospital, Naples, Italy. [25]RSE, Medical Centre Hospital of the President's Affairs Administration of the Republic of Kazakhstan, Astana, Kazakhstan. [26]Cardiology Hospital, Policlinico of Bari, Bari, Italy.

References
1. Picano E. Stress echocardiography. From pathophysiological toy to diagnostic tool. Point of view. Circulation. 1992;85:1604–12.
2. Pellikka PA. Stress echocardiography in the evaluation of chest pain and accuracy in the diagnosis of coronary artery disease. Prog Cardiovasc Dis. 1997;39:523–32.
3. Picano E, Pibarot P, Lancellotti P, Monin JL, Bonow RO. The emerging role of exercise testing and stress echocardiography in valvular heart disease. J Am Coll Cardiol. 2009;54:2251–60.
4. Picano E, Pellikka PA. Stress echo applications beyond coronary artery disease. Eur Heart J. 2014;35:1033–40.
5. Pellikka PA, Nagueh SF, Elhendy AA, Kuehl CA, Sawada SG. American Society of Echocardiography recommendations for performance, interpretation, and application of stress echocardiography. J Am Soc Echocardiogr. 2007;20:1021–4.

6. Sicari R, Nihoyannopoulos P, Evangelista A, Kasprzak J, Lancellotti P, Poldermans D, Voigt JU, Zamorano JL, on behalf of the European Association of Echocardiography. Stress echocardiography expert consensus statement. European Association of Echocardiography (EAE) (a registered branch of the ESC). Eur J Echocardiogr. 2008;9:415–37.

7. Montalescot G, Sechtem U, Achenbach S, Andreotti F, Arden C, Budaj A, Bugiardini R, Crea F, Cuisset T, Di Mario C, Ferreira JR, Gersh BJ, Gitt AK, Hulot JS, Marx N, Opie LH, Pfisterer M, Prescott E, Ruschitzka F, Sabaté M, Senior R, Taggart DP, van der Wall EE, Vrints CJ, ESC Committee for Practice Guidelines, Hoes AW, Kirchhof P, Knuuti J, Kolh P, Lancellotti P, Linhart A, Nihoyannopoulos P, Piepoli MF, Ponikowski P, Sirnes PA, Tamargo JL, Tendera M, Torbicki A, Wijns W, Windecker S, Knuuti J, Valgimigli M, Bueno H, Claeys MJ, Donner-Banzhoff N, Erol C, Frank H, Funck-Brentano C, Gaemperli O, Gonzalez-Juanatey JR, Hamilos M, Hasdai D, Husted S, James SK, Kervinen K, Kolh P, Kristensen SD, Lancellotti P, Maggioni AP, Piepoli MF, Pries AR, Romeo F, Rydén L, Simoons ML, Sirnes PA, Steg PG, Timmis A, Wijns W, Windecker S, Yildirir A, Zamorano JL. 2013 ESC guidelines on the management of stable coronary artery disease: the Task Force on the management of stable coronary artery disease of the European Society of Cardiology. Eur Heart J. 2013;34:2949–3003.

8. Wolk MJ, Bailey SR, Doherty JU, Douglas PS, Hendel RC, Kramer CM, Min JK, Patel MR, Rosenbaum L, Shaw LJ, Stainback RF, Allen JM, Technical Panel, Brindis RG, Kramer CM, Shaw LJ, Cerqueira MD, Chen J, Dean LS, Fazel R, Hundley WG, Itchhaporia D, Kligfield P, Lockwood R, Marine JE, McCully RB, Messer JV, O'Gara PT, Shemin RJ, Wann LS, Wong JB, Appropriate Use Criteria Task Force, Patel MR, Kramer CM, Bailey SR, Brown AS, Doherty JU, Douglas PS, Hendel RC, Lindsay BD, Min JK, Shaw LJ, Stainback RF, Wann LS, Wolk MJ, Allen JM. American College of Cardiology Foundation Appropriate Use Criteria Task Force ACCF/AHA/ASE/ASNC/HFSA/HRS/SCAI/SCCT/SCMR/STS 2013 multimodality appropriate use criteria for the detection and risk assessment of stable ischemic heart disease: a report of the American College of Cardiology Foundation Appropriate Use Criteria Task Force, American Heart Association, American Society of Echocardiography, American Society of Nuclear Cardiology, Heart Failure Society of America, Heart Rhythm Society, Society for Cardiovascular Angiography and Interventions, Society of Cardiovascular Computed Tomography, Society for Cardiovascular Magnetic Resonance, and Society of Thoracic Surgeons. J Am Coll Cardiol. 2014;63:380–406.

9. Yancy CW, Jessup M, Bozkurt B, Butler J, Casey Jr DE, Colvin MM, Drazner MH, Filippatos G, Fonarow GC, Givertz MM, Hollenberg SM, Lindenfeld J, Masoudi FA, McBride PE, Peterson PN, Stevenson LW, American WC. College of Cardiology Foundation; American Heart Association Task Force on Practice Guidelines 2013 ACCF/AHA guideline for the management of heart failure: a report of the American College of Cardiology Foundation/American Heart Association Task Force on Practice Guidelines. J Am Coll Cardiol. 2013;62:e147–239.

10. Ponikowski P, Voors AA, Anker SD, Bueno H, Cleland JG, Coats AJ, Falk V, González-Juanatey JR, Harjola VP, Jankowska EA, Jessup M, Linde C, Nihoyannopoulos P, Parissis JT, Pieske B, Riley JP, Rosano GM, Ruilope LM, Ruschitzka F, Rutten FH, van der Meer P, et al. ESC guidelines for the diagnosis and treatment of acute and chronic heart failure: the Task Force for the diagnosis and treatment of acute and chronic heart failure of the European Society of Cardiology. Eur J Heart Fail. 2016;18:891–975.

11. Picano E, Vañó E, Rehani MM, Cuocolo A, Mont L, Bodi V, Bar O, Maccia C, Pierard L, Sicari R, Plein S, Mahrholdt H, Lancellotti P, Knuuti J, Heidbuchel H, Di Mario C, Badano LP. The appropriate and justified use of medical radiation in cardiovascular imaging: a position document of the ESC Associations of Cardiovascular Imaging, Percutaneous Cardiovascular Interventions and Electrophysiology. Eur Heart J. 2014;35:665–72.

12. Lancellotti P, Pellikka PA, Budts W, Chaudry F, Donal E, Dulgheru R, Edvarsen T, Garbi M, Ha JW, Kane G, Kreeger J, Mertens L, Pibarot P, Picano E, Ryan T, Tsutsui J, Varga A. Recommendations for the clinical use of stress echocardiography in non-ischemic heart disease: joint document of the European Association of Cardiovascular imaging and the American Society of Echocardiography. Eur Heart J Cardiov Imaging. 2016;190:1191–229.

13. Ciampi Q, Citro R, Severino S, Labanti G, Cortigiani L, Sicari R, Gaibazzi N, Galderisi M, Bossone E, Colonna P, Picano E. Stress echo in Italy: state of the art 2015. Eur Heart J Cardiovasc Imaging. 2016;17:23 (abstract).

14. Ciampi Q, Paterni M, Cortigiani L, Citro R, Sicari R, Galderisi M, Bossone E, Colonna P, Picano E. Next generation stress echo computerized software. Eur Heart J Cardiovasc Imaging. 2016;17:24 (abstract).

15. Hoffmann R, Lethen H, Marwick T, Arnese M, Fioretti P, Pingitore A, Picano E, Buck T, Erbel R, Flachskampf FA, Hanrath P. Analysis of interinstitutional observer agreement in interpretation of dobutamine stress echocardiograms. J Am Coll Cardiol. 1996;27:330–6.

16. Picano E, Lattanzi F, Orlandini A, Marini C, L'Abbate A. Stress echocardiography and the human factor: the importance of being expert. J Am Coll Cardiol. 1991;17:666–9.

17. Varga A, Picano E, Dodi C, Barbieri A, Pratali L, Gaddi O, et al. Madness and method in stress echo reading. Eur Heart J. 1999;20:1271–5.

18. Popescu BA, Stefanidis A, Nihoyannopoulos P, Fox KF, Ray S, Cardim N, Rigo F, Badano LP, Fraser AG, Pinto F, Zamorano JL, Habib G, Maurer G, Lancellotti P, Andrade MJ, Donal E, Edvardsen T, Varga A. Updated standards and processes for accreditation of echocardiographic laboratories from The European Association of Cardiovascular Imaging. Eur Heart J Cardiovasc Imaging. 2014;15:717–27.

19. Picano E, Pingitore A, Sicari R, Minardi G, Gandolfo N, Seveso G, Chiarella F, Bolognese L, Chiarandà G, Sclavo MG, Previtali M, Margaria F, Magaia O, Bianchi F, Pirelli S, Severi S, Raciti M, Landi P, Vassalle C, Sousa BMJ, Felipe L, Duarte M, on behalf of the Echo Persantine International (EPIC) study group. Stress echocardiographic results predict risk of reinfarction early after uncomplicated acute myocardial infarction: Large-scale multicenter study. J Am Coll Cardiol. 1995;26:908–13.

20. Gottdiener JS, Bednarz J, Devereux R, Gardin J, Klein A, Manning WJ. American Society of Echocardiography. American Society of Echocardiography recommendations for use of echocardiography in clinical trials. J Am Soc Echocardiogr. 2004;17:1086–119.

21. Gargani L, Sicari R, Raciti M, Serasini L, Passera M, Torino C, Letachowicz K, Ekart R, Fliser D, Covic A, Balafa O, Stavroulopoulos A, Massy ZA, Fiaccadori E, Caiazza A, Bachelet T, Slotki I, Shavit L, Martinez-Castelao A, Coudert-Krier MJ, Rossignol P, Kraemer TD, Hannedouche T, Panichi V, Wiecek A, Pontoriero G, Sarafidis P, Klinger M, Hojs R, Seiler-Mußler S, Lizzi F, Onofriescu M, Zarzoulas F, Tripepi R, Mallamaci F, Tripepi G, Picano E, London GM, Zoccali C. Efficacy of a remote web-based lung ultrasound training for nephrologists and cardiologists: a LUST trial sub-project. Nephrol Dial Transplant. 2016;31:1982-1988.

22. Lang RM, Badano LP, Mor-Avi V, Afilalo J, Armstrong A, Ernande L, Flachskampf FA, Foster E, Goldstein SA, Kuznetsova T, Lancellotti P, Muraru D. Recommendations for Cardiac Chamber Quantification by Echocardiography in Adults: An Update from the American Society of Echocardiography and the European Association of Cardiovascular Imaging. Eur Heart J Cardiovasc Imaging. 2015;16:233–70.

23. Chung ES, Leon AR, Tavazzi L, Sun JP, Nihoyannopoulos P, Merlino J, Abraham WT, Ghio S, Leclercq C, Bax JJ, Yu CM, John Gorcsan IIIJ, St John Sutton M, De Sutter J, Murillo J. Results of the Predictors of Response to CRT (PROSPECT) Trial. Circulation. 2008;117:2608–16.

24. Ciampi Q, Carpeggiani C, Michelassi C, Picano E. Left ventricular contractile reserve by stress echocardiography as a predictor of response to cardiac resynchronization therapy. A meta-analysis. Eur Heart J- Cardiovasc Imaging. 2016;17:52 (abstract)

25. Sénéchal M, Lancellotti P, Magne J, Garceau P, Champagne J, Blier L, Molin F, Philippon F, Marie M, O'Hara G, Dubois M. Contractile reserve assessed using dobutamine echocardiography predicts left ventricular reverse remodeling after cardiac resynchronization therapy: prospective validation in patients with left ventricular dyssynchrony. Echocardiography. 2010;27: 668–76.

26. Chaudhry FA, Shah A, Bangalore S, DeRose J, Steinberg JS. Inotropic contractile reserve and response to cardiac resynchronization therapy in patients with markedly remodeled left ventricle. J Am Soc Echocardiogr. 2011;24:91–7.

27. Gasparini M, Muto C, Iacopino S, Zanon F, Dicandia C, Distefano G, Favale S, Peraldo Neja C, Bragato R, Davinelli M, Mangoni L, Denaro A. Low-dose dobutamine test associated with interventricular dyssynchrony: a useful tool to identifycardiac resynchronization therapy responders: data from the LOw dose DObutamine stress-echo test in Cardiac Resynchronization Therapy (LODO-CRT) phase 2 study. Am Heart J. 2012;163:422–9.

28. Ciampi Q, Pratali L, Citro R, Villari B, Picano E, Sicari R. Clinical and Prognostic Role of Pressure-Volume Relationship in the Identification of Responders to Cardiac Resynchronization Therapy. Am Heart J. 2010;160:906–14.

29. Picano E, Frassi F, Agricola E, Gligorova S, Gargani L, Mottola G. Ultrasound lung comets: a clinically useful sign of extravascular lung water. J Am Soc Echocardiogr. 2006;19:356–63.

30. Agricola E, Picano E, Oppizzi M, Pisani M, Meris A, Fragasso G, Margonato A. Assessment of stress-induced pulmonary interstitial edema by chest ultrasound during exercise echocardiography and its correlation with left ventricular function. J Am Soc Echocardiogr. 2006;19:457–63.

31. Scali MC, Cortigiani L, Simionuc A, Gregori D, Marzilli M, Picano E. Exercise-induced B-lines identify worse functional and prognostic stage in heart failure patients with depressed left ventricular function. Eur J Heart Fail. 2017;19. doi:10.1002/ejhf.776

32. Picano E, Pellikka PA. Ultrasound of extravascular lung water: a new standard for pulmonary congestion. Eur Heart J. 2016;14:2091–104.

33. Elliott PM, Anastasakis A, Borger MA, Borggrefe M, Cecchi F, Charron P, Hagege AA, Lafont A, Limongelli G, Mahrholdt H, McKenna WJ, Mogensen J, Nihoyannopoulos P, Nistri S, Pieper PG, Pieske B, Rapezzi C, Rutten FH, Tillmanns C, Watkins H. 2014 ESC Guidelines on diagnosis and management of hypertrophic cardiomyopathy: the Task Force for the Diagnosis and Management of Hypertrophic Cardiomyopathy of the European Society of Cardiology (ESC). Eur Heart J. 2014;35:2733–79.

34. Ciampi Q, Olivotto I, Gardini C, Mori F, Peteiro J, Monserrat L, Fernandez X, Cortigiani L, Rigo F, Lopes LR, Cruz I, Cotrim C, Losi M, Betocchi S, Beleslin B, Tesic M, Dikic AD, Lazzeroni E, Lazzeroni D, Sicari R, Picano E. Prognostic role of physical and pharmacological stress echocardiography in hypertrophic cardiomyopathy. The International Stress echo registry. Int J Cardiol. 2016;219:331–8.

35. Cardim N, Galderisi M, Edvardsen T, Plein S, Popescu BA, D'Andrea A, Bruder O, Cosyns B, Davin L, Donal E, Freitas A, Habib G, Kitsiou A, Petersen SE, Schroeder S, Lancellotti P, Camici P, Dulgheru R, Hagendorff A, Lombardi M, Muraru D, Sicari R. Role of multimodality cardiac imaging in the management of patients with hypertrophic cardiomyopathy: an expert consensus of the European Association of cardiovascular imaging endorsed by the Saudi Heart Association. Eur Heart J Cardiovasc Imaging. 2015;16:280.

36. Nagueh SF, Smiseth OA, Appleton CP, Byrd BF 3rd, Dokainish H, Edvardsen T, Flachskampf FA, Gillebert TC, Klein AL, Lancellotti P, Marino P, Oh JK, Alexandru Popescu B, Waggoner AD. Recommendations for the evaluation of left ventricular diastolic function by echocardiography:an update from the American Society of Echocardiography and the European Association of Cardiovascular Imaging. Eur Heart J Cardiovasc Imaging 2016; doi:10.1093/ehjci/jew082

37. Donal E, Lund LH, Oger E, Reynaud A, Schnell F, Persson H, Drouet E, Linde C, Daubert C, KaRen investigators. Value of exercise echocardiography in heart failure with preserved ejection fraction : a substudy from the Karen study. Eur Heart J Cardiovasc Imaging. 2016;17:106–13.

38. Shimiaie J, Sherez J, Aviram G, Megidish R, Viskin S, Halkin A, Ingbir M, Nesher N, Biner S, Keren G, Topilsky Y. Determinants of effort intolerance in patients with heart failure. JACC Heart Fail. 2015;3:803–14.

39. Mor-Avi V, Lang RM, Badano LP, Belohlavek M, Cardim NM, Derumeaux G, Galderisi M, Marwick T, Nagueh SF, Sengupta PP, Sicari R, Smiseth OA, Smulevitz B, Takeuchi M, Thomas JD, Vannan M, Voigt JU, Zamorano JL. Current and evolving echocardiographic techniques for the quantitative evaluation of cardiac mechanics. Eur J Echocardiogr. 2011;12:325–37.

40. Chakravarty T, Van Belle E, Jilaihawi H, Noheria A, Testa L, Bedogni F, Rück A, Barbanti M, Toggweiler S, Thomas M, Khawaja MZ, Huttern A, Abramowitz Y, Siegel RJ, Cheng W, Webb J, Leon MB, Makkar RR. Meta-analysis of the impact of mitral regurgitation on outcomes after transcatheter aortic valve implantation. Am J Cardiol. 2015;115:942–9.

41. Garbi M, Chambers J, Vannan M, Lancellotti P. Valve stress echocardiography: a practical guide for referral, procedure, reporting, and clinical implementation of results from the HAVEC group. JACC Cardiovasc Imaging. 2015;8:724–36.

42. Fagenholz PJ, Gutman JA, Murray AF, Noble VE, Thomas SH, Harris NS. Chest ultrasonography for the diagnosis and monitoring of high-altitude pulmonary edema. Chest. 2007;131:1013–8.

43. Pratali L, Cavana M, Sicari R, Picano E. Frequent subclinical high- altitude pulmonary edema detected by chest sonography as ultrasound lung comets in recreational climbers. Crit Care Med. 2010;38:1818–23.

44. Frassi F, Pingitore A, Cialoni D, Picano E. Chest sonography detects lung water accumulation in healthy elite apnea divers. J Am Soc Echocardiogr. 2008;21:1150–5.

45. Pingitore A, Garbella E, Piaggi P, Menicucci D, Frassi F, Lionetti V, Piarulli A, Catapano G, Lubrano V, Passera M, Di Bella G, Castagnini C, Pellegrini S, Metelli MR, Bedini R, Gemignani A, L'Abbate A. Early subclinical increase in pulmonary water content in athletes performing sustained heavy exercise at sea level: ultrasound lung comet tail evidence. Am J Physiol Heart Circ Physiol. 2011;301:H2161–7.

46. Gurvitz M, Burns KM, Brindis R, Broberg CS, Daniels CJ, Fuller SM, Honein MA, Khairy P, Kuehl KS, Landzberg MJ, Mahle WT, Mann DL, Marelli A, Newburger JW, Pearson GD, Starling RC, Tringali GR, Valente AM, Wu JC, Califf RM. Emerging research directions in adult congenital heart disease. A report from the NHLBI/ACHA working group. J Am Coll Cardiol. 2016;673: 1956–64.

47. Sarubbi B, Pacileo G, Pisacane C, Ducceschi V, Iacono C, Russo MG, Iacono A, Calabrò R. Exercise capacity in young patients after total repair of tetralogy of Fallot. Pediatr Cardiol. 2000;21:211–5.

48. Apostolopoulou SC, Laskari CV, Tsoutsinos A, Rammos S. Doppler tissue imaging evaluation of right ventricular function at rest and during dobutamine infusion in patients after repair of tetralogy of Fallot. Int J Cardiovasc Imaging. 2007;23:25–31.

49. Brili S, Stamatopoulos I, Barbetseas J, Chrysohoou C, Alexopoulos N, Misailidou M, Bratsas A, Stefanadis C. Usefulness of dobutamine stress echocardiography with tissue Doppler imaging for the evaluation and follow-up of patients with repaired tetralogy of Fallot. J Am Soc Echocardiogr. 2008;21:1093–8.

50. Ait-Ali L, Siciliano V, Passino C, Molinaro S, Pasanisi E, Sicari R, Pingitore A, Festa P. Role of stress echocardiography in operated Fallot: feasibility and detection of right ventricular response. J Am Soc Echocardiogr. 2014;142: 1158–65.

51. Cifra B, Dragulescu A, Border WL, Mertens L. Stress echocardiography in paediatric cardiology. Eur Heart J Cardiovasc Imaging. 2014;16:1051–9.

52. Claessen G, La Gerche A, Voigt JU, Dymarkowski S, Schnell F, Petit T, Willems R, Claus P, Delcroix M, Heidbuchel H. Accuracy of echocardiography to evaluate pulmonary vascular and right ventricular function during exercise. JACC Cardiovasc Imaging. 2016;9:532–43.

53. Codullo V, Caporali R, Cuomo G, Ghio S, D'Alto M, Fusetti C, Borgogno E, Montecucco C, Valentini G. Stress Doppler echocardiography in systemic sclerosis:evidence for a role in the prediction of pulmonary hypertension. Arthritis Rheum. 2013;65:2403–11.

54. Kusunose K, Yamada H, Hotchi J, Bando M, Nishio S, Hirata Y, Ise T, Yamaguchi K, Yagi S, Soeki T, Wakatsuki T, Kishi J, Sata M. Prediction of future overt pulmonary hypertension by 6-min walk stress echocardiography in patients with connective tissue disease. J Am Coll Cardiol. 2015;66:376–84.

55. Grünig E, Tiede H, Enyimayew EO, Ehlken N, Seyfarth HJ, Bossone E, D'Andrea A, Naeije R, Olschewski H, Ulrich S, Nagel C, Halank M, Fischer C. Assessment and prognostic relevance of right ventricular contractile reserve in patients with severe pulmonary hypertension. Circulation. 2013;29(128): 2005–15.

56. Galiè N, Humbert M, Vachiery J-L, Gibbs S, Lang I, Torbicki A, Simonneau G, Peacock A, Vonk Noordegraaf A, Beghetti M, Ghofrani A, Gomez Sanchez MA, Hansmann G, Klepetko W, Lancellotti P, Matucci M, McDonagh T, Pierard LA, Trindade PT, Zompatori M, Hoeper M. 2015 ESC/ERS Guidelines for the diagnosis and treatment of pulmonary hypertension. Eur Heart J. 2016;37:67–119.

57. Rudski LG, Lai WW, Afilalo J, Hua L, Handschumacher MD, Chandrasekaran K, Solomon SD, Louie EK, Schiller NB, et al. Guidelines for the echocardiographic assessment of the right heart in adults: a report from the American Society of Echocardiography endorsed by the European Association of Echocardiography, a registered branch of the European Society of Cardiology, and the Canadian Society of Echocardiography. J Am Soc Echocardiogr. 2010;23:685–713.

58. Chemla D, Castelain V, Humbert M, Hébert JL, Simonneau G, Lecarpentier Y, Hervé P. New formula for predicting mean pulmonary artery pressure using systolic pulmonary artery pressure. Chest. 2004;126:1313–7.

59. Lewis GD, Bossone E, Naeije R, Grünig E, Saggar R, Lancellotti P, Ghio S, Varga J, Rajagopalan S, Oudiz R, Rubenfire M. Pulmonary vascular hemodynamic response to exercise in cardiopulmonary diseases. Circulation. 2013;128:1470–9.

60. Bossone E, Ferrrara F, Grunig E. Echocardiography in pulmonary hypertension. Curr Opin Cardiol. 2015;30:574–86.

61. Rigo F, Cortigiani L, Pasanisi E, Richieri M, Cutaia V, Celestre M, Raviele A, Picano E. The additional prognostic value of coronary flow reserve on left anterior descending artery in patients with negative stress echo by wall motion criteria. A Transthoracic Vasodilator Stress Echocardiography Study. Am Heart J. 2006;151:124–30.

62. Cortigiani L, Rigo F, Gherardi S, Bovenzi F, Molinaro S, Picano E, Sicari R. Coronary flow reserve during dipyridamole stress echocardiography predicts mortality. JACC Cardiov Imaging. 2012;5:1079–85.

63. Zagatina A, Zhuravskaya A. The additive prognostic value of coronary flow velocity reserve during exercise echocardiography. Eur Heart J Cardiovasc Imaging. 2016;18 (in press).

64. Bombardini T, Gherardi S, Marraccini P, Schlueter MC, Sicari R, Picano E. The incremental diagnostic value of coronary flow reserve and left ventricular elastance during high-dose dipyridamole stress echocardiography in patients with normal wall motion at rest. Int J Cardiol. 2013;168:1683–4.

65. Grosu A, Bombardini T, Senni M, Duino V, Gori M, Picano E. End-systolic pressure/volume relationship during dobutamine stress echo: a prognostically useful non-invasive index of left ventricular contractility. Eur Heart J. 2005;26:2404–12.

66. Lopes LR, Cotrim C, Cruz I, Picano E, Pinto F, Pereira H. Left ventricular outflow tract obstruction as a primary phenotypic expression of hypertrophic cardiomyopathy in mutation carriers without hypertrophy. Int J Cardiol. 2014;176:1264–7.

67. Grünig E, Weissmann S, Ehlken N, Fijalkowska A, Fischer C, Fourme T, Galié N, Ghofrani A, Harrison RE, Huez S, Humbert M, Janssen B, Kober J, Koehler R, Machado RD, Mereles D, Naeije R, Olschewski H, Provencher S, Reichenberger F, Retailleau K, Rocchi G, Simonneau G, Torbicki A, Trembath R, Seeger W. Stress Doppler echocardiography in relatives of patients with idiopathic and familial pulmonary arterial hypertension. Results of a multicenter European analysis of pulmonary artery pressure response to exercise and hypoxia. Circulation. 2009;119:1747–57.

68. Fatkin D, Yeoh T, Hayward CS, Benson V, Sheu A, Richmond Z, Feneley MP, Keogh AM, Mc Donald PS. Evaluation of left ventricular enlargement as a marker of early disease in familial dilated cardiomyopathy. Circ Cardiov Genet. 2011;4:341–8.

69. Picano E. Stress echocardiography: a historical perspective, Special article. Am J Med. 2003;114:126–30.

70. Picano E. Sustainability of medical imaging. Education and debate. BMJ. 2004;328:578–80.

71. Picano E, Marini C, Pirelli S, Maffei S, Bolognese L, Chiriatti GP, Chiarella F, Orlandini A, Seveso G, Quarta Colosso M, Sclavo MG, Magaia O, Agati L, Previtali M, Lowenstein J, Torre F, Rosselli P, Ciuti M, Ostojic M, Gandolfo N, Margaria F, Giannuzzi P, Di Bello V, Lombardi M, Gigli G, Ferrara N, Santoro F, Lusa AM, Chiarandà G, Papagna D, Coletta C, Boccardi L, De Cristofaro M, Papi L, Landi P, on behalf of the EPIC study group. Safety of intravenous high-dose dipyridamole echocardiography. Am J Cardiol. 1992;70:252–6.

72. Picano E, Mathias Jr W, Pingitore A, Bigi R, Previtali M, on behalf of the EDIC study group. Safety and tolerability of dobutamine-atropine stress echocardiography: a prospective, large scale, multicenter trial. Lancet. 1994; 344:1190–2.

73. Picano E, Landi P, Bolognese L, Chiarandà G, Chiarella F, Seveso G, Sclavo MG, Gandolfo N, Previtali M, Orlandini A, Margaria F, Pirelli S, Magaja O, Minardi G, Bianchi F, Marini C, Raciti M, Michelassi C, Severi S, Distante A, on behalf of the EPIC study group. Prognostic value of dipyridamole-echocardiography early after uncomplicated myocardial infarction: a large scale multicenter trial. Am J Med. 1993;11:608–18.

74. Sicari R, Cortigiani L, Bigi R, Landi P, Raciti M, Picano E, on behalf of the Echo-Persantine International Cooperative (EPIC) and Echo-Dobutamine International Cooperative (EDIC) Study Groups. The prognostic value of pharmacological stress echo is affected by concomitant anti-ischemic therapy at the time of testing. Circulation. 2004;109:2428–31.

75. Braunwald E. Happy Birthday, GISSI! Am Heart J. 2004;148:187.

76. Pellikka PA, Douglas PS, Miller JG, Abraham TP, Baumann R, Buxton DB, Byrd BF 3rd, Chen P, Cook NL, Gardin JM, Hansen G, Houle HC, Husson S, Kaul S, Klein AL, Lang RM, Leong-Poi H, Lopez H, Mahmoud TM, Maslak S, McCulloch ML, Metz S, Nagueh SF, Pearlman AS, Pibarot P, Picard MH, Porter TR, Prater D, Rodriguez R, Sarano ME, Scherrer-Crosbie M, Shirali GS, Sinusas A, Slosky JJ, Sugeng L, Tatpati A, Villanueva FS, von Ramm OT, Weissman NJ, Zamani S. American society of echocardiography cardiovascular technology and research summit: a roadmap for 2020. J Am Soc Echocardiogr. 2013;26:325–37.

4

Right ventricular ejection fraction measurements using two-dimensional transthoracic echocardiography by applying an ellipsoid model

Stina Jorstig[1,5*], Micael Waldenborg[1,2], Mats Lidén[1,3] and Per Thunberg[1,4]

Abstract

Background: There is today no established approach to estimate right ventricular ejection fraction (RVEF) using 2D transthoracic echocardiography (TTE). The aim of this study was to evaluate a new method for RVEF calculations using 2D TTE and compare the results with cardiac magnetic resonance (CMR) imaging and tricuspid annular plane systolic excursion (TAPSE).

Methods: A total of 37 subjects, 25 retrospectively included patients and twelve healthy volunteers, were included to give a wide range of RVEF. The right ventricle (RV) was modeled as a part of an ellipsoid enabling calculation of the RV volume by combining three distance measurements. RVEF calculated according to the model, $RVEF_{TTE}$, were compared with reference CMR-derived RVEF, $RVEF_{CMR}$. Further, TAPSE was measured in the TTE images and the correlations were calculated between $RVEF_{TTE}$, TAPSE and $RVEF_{CMR}$.

Results: The mean values were $RVEF_{CMR} = 43 \pm 12\%$ (range 20–66%) and $RVEF_{TTE} = 50 \pm 9\%$ (range 34–65%). There was a high correlation ($r = 0.80$, $p < 0.001$) between $RVEF_{TTE}$ and $RVEF_{CMR}$. Bland-Altman analysis showed a mean difference between $RVEF_{CMR}$ and $RVEF_{TTE}$ of 6 percentage points (ppt) with limits of agreement from −11 to 23 ppt. The mean value for TAPSE was 19 ± 5 mm and the correlation between TAPSE and $RVEF_{CMR}$ was moderate ($r = 0.54$, $p < 0.001$). The correlation between $RVEF_{TTE}$ and $RVEF_{CMR}$ was significantly higher ($p < 0.05$) than the correlation between TAPSE and $RVEF_{CMR}$.

Conclusions: The ellipsoid model shows promise for RVEF calculations using 2D TTE for a wide range of RVEF, providing RVEF estimates that were significantly better correlated to RVEF obtained from CMR compared to TAPSE.

Keywords: Right ventricle, Right ventricular function, Echocardiography, Cardiac magnetic resonance imaging

Background

Right ventricular (RV) function is an important predictor of survival in cardiopulmonary disease [1]. Evaluation of RV function is therefore essential in both congenital and acquired heart diseases, such as atrial septal defect, pulmonary and tricuspid regurgitation, pulmonary hypertension (PH) and arrhythmogenic right ventricular cardiomyopathy [2–4].

The complex shape of the RV, and the relatively large element of trabeculations, makes its function more challenging to assess as compared to the left ventricle (LV), when using echocardiography. Cardiac magnetic resonance (CMR) imaging is considered to be the reference method for RV evaluation allowing full ventricular coverage. In CMR, right ventricular ejection fraction (RVEF) is often used as a measure of RV function. RVEF can be determined by calculating the end-diastolic and end-systolic volumes of the RV in the short-axis (SA) plane [5]. Previous studies have shown that RVEF predicts long-term outcome in PH patients for both children and adults [6, 7].

* Correspondence: stina.jorstig@regionorebrolan.se
[1]School of Medical Sciences, Faculty of Medicine and Health, Örebro University, 70182 Örebro, Sweden
[5]Biomedical Engineering, Örebro University Hospital, 70185 Örebro, Sweden
Full list of author information is available at the end of the article

The most common method for RV assessment is, however, transthoracic echocardiography (TTE) due to its high availability compared to CMR. A challenge when using TTE for RV evaluation is the position of the RV behind the sternum [8]. When imaging the RV in standard apical four-chamber (4CH) view shadows caused by a rib or lung often make the RV free wall hard to visualize, particularly the most apical parts. The absence of a distinct RV free wall in the TTE image makes following area and volume estimations very uncertain by both 2D and 3D TTE. For this reason tricuspid annular plane systolic excursion (TAPSE), also known as tricuspid annulus motion (TAM), is often used as a substitute for RVEF. There are, however, contradictory conclusions in the literature how well TTE-derived TAPSE correlates to CMR-derived RVEF. There are examples where the correlation between TAPSE and RVEF varies from no correlation [9, 10] to statistically significant correlation (range 0.45-0.86) [11–13]. Recent guidelines for echocardiography still recommend RV assessment by 2D TTE using multiple acoustic windows, while 3D TTE is only recommended for laboratories with experience in this area [14].

Evaluation of the RV using TTE is often made by the one-dimensional measure of TAPSE along with quantification of the RV size, often by measuring the RV diameter, and a visual evaluation of the concentric movement of the RV free wall. The fact that TTE provides a real time image of the ventricle function is an advantage, but the visual assessment might imply risk of subjectivity. Also, when using TAPSE the objective evaluation of the RV is only one-dimensional with a focus on longitudinal movement of the free wall and potential information may be left out in terms of global function. The inclusion of more than one distance measurement in the evaluation of the RVEF using TTE is a conceivable alternative for achieving a more consistent measure of RVEF which relies on a three-dimensional property (volume).

In a previous study, on healthy individuals, we have presented and evaluated a model for RV volume estimations [15], where the RV is approximated by an ellipsoid composed of three distances easily measured by TTE. The results from that study showed that the ellipsoid model underestimates RV volumes compared to reference CMR-derived RV volumes, due to underestimation of distance measurements in TTE compared to CMR. There was however a good agreement between the ellipsoid model derived RVEF and RVEF obtained from CMR. Since RVEF is calculated as a quota, it is still possible that this value can be estimated accurately even though the volumes are underestimated.

The aim of the present study was to evaluate whether the ellipsoid model can be an alternative to TAPSE for RVEF estimations by i) estimating the agreement between RVEF obtained by the ellipsoid model (RVEF$_{TTE}$) and reference CMR-derived RVEF (RVEF$_{CMR}$) and ii) comparing the correlation for RVEF$_{TTE}$ and TAPSE to RVEF$_{CMR}$ for a group of subjects with a wide range of RVEF.

Methods

Sample size

A power analysis was performed to calculate the sample size needed to detect differences in RVEF of 5 percentage points (ppt) between the ellipsoid model and the reference, with an estimated standard deviation (SD) of 10, power 80% and $\alpha = 0.05$. The power analysis concluded a minimum of 34 subjects.

Study population

Twenty-five patients with reduced RV function, and examined with both TTE and CMR, were retrospectively included in the study. Patients were identified in the radiology information system (RIS) using a list of all CMR examinations performed between January 2012 and May 2015. A subject was included if there was an entry of a reduced RV function in the clinical CMR report and a TTE examination had been performed within three months from the CMR examination. All subjects younger than 18 years were excluded. The criteria for inclusion in the study was met if there was a notification of reduced RV function in the CMR report defined as RVEF <50%, TAPSE <20 mm or based on visual assessment. The exact degree of reduced RV function for a specific patient was not crucial, since to the aim was to get a variety RVEF. Care was taken to ensure that the patients had not undergone any cardiac intervention of significance during the time between CMR and TTE, such as surgery and treatments including electrophysiology or potent drugs, which could have influenced on cardiac function. In this regard, care was also taken to ensure that the loading and filling conditions did not differ significantly between the two examinations such as heart rate, presence of severe valve dysfunctions and/or pericardial effusion.

In addition to the 25 patients, the twelve healthy volunteers from the previous ellipsoid study [15] were included to ensure a wide range of RVEF. These twelve examinations were consequently used in both studies. Characteristics of the subjects are presented in Table 1.

The Regional Ethical Review Board approved the study and waived the informed consent requirement for the retrospectively included patients, while written informed consent was obtained from the healthy subjects.

Table 1 Subject characteristics. Parameter values are presented as mean ± SD. Number of subjects is given as a quantity with the proportion (%) relative all subjects within brackets. Abbreviations: ARVC = arrhythmogenic right ventricular cardiomyopathy, BMI = body mass index, CMR = cardiac magnetic resonance, n = number, n.a. = not applicable, PH = pulmonary hypertension, RVEF = right ventricular ejection fraction, TAPSE = tricuspid annular plane systolic excursion, TTE = transthoracic echocardiography

Variables	Patients (n = 25)	Healthy subjects (n = 12)	Overall (n = 37)
Age (year)	55 ± 11	36 ± 12	49 ± 15
BMI [weight(kg)/length(m)^2]	27 ± 4	24 ± 4	26 ± 4
Women	5 (20%)	4 (33%)	9 (24%)
RVEF by TTE (ellipsoid model), %	45 ± 7	59 ± 3	50 ± 9
TAPSE by TTE, mm	17 ± 5	22 ± 3	19 ± 5
RVEF by CMR (endocardial delineation in short-axis images and summation of subvolumes), %	38 ± 10	56 ± 4	43 ± 12
Time difference between CMR and TTE, days	29 ± 26	n.a.[a]	n.a.[a]
Absence of significant heart valve disease at TTE[b]	20 (80%)	12 (100%)	32 (86%)
Absence of significant pericardial effusion at TTE[c]	25 (100%)	12 (100%)	37 (100%)
Diagnosed with or suspected primarily right-sided pathology before or during the current time of study entry[d]	7 (28%)	0 (0%)	7 (19%)

[a] All healthy subjects had CMR and TTE at the same visit (separated by <30 min)
[b] Valve disease defined as significant stenosis and-/or regurgitation (≥ grade 2/3)
[c] Pericardial effusion defined as being recognized with a clear hemodynamic influence
[d] One patient was diagnosed with ARVC, five patients had suspected primarily right-sided pathology and one patient had biventricular dilated cardiomyopathy

Examinations

The healthy subjects were examined by TTE and CMR at the same day and location, separated by less than 30 min.

All CMR examinations were performed on a clinical 1.5 T Philips Achieva system (Philips Healthcare, Best, the Netherlands). A retrospectively triggered balanced turbo field echo (b-TFE) pulse sequence was used for the acquisition of conventional images. The following parameters were applied; TR/TE shortest (typical 3.5 ms/1.7 ms), pixel size typically 1.5x1.5 mm2, flip angle 60°, 1 NSA. For the retrospectively included patients an acceleration factor (SENSE) of 2 was used, while no acceleration factor was used for the healthy subjects (SENSE = 1). For the retrospectively included patients the slice thickness/slice spacing was 5/8 mm and 30 consecutive heart phases were used for the SA images for all patients but one where 13 consecutive heart phases were used for the SA images. For the healthy subjects the slice thickness/slice spacing was 8/8 mm and 20 consecutive heart phases were used for the SA images. The protocol applied for examination of patients was slightly different from the protocol used for the healthy volunteers. The main reason for this difference is the adaptation of the protocol to a lower breath hold ability of the patients compared to healthy volunteers.

The TTE examinations of the group of patients were performed using three different types of commercial ultrasound scanners: General Electric Vivid E9 (GE Vingmed Ultrasound A/S Horten, Norway), Siemens ACUSON SC2000 (Siemens AG, Germany) or Philips iE33 (Philips Medical Systems, Andover, MA, USA).

Each system was equipped with a compatible transducer (phased array and multi-frequency based). The examinations had been carried out as in clinical routine, with the subjects in the left lateral recumbent position and ECG-triggering, thus, including digital storage of moving clips (i.e. cine-loops) from standardized views, allowing offline measurements. The TTE examinations of the healthy group were performed solely using one kind of ultrasound system (GE Vivid E9). As in clinical routine, these examinations also included standardized collection procedure and digital storage of cine-loops (from standardized views).

Ellipsoid model

The RV was approximated by an ellipsoid as previously described [15]. In short, the ellipsoid model represents the RV by an ellipsoid composed of three distance measurements available in TTE images; right ventricular inflow tract ($RVIT_3$), right ventricular long axis (RVLAX) and the left ventricular maximum outer basal diameter (LVD). The right ventricular volume (RVV) is then approximated as:

$$RVV = \frac{\pi}{6} \times RVIT_3 \times RVLAX \times LVD$$

For a detailed derivation of the equation see Appendix. By using this estimate of the RVV, for both diastolic and systolic measurements, RVEF can be calculated.

Measurements

The distances needed for the ellipsoid model, i.e. $RVIT_3$, RVLAX and LVD, were measured in diastole and systole in the stored TTE images (i.e. 2D cine-loops). $RVIT_3$ and RVLAX were measured in apical 4CH view, while LVD was measured in apical two-chamber (2CH) view (Fig. 1).

In addition, TAPSE was measured from M-mode TTE images as obtained in the 4CH view, for all subjects but one; where M-mode was not available. For this subject, however, TAPSE was measured in a corresponding 2D image (by so-called anatomic M-mode feature).

Offline analysis, regarding all of the TTE examinations, was done using dedicated software (EchoPAC PC, GE Vingmed Ultrasound). All TTE measurements were calculated as the average of up to three different cardiac cycles, as in clinical routine, with regard to image quality and the amount of images per view.

In SA CMR images the end-diastolic and end-systolic volumes were achieved by manually delineating the endocardium of the right ventricle using the freely available software Segment version 2.0 R4800 (http://www.segment.heiberg.se/ [16]. All available stacks with information of the tricuspid and the pulmonary valves were used to add information about the valves position in the SA images to improve the decision of which parts of the most basal slices to include in the ventricle volume. Using these end-diastolic and end-systolic volumes the RVEF was calculated.

The TTE measurements were performed by one biomedical scientist with 8 years of experience (observer 1), and one master of science in biomedical engineering with 3 years' of experience in the scientific TTE field but limited clinical experience (observer 2). The CMR measurements were performed by one radiologist with 4 years of experience (observer3), and one master of science in biomedical engineering with 5 years' experience in the scientific CMR field but limited clinical experience (observer 2).

Inter-observer (intra-modality) agreement for each modality was performed.

The mean value for the two observers for each method was calculated to give $RVEF_{TTE}$ and $RVEF_{CMR}$. These mean values were used for the inter-modality agreement evaluation.

Statistics

Shapiro-Wilk's test was used to determine normality of the data. Paired Student's t-test was used to test the significance for normally distributed differences, while Wilcoxon signed-rank test was used for non-normally distributed differences. Bland-Altman limits of agreement method were used to evaluate the differences [17] for both normally and non-normally distributed differences as non-normality does not have a great impact on the limits of agreement [18]. Pearson's correlation coefficient was used to test the correlation between the two different methods for calculating RVEF and interpreted as negligible $(0 < r < 0.3)$, low $(0.3 < r < 0.5)$, moderate

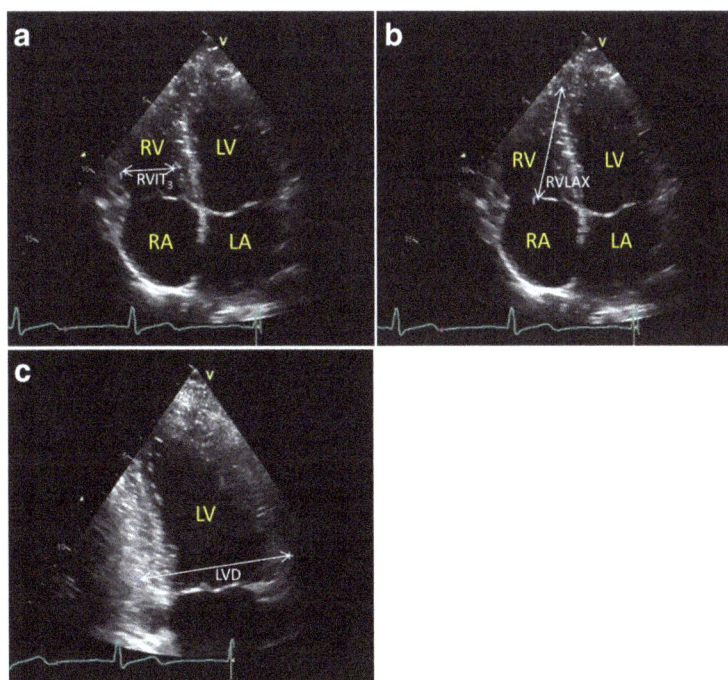

Fig. 1 Transthoracic echocardiography distances. Images showing the transthoracic echocardiography distances for a healthy 33 year old male subject in **a**) and **b**) apical 4CH view and in **c**) apical 2CH view. LA = left atrium, LV = left ventricle, LVD = left ventricular diameter, RA = right atrium, RV = right ventricle, $RVIT_3$ = right ventricular inflow tract, RVLAX = right ventricular long axis

$(0.5 < r < 0.7)$, high $(0.7 < r < 0.9)$ and very high $(r > 0.9)$ [19]. Steiger's z-test was used to decide whether two correlation coefficients were significantly different or not [20]. Statistical analyzes were performed using IBM SPSS Statistics version 22 (IBM Corp., Armonk, NY, USA) and Stata (version 14.1, StataCorp LP, College Station, Texas, USA). All values are presented as mean ± 1 SD. $p < 0.05$ was considered to indicate statistical significance.

Results

The 25 retrospectively included patients had a mean age of 55 years (range 27–72 years, 20% women), while the twelve healthy subjects had a mean age of 36 years (range 18–65 years, 33% women). The TTE and CMR examinations for the 25 patients were separated by a maximum of 77 days (mean 29 days, range 0–77 days) (Table 1).

There was a high correlation $r = 0.80$ $(p < 0.001)$ between $RVEF_{TTE}$ and $RVEF_{CMR}$, while the correlation between TAPSE and $RVEF_{CMR}$ was moderate $r = 0.54$ $(p < 0.001)$ (Fig. 2). The correlation between TAPSE and $RVEF_{CMR}$ was significantly lower than the correlation between $RVEF_{TTE}$ and $RVEF_{CMR}$ $(p < 0.05)$. $RVEF_{TTE}$ obtained from the ellipsoid model was 50 ± 9% (range 34–65) and $RVEF_{CMR}$ was 43 ± 12% (range 20–66). There was a significant difference between $RVEF_{TTE}$ and $RVEF_{CMR}$ using Wilcoxon signed rank test (Z = −4.1, $p < 0.001$). The mean value for TAPSE was 19 ± 5 mm. Figure 3 shows the Bland-Altman plot for the difference between $RVEF_{TTE}$ and $RVEF_{CMR}$. The standard deviation

for the differences of the mean values in the Bland-Altman analysis was calculated according to the recommendation for analyzes based on mean values [17].

When the healthy subjects were excluded, the correlation between $RVEF_{TTE}$ and $RVEF_{CMR}$ for the remaining subgroup of 25 patients was moderate, $r = 0.62$ $(p < 0.01)$, while the correlation between TAPSE and $RVEF_{CMR}$ was low, $r = 0.34$, and could not be statistically verified. There was a significant difference $(p < 0.001)$ between $RVEF_{TTE}$ and $RVEF_{CMR}$ for this subgroup of 8 ± 8 ppt (95% CI: 4.1-11).

The results for the RVEF calculations of each observer were $RVEF_{TTE\ obs1} = 47 \pm 10$ (range 30–65), $RVEF_{TTE\ obs2} = 52 \pm 9$ (range 34–70), $RVEF_{CMR\ obs2} = 42 \pm 14$ (range 17–68) and $RVEF_{CMR\ obs3} = 45 \pm 12$ (range 18–63). An additional file contains the RVEF values for each subject (see Additional file 1). The mean difference between $RVEF_{TTE\ obs1}$ and $RVEF_{TTE\ obs2}$ was 6 ± 7 ppt, while the mean difference between $RVEF_{CMR\ obs2}$ and $RVEF_{CMR\ obs3}$ was 2 ± 6 ppt. Both differences were normally distributed and statistically significant $(p < 0.05)$. This inter-observer agreement can also be considered as an intra-modality agreement since they rely on data from the same modality. The correlation between $RVEF_{TTE\ obs1}$ and $RVEF_{TTE\ obs2}$ was high $r = 0.73$ $(p < 0.001)$, while the correlation between $RVEF_{CMR\ obs2}$ and $RVEF_{CMR\ obs3}$ was very high $r = 0.91$ $(p < 0.001)$.

Discussion

Determination of RVEF is an important parameter in the assessment of cardiovascular diseases. There is

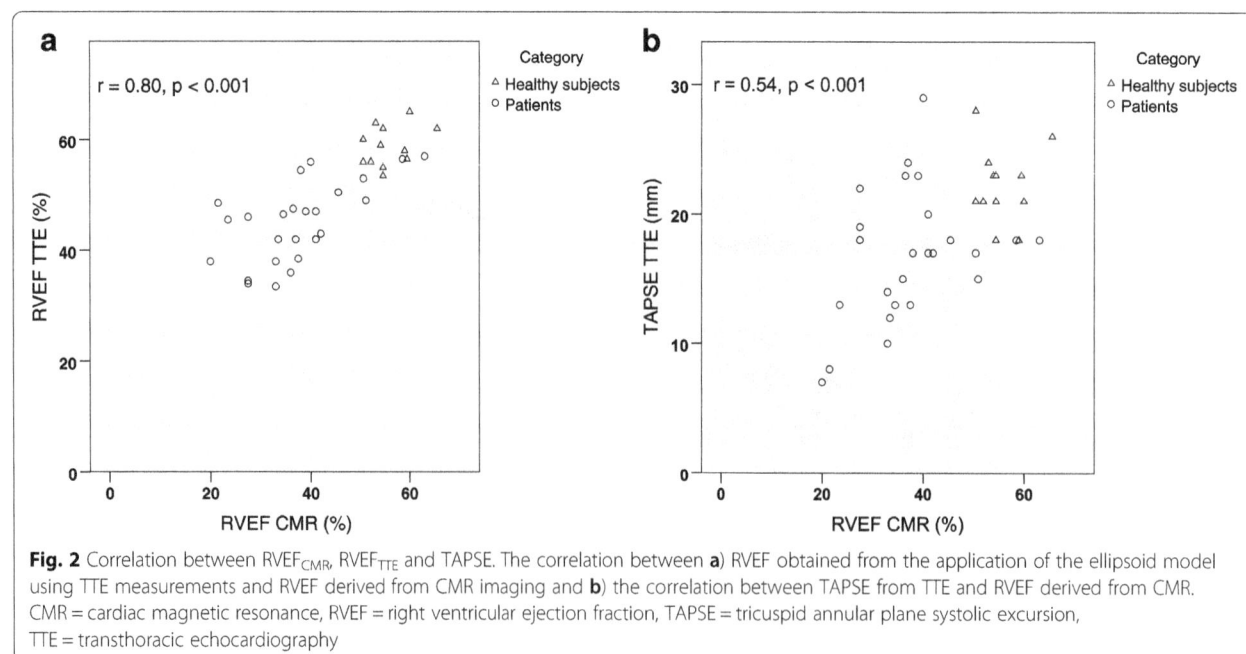

Fig. 2 Correlation between $RVEF_{CMR}$, $RVEF_{TTE}$ and TAPSE. The correlation between **a**) RVEF obtained from the application of the ellipsoid model using TTE measurements and RVEF derived from CMR imaging and **b**) the correlation between TAPSE from TTE and RVEF derived from CMR. CMR = cardiac magnetic resonance, RVEF = right ventricular ejection fraction, TAPSE = tricuspid annular plane systolic excursion, TTE = transthoracic echocardiography

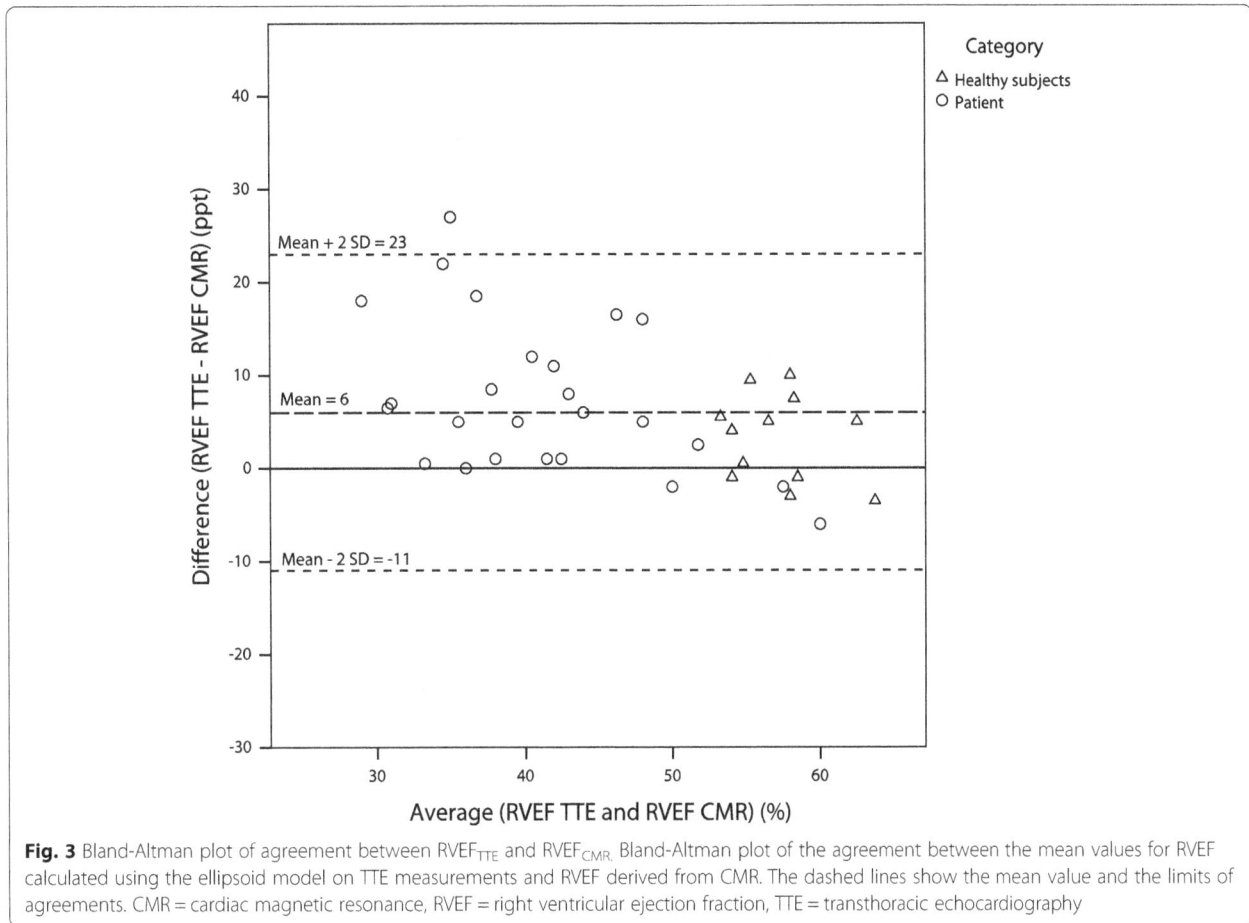

Fig. 3 Bland-Altman plot of agreement between RVEF$_{TTE}$ and RVEF$_{CMR}$. Bland-Altman plot of the agreement between the mean values for RVEF calculated using the ellipsoid model on TTE measurements and RVEF derived from CMR. The dashed lines show the mean value and the limits of agreements. CMR = cardiac magnetic resonance, RVEF = right ventricular ejection fraction, TTE = transthoracic echocardiography

today no established method for measurement of RVEF based on volume estimations using 2D TTE. The results in this study show that a combination of three conventional distance measurements in 2D TTE provides volume-based estimations of RVEF that strongly correlates to CMR for a clinically relevant range of RVEFs. The distances can easily be measured in the 2D TTE images and is not dependent on a complete visualization of the RV free wall which remains as a challenge in echocardiography. The time for measuring the distances necessary for the ellipsoid model is, after some initial testing at our department, considerably shorter compared to RVEF calculations using 3D TTE data with post processing software. The ellipsoid model is not necessarily less time-consuming compared to other conventional 2D parameters (such as TAPSE, fractional area change, longitudinal strain and strain rate by Doppler tissue imaging and speckle-tracking echocardiography (STE)), although it may be recognized with relatively high applicability in this regard; since it does not require full visualization of the entire RV free wall. The moderate correlation between TAPSE and RVEF$_{CMR}$ was significantly lower

compared to the high correlation between RVEF$_{CMR}$ and the RVEF obtained using the ellipsoid model. This difference in correlation might seem reasonable since the ellipsoid model combines distances expanding a volume while TAPSE provides a one-directional estimate.

An upcoming method for RV evaluation is longitudinal STE strain for regional or global analysis of the RV free wall. STE strain enables quantification of the RV free wall which, compared to Doppler tissue imaging strain, is less angle dependent but the need for good image quality and full visualization of the RV free wall is still present [14]. A recent study provided reference values for RV longitudinal strain (RVLS) by STE [21]. These reference values for RVLS showed a weak correlation to RVEF by 3D TTE (0.27 for 6-segment RVLS and 0.28 for 3-segment RVLS). The authors discuss the fact that RVLS does not take into account the radial movement of the RV and that RV radial strain is difficult to measure by 2D STE [21]. Thus, at the moment this technique does not seem to add any extra value in this context (in addition to measuring TAPSE). A comparison between STE strain and the proposed ellipsoid model, regarding the assessment of the RV function, would be of interest for future studies.

There was a small but significant mean difference regarding RVEF as estimated with the ellipsoid model compared to CMR, where the ellipsoid overestimates the RVEF. As seen in Figs. 2 and 3 there are larger differences for low RVEF values compared to higher values. The limits of agreement in the Bland Altman analysis are −11 to 23 ppt. This is a rather wide range for the limits of agreement, but as shown in Fig. 3 there are six out of the 25 patients which mainly contribute to the increased mean difference and limits of agreements. Among these six patients one was diagnosed with ARVC, while four of them (of which one was recognized with severe PH) showed signs of more or less regional RV dilatation; despite not fulfilling the criteria for ARVC (Table 1). Thus, the majority of these outliers had a clearly abnormal RV morphology, indicating that the ellipsoid model is less suitable for this category of patients. However, the ellipsoid model might be used to detect RV dysfunction before it results in RV deformation. For the remaining 31 subjects however, among which there were no diagnoses of ARVC, severe PH or signs of abnormal morphology, the difference is about 10 ppt or lower, which could be considered as clinically acceptable differences.

The correlation between RVEF estimated by the ellipsoid model and CMR was lower for the subgroup of 25 patients compared to the correlation for all subjects, but still at a moderate level, while there was no correlation between TAPSE and CMR for this subgroup. This indicates that the ellipsoid model provides a better estimate of global RV function compared to TAPSE. The fact that there were up to three months between the TTE and CMR examinations for the patient group is a possible reason for the greater differences and lower correlation, along with the issue of abnormal RV morphology discussed above. Also, the number of subjects and the distribution of the RVEF-values differ when comparing the correlation coefficient for the subgroup of 25 patients to the correlation coefficient for all 37 subjects. A prospective study, performing CMR and TTE examinations on the same day for a group of subjects with a wide range of RVEF values, is needed to further evaluate the ellipsoid model.

In TTE, according to our experience, RVEF is quite often determined by visual estimation of the concentric movement of the RV free wall, along with TAPSE measurements. We believe that this new method for RVEF calculations is a way to improve the RVEF estimations using TTE, and making it less subjective.

Looking at the intra-modality agreement there was a high correlation for TTE compared to a very high for CMR. There was a slightly smaller bias and more narrow limits of agreements for CMR compared to TTE. This indication, that CMR measurements are more reproducible, agrees with CMR being considered to be the reference for such measurements. Also, the inter-observer variability may be affected by the difference in clinical experience between the observers.

CMR and TTE complement each other and a multimodality approach is often a good alternative when possible. We believe, however, that this new method proposed for RVEF calculations using TTE may be of value when CMR is not possible.

Limitations

One of the dimensions in the ellipsoid model is based on a left ventricular measure (LVD) and is not a direct right ventricular measure. This could influence the accuracy for groups of patients, such as patients with arrhythmogenic right ventricular cardiomyopathy (ARVC), due to the risk of an increase of the right ventricle width in this direction, which not necessarily leads to an increase of the left ventricular diameter. Further evaluation of the model's applicability for this group of patients is necessary. An alternative to using the LVD measure in the equation, could be to replace it with the corresponding measure of the RV in a basal parasternal short-axis view, possibly resulting in better agreement also for patients with abnormal RV morphology.

When measuring $RVIT_3$, the apical 4CH view should be focused on the RV, as recommended in the guidelines [14]. For the healthy subjects the RV focused apical 4CH view was used, while it is not certain that this was the case for the retrospectively included patients. This means that there is a risk of volumetric underestimation regarding the group of retrospectively included patients. However, since the RVEF is a quota, this aspect may be considered to be less significant in the context.

The fact that it was up to three months between the examinations for the retrospectively included patients might influence the results.

In this study, CMR is used as reference method. It is the method commonly used as reference method for ventricular volume calculations, but it is however important to remember that the calculations by CMR also are estimations. In particular for the RV, delineation of the endocardium is a difficult task and the true value remains unknown.

Conclusions

The ellipsoid model provides an alternative for RVEF calculations using 2D TTE that gives a higher correlation to CMR compared to TAPSE for a wide range of RVEF. An incomplete visualization of the RV free wall, which is a common challenge in TTE, is not a restriction for the application of the method.

Appendix

The area of an ellipse and volume of an ellipsoid is expressed as:

$$A = \pi ab$$

$$V = \frac{4\pi abc}{3}$$

where a, b and c are the radiuses of the ellipse or ellipsoid.

Figure 4 shows parts of two ellipsoids with two common radiuses, b and c. The third radius, a_1 and a_2 are not equal. The volume of grey region can be expressed as the difference between a quarter of the volume of the larger ellipsoid and a quarter of the volume of the smaller ellipsoid, i.e.:

$$V_{grey} = \frac{\pi bc}{3}(a_2 - a_1)$$

If $a_2 - a_1$ is approximated by $RVIT_3$, b approximated by LVD/2 and c approximated by RVLAX, an estimate of RVV is given by:

$$RVV = \frac{\pi}{6} \times RVIT_3 \times RVLAX \times LVD$$

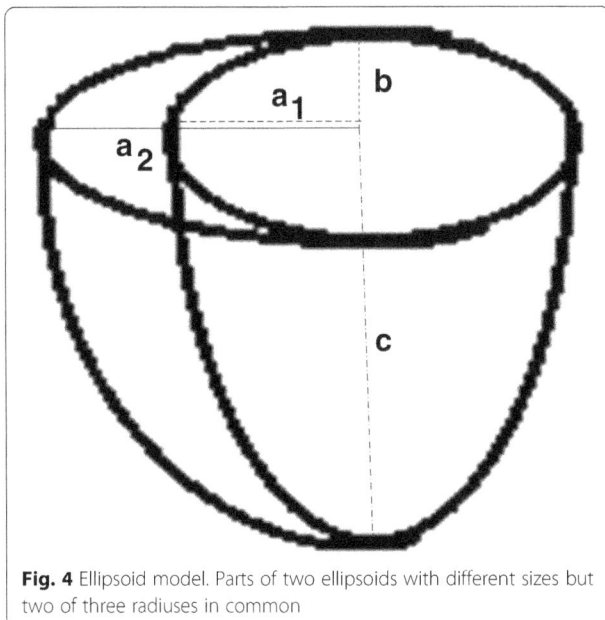

Fig. 4 Ellipsoid model. Parts of two ellipsoids with different sizes but two of three radiuses in common

Abbreviations
4CH: Four-chamber; b-TFE: Balanced turbo field echo; CMR: Cardiac magnetic resonance; LA: Left atrium; LV: Left ventricle; LVD: Left ventricular maximum outer basal diameter; PH: Pulmonary hypertension; PPT: Percentage points; RA: Right atrium; RV: Right ventricle; RVEF: Right ventricular ejection fraction; $RVIT_3$: Right ventricular inflow tract; RVLAX: Right ventricular long axis; RVLS: Right ventricular longitudinal strain; RVV: Right ventricular volume; SA: Short-axis; SD: Standard deviation; STE: Speckle-tracking echocardiographic; TAM: Tricuspid annulus motion; TAPSE: Tricuspid annular plane systolic excursion; TTE: Transthoracic echocardiography

Acknowledgement
The authors wish to thank Yang Cao for statistical advice.

Funding
This work has been supported by the Research Committee of Region Örebro County (OLL-573211). The funding source had no role in the research or preparation of the article.

Authors' contributions
SJO: Concept/design of the study, acquisition of data, analyses/interpretation of the data, drafting the article, final approval of the submitted version. MWA: Acquisition of data, critical revision of article, final approval of the submitted version. MLI: Acquisition of data, critical revision of article, final approval of the submitted version. PTH: Concept/design of the study, critical revision of article, final approval of the submitted version.

Competing interests
The authors declare that they have no competing interests.

Author details
[1]School of Medical Sciences, Faculty of Medicine and Health, Örebro University, 70182 Örebro, Sweden. [2]Department of Clinical Physiology, Faculty of Medicine and Health, Örebro University, 70182 Örebro, Sweden. [3]Department of Radiology, Faculty of Medicine and Health, Örebro University, 70182 Örebro, Sweden. [4]Department of Medical Physics, Faculty of Medicine and Health, Örebro University, 70182 Örebro, Sweden. [5]Biomedical Engineering, Örebro University Hospital, 70185 Örebro, Sweden.

References
1. Haddad F, Doyle R, Murphy DJ, Hunt SA. Right ventricular function in cardiovascular disease, part II: pathophysiology, clinical importance, and management of right ventricular failure. Circulation. 2008;117:1717–31.
2. Davlouros PA, Niwa K, Webb G, Gatzoulis MA. The right ventricle in congenital heart disease. Heart. 2006;92 Suppl 1:i27–38.
3. Chin KM, Kim NH, Rubin LJ. The right ventricle in pulmonary hypertension. Coron Artery Dis. 2005;16:13–8.
4. Hulot JS, Jouven X, Empana JP, Frank R, Fontaine G. Natural history and risk stratification of arrhythmogenic right ventricular dysplasia/cardiomyopathy. Circulation. 2004;110:1879–84.
5. Alfakih K, Reid S, Jones T, Sivananthan M. Assessment of ventricular function and mass by cardiac magnetic resonance imaging. Eur Radiol. 2004;14: 1813–22.
6. Moledina S, Pandya B, Bartsota M, Mortensen KH, McMillan M, Quyam S, et al. Prognostic significance of cardiac magnetic resonance imaging in children with pulmonary hypertension. Circ Cardiovasc Imaging. 2013;6: 407–14.
7. Kawut SM, Horn EM, Berekashvili KK, Garofano RP, Goldsmith RL, Widlitz AC, et al. New predictors of outcome in idiopathic pulmonary arterial hypertension. Am J Cardiol. 2005;95:199–203.
8. Ho SY, Nihoyannopoulos P. Anatomy, echocardiography, and normal right ventricular dimensions. Heart. 2006;92 Suppl 1:i2–13.
9. Kuhn A, Meierhofer C, Rutz T, Rondak IC, Rohlig C, Schreiber C, et al. Non-volumetric echocardiographic indices and qualitative assessment of right ventricular systolic function in Ebstein's anomaly: comparison with CMR-derived ejection fraction in 49 patients. Eur Heart J Cardiovasc Imaging. 2016;17;930-5.

10. Li YD, Wang YD, Zhai ZG, Guo XJ, Wu YF, Yang YH, et al. Relationship between echocardiographic and cardiac magnetic resonance imaging-derived measures of right ventricular function in patients with chronic thromboembolic pulmonary hypertension. Thromb Res. 2015;135:602–6.

11. Vizzardi E, Bonadei I, Sciatti E, Pezzali N, Farina D, D'Aloia A, et al. Quantitative analysis of right ventricular (RV) function with echocardiography in chronic heart failure with no or mild RV dysfunction: comparison with cardiac magnetic resonance imaging. J Ultrasound Med. 2015;34:247–55.

12. Focardi M, Cameli M, Carbone SF, Massoni A, De Vito R, Lisi M, et al. Traditional and innovative echocardiographic parameters for the analysis of right ventricular performance in comparison with cardiac magnetic resonance. Eur Heart J Cardiovasc Imaging. 2015;16:47–52.

13. Sato T, Tsujino I, Oyama-Manabe N, Ohira H, Ito YM, Sugimori H, et al. Simple prediction of right ventricular ejection fraction using tricuspid annular plane systolic excursion in pulmonary hypertension. Int J Cardiovasc Imaging. 2013;29:1799–805.

14. Lang RM, Badano LP, Mor-Avi V, Afilalo J, Armstrong A, Ernande L, et al. Recommendations for cardiac chamber quantification by echocardiography in adults: an update from the American Society of Echocardiography and the European Association of Cardiovascular Imaging. J Am Soc Echocardiogr. 2015;28:1–39. e14.

15. Jorstig S, Waldenborg M, Liden M, Wodecki M, Thunberg P. Determination of Right Ventricular Volume by Combining Echocardiographic Distance Measurements. Echocardiography. 2016;33:844–53.

16. Heiberg E, Sjogren J, Ugander M, Carlsson M, Engblom H, Arheden H. Design and validation of Segment–freely available software for cardiovascular image analysis. BMC Med Imaging. 2010;10:1.

17. Bland JM, Altman DG. Statistical methods for assessing agreement between two methods of clinical measurement. Lancet. 1986;1:307–10.

18. Bland JM, Altman DG. Measuring agreement in method comparison studies. Stat Methods Med Res. 1999;8:135–60.

19. Mukaka MM. Statistics corner: A guide to appropriate use of correlation coefficient in medical research. Malawi Med J. 2012;24:69–71.

20. Cohen J, Cohen P, West S, Aiken L. Bivariate Correlation and Regression. In: Riegert D, editor. Applied Multiple Regression/Correlation Analysis for the Behavioral Sciences. 3rd ed. Mahwah: Lawrence Erlbaum Associates; 1983. p. 19–31.

21. Muraru D, Onciul S, Peluso D, Soriani N, Cucchini U, Aruta P, et al. Sex- and Method-Specific Reference Values for Right Ventricular Strain by 2-Dimensional Speckle-Tracking Echocardiography. Circ Cardiovasc Imaging. 2016;9:e003866.

5

The clinical use of stress echocardiography in ischemic heart disease

Rosa Sicari[1*] [iD] and Lauro Cortigiani[2]

Abstract

Stress echocardiography is an established technique for the assessment of extent and severity of coronary artery disease. The combination of echocardiography with a physical, pharmacological or electrical stress allows to detect myocardial ischemia with an excellent accuracy. A transient worsening of regional function during stress is the hallmark of inducible ischemia. Stress echocardiography provides similar diagnostic and prognostic accuracy as radionuclide stress perfusion imaging or *magnetic* resonance, but at a substantially lower cost, without environmental impact, and with no biohazards for the patient and the physician.

The evidence on its clinical impact has been collected over 35 years, based on solid experimental, pathophysiological, technological and clinical foundations. There is the need to implement the combination of wall motion and coronary flow reserve, assessed in the left anterior descending artery, into a single test. The improvement of technology and in imaging quality will make this approach more and more feasible. The future issues in stress echo will be the possibility of obtaining quantitative information translating the current qualitative assessment of regional wall motion into a number. The next challenge for stress echocardiography is to overcome its main weaknesses: dependance on operator expertise, the lack of outcome data (a widesperad problem in clinical imaging) to document the improvement of patient outcomes. This paper summarizes the main indications for the clinical applications of stress echocardiography to ischemic heart disease.

Background

Pathophysiologic mechanisms

Stress echocardiography is the combination of 2D echocardiography with a physical, pharmacological, or electrical stress [1]. The diagnostic endpoint for the detection of myocardial ischaemia is the induction of a transient change in regional function during stress. A transient regional imbalance between oxygen demand and supply usually results in myocardial ischaemia, the signs and symptoms of which can be used as a diagnostic tool [1]. Myocardial ischaemia results in a typical 'cascade' of events in which the various markers are hierarchically ranked in a well-defined time sequence [2]. Flow heterogeneity, especially between the subendocardial and subepicardial perfusion, is the forerunner of ischaemia, followed by metabolic changes, alteration in regional mechanical function, and only at a later stage by electrocardiographic changes, and pain. The pathophysiological concept of the ischaemic cascade is translated clinically into a gradient of sensitivity of different available clinical markers of ischaemia, with chest pain being the least and regional malperfusion the most sensitive. The reduction of coronary flow reserve (CFR) is the common pathophysiological mechanism. Regardless of the stress used and the morphological substrate, ischaemia tends to propagate centrifugally with respect to the ventricular cavity: [3, 4] it involves primarily the subendocardial layer, whereas the subepicardial layer is affected only at a later stage if the ischaemia persists [4]. In fact, extravascular pressure is higher in the subendocardial than in the subepicardial layer; this provokes a higher metabolic demand (wall tension being among the main determinants of myocardial oxygen consumption) and an increased resistance to flow. In the absence of coronary artery disease (CAD), CFR can be reduced in microvascular disease (e.g. in syndrome X) or left ventricular (LV) hypertrophy (e.g. arterial hypertension). In this condition, angina with ST-segment depression can occur with regional perfusion changes, typically in the absence of any regional wall motion abnormalities during stress. Wall

* Correspondence: rosas@ifc.cnr.it
[1]CNR, Institute of Clinical Physiology, Via G. Moruzzi, 1, 56124 Pisa, Italy
Full list of author information is available at the end of the article

motion abnormalities are more specific than CFR and/or perfusion changes for the diagnosis of CAD [5–10].

Diagnostic criteria

All stress echocardiographic diagnoses can be summarized into four equations centered on regional wall function and describing the fundamental response patterns: normal, ischemic, necrotic, and viable.

Normal response

A segment is normokinetic at rest and normal or hyperkinetic during stress.

Ischemic response

The function of a segment worsens during stress from normokinesia to hypokinesia (decrease of endocardial movement and systolic thickening), akinesia (absence of endocardial movement and systolic thickening), or dyskinesia (paradoxical outward movement and possible systolic thinning). However, a resting akinesia becoming dyskinesia during stress reflects purely passive phenomenon of increased intraventricular pressure developed by normally contracting walls and should not be considered a true active ischemia [1].

Necrotic response

A segment with resting dysfunction remains fixed during stress.

Viability response

A segment with resting dysfunction may show either a sustained improvement during stress indicating a non-jeopardized myocardium (stunned) or improve during early stress with subsequent deterioration at peak (biphasic response). The biphasic response is suggestive of viability and ischemia, with jeopardized myocardium fed by a critically coronary stenosis [1] Table 1.

Ischaemic stressors

Exercise, dobutamine, and dipyridamole are the most frequently used stressors for echocardiographic test [11]. There are distinct advantages and disadvantages to exercise versus pharmacological stress. In Table 2 the stress echo protocols are reported.

Table 1 Stress echocardiography in 4 equations

Rest	+	Stress	=	Diagnosis
Normokinesis	+	Normo-Hyperkinesis	=	Normal
Normokinesis	+	Hypo, A, Dyskinesis	=	Ischaemia
Akinesis	+	Hypo, Normokinesis	=	Viable
A-, Dyskinesis	+	A-, Dyskinesis	=	Necrosis

Table 2 Stress echo protocols

Test	Equipment	Protocols
Exercise	Semi-supine bycicle ergometer	25 W x 2' with incremental loading
Dobutamine	Infusion Pump	5 mcg/Kg/min 10-20-30-40 + atropine (0.25 x 4) up to 1 mg
Dipyridamole	Syringe	0.84 mg/Kg in 6' or 0.84 mg/Kg in 10' + atropine (0.25 x 4) up to 1 mg
Adenosine	Syringe	140 mcg/Kg/min in 6'
Pacing	External Pacing	From 100 bpm with increments of 10 beats/min up to target heart rate

Exercise

Exercise echocardiography can be performed using either a treadmill or bicycle protocol. When a treadmill test is performed, post-exercise imaging is evaluated. Regional wall motion abnormalities would persist long enough into recovery to be detected but when recovery is rapid false-negative results occur [11]. Some Authors [12], perform peak-exercise imaging also during treadmill by keeping the patient standing still. Although challenging such an approach avoid false negative results in case of a rapid recovery to resting conditions. Information on exercise capacity, heart rate response, and rhythm and blood pressure changes are analysed and, together with wall motion analysis, become part of the final interpretation [11]. Bicycle exercise echocardiography is performed during either an upright or a recumbent posture. Unlike treadmill test, bicycle exercise allows to obtain images during the various levels of exercise. The supine position is the most suited for exercise echocardiography due to its ease of image acquisition in all views through the steps of the graded exercise [13]. In the upright posture, imaging is generally limited to apical views.

Dobutamine

The standard dobutamine stress protocol consists of continuous intravenous infusion of dobutamine in 3 min increments, starting with 5 µg/kg/min and increasing to 10, 20, 30, and 40 µg/kg/min. If no endpoint is reached, atropine (up to 1 mg) is added to the 40 µg/kg/min dobutamine infusion [11, 14, 15].

Dipyridamole

The standard dipyridamole protocol consists of an intravenous infusion of 0.84 mg/kg over 10 min, in two separate infusions: 0.56 mg/kg over 4 min, followed by 4 min of no dose and, if still negative, and additional 0.28 mg/kg over 2 min [11, 16, 17]. If no endpoint is reached, atropine (up to 1 mg) is added [18]. The same overall dose of 0.84 mg/kg can be given over 6 min [11, 19]. Aminophylline should be available for immediate use in case an adverse dipyridamole-related event occurs and routinely infused at the end of the test independent of the result [1, 11].

Adenosine

Adenosine is usually infused at a maximum dose of 140 µg/kg/min over 6 min [3, 20]. When side-effects are intolerable, down-titration of the dose is also possible.

Pacing

The presence of a permanent pacemaker can be exploited to conduct a pacing stress test in a totally non-invasive manner by externally programming the pacemaker to increasing frequencies. Pacing is started at 100 bpm and increased every 2 min by 10 bpm until the target heart rate or other standard endpoints are achieved [3, 21]. A limiting factor is, however, that several pacemakers cannot be programmed to the target heart rate.

Indications to stress echo

Indications for stress echocardiography can be grouped in very broad categories which can encompass the majority of patients (see Table 3) [11]:

(i) CAD diagnosis;
(ii) prognosis and risk stratification in patients with established diagnosis (e.g. after myocardial infarction);
(iii) preoperative risk assessment;
(iv) evaluation for cardiac aetiology of exertional dyspnoea;
(v) evaluation after revascularization;
(vi) ischaemia localization;

As a rule, the less informative the exercise ECG test is, the stricter the indication for stress echocardiography will be. Out of five patients, one is unable to exercise, one exercises submaximally, and one exercises maximally but the ECG is uninterpretable.

Table 3 Indications to stress echocardiography

Diagnosis of CAD in patients in whom exercise ECG is contraindicated, not feasible, uninterpretable, non-diagnostic or gives ambiguous results
Risk stratification in patients with established diagnosis
Pre-operative risk assessment (high-risk non emergent, poor exercise tolerance)
Evaluation after revascularization (not in the early post-procedure period, with change in symptoms)
Search for viability in patients with ischemic cardiomyopathy eligible for revascularization
Coronary artery disease of unclear significance at angiography or computed tomography

The three main specific indications for pharmacologic stress echocardiography can be summarized as follows:

(i) patients in whom the exercise stress test is contraindicated (e.g. patients with severe arterial hypertension);
(ii) patients in whom the exercise stress test is not feasible (e.g. those with intermittent claudication);
(iii) patients in whom the exercise stress test was nondiagnostic or yielded ambiguous results: inability to achieve the target heart rate response, presence of chest pain in the absence of significant electrocardiographic changes, and a concomitance of conditions lowering the reliability of the ECG marker of ischemia (female gender, arterial hypertension, repolarization abnormalities on ECG under resting conditions or after hyperventilation, and the need to continue drugs such as digitalis or anti-arrhythmic that potentially induce ST-segment and T wave changes). Tables 4 and 5 report the main reasons for test interruption.

2013 ESC guidelines on stable CAD have posed a new emphasis on the use of non-invasive imaging due to its significantly higher diagnostic accuracy [22]. However, the real impact of non-invasive imaging as a gate-keeper to coronary angiography need to to be tested on outcomes studies. The reported indications may change over time due to the evidence accumulating on survival impact. Exercise ECG remains a first-line in patients with interpretable ECG due to its simplicity, safety, availability, low cost, and high negative predictive value. Appropriateness criteria that may shed light on the use of stress echocardiography are derived from a balance between hard evidence, expert opinion, clinical experience and common sense.

Diagnostic accuracy

In a meta-analysis of 55 studies with 3,714 patients, exercise, dobutamine, dipyridamole, and adenosine echocardiography showed a sensitivity, respectively, of 83, 81, 72, and 79%, and a specificity of 84, 84, 95, and 91% [23]. In another meta-analysis of 5 studies adopting state of the art protocols for dipyridamole (fast or atropine-potentiated) and dobutamine (atropine-potentiated) test,

Table 4 Stress echocardiographic diagnostic criteria

Maximal dose or workload
Target heart rate
Echocardiographic Positivity (new or worsening of wall motion abnormality)
Chest Pain
ECG modification (ST Segment Shift > 2 mm)

Table 5 Submaximal non diagnostic criteria for test interruption

Intolerable symptoms
Hypertension: Systolic Blood Pressure >220 mmHg; Diastolic Blood Pressure > 120 mmHg
Hypotension (Absolute or Relative): Blood Pressure Fall > 30 mmHg
Supraventricular Arrhythmias: Tachycardia; Atrial Fibrillation
Ventricular Arrhythmias: Ventricular Tachycardia; Polymorphous PVCs

the two stresses had identical sensitivity (84%) and comparable specificity (92% vs 87%) [24]. When compared to standard exercise electrocardiography, stress echocardiography has a particularly impressive advantage in terms of specificity [25]. Compared to nuclear perfusion imaging, stress echocardiography at least has similar accuracy, with a moderate sensitivity gap that is more than balanced by a markedly higher specificity [23]. Familiarity with all forms of stress is an index of the quality of the echo lab. In this way, indications in the individual patient can be optimised, thereby avoiding the relative and absolute contraindications of each test. For instance, a patient with severe hypertension and/or a history of significant atrial or ventricular arrhythmias can more reasonably undergo to the dipyridamole stress test which, unlike dobutamine, has no arrhythmogenic or hypertensive effect. In contrast, a patient with severe conduction disturbances or advanced asthmatic disease should undergo the dobutamine stress test, since adenosine has a negative chronotropic and dromotropic effect, as well as a documented bronchoconstrictor activity. Patients either taking xanthine medication or under the effect of caffeine contained in drinks (tea, coffee, cola) should undergo the dobutamine test. Both dipyridamole and dobutamine have overall good tolerance and feasibility. The choice of one test over the other depends on patient characteristics, local drug cost and the physician's preference. It is important for all stress echocardiography laboratories to become familiar with all stresses to achieve a flexible and versatile diagnostic approach that enables the best stress to be tailored to individual patient needs. Antianginal medical therapy (in particular, beta-blocking agents) significantly affects the diagnostic accuracy of all forms of stress; therefore, it is recommended, whenever possible, to withhold medical therapy at the time of testing to avoid a false-negative result [11, 26].

Prognostic value

The presence (or absence) of inducible wall motion abnormalities separates patients with different prognoses. Information has been obtained from data banks of thousands of patients - also with multicentre design - for exercise [27–43], dobutamine [44–52], and dipyridamole [25, 47, 53–57]. A normal stress echocardiogram yields

an annual risk of 0.4–0.9% based on a total of >11000 patients [43], the same as for a normal stress myocardial perfusion scan (Fig. 1). Thus in patients with suspected CAD, a normal stress echocardiogram implies excellent prognosis and coronary angiography can safely be avoided. The positive and the negative response can be further stratified with interactions with clinical parameters (diabetes, renal dysfunction, and therapy at the time of test), resting echo (global LV function), and additive stress echo parameters (LV cavity dilatation, CFR, and previous revascularization). While the ischemic or necrotic pattern are associated with markedly increased risk of death or myocardial infarction, a normal test is predictive of a generally favorable outcome particularly in nondiabetic patients [58]. The ischemic response can be further stratified with additive stress echo parameters, such as the extent of inducible wall motion abnormalities and the workload/dose [47]. The higher the wall motion score index and the shorter the ischemia-free stress time are, the lower is the survival rate [47] (Fig. 2). As for the prognostic implication of the different pharmacological stress modalities, a similar prognostic value has been reported for dobutamine and dipyridamole testing [49]. Antiischemic therapy heavily modulates the prognostic impact of pharmacological stress echocardiography [59]. Inducible myocardial ischemia in patients on medical therapy identifies the subset of patients at highest risk of death. On the opposite end, the incidence of death in patients with a negative test off therapy is very low. At intermediate risk are those patients with a negative test on medical therapy or a positive test off medical therapy [59] (Fig. 3). The established prognostic stress echo parameters with their relative event rate are shown in Tables 6 and 7.

Stress echo in special subsets of patients
Hypertensive patients

In hypertensive patients CFR may be significantly reduced independent of the presence of significant CAD. CFR impairment reduces the diagnostic value of exercise electrocardiography and nuclear techniques in the

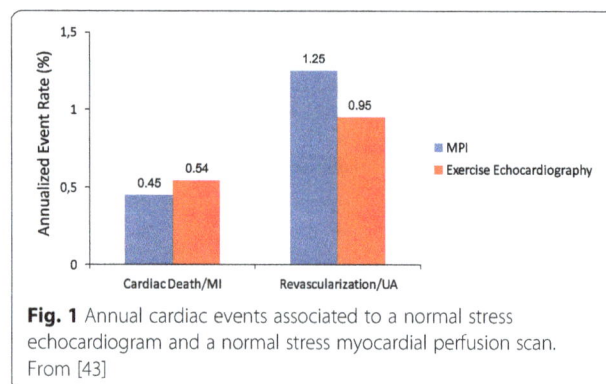

Fig. 1 Annual cardiac events associated to a normal stress echocardiogram and a normal stress myocardial perfusion scan. From [43]

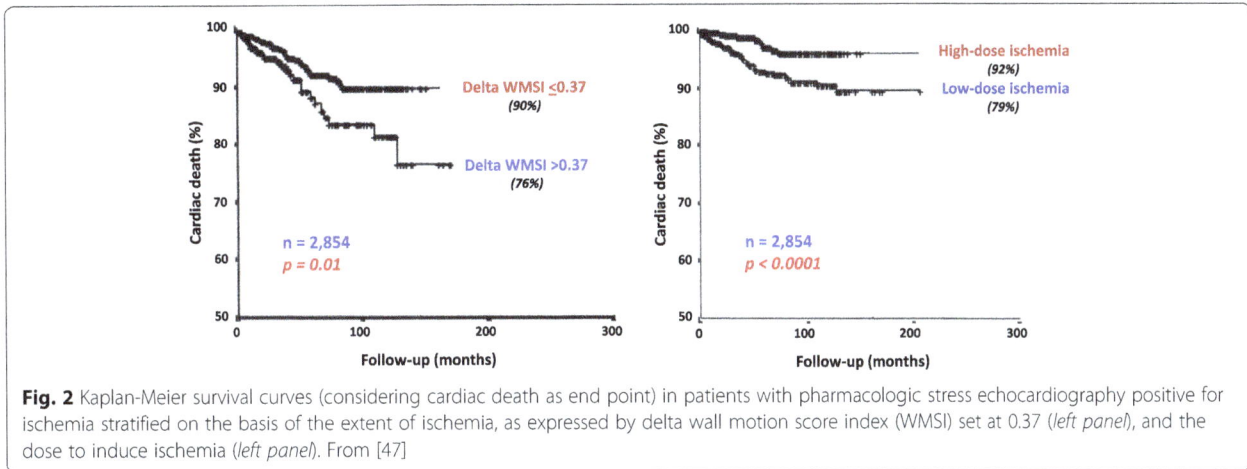

Fig. 2 Kaplan-Meier survival curves (considering cardiac death as end point) in patients with pharmacologic stress echocardiography positive for ischemia stratified on the basis of the extent of ischemia, as expressed by delta wall motion score index (WMSI) set at 0.37 (*left panel*), and the dose to induce ischemia (*left panel*). From [47]

hypertensive population, due to high rate of false-positive responses [10]. In hypertensive patients, stress echocardiography provides superior diagnostic specificity than exercise electrocardiography with no differences in sensitivity [60–62]. Moreover, dipyridamole stress echocardiography is most accurate than perfusion scintigraphy to assess coronary artery disease in patients with exercise electrocardiography positive for ischemia [63]. The prognostic assessment of hypertensive patients is of primary clinical importance since hypertension is associated with almost double risk of developing CAD [64]. Stress-induced wall motion abnormality during pharmacological testing is a strong multivariable predictor of future cardiac events in hypertensive patients with chest pain of unknown origin [65], including those with LV hypertrophy [66], and added prognostic information on top of clinical and exercise electrocardiography [67]. Moreover, the result of test is independently associated with cardiac death in an unselected cohort of hypertensive patients with known or suspected CAD [68].

However, mortality is predicted by inducible ischemia in exercise-tested patients and by the presence of any stress echocardiographic abnormality in those undergoing dobutamine challenge [69]. Inducible ischemia at inotropic stress is also associated with unfavourable outcome in the high-risk population of hypertensive patients unable to exercise [69]. Exercise-induced change in LV ejection fraction proved to be a multivariable predictor of mortality incremental to clinical findings, LV mass index, and resting LV function among hypertensive patients with LV hypertrophy [70]. Finally, echocardiographic LV wall motion abnormalities in adults without overt cardiovascular disease is associated with 2.4 to 3.4 fold higher risks of cardiovascular morbidity and mortality, independent of established risk factors [71]. It has been demonstrated in a large sample of 11.542 patients, that a normal study with any type of stressor is a marker of low risk; however in the hypertensive group the risk is higher [72]. Inducible ischemia at stress echocardiography is an independent predictor of hard cardiac events, and the level of risk is related to the extent of the inducible abnormality as expressed by peak wall motion score index [72] (Fig. 4).

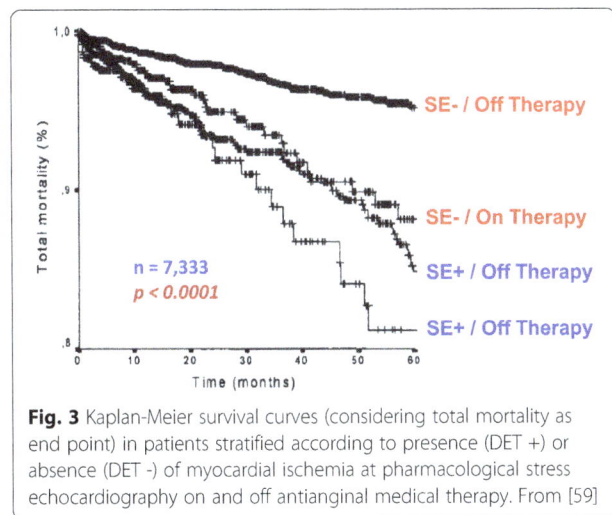

Fig. 3 Kaplan-Meier survival curves (considering total mortality as end point) in patients stratified according to presence (DET +) or absence (DET -) of myocardial ischemia at pharmacological stress echocardiography on and off antianginal medical therapy. From [59]

Table 6 Risk stratification for a positive test

1-year Risk (hard events)	Intermediate (1-3% year)	High (>10% year)
Dose/workload	High	Low
Resting EF	>50%	<40%
Anti-ischaemic therapy	Off	On
Coronary territory	LCx/RCA	LAD
Peak WMSI	Low	High
Recovery	Fast	Slow
Positivity or baseline dyssynergy	Homozonal	Heterozonal
CFR	>2.0	<2.0

Table 7 Risk stratification for a negative test

1-year Risk (hard events)	Very low (<0.5% year)	Low (1-3% year)
Stress	Maximal	Submaximal
Resting EF	>50%	<40%
Anti-ischaemic therapy	Off	On
CFR	>2.0	<2.0

Diabetic patients

Exercise electrocardiography is of limited value in diabetic patients because exercise capacity is often impaired by peripheral vascular disease, neuropathic disease, and obesity. In addition, test specificity on electrocardiographic criteria is less than ideal due to high prevalence of hypertension and microvascular disease. Stress echocardiography can play a key role in the optimal identification of high risk diabetic patients, also minimizing the economic and biologic costs of diagnostic screening [1]. The coexistence of epicardial coronary artery stenosis with microangiopathy can explain the low specificity of perfusion imaging compared to stress echocardiography in the detection of CAD in asymptomatic and symptomatic diabetic patients [73, 74]. In diabetic patients, stress echocardiography has shown a higher specificity than perfusion imaging but suffers from higher rate of false-positive results, possibly due to the coexistence of cardiomyopathy in many patients [75]. Risk stratification of diabetic patients is a major objective for the clinical cardiologist, given their increased risk for coronary artery disease [76]. Several studies have addressed the prognostic ability of stratification of non-invasive imaging in patients with and without diabetes. In particular, in patients with overt resting ischemic cardiomyopathy, the presence of myocardial viability recognized by dobutamine stress echocardiography independently predicted improved outcome following revascularization in nondiabetics as well as in diabetic patients following revascularization [77]. Also in unselected patient populations with proven or suspected CAD, a clear refinement of

prognosis can be obtained with stress echocardiography, first and foremost on the basis of classical wall motion abnormalities [58, 78–83], which place the patients in a high-risk subset for cardiovascular events. The incremental prognostic information provided by stress echocardiography is highest in patients with intermediate-to-high threshold positive exercise electrocardiography test results [84]. However, in diabetic patients – differently from nondiabetic subjects – a negative test result based solely on wall motion criteria is associated with less benign outcome [58] (Fig. 5). In a study on 2,349 diabetic patients investigated with dobutamine stress echocardiography, the mortality and cardiovascular morbidity were significantly higher in subjects with abnormal or ischemic test results [82]. Also, failure to achieve target heart rate and percentage of ischemic segments, an indicator of the extent of inducible ischemia, were independent predictors and incremental to clinical and rest echocardiographic variables for predicting adverse long-term outcomes [82]. In a more recent study assessing the long-term follow-up of stress echocardiography, dobutamine stress echocardiography provided restricted predictive value of adverse outcome in patients with diabetes who were unable to perform an adequate exercise stress test [83]. The Authors also identified a "warranty" period of the test which provided optimal risk stratification up to 7 years after initial testing. Repeated dobutamine stress echocardiography at that time might add to its prognostic value [83]. In a recent study enrolling a large sample of 14.000 diabetic and nondiabetic patients, stress echocardiography showed that a normal study with any type of stressor is a marker of low risk; however in the diabetic group the risk is higher [85] (Fig. 5). Inducible ischemia at stress echocardiography is an independent predictor of mortality, and the level of risk is related to the extent of the inducible abnormality as expressed by peak wall motion score index. However, the presence of rest wall motion abnormalities is an independent predictor of mortality in both patient groups [85]. Medical therapy at time of testing confers a higher risk of mortality in nondiabetics

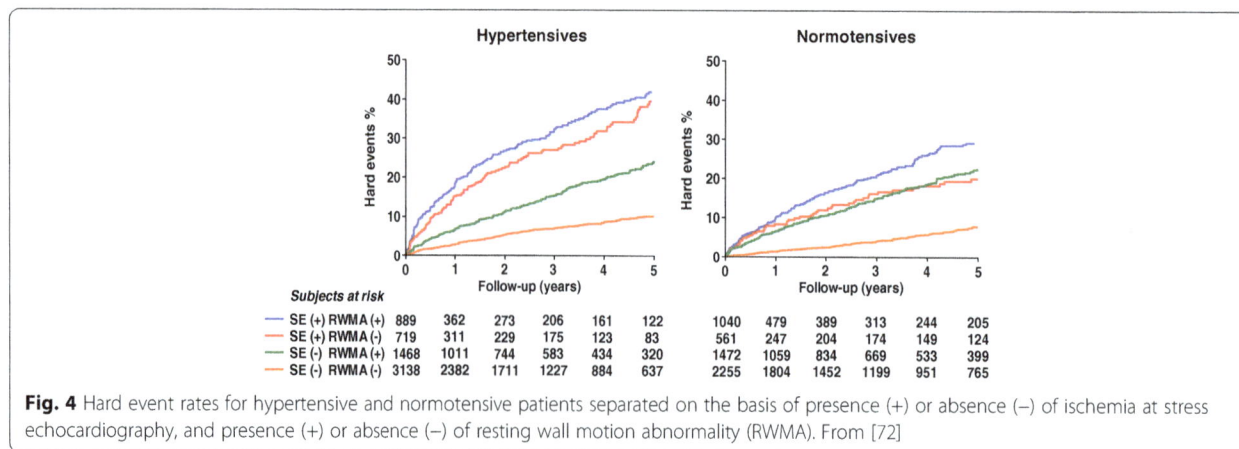

Fig. 4 Hard event rates for hypertensive and normotensive patients separated on the basis of presence (+) or absence (−) of ischemia at stress echocardiography, and presence (+) or absence (−) of resting wall motion abnormality (RWMA). From [72]

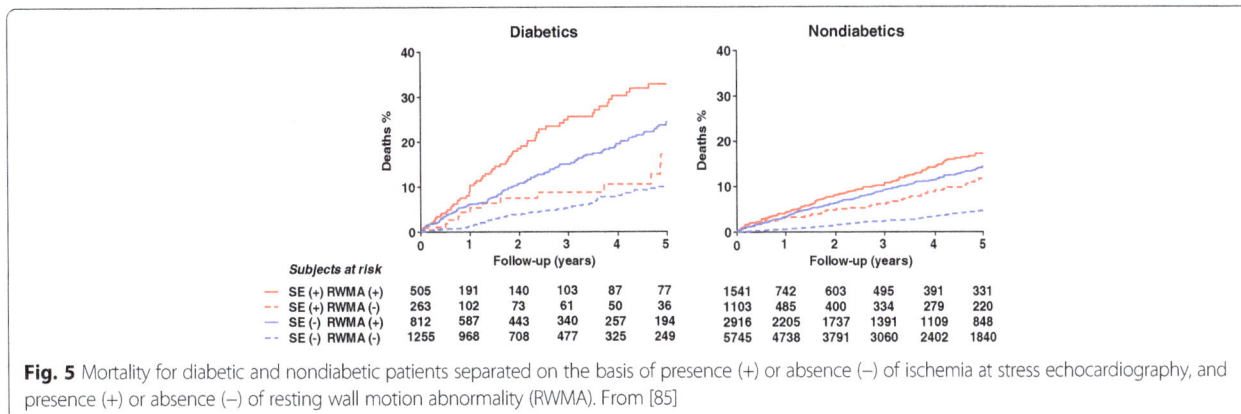

Fig. 5 Mortality for diabetic and nondiabetic patients separated on the basis of presence (+) or absence (−) of ischemia at stress echocardiography, and presence (+) or absence (−) of resting wall motion abnormality (RWMA). From [85]

but did not appear to impact on outcome in the diabetic group [85]. The lack of modulation of stress testing by medical therapy suggest that inducible ischemia is more severe in the diabetic population. Stress myocardial perfusion imaging can be considered a viable alternative to stress echocardiography with the limitation of being less available, more expensive and with potential long-term downstream detrimental effect due to ionizing radiations [86]. Stress myocardial perfusion imaging has been shown to have significant prognostic power for future cardiac events in the symptomatic diabetic population. In a large multicenter study enrolling 4,755 patients (20% diabetic patients) who underwent exercise of pharmacologic myocardial perfusion imaging for symptomatic CAD, abnormal stress myocardial perfusion imaging was found to be an independent predictor of cardiac events in both diabetic and nondiabetic sample [87]. Moreover, the number of abnormal segments (fixed or ischemic) was related to worse outcome [87] and this is consistent with the stress echocardiographic findings showing an ominous outcome for higher values of wall motion score index.

Women

The diagnostic specificity of exercise electrocardiography and myocardial perfusion scintigraphy is definitely lower in women than in men. Reduction of coronary flow reserve in syndrome X (mostly affecting female patients), hormonal influences for exercise testing, and breast attenuation for nuclear technique are potential explanations. In contrast, echocardiography combined with exercise or pharmacologic agents provides similar sensitivity but a better specificity as compared to exercise electrocardiography [88, 89] and perfusion scintigraphy [90]. In women the prognostic value of stress echocardiography is high, similar to that in men [91]. In patients with chest pain of unknown origin, a normal test is associated with <1% event-rate at 3 years of follow-up, while an ischemic test is a strong and independent predictor of future events [92]. Moreover, stress-induced ischemia adds prognostic information on top of clinical and

exercise electrocardiography data [93] (Fig. 6). In contrast to ECG stress test and perfusion imaging, stress echocardiography is an "equal opportunity" test, with no difference in diagnostic and prognostic accuracy between males and females. When exercise electrocardiography gives positive or ambiguous results, stress echocardiography is warranted [94]. The choice of an imaging test in this setting should take into account the radiologic burden. Recommendations from the European Society of Cardiology suggest to use non-ionising imaging techniques especially in highly vulnerable subjects such as younger women [87].

Left bundle branch block

The presence of left bundle branch block makes the electrocardiogram uninterpretable for ischemia and, therefore, a stress imaging is necessary. The abnormal sequence of LV activation determines increased diastolic extravascular resistance, with lower and slower diastolic coronary flow, accounting for the stress-induced defect often observed by perfusion imaging in patients with normal coronary arteries [95]. In spite of the difficulty posed by abnormal wall motion, stress echocardiography is the

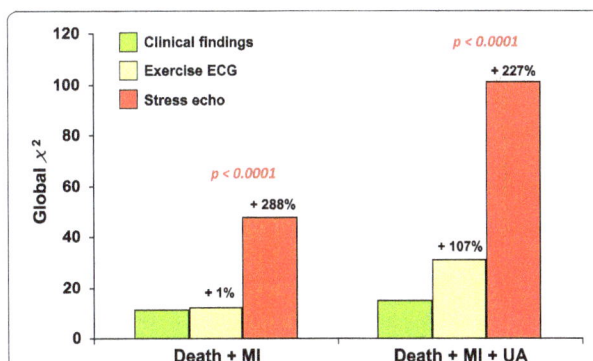

Fig. 6 Incremental prognostic value of pharmacological stress echocardiography to clinical and exercise electrocardiography data, as determined by the comparison of the global chi-square at each step. From [93]

best diagnostic option in patients with left bundle branch block. It is more specific than perfusion imaging [95], and its sensitivity is good, albeit reduced in the left anterior descending territory in the presence of a dyskinetic septum in resting conditions [96]. Moreover, myocardial ischemia by pharmacologic stress echocardiography has a strong and independent power in the prediction of future hard events in left bundle branch block patients, providing a prognostic contribution that is incremental to that of clinical and resting echo findings in the group without previous myocardial infarction [97].

Noncardiac vascular surgery

Perioperative ischemia is a frequent event in patients undergoing major noncardiac vascular or general surgery and coronary disease is known to be the leading cause of perioperative mortality and morbidity following vascular and general surgery [98, 99]. The diagnostic/therapeutic corollary of these considerations is that CAD – and therefore the perioperative risk – in these patients has to be identified in an effective way preoperatively. This is not feasible in an accurate way with either clinical scores (such as Detsky's or Goldman's score) or rest echocardiography, only. The updated ESC guidelines recommend an imaging stress testing before high-risk surgery in patients with more than two clinical risk factors and poor functional capacity (Class I, Evidence C) [98]. Pharmacological stress echocardiography has been proven to be an effective tool for risk stratification when compared to perfusion scintigraphy [100–112]. Its advantages are due to lower costs and the lack of ionising radiations and in this particular setting it is more feasible than exercise stress echo. The experience with either dipyridamole and dobutamine indicates that these tests have a very high and comparable negative predictive value (between 90 and 100%) [113]. A negative test result is associated with a very low incidence of cardiac events allowing a safe surgical procedure [113–115]. The positive predictive value is relatively low (between 25 and 45%): this means that the post-surgical probability of events is low. Stress echocardiography shows a comparable diagnostic and prognostic accuracy when compared to perfusion imaging. The risk stratification capability is high for perioperative events and also remains excellent for long-term follow-up [116, 117]. Other techniques such as CMR and CCTA are available but the evidence is too scant to be recommended. Moreover, costs and risks should be weighed in the model of stratification and high tech imaging techniques do not seem to be adequate for a large scale assessment. Stress testing should be used in the diagnostic algorithm only when its result might influence peri-operative management and outcome. To date, it appears reasonable to perform coronary revascularization before peripheral vascular surgery in the presence of a markedly positive result of stress echocardiography in which standard medical therapy appears insufficient to prevent a peri-operative cardiac event. A more conservative approach – with watchful cardiological surveillance coupled with pharmacological cardioprotection with β-blockers – can be adopted in patients with less severe ischemic responses during stress [99]. Concerns have been raised on the initiation of betablockers before surgery without titration (to avoid hypotension and bradychardia) and in low risk patients [118]. Interestingly, clearly inappropriate indications for preoperative risk stratification before noncardiac surgery (intermediate risk surgery in patients with good exercise capacity, and low risk surgery) account for 25% of all inappropriate testing in large-volume stress echocardiography laboratories [119–122], and therefore this field provides a key opportunity for quality improvement and targeted educational programs to achieve measurable improvements in results.

Myocardial viability

The stress echo sign of myocardial viability is a stress-induced improvement of function during low levels of stress in a region that is abnormal at rest. By far, the widest experience is available with low-dose dobutamine stress echocardiography [123–125] the preferred stressor for assessing myocardial viability. However, it is also possible to assess the presence of myocardial viability using low-dose dipyridamole [126–128] or low-level exercise [129] or enoximone [130, 131].

In patients with dysfunctional but viable myocardium, regional function can be improved by the inotropic effect of low-dose (5–10 µg/kg/min.) dobutamine stress echocardiography [11]. Sensitivity and specificity of low-dose dobutamine test are, respectively, 86 and 90% for predicting spontaneous functional recovery after an acute myocardial infarction (stunning) [123], and 84 and 81% for predicting functional recovery following revascularization in patients with chronic CAD (hibernation) [124]. Compared to nuclear techniques, dobutamine stress echocardiography has lower sensitivity, but higher specificity, with similar overall accuracy regarding recovery of function [124, 125]. In quantitative terms, contractile reserve evidenced by a positive dobutamine requires at least 50% viable myocytes in a given segment, whereas scintigraphic methods also identify segments with less viable myocytes [132]. Minor levels of viability, characterized by scintigraphic positivity and dobutamine echocardiography negativity, are often unable to translate into functional recovery. This explains the different diagnostic performance of the two methods.

Observational studies have indeed suggested that patients with ischaemic LV dysfunction and a significant amount of viable myocardium (at least five segments or a wall motion score index >0.25) [133–142] have lower perioperative mortality, greater improvements in regional and global LV function, fewer heart failure symptoms, and improved long-term survival after revascularization than patients with large areas of non-viable myocardium. On the other hand, viability has no impact on survival in patients with preserved or just moderately depressed LV function; in this case, it can rather predict the occurrence of acute coronary events, representing a substrate for unstable ischemic episodes [50].

Viability at dobutamine stress echocardiography predicts an improved outcome following revascularization both in diabetic and nondiabetic patients with ischemic cardiomyopathy [77]. No measurable performance difference for predicting revascularization benefit between stress echocardiography and nuclear methods has been reported [141]. The documentation of viable myocardium at dobutamine test also predicts responders to resynchronization therapy: patients with contractile reserve show a favourable clinical and reverse LV remodelling response to resynchronization therapy [143, 144].

Coronary flow reserve

In recent years the evaluation of CFR by combining transthoracic Doppler assessment of coronary flow velocities with vasodilator stress has entered the echo lab as an effective modality for both diagnostic and prognostic purposes [1]. The use of CFR as a stand-alone diagnostic criterion suffers from two main limitations. In fact, only left anterior descending artery is sampled with very high success rate. Moreover, CFR cannot distinguish between microvascular and macrovascular coronary disease [1]. Therefore it is much more interesting to assess the additional diagnostic value over conventional wall motion analysis. CFR of left anterior descending artery is a strong and independent indicator of mortality, conferring additional prognostic value over wall motion analysis in patients with known or suspected CAD [145] (Fig. 7). A negative result on stress echocardiography with a normal CFR confers an annual risk of death <1% [145] (Fig. 7). Moreover, CFR yields useful prognostic information in several clinical subsets, such as diabetics with unchanged wall motion during stress [146] (Fig. 8), hypertensives [147], patients with intermediate coronary stenosis [148], left bundle branch block [149], and normal or near normal coronary arteries [147, 149–151] (Fig. 9). A CFR <2.0 is an additional parameter of ischemia severity in the risk stratification of the stress echocardiographic response whereas patients with a negative test for wall motion criteria and CFR >2.0 during dipyridamole stress echocardiography have a favorable outcome. Similar results have been obtained when perfusion imaging was added to wall motion analysis [152] (Fig. 10). In diabetic patients, a normal CFR is associated with tighter glycemic control [153] and better

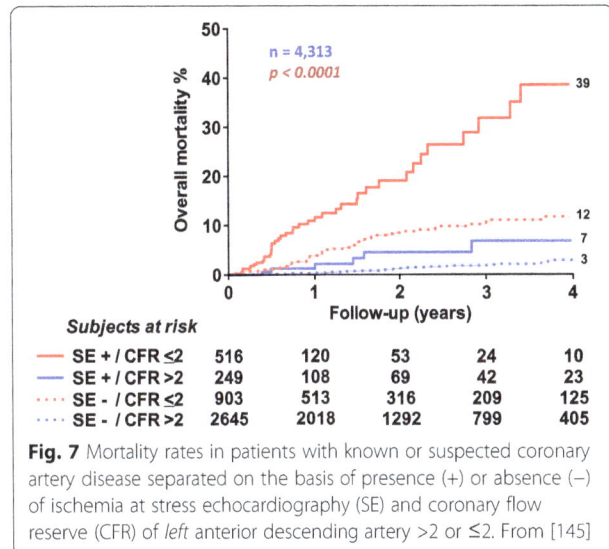

Fig. 7 Mortality rates in patients with known or suspected coronary artery disease separated on the basis of presence (+) or absence (−) of ischemia at stress echocardiography (SE) and coronary flow reserve (CFR) of *left* anterior descending artery >2 or ≤2. From [145]

Subjects at risk					
SE + / CFR ≤2	516	120	53	24	10
SE + / CFR >2	249	108	69	42	23
SE − / CFR ≤2	903	513	316	209	125
SE − / CFR >2	2645	2018	1292	799	405

long-term event-free survival both considering unselected patients [146, 154] and patients with angiographically normal coronary arteries [151] (Fig. 9). Within the subset of chest pain hypertensive patients with normal coronary arteries an effective risk stratification has been obtained according to quartiles of CFR [147] (Fig. 9). Anti-ischemic medication at the time of testing does not modulate the prognostic value of CFR, which is per se a prognostic marker independent of therapy [155] (Fig. 11). Specialist guidelines endorse an extensive application of CFR in the stress echo lab, suggesting that "whenever possible, it is recommended to perform dual imaging (flow and function) vasodilator stress echo [11].

The shift from qualitative to quantitative reading

The search for a totally operator-independent quantitative tool for stress echocardiography is still on-going. The state-of-the art diagnosis of ischaemia in stress echocardiography remains the eyeballing interpretation of regional wall motion in black and white cine-loops. Several ultrasound technologies have been proposed in the last few years in order to overcome the qualitative interpretation of stress echocardiography: tissue characterization, Tissue Doppler imaging, strain rate and speckle tracking. However, none of these technologies has a place in the routine clinical practice of stress echo. EACVI/ASE Guidelines do not recommend its rotine clinical use unless some major limitations and pitfalls are solved [156]: "While the published research provides the evidence basis for potential clinical applications of these techniques in multiple clinical scenarios, the writing group believes that in the majority of areas, this methodology is not yet ready for routine clinical use. The consensus is that: (1) additional testing is needed in multicenter settings to better establish the diagnostic accuracy of the

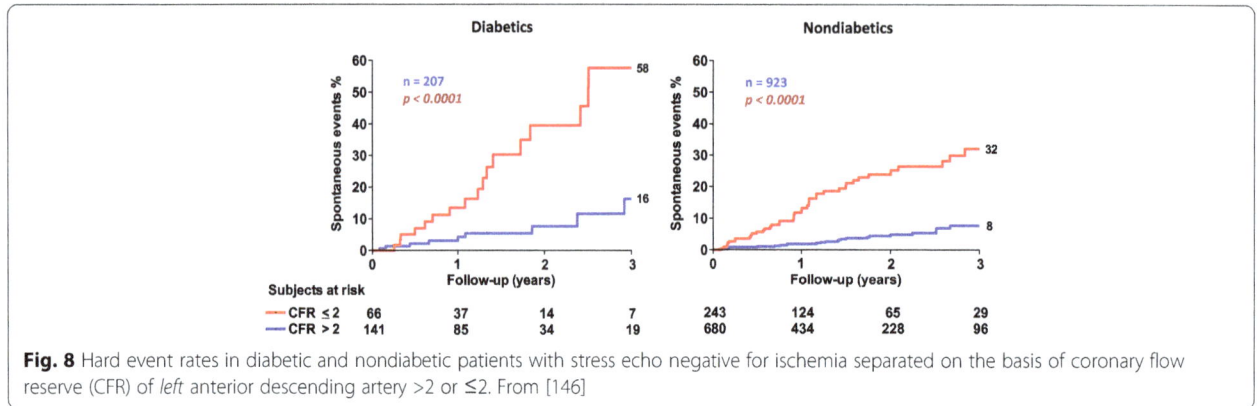

Fig. 8 Hard event rates in diabetic and nondiabetic patients with stress echo negative for ischemia separated on the basis of coronary flow reserve (CFR) of *left* anterior descending artery >2 or ≤2. From [146]

different parameters and their reproducibility in various disease states, (2) standardization is needed for what should be measured and how measurements should be performed, and (3) standardization among manufacturers is essential, as clinicians should be able to interpret data generated by different equipment irrespective of vendor". It is conceivable that once the inter-vendor comparability is solved, speckle tracking would play a relevant role in determining forms of subtle LV dysfunction and minor degrees of subendocardial ischemia, otherwise non detectable with wall motion analysis. Real-time three

dimensional echocardiography has also proven to be accurate and reproducible, but it remains time consuming and frame rates are too low for stress echocardiography [1]. The EACVI/ASE consensus document states that 3D stress transthoracic echocardiography holds promise for incorporation into clinical practice in the future [157]. Its advantages are: 1. Better visualization of the LV apex, which is frequently foreshortened on standard 2D apical images; 2. Rapid acquisition of peak stress images before the heart declines in recovery; and 3. Evaluation of multiple segments from different planes from a single data set.

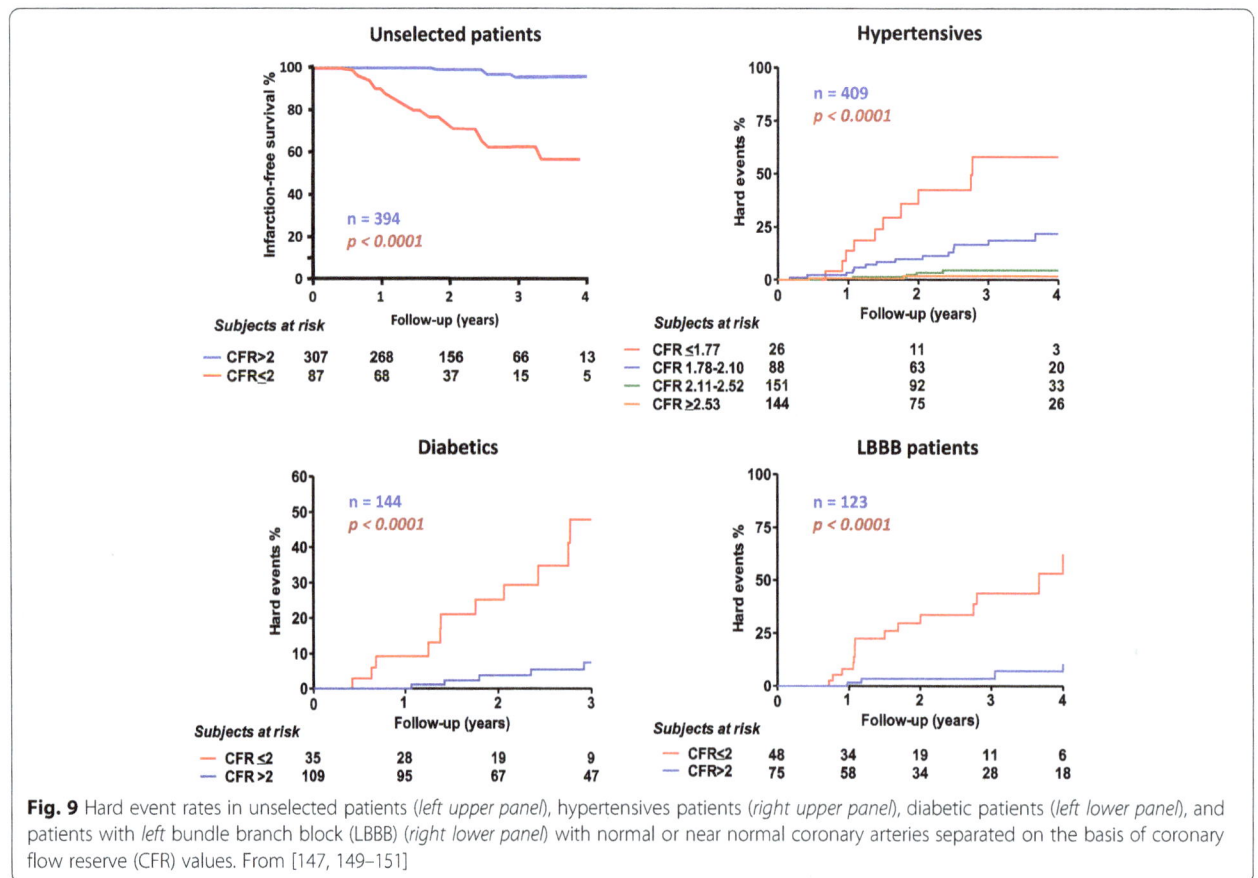

Fig. 9 Hard event rates in unselected patients (*left upper panel*), hypertensives patients (*right upper panel*), diabetic patients (*left lower panel*), and patients with *left* bundle branch block (LBBB) (*right lower panel*) with normal or near normal coronary arteries separated on the basis of coronary flow reserve (CFR) values. From [147, 149–151]

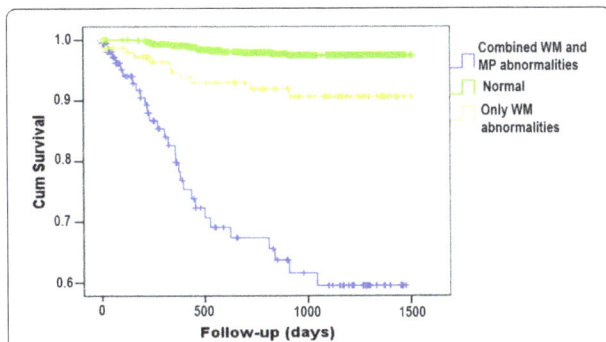

Fig. 10 Kaplan-Meier curves based on the combination of presence or absence of wall motion (WM) abnormalities and myocardial perfusion (MP) abnormalities. From [152]

Disadvantages include lower spatial resolution and lower frame rates [157].

Myocardial contrast echocardiography (MCE) has undergone rapid development in the past 5 years. With the advent of newer-generation microbubbles, intravenous agents can now be used to both improve endocardial border delineation and, detect myocardial perfusion. Along with the development of microbubbles which consistently opacify the left heart from a venous injection, newer imaging modalities have evolved which permit the detection of myocardial perfusion abnormalities in real time, at frame rates which are greater than 25Hz. In order to accurately detect wall motion abnormalities during stress echocardiography, a clear definition of endocardial borders is of particularly importance. The approved indication for the use of contrast echocardiography currently lies in improving endocardial border delineation in patients in whom adequate imaging is difficult or suboptimal [158].

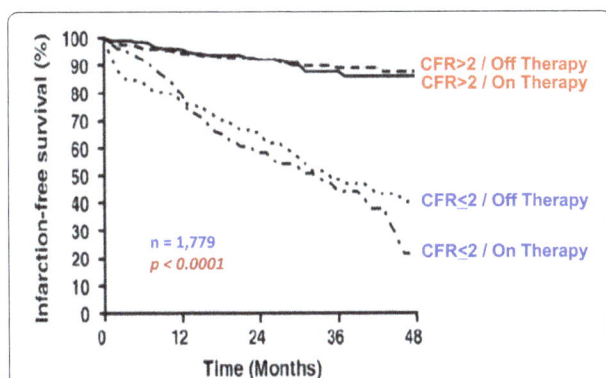

Fig. 11 Kaplan-Meier survival curves (considering hard events as end point) in patients stratified on the basis of coronary flow reserve (CFR) of *left* anterior descending artery >2 or ≤2 on and off antianginal medical therapy. From [155]

Safety of pharmacologic stress echocardiography

Stress echocardiography is a safe technique but minor, limiting, side effects may preclude the achievement of maximal testing. Safety profile of stress echocardiography depends on the stressor used. Exercise is the safest stressor as shown in large samples with the long – lasting experience of ECG stress test [159]. Stress echo registries collecting data on thousands of patients [160–163] have shown that exercise is the safest test. Death has an incidence rate of 1 in 10,000 tests. Major life-threatening effects (myocardial infarction, ventricular fibrillation, sustained ventricular tachycardia, stroke) occur in about 1 in 6000 patients with exercise in the international stress echocardiography registry – fivefold less than with dipyridamole echocardiography and tenfold less than with dobutamine echocardiography. Exercise, whenever feasible, should be the preferred stressor due to its safety profile. Exercise is safer than pharmacological stress echocardiography and dipyridamole is safer than dobutamine . Not all stress tests carry the same risk of major adverse reactions and the choice of one test over the other should take into account the safety profile.

Conclusions

Stress echocardiography is an established technique for the assessment of known or suspected CAD. It is recommended in all major cardiology guidelines in several clinical settings. However, its status of established technology, should prompt its clinical use as the preferred non-invasive imaging technique due to its low cost, wide availability and lack of radiation exposure. Though these unique features, an utilization gap remains with nuclear techniques percevied as more objective in the face of a comparable diagnostic and prognostic accuracy. The flexible use of stressors (exercise, inotropic and vasodilating) maximazes the feasibility, avoids specific contra-indications and allows tailoring the exam on each individual patient. A paradigm shift will occur when from a highly expertise qualitative reading stress echocardiography will move to a quantitative approach that would make it easier also for less skilled readers. Technological premises are there at hand but they have not reached a fullblown status to be used on a routine clinical basis. Society recommendantions and guidelines are mostly based on consensus and level of evidence C. The gap of knowledge should be filled with prospective large scale studies to support evidence-based treatment strategies. Eugenio Picano and Patricia Pellikka, two pioneers of the technique invite the scientific community to design "prospective large scale and (when possible) randomised (medical vs. interventional treatment) outcome studies to support more evidence-based rather than consensus-based strategies, based on stress echo results, in CAD and non-CAD patients" [164].

Abbreviations

ASE: American Society of Echocardiography; CAD: Coronary artery disease; CFR: Coronary flow reserve; EACVI: European Association of Cardiovascular Imaging; ESC: European Society of Cardiology; LV: Left ventricle

Funding

No funding was needed to conduct the study.

Authors' contribution

RS Drafted the manuscript, reviewed literature; LC contributed with relevant criticism to the final draft of the manuscript. Both authors read and approved the final manuscript.

Competing interests

RS is the Editor-in-Chief of Cardiovascular but the manuscript was independently handled by an Associate Editor.

Author details

[1]CNR, Institute of Clinical Physiology, Via G. Moruzzi, 1, 56124 Pisa, Italy.
[2]Department of Cardiology, San Luca Hospital, Lucca, Italy.

References

1. Picano E. Stress echocardiography. 6th ed. Heidelberg: Springer Verlag; 2015.
2. Picano E. Dipyridamole-echocardiography test: historical background and physiologic basis. Eur Heart J. 1989;10:365–76.
3. Ross Jr J. Mechanisms of regional ischaemia and antianginal drug action during exercise. Prog Cardiovasc Dis. 1989;31:455–66.
4. Gallagher KP, Matsuzaki M, Koziol JA, Kemper WS, Ross Jr J. Regional myocardial perfusion and wall thickening during ischaemia in conscious dogs. Am J Physiol. 1984;247:H727–738.
5. Picano E, Lattanzi F, Masini M, Distante A, L'Abbate A. Usefulness of a high-dose dipyridamole-echocardiography test for diagnosis of syndrome X. Am J Cardiol. 1987;60:508–12.
6. Kaski JC, Rosano GM, Collins P, Nihoyannopoulos P, Maseri A, Poole-Wilson PA. Cardiac syndrome X: clinical characteristics and left ventricular function. Long-term follow-up study. J Am Coll Cardiol. 1995;25:807–14.
7. Palinkas A, Toth E, Amyot R, Rigo F, Venneri L, Picano E. The value of ECG and echocardiography during stress testing for identifying systemic endothelial dysfunction and epicardial artery stenosis. Eur Heart J. 2002;23:1587–95.
8. Camici PG, Gistri R, Lorenzoni R, Sorace O, Michelassi C, Bongiorni MG, Salvadori PA, L'Abbate A. Coronary reserve and exercise ECG in patients with chest pain and normal coronary angiograms. Circulation. 1992;86:179–86.
9. Nihoyannopoulos P, Kaski J-C, Crake T, Maseri A. Absence of myocardial dysfunction during stress in patients with syndrome X. J Am Coll Cardiol. 1991;18:1463–70.
10. Picano E, Palinkas A, Amyot R. Diagnosis of myocardial ischaemia in hypertensive patients. J Hypertens. 2001;19:1177–83.
11. Sicari R, Nihoyannopoulos P, Evangelista A, Kasprzak J, Lancellotti P, Poldermans D, Voigt J, Zamorano JL. Stress echocardiography expert consensus statement. Eur J Echocardiogr. 2008;9:415–37.
12. Peteiro J, Bouzas-Mosquera A, Estevez R, Pazos P, Piñeiro M, Castro-Beiras A. Head-to-head comparison of peak supine bicycle exercise echocardiography and treadmill exercise echocardiography at peak and at post-exercise for thedetection of coronary artery disease. J Am Soc Echocardiogr. 2012;25:319–26.
13. Piérard LA. Echocardiographic monitoring throughout exercise better than the post-treadmill approach? J Am Coll Cardiol. 2007;50:1864–6.
14. Berthe C, Pierard LA, Hiernaux M, Trotteur G, Lempereur P, Carlier J, Kulbertus HE. Predicting the extent and location of coronary artery disease in acute myocardial infarction by echocardiography during dobutamine infusion. Am J Cardiol. 1986;58:1167–72.
15. McNeill AJ, Fioretti PM, El-Said SM, Salustri A, Forster T, Roelandt JR. Enhanced sensitivity for detection of coronary artery disease by addition of atropine to dobutamine stress echocardiography. Am J Cardiol. 1992;70:41–6.
16. Picano E, Simonetti I, Masini M, Marzilli M, Lattanzi F, Distante A, De Nes M, L'Abbate A. Transient myocardial dysfunction during pharmacologic vasodilation as an index of reduced coronary reserve: a coronary hemodynamic and echocardiographic study. J Am Coll Cardiol. 1986;8(1):84–90.
17. Picano E, Lattanzi F, Masini M, Distante A, L'Abbate A. High dose dipyridamoleechocardiography test in effort angina pectoris. J Am Coll Cardiol. 1986;8:848–54.
18. Picano E, Pingitore A, Conti U, Kozàkovà M, Boem A, Cabani E, Ciuti M, Distante A, L'Abbate A. Enhanced sensitivity for detection of coronary artery disease by addition of atropine to dipyridamole echocardiography. Eur Heart J. 1993;14:1216–22.
19. Dal Porto R, Faletra F, Picano E, Pirelli S, Moreo A, Varga A. Safety, feasibility, and diagnostic accuracy of accelerated high-dose dipyridamole stress echocardiography. Am J Cardiol. 2001;87:520–4.
20. Zoghbi WA, Cheirif J, Kleiman NS, Verani MS, Trakhtenbroit A. Diagnosis ofischemic heart disease with adenosine echocardiography. J Am Coll Cardiol. 1991;18:1271–9.
21. Picano E, Alaimo A, Chubuchny V, Plonska E, Baldo V, Baldini U, Pauletti M, Perticucci R, Fonseca L, Villarraga HR, Emanuelli C, Miracapillo G, Hoffmann E, De Nes M. Noninvasive pacemaker stress echocardiography for diagnosis of coronary artery disease: a multicenter study. J Am Coll Cardiol. 2002;40: 1305–10.
22. Task Force Members, Montalescot G, Sechtem U, Achenbach S, Andreotti F, Arden C, Budaj A, Bugiardini R, Crea F, Cuisset T, Di Mario C, Ferreira JR, Gersh BJ, Gitt AK, Hulot JS, Marx N, Opie LH, Pfisterer M, Prescott E, Ruschitzka F, Sabaté M, Senior R, Taggart DP, van der Wall EE, Vrints CJ, ESC Committee for Practice Guidelines, Zamorano JL, Achenbach S, Baumgartner H, Bax JJ, Bueno H, Dean V, Deaton C, Erol C, Fagard R, Ferrari R, Hasdai D, Hoes AW, Kirchhof P, Knuuti J, Kolh P, Lancellotti P, Linhart A, Nihoyannopoulos P, Piepoli MF, Ponikowski P, Sirnes PA, Tamargo JL, Tendera M, Torbicki A, Wijns W, Windecker S, Document R, Knuuti J, Valgimigli M, Bueno H, Claeys MJ, Donner-Banzhoff N, Erol C, Frank H, Funck-Brentano C, Gaemperli O, Gonzalez-Juanatey JR, Hamilos M, Hasdai D, Husted S, James SK, Kervinen K, Kolh P, Kristensen SD, Lancellotti P, Maggioni AP, Piepoli MF, Pries AR, Romeo F, Rydén L, Simoons ML, Sirnes PA, Steg PG, Timmis A, Wijns W, Windecker S, Yildirir A, Zamorano JL. 2013 ESC guidelines on the management of stable coronary artery disease: the Task Force on the management of stable coronary artery disease of the European Society of Cardiology. Eur Heart J. 2013;34:2949–3003.
23. Heijenbrok-Kal MH, Fleischmann KE, Hunink MG. Stress echocardiography, stress single-photon-emission computed tomography and electron beam computed tomography for the assessment of coronary artery disease: a meta-analysis of diagnostic performance. Am Heart J. 2007;154:415–23.
24. Picano E, Molinaro S, Pasanisi E. The diagnostic accuracy of pharmacological stress echocardiography for the assessment of coronary artery disease: a meta-analysis. Cardiovasc Ultrasound. 2008;6:30.
25. Severi S, Picano E, Michelassi C, Lattanzi F, Landi P, Distante A, L'Abbate A. Diagnostic and prognostic value of dipyridamole echocardiography in patients with suspected coronary artery disease. Comparison with exercise electrocardiography. Circulation. 1994;89:1160–73.
26. Lattanzi F, Picano E, Bolognese L, Piccinino C, Sarasso G, Orlandini A, L'Abbate A. Inhibition of dipyridamole-induced ischemia by antianginal therapy in humans. Correlation with exercise electrocardiography. Circulation. 1991;83:1256–62.
27. Sawada SG, Ryan T, Conley M, Corya BC, Feigenbaum H, Armstrong W. Prognostic value of a normal exercise echocardiogram. Am Heart J. 1990;120:49–55.
28. Elhendy A, Shub C, McCully RB, Mahoney DW, Burger KN, Pellikka PA. Exercise echocardiography for the prognostic stratification of patients with low pretest probability of coronary artery disease. Am J Med. 2001;111:18–23.

29. Marwick TH, Case C, Vasey C, Allen S, Short L, Thomas JD. Prediction of mortality by exercise echocardiography: a strategy for combination with the duke treadmill score. Circulation. 2001;103:2566–71.

30. Arruda-Olson AM, Juracan EM, Mahoney DW, McCully RB, Roger VL, Pellikka PA. Prognostic value of exercise echocardiography in 5,798 patients: is there a gender difference? J Am Coll Cardiol. 2002;39:625–31.

31. McCully RB, Roger VL, Mahoney DW, Burger KN, Click RL, Seward JB, et al. Outcome after abnormal exercise echocardiography for patients with good exercise capacity: prognostic importance of the extent and severity of exercise-related left ventricular dysfunction. J Am Coll Cardiol. 2002;39:1345–52.

32. Jaarsma W, Visser C, Funke KA. Usefulness of two-dimensional exercise echocardiography shortly after myocardial infarction. Am J Cardiol. 1986;57:86–90.

33. Applegate RJ, Dell'italia LJ, Crawford MH. Usefulness of twodimensional echocardiography during low-level exercise testing early after uncomplicated myocardial infarction. Am J Cardiol. 1987;60:10–4.

34. Ryan T, Armstrong WF, O'Donnel JA, Feigenbaum H. Risk stratification following acute myocardial infarction during exercise two-dimensional echocardiography. Am Heart J. 1987;114:1305–16.

35. Quintana M, Lindvall K, Ryden L, Brolund F. Prognostic value of predischarge exercise stress echocardiography after acute myocardial infarction. Am J Cardiol. 1995;76:1115–21.

36. Hoque A, Maaieh M, Longaker RA, Stoddard MF. Exercise echocardiography and thallium-201 single-photon emission computed tomography stress test for 5- and 10-year prognosis of mortality and specific cardiac events. J Am Soc Echocardiogr. 2002;15:1326–34.

37. Elhendy A, Mahoney DW, Khandheria BK, Paterick TE, Burger KN, Pellikka PA. Prognostic significance of wall motion abnormalities during exercise echocardiography. J Am Coll Cardiol. 2002;40:1623–9.

38. Mazur W, Rivera JM, Khoury AF, Basu AG, Perez-Verdia A, Marks GF, Chang SM, Olmos L, Quiñones MA, Zoghbi WA. Prognostic value of exercise echocardiography: validation of a new risk index combining echocardiographic, treadmill, and exercise electrocardiographic parameters. J Am Soc Echocardiogr. 2003;16:318–25.

39. Marwick TH, Case C, Short L, Thomas JD. Prediction of mortality in patients without angina: use of an exercise score and exercise echocardiography. Eur Heart J. 2003;24:1223–30.

40. Peteiro J, Monserrat L, Vazquez E, Perez R, Garrido I, Vazquez N, Castro-Beiras A. Comparison of exercise echocardiography to exercise electrocardiographic testing added to echocardiography at rest for risk stratification after uncomplicated acute myocardial infarction. Am J Cardiol. 2003;92:373–6.

41. Elhendy A, Mahoney DW, Burger KN, McCully RB, Pellikka PA. Prognostic value of exercise echocardiography in patients with classic angina pectoris. Am J Cardiol. 2004;94:559–63.

42. Garrido IP, Peteiro J, García-Lara J, Montserrat L, Aldama G, Vázquez-Rodríguez JM, Alvarez N, Castro-Beiras A. Prognostic value of exercise echocardiography in patients with diabetes mellitus and known or suspected coronary artery disease. Am J Cardiol. 2005;96:9–12.

43. Metz LD, Beattie M, Hom R, Redberg RF, Grady D, Fleischmann KE. The prognostic value of normal exercise myocardial perfusion imaging and exercise echocardiography: a meta-analysis. J Am Coll Cardiol. 2007;49:227–37.

44. Mazeika PK, Nadazdin A, Oakley CM. Prognostic value of dobutamine echocardiography in patients with high pretest likelihood of coronary artery disease. Am J Cardiol. 1993;71:33–9.

45. Poldermans D, Fioretti PM, Boersma E, Cornel JH, Borst F, Vermeulen EG, Arnese M, el-Hendy A, Roelandt JR. Dobutamine–atropine stress echocardiography and clinical data for predicting late cardiac events in patients with suspected coronary artery disease. Am J Med. 1994;97:119–25.

46. Marwick TH, Case C, Sawada S, Rimmerman C, Brenneman P, Kovacs R, Short L, Lauer M. Prediction of mortality using dobutamine echocardiography. J Am Coll Cardiol. 2001;37:754–60.

47. Sicari R, Pasanisi E, Venneri L, Landi P, Cortigiani L, Picano E, Echo Persantine International Cooperative (EPIC) Study Group; Echo Dobutamine International Cooperative (EDIC) Study Group. Stress echo results predict mortality: a large scale multicenter prospective international study. J Am Coll Cardiol. 2003;41:589–5895.

48. Carlos ME, Smart SC, Wynsen JC, Sagar KB. Dobutamine stress echocardiography for risk stratication after myocardial infarction. Circulation. 1997;18:1402–10.

49. Pingitore A, Picano E, Varga A, Gigli G, Cortigiani L, Previtali M, Minardi G, Quarta Colosso M, Lowenstein J, Mathias Jr W, Landi P. Prognostic value of pharmacological stress echocardiography in patients with known or suspected coronary artery disease: a prospective, large scale, multicenter, head-to-head comparison between dipyridamole and dobutamine test. J Am Coll Cardiol. 1999;34:1769–77.

50. Sicari R, Picano E, Landi P, Pingitore A, Bigi R, Coletta C, Heyman J, Casazza F, Previtali M, Mathias Jr W, Dodi C, Minardi G, Lowenstein J, Garyfallidis X, Cortigiani L, Morales MA, Raciti M. Prognostic value of dobutamine-atropine stress echocardiography early after acute myocardial infarction. Echo Dobutamine International Cooperative (EDIC) Study. J Am Coll Cardiol. 1997;29:254–60.

51. Poldermans D, Fioretti PM, Boersma E, Bax JJ, Thomson IR, Roelandt JR, Simoons ML. Long-term prognostic value of dobutamine-atropine stress echocardiography in 1737 patients with known or suspected coronary artery disease: a single-center experience. Circulation. 1999;99:757–562.

52. Previtali M, Fetiveau R, Lanzarini L, Cavalotti C, Klersy C. Prognostic value of myocardial viability and ischemia detected by dobutamine stress echocardiography early after acute myocardial infarction treated with thrombolysis. J Am Coll Cardiol. 1998;32:380–6.

53. Picano E, Severi S, Michelassi C, Lattanzi F, Masini M, Orsini E, Distante A, L'Abbate A. Prognostic importance of dipyridamole-echocardiography test in coronary artery disease. Circulation. 1989;80:450–7.

54. Picano E, Landi P, Bolognese L, Chiarandà G, Chiarella F, Seveso G, Sclavo MG, Gandolfo N, Previtali M, Orlandini A. Prognostic value of dipyridamole echocardiography early after uncomplicated myocardial infarction: a large-scale, multicenter trial. The EPIC Study Group. Am J Med. 1993;95:608–18.

55. van Daele ME, Mcneill AJ, Fioretti PM, Salustri A, Pozzoli MM, el-Said ES, Reijs AE, Mcfalls EO, Slagboom T, Roelandt JR. Prognostic value of dipyridamole sestamibi single-photon emission computed tomography and dipyridamole stress echocardiography for new cardiac events after an uncomplicated myocardial infarction. J Am Soc Echocardiogr. 1994;7:370–80.

56. Neskovic AN, Popovic AD, Babic R, Marinkovic J, Obradovic V. Positive high-dose dipyridamole echocardiography test after acute myocardial infarction is an excellent predictor of cardiac events. Am Heart J. 1995;129:31–9.

57. Sicari R, Landi P, Picano E, Pirelli S, Chiaranda G, Previtali M, Seveso G, Gandolfo N, Margaria F, Magaia O, Minardi G, Mathias W, EPIC (Echo Persantine International Cooperative); EDIC (Echo Dobutamine International Cooperative) Study Group. Exercise-electrocardiography and/or pharmacological stress echocardiography for non-invasive risk stratication early after uncomplicated myocardial infarction.A prospective international large scale multicentre study. Eur Heart J. 2002;23:1030–7.

58. Cortigiani L, Bigi R, Sicari R, Landi P, Bovenzi F, Picano E. Prognostic value of pharmacological stress echocardiography in diabetic and nondiabetic patients with known or suspected coronary artery disease. J Am Coll Cardiol. 2006;47:605–10.

59. Sicari R, Cortigiani L, Bigi R, Landi P, Raciti M, Picano E. The prognostic value of pharmacologic stress echo is affected by concomitant anti-ischemic therapy at the time of testing. Circulation. 2004;109:1428–31.

60. Picano E, Lucarini AR, Lattanzi F, Distante A, Di Legge V, Salvetti A, L'Abbate A. Dipyridamole-echocardiography test in essential hypertensives with chest pain. Hypertension. 1988;12:238–43.

61. Cortigiani L, Bigi R, Rigo F, Landi P, Baldini U, Mariani PR, Picano E. Diagnostic value of exercise electrocardiography and dipyridamole stress echocardiography in hypertensive and normotensive chest pain patients with right bundle branch block. J Hypertens. 2003;21:2189–94.

62. Senior R, Basu S, Handler C, Raftery EB, Lahiri A. Diagnostic accuracy of dobutamine stress echocardiography for detection of coronary heart disease in hypertensive patients. Eur Heart J. 1996;17:289–95.

63. Astarita C, Palinkas A, Nicolai E, Maresca FS, Varga A, Picano E. Dipyridamole-atropine stress echocardiography versus exercise SPECT scintigraphy for detection of coronary artery disease in hypertensives with positive exercise test. J Hypertens. 2001;19:495–502.

64. Mancia G, De Backer G, Dominiczak A, Cifkova R, Fagard R, Germano G, Grassi G, Heagerty AM, Kjeldsen SE, Laurent S, Narkiewicz K, Ruilope L, Rynkiewicz A, Schmieder RE, Boudier HA, Zanchetti A, Vahanian A, Camm J, De Caterina R, Dean V, Dickstein K, Filippatos G, Funck-Brentano C, Hellemans I, Kristensen SD, McGregor K, Sechtem U, Silber S, Tendera M, Widimsky P, Zamorano JL, Erdine S, Kiowski W, Agabiti-Rosei E, Ambrosioni E, Lindholm LH, Viigimaa M, Adamopoulos S, Agabiti-Rosei E, Ambrosioni E, Bertomeu V, Clement D, Erdine S, Farsang C, Gaita D, Lip G, Mallion JM, Manolis AJ, Nilsson PM, O'Brien E, Ponikowski P, Redon J, Ruschitzka F, Tamargo J, van Zwieten P, Waeber B, Williams B. 2007 Guidelines for the management of arterial hypertension: The Task Force for the Management of Arterial Hypertension of the European Society of Hypertension (ESH) and of the European Society of Cardiology (ESC). Eur Heart J. 2007;28:1462–536.

65. Cortigiani L, Paolini EA, Nannini E. Dipyridamole stress echocardiography for risk stratification in hypertensive patients with chest pain. Circulation. 1998; 98:2855–9.

66. Mondillo S, Agricola E, Ammaturo T, Guerrini F, Barbati R, Focardi M, Picchi A, Ballo P, Nami R. Prognostic value of dipyridamole stress echocardiography in hypertensive patients with left ventricular hypertrophy, chest pain and resting electrocardiographic repolarization abnormalities. Can J Cardiol. 2001;17:571–7.

67. Cortigiani L, Coletta C, Bigi R, Amici E, Desideri A, Odoguardi L. Clinical, exercise electrocardiographic, and pharmacologic stress echocardiographic findings for risk stratification of hypertensive patients with chest pain. Am J Cardiol. 2003;9:941–5.

68. Marwick TH, Case C, Sawada S, Vasey C, Thomas JD. Prediction of outcomes in hypertensive patients with suspected coronary disease. Hypertension. 2002;39:1113–8.

69. Bigi R, Bax JJ, van Domburg RT, Elhendy A, Cortigiani L, Schinkel AFL, Fiorentini C, Poldermans D. Simultaneous echocardiography and myocardial perfusion single photon emission computed tomography associated with dobutamine stress to predict long-term cardiac mortality in normotensive and hypertensive patients. J Hypertens. 2005;23:1409–15.

70. Sozzi FB, Elhendy A, Rizzello V, van Domburg RT, Kertai M, Vourvouri E, Schinkel AF, Bax JJ, Roelandt JR, Poldermans D. Prognostic value of dobutamine stress echocardiography in patients with systemic hypertension and known or suspected coronary artery disease. Am J Cardiol. 2004;94:733–9.

71. Cicala S, de Simone G, Roman MJ, Best LG, Lee ET, Wang W, Welty TK, Galloway JM, Howard BV, Devereux RB. Prevalence and prognostic significance of wall-motion abnormalities in adults without clinically recognized cardiovascular disease: the strong heart study. Circulation. 2007;116:143–50.

72. Cortigiani L, Bigi R, Landi P, Bovenzi F, Picano E, Sicari R. Prognostic implication of stress echocardiography in 6214 hypertensive and 5328 normotensive patients. Eur Heart J. 2011;32:1509–18.

73. Hennessy TG, Codd MB, Kane G, McCarthy C, McCann HA, Sugrue DD. Evaluation of patients with diabetes mellitus for coronary artery disease using dobutamine stress echocardiography. Coron Artery Dis. 1997;8:171–4.

74. Elhendy A, van Domburg RT, Poldermans D, Bax JJ, Nierop PR, Geleijnse ML, Roelandt JR. Safety and feasibility of dobutamine-atropine stress echocardiography for the diagnosis of coronary artery disease in diabetic patients unable to perform an exercise stress test. Diabetes Care. 1998;21:1797–802.

75. Griffin ME, Nikookam K, Teh MM, McCann H, O'Meara NM, Firth RG. Dobutamine stress echocardiography: false positive scans in proteinuric patients with type 1 diabetes mellitus at high risk of ischaemic heart disease. Diabet Med. 1998;15:427–30.

76. Young LH, Wackers FJ, Chyun DA, Davey JA, Barrett EJ, Taillefer R, Heller GV, Iskandrian AE, Wittlin SD, Filipchuk N, Ratner RE, Inzucchi SE. Cardiac outcomes after screening for asymptomatic coronary artery disease in patients with type 2 diabetes: the DIAD study: a randomized controlled trial. JAMA. 2009;301:1547–55.

77. Cortigiani L, Sicari R, Desideri A, Bigi R, Bovenzi F, Picano E, VIDA (Viability Identification With Dobutamine Administration) Study Group. Dobutamine stress echocardiography and the effect of revascularization on outcome in diabetic and non-diabetic patients with chronic ischaemic left ventricular dysfunction. Eur J Heart Fail. 2007;9:1038–43.

78. Elhendy A, Arruda AM, Mahoney DW, Pellikka PA. Prognostic stratification of diabetic patients by exercise echocardiography. J Am Coll Cardiol. 2001;37: 1551–7.

79. Bigi R, Desideri A, Cortigiani L, Bax JJ, Celegon L, Fiorentini C. Stress echocardiography for risk stratification of diabetic patients with known or suspected coronary artery disease. Diabetes Care. 2001;24:1596–601.

80. Kamalesh M, Matorin R, Sawada S. Prognostic value of a negative stress echocardiographic study in diabetic patients. Am Heart J. 2002;143:163–8.

81. Marwick TH, Case C, Sawada S, Vasey C, Short L, Lauer M. Use of stress echocardiography to predict mortality in patients with diabetes and known or suspected coronary artery disease. Diabetes Care. 2002;25:1042–8.

82. Chaowalit N, Arruda AL, McCully RB, Bailey KR, Pellikka PA. Dobutamine stress echocardiography in patients with diabetes mellitus: enhanced prognostic prediction using a simple risk score. J Am Coll Cardiol. 2006;47:1029–36.

83. van der Sijde JN, Boiten HJ, Sozzi FB, Elhendy A, van Domburg RT, Schinkel AF. Long-term prognostic value of dobutamine stress echocardiography in diabetic patients with limited exercise capability: a 13-year follow-up study. Diabetes Care. 2012;35:634–9.

84. Cortigiani L, Bigi R, Sicari R, Rigo F, Bovenzi F, Picano E. Comparison of prognostic value of pharmacologic stress echocardiography in chest pain patients with versus without diabetes mellitus and positive exercise electrocardiography. Am J Cardiol. 2007;100:1744–9.

85. Cortigiani L, Borelli L, Raciti M, Bovenzi F, Picano E, Molinaro S, Sicari R. Prediction of mortality by stress echocardiography in 2835 diabetic and 11 305 nondiabetic patients. Circ Cardiovasc Imaging. 2015;8(5). doi: 10.1161/CIRCIMAGING.114.002757

86. Picano E, Vañó E, Rehani MM, Cuocolo A, Mont L, Bodi V, Bar O, Maccia C, Pierard L, Sicari R, Plein S, Mahrholdt H, Lancellotti P, Knuuti J, Heidbuchel H, Di Mario C, Badano LP. The appropriate and justified use of medical radiation in cardiovascular imaging: a position document of the ESC Associations of Cardiovascular Imaging, Percutaneous Cardiovascular Interventions and Electrophysiology. Eur Heart J. 2014;35:665–72.

87. Giri S, Shaw LJ, Murthy DR, Travin MI, Miller DD, Hachamovitch R, Borges-Neto S, Berman DS, Waters DD, Heller GV. Impact of diabetes on the risk stratification using stress single-photon emission computed tomography myocardial perfusion imaging in patients with symptoms suggestive of coronary artery disease. Circulation. 2002;105:32–40.

88. Masini M, Picano E, Lattanzi F, Distante A, L'Abbate A. High-dose dipyridamole echocardiography test in women: correlation with exercise-electrocardiography test and coronary arteriography. J Am Coll Cardiol. 1998;12:682–5.

89. Marwick TH, Anderson T, Williams MJ, Haluska B, Melin JA, Pashkow F, Thomas JD. Exercise echocardiography is an accurate and cost-efficient technique for detection of coronary artery disease in women. J Am Coll Cardiol. 1995;26:335–41.

90. Elhendy A, van Domburg RT, Bax JJ, Nierop PR, Geleijnse ML, Ibrahim MM, Roelandt JR. Noninvasive diagnosis of coronary artery stenosis in women with limited exercise capacity: comparison of dobutamine stress echocardiography and 99mTc sestamibi single-photon emission CT. Chest. 1998;114:1097–104.

91. Cortigiani L, Sicari R, Bigi R, Landi P, Bovenzi F, Picano E. Impact of gender on risk stratification by stress echocardiography. Am J Med. 2009;122:301–9.

92. Cortigiani L, Dodi C, Paolini EA, Bernardi D, Bruno G, Nannini E. Prognostic value of pharmacological stress echocardiography in women with chest pain and unknown coronary artery disease. J Am Coll Cardiol. 1998;32:1975–81.

93. Dodi C, Cortigiani L, Masini M, Olivotto I, Azzarelli A, Nannini E. The incremental prognostic value of stress echo over exercise electrocardiography in women with chest pain of unknown origin. Eur Heart J. 2001;22:145–52.

94. Cortigiani L, Gigli G, Vallebona A, Mariani PR, Bigi R, Desideri A. The stress echo prognostic gender gap. Eur J Echocardiogr. 2001;2:132–8.

95. Mairesse GH, Marwick TH, Arnese M, Vanoverschelde JL, Cornel JH, Detry JM, Melin JA, Fioretti PM. Improved identification of coronary artery disease in patients with left bundle branch block by the use of dobutamine stress echocardiography and comparison with myocardial perfusion tomography. Am J Cardiol. 1995;76:321–5.

96. Geleijnse ML, Vigna G, Kasprzak JD, Rambaldi R, Salvatori MP, Elhendy A, Cornel JH, Fioretti PM, Roelandt JR. Usefulness and limitations of dobutamine-atropine stress echocardiography for the diagnosis of coronary artery disease in patients with left bundle branch block. Eur Heart J. 2000;21:1666–73.

97. Cortigiani L, Picano E, Vigna C, Lattanzi F, Coletta C, Mariotti E, Bigi R. Prognostic value of pharmacologic stress echocardiography in patients with left bundle branch block. Am J Med. 2001;110:361–9.

98. Fleisher LA, Fleischmann KE, Auerbach AD, Barnason SA, Beckman JA, Bozkurt B, Davila-Roman VG, Gerhard-Herman MD, Holly TA, Kane GC, Marine JE, Nelson MT, Spencer CC, Thompson A, Ting HH, Uretsky BF, Wijeysundera DN. 2014 ACC/AHA guideline on perioperative cardiovascular evaluation and management of patients undergoing noncardiac surgery: a report of the American College of Cardiology/American Heart Association Task Force on practice guidelines. J Am Coll Cardiol. 2014;64:e77–137.

99. Kristensen SD, Knuuti J, Saraste A, Anker S, Bøtker HE, Hert SD, Ford I, Gonzalez-Juanatey JR, Gorenek B, Heyndrickx GR, Hoeft A, Huber K, Iung B, Kjeldsen KP, Longrois D, Lüscher TF, Pierard L, Pocock S, Price S, Roffi M, Sirnes PA, Sousa-Uva M, Voudris V, Funck-Brentano C, Authors/Task Force Members. 2014 ESC/ESA guidelines on non-cardiac surgery: cardiovascular assessment and management: the Joint Task Force on non-cardiac surgery: cardiovascular assessment and management of the European Society of Cardiology (ESC) and the European Society of Anaesthesiology (ESA). Eur Heart J. 2014;35:2383–431.

100. Tischler MD, Lee TH, Hirsch AT, et al. Prediction of major cardiac events after peripheral vascular surgery using dipyridamole echocardiography. Am J Cardiol. 1991;68:593–7.

101. Sicari R, Picano E, Lusa AM, et al. The value of dipyridamole echocardiography in risk stratification before vascular surgery. A multicenter study. The EPIC (Echo Persantine International Study) Group-Subproject: risk stratification before major vascular surgery. Eur Heart J. 1995;16:842–7.

102. Rossi E, Citterio F, Vescio MF, et al. Risk stratification of patients undergoing peripheral vascular revascularization by combined resting and dipyridamole echocardiography. Am J Cardiol. 1998;82:306–10.

103. Pasquet A, D'Hondt AM, Verhelst R, et al. Comparison of dipyridamole stress echocardiography and perfusion scintigraphy for cardiac risk stratification in vascular surgery patients. Am J Cardiol. 1998;82:1468–74.

104. Sicari R, Ripoli A, Picano E, on behalf of the EPIC study group, et al. Perioperative prognostic value of dipyridamole echocardiography in vascular surgery: a large-scale multicenter study on 509 patients. Circulation. 1999;100 Suppl 19:II269–74.

105. Zamorano J, Duque A, Baquero M, et al. Stress echocardiography in the pre-operative evaluation of patients undergoing major vascular surgery. Are results comparable with dipyridamole versus dobutamine stress echo? Rev Esp Cardiol. 2002;55:121–6.

106. Lane RT, Sawada SG, Segar DS, et al. Dobutamine stress echocardiography for assessment of cardiac risk before noncardiac surgery. Am J Cardiol. 1991;68:976–7.

107. Lalka SG, Sawada SG, Dalsing MC, et al. Dobutamine stress echocardiography as a predictor of cardiac events associated with aortic surgery. J Vasc Surg. 1992;15:831–42.

108. Davila-Roman VG, Waggoner AD, Sicard GA, et al. Dobutamine stress echocardiography predicts surgical outcome in patients with an aortic aneurysm and peripheral vascular disease. J Am Coll Cardiol. 1993;21:957–63.

109. Eichelberger JP, Schwarz KQ, Black ER, et al. Predictive value of dobutamine echocardiography just before noncardiac vascular surgery. Am J Cardiol. 1993;72:602–7.

110. Poldermans D, Fioretti PM, Forster T, et al. Dobutamine stress echocardiography for assessment of perioperative cardiac risk in patients undergoing major vascular surgery. Circulation. 1993;87:1506–12.

111. Karagiannis SE, Feringa HH, Vidakovic R, et al. Value of myocardial viability estimation using dobutamine stress echocardiography in assessing risk preoperatively before noncardiac vascular surgery in patients with left ventricular ejection fraction < 35%. Am J Cardiol. 2007;99:1555–9.

112. Das MK, Pellikka PA, Mahoney DW, Roger VL, Ohjk MCRB, et al. Assessment of cardiac risk before nonvascular surgery: dobutamine stress echocardiography in 530 patients. J Am Coll Cardiol. 2000;35:1647–53.

113. Beattie WS, Abdelnaem E, Wijeysundera DN, Buckley DN. A meta-analytic comparison of preoperative stress echocardiography and nuclear scintigraphy imaging. Anesth Analg. 2006;102:8–16.

114. Shaw LJ, Eagle KA, Gersh BJ, et al. Meta-analysis of intravenous dipyridamole-thallium-201 imaging (1985 to 1994) and dobutamine echocardiography (1991 to 1994) for risk stratification before vascular imaging. J Am Coll Cardiol. 1996;27:787–98.

115. Kertai MD, Boersma E, Bax JJ, et al. A meta-analysis comparing the prognostic accuracy of six diagnostic tests for predicting perioperative cardiac risk in patients undergoing major vascular surgery. Heart. 2003;89:1327–34.

116. Poldermans D, Arnese M, Fioretti PM, et al. Sustained prognostic value of dobutamine stress echocardiography for late cardiac events after major noncardiac vascular surgery. Circulation. 1997;195:53–8.

117. Sicari R, Ripoli A, Picano E, on behalf of the EPIC (Echo Persantine International Cooperative) Study Group, et al. Long-term prognostic value of dipyridamole echocardiography in vascular surgery: a large-scale multicenter study. Coron Artery Dis. 2002;13:49–55.

118. Luscher TF, Gersh B, Landmesser U, Ruschitzka F. Is the panic about beta-blockers in peri-operative care justified? Eur Heart J. 2014;35:2442–4.

119. Picano E, Pasanisi E, Brown J, et al. A gatekeeper for the gatekeeper: inappropriate referrals to stress echocardiography. Am Heart J. 2007;154:285–90.

120. Gibbons RJ, Miller TD, Hodge D, et al. Application of appropriateness criteria to stress single-photon emission computed tomography sestamibi studies and stress echocardiograms in an academic medical center. J Am Coll Cardiol. 2008;51:1283–9.

121. Mansour IN, Lang RM, Aburuwaida WM, Bhave NM, Ward RP. Evaluation of the clinical application of the ACCF/ASE appropriateness criteria for stress echocardiography. J Am Soc Echocardiogr. 2010;23:1199–204.

122. Cortigiani L, Bigi R, Bovenzi F, Molinaro S, Picano E, Sicari R. Prognostic implication of appropriateness criteria for pharmacologic stress echocardiography performed in an outpatient clinic. Circ Cardiovasc Imaging. 2012;5:298–305.

123. Smart SC, Sawada S, Ryan T, Segar D, Atherton L, Berkovitz K, Bourdillon PD, Feigenbaum H. Low-dose dobutamine echocardiography detects reversible dysfunction after thrombolytic therapy of acute myocardial infarction. Circulation. 1993;88:405–15.

124. Bax JJ, Cornel JH, Visser FC, Fioretti PM, van Lingen A, Reijs AE, Boersma E, Teule GJ, Visser CA. Prediction of recovery of myocardial dysfunction after revascularization. Comparison of fluorine-18 fluorodeoxyglucose/thallium-201 SPECT, thallium-201 stress-reinjection SPECT and dobutamine echocardiography. J Am Coll Cardiol. 1996;28:558–64.

125. Bax JJ, Wijns W, Cornel JH, Visser FC, Boersma E, Fioretti PM. Accuracy of currently available techniques for prediction of functional recovery after revascularization in patients with left ventricular dysfunction due to chronic coronary artery disease: comparison of pooled data. J Am Coll Cardiol. 1997;30:1451–60.

126. Picano E, Marzullo P, Gigli G, Reisenhofer B, Parodi O, Distante A, L'Abbate A. Identification of viable myocardium by dipyridamole-induced improvement in regional left ventricular function assessed by echocardiography in myocardial infarction and comparison with thallium scintigraphy at rest. Am J Cardiol. 1992;70:703–10.

127. Varga A, Ostojic M, Djordjevic-Dikic A, Sicari R, Pingitore A, Nedeljkovic I, Picano E. Infra-low dose dipyridamole test. A novel dose regimen for selective assessment of myocardial viability by vasodilator stress echocardiography. Eur Heart J. 1996;17:629–34.

128. Picano E, Ostojic M, Varga A, Sicari R, Djordjevic-Dikic A, Nedeljkovic I, Torres M. Combined low dose dipyridamole-dobutamine stress echocardiography to identify myocardial viability. J Am Coll Cardiol. 1996;27:1422–8.

129. Hoffer EP, Dewe W, Celentano C, Pierard LA. Low-level exercise echocardiography detects contractile reserve and predicts reversible dysfunction after acute myocardial infarction: comparison with low-dose dobutamine echocardiography. J Am Coll Cardiol. 1999;34:989–97.

130. Lu C, Carlino M, Fragasso G, Maisano F, Margonato A, Cappelletti A, Chierchia SL. Enoximone echocardiography for predicting recovery of left ventricular dysfunction after revascularization: a novel test for detecting myocardial viability. Circulation. 2000;101:12551260.

131. Ghio S, Constantin C, Raineri C, Fontana A, Klersy C, Campana C, Tavazzi L. Enoximone echocardiography: a novel test to evaluate left ventricular contractile reserve in patients with heart failure on chronic betablocker therapy. Cardiovasc Ultrasound. 2003;1:13.

132. Baumgartner H, Porenta G, Lau YK, Wutte M, Klaar U, Mehrabi M, Siegel RJ, Czernin J, Laufer G, Sochor H, Schelbert H, Fishbein MC, Maurer G. Assessment of myocardial viability by dobutamine echocardiography, positron emission tomography and thallium-201 SPECT: correlation with histopathology in explanted hearts. J Am Coll Cardiol. 1998;32:1701–8.

133. Williams MJ, Odabashian J, Lauer MS, Thomas JD, Marwick TH. Prognostic value of dobutamine echocardiography in patients with left ventricular dysfunction. J Am Coll Cardiol. 1996;27:132–9.

134. Bax JJ, Poldermans D, Elhendy A, Cornel JH, Boersma E, Rambaldi R, Roelandt JR, Fioretti PM. Improvement of left ventricular ejection fraction, heart failure symptoms and prognosis after revascularization in patients with chronic coronary artery disease and viable myocardium detected by dobutamine stress echocardiography. J Am Coll Cardiol. 1999;34:163–9.

135. Meluzín J, Cerný J, Frélich M, Stetka F, Spinarová L, Popelová J, Stípal R. Prognostic value of the amount of dysfunctional but viable myocardium in revascularized patients with coronary artery disease and left ventricular dysfunction. J Am Coll Cardiol. 1998;32:912–20.

136. Marwick TH, Zuchowski C, Lauer MS, Secknus MA, Williams J, Lytle BW. Functional status and quality of life in patients with heart failure undergoing coronary bypass surgery after assessment of myocardial viability. J Am Coll Cardiol. 1999;33:750–8.

137. Chaudry FA, Tauke JT, Alessandrini RS, Vardi G, Parker MA, Bonow RO. Prognostic implications of myocardial contractile reserve in patients with coronary artery disease and left ventricular dysfunction. J Am Coll Cardiol. 1999;34:730–8.

138. Sicari R, Ripoli A, Picano E, Borges AC, Varga A, Mathias W, Cortigiani L, Bigi R, Heyman J, Polimeno S, Silvestri O, Gimenez V, Caso P, Severino S, Djordjevic-Dikic A, Ostojic M, Baldi C, Seveso G, Petix N, VIDA (Viability Identification With Dipyridamole Administration) Study Group. The

prognostic value of myocardial viability recognized by low dose dipyridamole echocardiography in patients with chronic ischaemic left ventricular dysfunction. Eur Heart J. 2001;22:837–44.

139. Sicari R, Picano E, Cortigiani L, Borges AC, Varga A, Palagi C, Bigi R, Rossini R, Pasanisi E, VIDA (Viability Identification with Dobutamine Administration) Study Group. Prognostic value of myocardial viability recognized by low-dose dobutamine echocardiography in chronic ischaemic left ventricular dysfunction. Am J Cardiol. 2003;92:1263–6.

140. Senior R, Kaul S, Lahiri A. Myocardial viability on echocardiography predicts long-term survival after revascularization in patients with ischaemic congestive heart failure. J Am Coll Cardiol. 1999;33:1848–54.

141. Allman KC, Shaw LJ, Hachamovitch R, Udelson JE. Myocardial viability testing and impact of revascularization on prognosis inpatients with coronary artery disease and left ventricular dysfunction: a meta-analysis. J Am Coll Cardiol. 2002;39:1151–8.

142. Rizzello V, Poldermans D, Schinkel AF, Biagini E, Boersma E, Elhendy A, Sozzi FB, Maat A, Crea F, Roelandt JR, Bax JJ. Long term prognostic value of myocardial viability and ischaemia during dobutamine stress echocardiography in patients with ischaemic cardiomyopathy undergoing coronary revascularisation. Heart. 2006;92:239–44.

143. Ciampi Q, Pratali L, Citro R, Piacenti M, Villari B, Picano E. Identification of responders to cardiac resynchronization therapy by contractile reserve during stress echocardiography. Eur J Heart Fail. 2009;11:489–96.

144. Moonen M, Senechal M, Cosyns B, Melon P, Nellessen E, Pierard L, Lancellotti P. Impact of contractile reserve on acute response to cardiac resynchronization therapy. Cardiovasc Ultrasound. 2008;6:65.

145. Cortigiani L, Rigo F, Gherardi S, Bovenzi F, Molinaro S, Picano E, Sicari R. Coronary flow reserve during dipyridamole stress echocardiography predicts mortality. JACC Cardiovasc Imaging. 2012;5:1079–85.

146. Cortigiani L, Rigo F, Gherardi S, Sicari R, Galderisi M, Bovenzi F, Picano E. Additional prognostic value of coronary flow reserve in diabetic and nondiabetic patients with negative dipyridamole stress echocardiography by wall motion criteria. J Am Coll Cardiol. 2007;50:1354–61.

147. Cortigiani L, Rigo F, Gherardi S, Galderisi M, Bovenzi F, Picano E, Sicari R. Diagnostic and prognostic value of Doppler echocardiographic coronary flow reserve in left anterior descending artery in hypertensive and normotensive patients. Heart. 2011;97:1758–65.

148. Rigo F, Sicari R, Gherardi S, Djordjevic-Dikic A, Cortigiani L, Picano E. Prognostic value of coronary flow reserve in medically treated patients with left anterior descending coronary disease with stenosis 51%-75% in diameter. Am J Cardiol. 2007;100:1527–31.

149. Cortigiani L, Rigo F, Gherardi S, Bovenzi F, Molinaro S, Picano E, Sicari R. Prognostic implication of Doppler echocardiographic derived coronary flow reserve in patients with left bundle branch block. Eur Heart J. 2013;34:364–73.

150. Sicari R, Rigo F, Cortigiani L, Gherardi S, Galderisi M, Picano E. Long-term survival of patients with chest pain syndrome and angiographically normal or near normal coronary arteries: the additional prognostic value of coronary flow reserve. Am J Cardiol. 2009;103:626–31.

151. Cortigiani L, Rigo F, Gherardi S, Galderisi M, Bovenzi F, Picano E, Sicari R. Prognostic meaning of coronary microvascular disease in type 2 diabetes mellitus. A transthoracic Doppler echocardiographic study. J Am Soc Echocardiogr. 2014;27:742–8.

152. Gaibazzi N, Reverberi C, Lorenzoni V, Molinaro S, Porter TR. Prognostic value of high-dose dipyridamole stress myocardial contrast perfusion echocardiography. Circulation. 2012;126:1217–24.

153. Huang R, Abdelmoneim SS, Nhola LF, Mulvagh SL. Relationship between HbA1c and myocardial blood flow reserve in patients with type 2 diabetes mellitus: noninvasive assessment using real-time myocardial perfusion echocardiography. J Diabetes Res. 2014;2014:243518. doi:10.1155/2014/243518. Epub 2014 Jul 2.

154. Lowenstein JA, Caniggia C, Rousse G, Amor M, Sánchez ME, Alasia D, Casso N, García A, Zambrana G, Lowenstein Haber DM, Darú V. Coronary flow velocity reserve during pharmacologic stress echocardiography with normal contractility adds important prognostic value in diabetic and nondiabetic patients. J Am Soc Echocardiogr. 2014;27:1113–9.

155. Sicari R, Rigo F, Gherardi S, Galderisi M, Cortigiani L, Picano E. The prognostic value of Doppler echocardiographic-derived coronary flow reserve is not affected by concomitant antiischemic therapy at the time of testing. Am Heart J. 2008; 156:573–9.

156. Mor-Avi V, Lang RM, Badano LP, Belohlavek M, Cardim NM, Derumeaux G, Galderisi M, Marwick T, Nagueh SF, Sengupta PP, Sicari R, Smiseth OA,

Smulevitz B, Takeuchi M, Thomas JD, Vannan M, Voigt JU, Zamorano JL. Current and evolving echocardiographic techniques for the quantitative evaluation of cardiac mechanics: ASE/EAE consensus statement on methodology and indications endorsed by the Japanese Society of Echocardiography. Eur J Echocardiogr. 2011;12:167–205.

157. Lang RM, Badano LP, Tsang W, Adams DH, Agricola E, Buck T, Faletra FF, Franke A, Hung J, de Isla LP, Kamp O, Kasprzak JD, Lancellotti P, Marwick TH, McCulloch ML, Monaghan MJ, Nihoyannopoulos P, Pandian NG, Pellikka PA, Pepi M, Roberson DA, Shernan SK, Shirali GS, Sugeng L, Ten Cate FJ, Vannan MA, Zamorano JL, Zoghbi WA, American Society of Echocardiography; European Association of Echocardiography. EAE/ASE recommendations for image acquisition and display using three-dimensional echocardiography. Eur Heart J Cardiovasc Imaging. 2012;13:1–46.

158. Crouse LJ, Cheirif J, Hanly DE, Kisslo JA, Labovitz AJ, Raichlen JS, et al. Opacification and border delineation improvement in patients with suboptimal endocardial border definition in routine echocardiography: results of phase III Albunex multicenter trial. J Am Coll Cardiol. 1993;22:1494–500.

159. Fletcher GF, Balady GJ, Amsterdam EA, et al. Exercise standards for testing and training: a statement for healthcare professionals from the American Heart Association. Circulation. 2001;104:1694–740.

160. Varga A, Garcia MA, Picano E, et al. Safety of stress echocardiography (from the International Stress Echo Complication Registry). Am J Cardiol. 2006;98:541–3.

161. Picano E, Marini C, Pirelli S, et al. Safety of intravenous high-dose dipyridamole echocardiography. The Echo-Persantine International Cooperative Study Group. Am J Cardiol. 1992;70:252–8.

162. Picano E, Mathias Jr W, Pingitore A, et al. Safety and tolerability of dobutamine-atropine stress echocardiography: a prospective, multicentre study. Echo Dobutamine International Cooperative Study Group. Lancet. 1994;344:1190–2.

163. Beckmann S, Haug G. National registry 1995–1998 on 150,000 stress echo examinations side effects and complications in 60,448 examinations of the registry 1997–1998. Circulation. 1999;100(Suppl):3401A.

164. Picano E, Pellikka PA. Stress echo applications beyond coronary artery disease. Eur Heart J. 2014;35:1033–40.

6

Limitations and difficulties of echocardiographic short-axis assessment of paravalvular leakage after corevalve transcatheter aortic valve implantation

Marcel L. Geleijnse[1][*], Luigi F. M. Di Martino[2], Wim B. Vletter[1], Ben Ren[1], Tjebbe W. Galema[1], Nicolas M. Van Mieghem[1], Peter P. T. de Jaegere[1] and Osama I. I. Soliman[1,3]

Abstract

To make assessment of paravalvular aortic leakage (PVL) after transcatheter aortic valve implantation (TAVI) more uniform the second Valve Academic Research Consortium (VARC) recently updated the echocardiographic criteria for mild, moderate and severe PVL. In the VARC recommendation the assessment of the circumferential extent of PVL in the short-axis view is considered critical. In this paper we will discuss our observational data on the limitations and difficulties of this particular view, that may potentially result in overestimation or underestimation of PVL severity.

Keywords: Aortic valve, Regurgitation, Paravalvular, Echocardiography

Abbreviations: 2D, Two dimensional; 3D, Three dimensional; AR, Aortic regurgitation; AS, Aortic stenosis; LV, Left ventricle; PVL, Paravalvular regurgitation; SAX, Short-axis; TAVI, Transcatheter aortic valve implantation; VARC, Valve Academic Research Consortium

Background

Transcatheter aortic valve implantation (TAVI) is a relatively new therapeutic option in patients with aortic stenosis (AS) who are at high-operative risk or inoperable [1, 2]. Despite its favourable hemodynamics, [2] paravalvular aortic regurgitation (AR) or leakage (PVL) after TAVI is common and is considered by many the Achilles' heel of TAVI because there is growing evidence suggesting a significant association of PVL with short- and long-term mortality [3]. This may even become more troublesome as these therapies are offered to progressively younger patients. Unfortunately, the transthoracic echocardiographic assessment of PVL severity is extremely challenging. In contrast to AR in native valves, a zone of flow convergence and vena contracta, the single most important parameters in assessment of AR severity, [4, 5] do not exist or are difficult to image in patients with PVL. In contrast, the PVL is of variable size, starting somewhere at the level of the aortic annulus, running a poor to visualize course next to the stent frame with an exit of the flow into the left ventricle (LV) next to the inflow-end of the stent frame or into the LV "outflow tract", in case of an eccentric jet passing through the stent frame before its end. In addition, even in native valves there has been no validation for adding multiple jets as may be frequently encountered in TAVI patients (Fig. 1). In the presence of a surgical aortic valve prosthesis it has been suggested that careful imaging of the neck of the jet in a short-axis (SAX) view, at the level of the prosthesis sewing ring, allows determination of the circumferential extent of PVL serving as a semi-quantitative measure of severity. According to this method a circumferential extent less than 10 % suggests mild PVL, 10 % to 20 % moderate PVL, and more than 20 % severe PVL (Fig. 2) [5, 6]. However, it should be noticed that this is only an approximate guide and its classification is strictly arbitrary, without any validation (the PVL volume of a given circumferential extent is unknown). Despite all the mentioned limitations and

* Correspondence: m.geleijnse@erasmusmc.nl
[1]From the department of Cardiology, Thoraxcenter, Erasmus University Medical Center, Thoraxcenter, Ba304, 's-Gravendijkwal 230, 3015, CE, Rotterdam, The Netherlands
Full list of author information is available at the end of the article

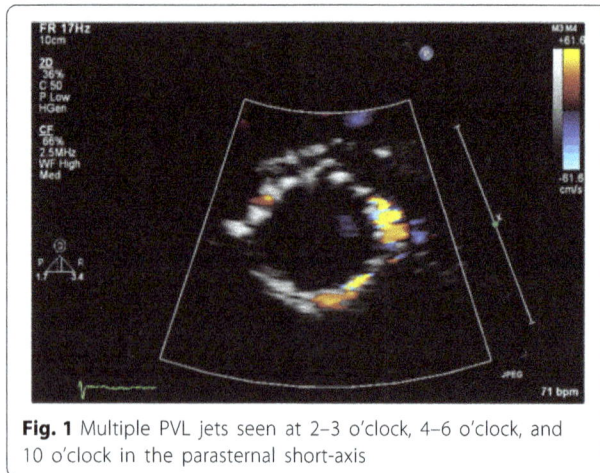

Fig. 1 Multiple PVL jets seen at 2–3 o'clock, 4–6 o'clock, and 10 o'clock in the parasternal short-axis

Data acquisition and analysis/Clinical characteristics

In total 554 transthoracic echocardiograms up to one year after implantation of a CoreValve Revalving System$^{©}$ because of severe AS were analysed. These echocardiograms were acquired according to VARC recommendations in the period 2007–2013 [8]. More specifically, SAX images were scored for the presence of PVL jets according to a clock model [10]. Median age of the patients was 83 years, 46 % were males and body mass index was 26 ± 4. NYHA class 2, 3 and 4 before TAVI was present in 17 %, 63 % and 14 % of patients, respectively (the remaining patients were asymptomatic patients scheduled for cancer surgery). Consent was obtained obtained in all patients for anonymised prospective data collection for research purposes.

False negative parasternal SAX imaging

One of the major limitations in parasternal SAX analysis of the circumferential extent of PVL is the relatively high incidence of false negative studies, which may also imply underestimation of PVL in positive studies. In our series, 79 (14 %) of the SAX images were false negative, defined as absence of PVL in the SAX view but presence of PVL in the apical 3-chamber and/or 5-chamber views. Interestingly, in a recently published study it was shown that echocardiography (in contrast to angiography) did not correlate well with magnetic resonance in the assessment of PVL [11]. Echocardiographic analysis from a parasternal (long-axis) window underestimated AR with approximately 25 % of patients having a false negative study and 25 % having a positive but underestimated study. Also, in studies in which post-implantation angiographic and transthoracic parasternal echocardiographic data were compared the number of patients without PVL was clearly (up to three times) lower for echocardiography [12]. One of the inherent problems of parasternal imaging in post-TAVI patients is the imperfect imaging of the PVL jets due to acoustic shadowing by the stent or the crushed native material between the stent frame and the native aortic root or left ventricular outflow tract. In the normally positioned CoreValve prosthesis the

recognizing that all imaging windows should be used, the updated Valve Academic Research Consortium (VARC) adopted the SAX criterion as "critical" in assessing the number and severity of paravalvular jets in patients who underwent TAVI [7]. Surprisingly, in the most recent VARC-2 publication [8] the arbitrary cut-off value to define severe PVL was changed to more than 30 % (rather than the earlier published 20 %) [5–7] without any argument or reference given. This cut-off seems to be derived from a study published a year later, performed by some of the authors involved in the VARC2 publication [9]. Although we agree with the VARC-2 authors that – in absence of other simple and useful parameters – the SAX analysis is of vital importance in assessment of PVL it may result in significant underestimation or overestimation of PVL because of various reasons. Because we could in the literature not identify any detailed information on the specific problems of the SAX analysis we will in this expert opinion manuscript review the inherent limitations and difficulties of the SAX analysis in the estimation of PVL severity based on our observations.

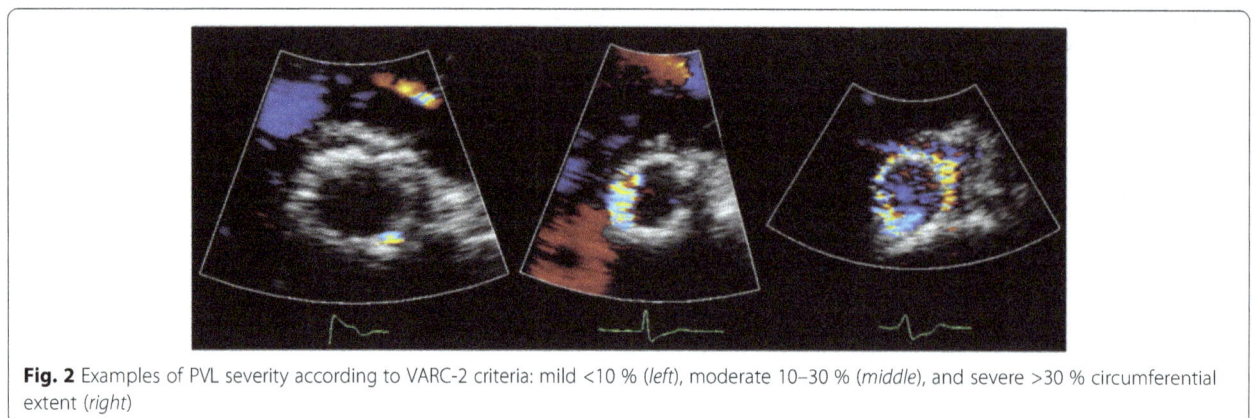

Fig. 2 Examples of PVL severity according to VARC-2 criteria: mild <10 % (*left*), moderate 10–30 % (*middle*), and severe >30 % circumferential extent (*right*)

new valve is positioned supra-annular, so the crushed native material will interfere with imaging of PVL jets distal to the new leaflet plane. In our series other clear reasons for false negative studies included poor quality in 5 % of the false negatives, SAX recorded at a too high level (valvular or supravalvular) in 8 % of the false negatives, and minor (trace) PVL (seen in apical views) in 43 % of the false negatives. Poor image quality due to patient characteristics like pulmonary disease (frequently present in the elderly referred for TAVI) or patient habitus and operator dependence (experience) are the Achilles' heels of transthoracic echocardiography. Importantly, sonographers tend to increase the overall 2D gain in poor quality echocardiograms that further negatively influences colour Doppler imaging (Fig. 3). Interestingly, in patients with both a pre-discharge echocardiogram and follow-up study available, false negative studies occurred more often in the pre-discharge echocardiograms (28 % vs. 20 % at 6 months and 21 % at 12 months). One of the reasons for this difference may be the relative immobility of the patient shortly after TAVI precluding recordings in the left decubitus position.

Localization of PVL

The localization of PVL jets in the SAX view has not been investigated in detail. According to Schultz et al.

the localization of PVL is inversely related to the site of force of apposition of the stent frame to the adjacent tissue [13]. Thus, less PVL is seen at the outside curvature of the aorta because of higher apposition force, that may even be increased by a transfemoral route that may push the device toward the outside curvature of the aorta. In Fig. 4, the PVL localization in our series of consecutive pre-discharge echocardiograms can be seen. Most PVL jets were indeed seen at the site of lower force of apposition of the stent frame to the adjacent tissue at the inside curvature of the aorta, that is from 1 to 6 o'clock in the SAX image. Interestingly, PVL jets were most frequently seen at the commissures between the right and left coronary cusps (2 o'clock) and between the left and non-coronary cusps (5 to 6 o'clock). This may be caused by calcification nearby the commissures and subsequent creation of paravalvular commissural spaces next to the sites where the stent frame is sitting on the calcium ridges. Indeed, in one study it was shown that calcification in the area of the commissures predicted the site of PVL [14].

Defining jet origin by the localization of the jet as seen just below the valve stent frame (as defined in the VARC paper) is prone to specific pitfalls. Firstly, the PVL jet origin at the level of the aortic annulus may be difficult to assess because we are actually imaging only the exit of the flow into the LV at the inflow-end of the stent frame. Secondly, many jets are eccentric, often passing through the stent before the inflow-end of the stent frame and some may even totally crossover to the other side of the inflow part of the stent frame (Fig. 5). Jets may at one extreme thus originate from the opposite site of the stent frame, although the incidence of totally

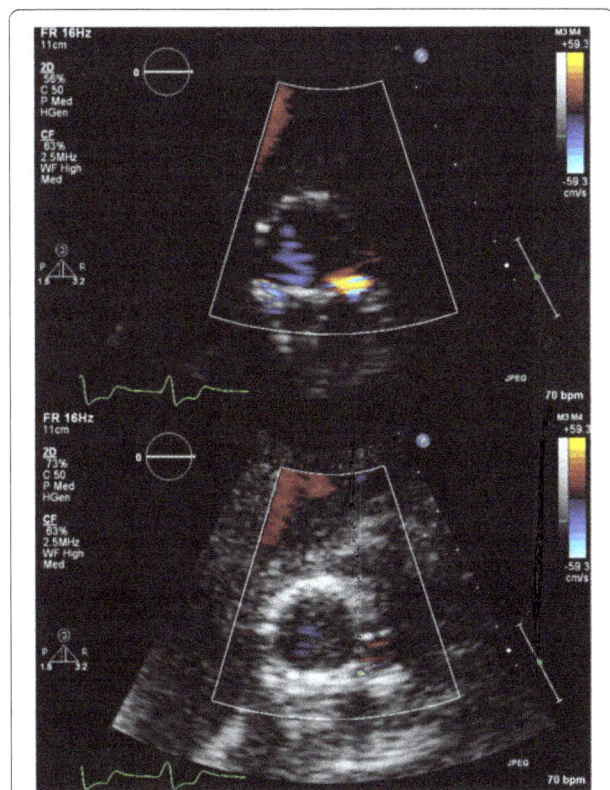

Fig. 3 The destructive effect of 2D gain on colour Doppler. Top image gain 56 % and a clear jet seen at 5 o'clock, bottom image gain at 73 % with the same jet now barely visible

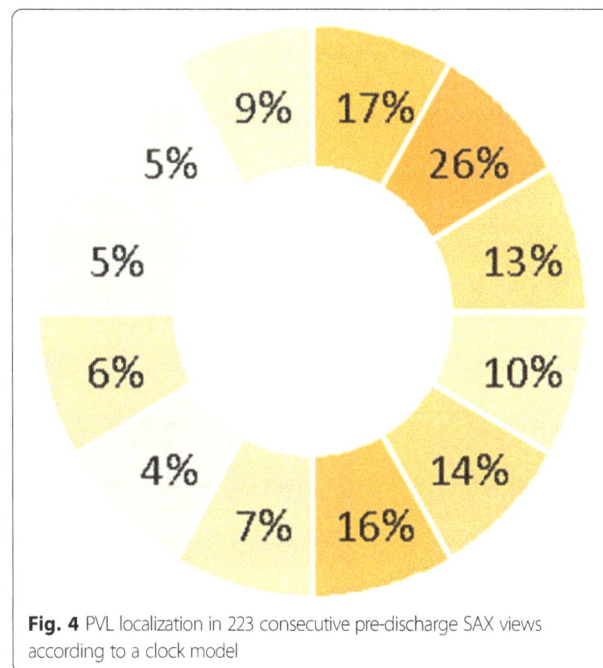

Fig. 4 PVL localization in 223 consecutive pre-discharge SAX views according to a clock model

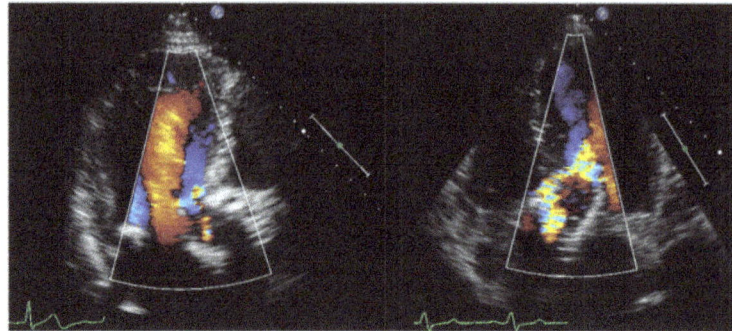

Fig. 5 Two examples of eccentric PVL jets totally crossing over to the other side of the inflow part of the stent frame

crossover jets in our series was low (approximately 2 %). Also, *valvular* regurgitant jets may sometimes be eccentric and wall-hugging thus entering the LV from the inflow-end of the stent frame and falsely regarded as a localized PVL. These jets may in most cases be recognised because they follow a course along the inside of the stent frame. However, an isolated SAX view recorded just below the stent frame may make any eccentric jet, whether valvular or paravalvular, almost look similar.

The level of SAX acquisition – "Flying jets"

As mentioned earlier, according to the VARC recommendations colour Doppler evaluation of PVL should be performed just below the valve stent [8]. However, such an evaluation harbours apart from the earlier described problems in localizing the origin of PVL some other pitfalls. PVL jets are not simple jets running a straight course alongside the stent frame to the inflow part of the frame and the LV. In contrast, the jet will on its way towards the LV frequently encounter variously sized gaps or spaces, calcium ridges and crushed parts of the native aortic root and thus runs an unpredictable, variable (and difficult to visualise) course, and at certain levels it may even run

in a more or less circumferential direction. In addition, as mentioned before, a substantial number of jets may pass through the stent frame before the inflow-end of the stent frame, and such an eccentric jet may spread out in all directions into the inflow area of the stent frame. Overestimation of PVL severity is therefore possible because obviously the true neck of the jet is in such cases not imaged at the recommended SAX level just below the stent frame (Fig. 6). Therefore, it should be recommended to start the SAX colour Doppler evaluation of PVL in a plane just below the valve stent *but always followed by* a more cranial scan to better detect the "origin" or "neck" of the PVL (Fig. 7).

Still it may not be possible to image the origin and neck of the jet in some patients, in particular in those with extremely eccentric jets that pass through the stent frame. In such cases the Doppler velocity may help to locate the origin of the jet (Fig. 8) and it may be better to estimate the circumferential extent of the jet by extrapolating its radius onto the circumference of the stent. In some cases the eccentric PVL jet is not mosaic coloured but red or blue coloured (Fig. 8); this will make the localization of the origin of the jet easy since a red

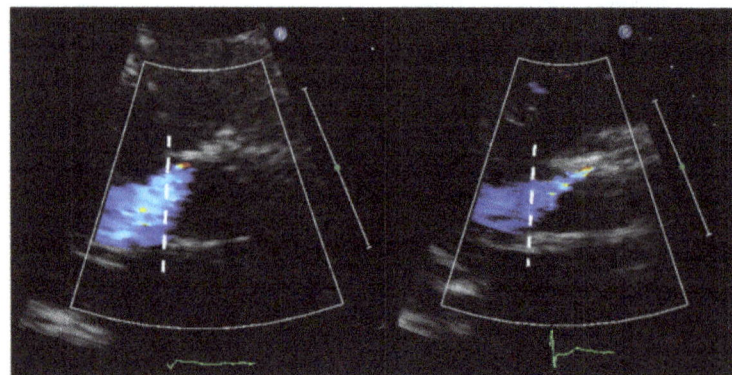

Fig. 6 Two examples of eccentric PVL jets spreading out in all directions into the inflow area of the stent frame as seen in a parasternal long-axis view. Recording an image just below the stent frame (see dashed line) as recommended in the VARC publication will not show the "origin" or "neck" of the jet

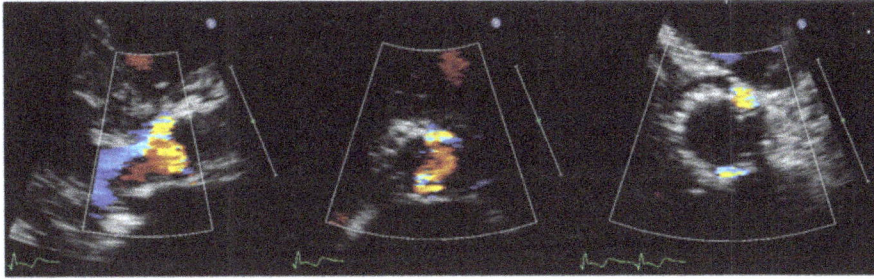

Fig. 7 Parasternal long-axis showing two jets (*left*). Short-axis colour Doppler evaluation of PVL should start just below the valve stent (*middle*) *but should always be followed by* scanning more cranial to better detect the "origin" or "neck" of the PVL (*right*)

jet will be directed towards the transducer (positive velocity on Doppler) and a blue jet will be directed away from the transducer, (negative velocity on Doppler). Problematic may, however, be that these low-velocity jets may contain less volume compared to a high-velocity jet giving an extra dimension to the difficulty in assessment of PVL severity. Another problem in eccentric jets that pass the stent frame is that occasionally they run a course into but directly next to the inflow part of the stent frame, giving the impression of a jet with an extensive circumferential area (Fig. 9). Again, the jet circumferential extent should be estimated by extrapolating the radial extent of the jet onto the circumference of the stent.

Even more challenging may be the identification of parts of the jet in the SAX view that are actually not representative for the circumferential extent because the jet follows a (partly) circumferential course (Fig. 10). In such cases the circumferential extent of the PVL may be overestimated by giving in a SAX analysis the impression of an extensive jet. It is our practice to focus measurement on the mosaic part of the jet (Fig. 10). Typically red (jet directed towards the transducer, positive velocity on Doppler) or blue (jet directed away form the transducer, negative velocity on Doppler) parts are discarded. This should also be done in jets flying away from the stent (Fig. 10).

Other problems in variability in jet numbers, localization and size

Another pitfall associated with the level of SAX imaging is the moment to measure the diastolic PVL because of the through-plane motion of the CoreValve prosthesis. In a normal contractile heart the longitudinal-orientated cardiac fibres of the heart cause the base of the heart to move towards the apex in systole whereas in diastole the reverse will occur: a motion of the base of the heart

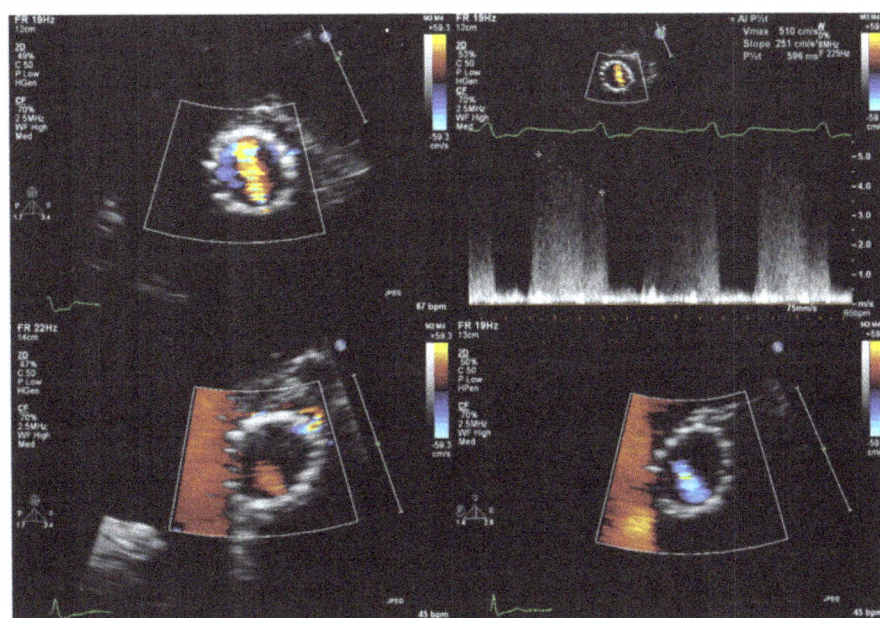

Fig. 8 The origin of the PVL jet may be identified by Doppler imaging (*top images*) or the colour of the jet: red jet moving towards the transducer (*left, bottom image*) and blue jet moving away from the transducer (*right, bottom image*)

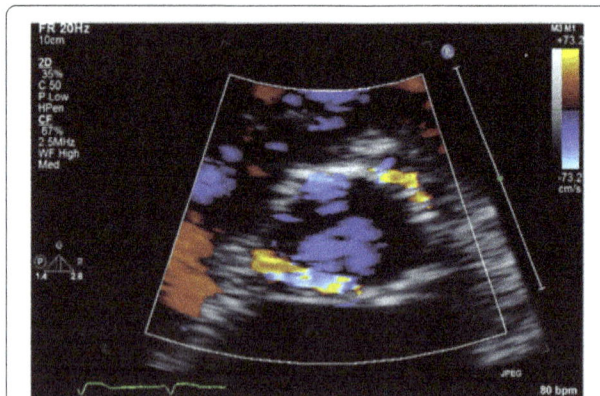

Fig. 9 An extremely eccentric jet crossing the stent frame and mimicking a jet with an extensive circumferential extent. Note that it is actually a high velocity jet with a direction ("flying") independent of the stent shape

away from the apex [15]. Since the transducer is in a fixed position it means that in early diastole a relatively small jet may be captured but later in diastole maybe more colours are picked up because it represents a more distal level of the jet when it has spread in radial and circumferential directions (see Fig. 11). Also, the circumferential PVL extent on SAX imaging may be quite variable between cardiac beats and even within one beat independent on the longitudinal motion of the heart (Fig. 12). There is currently no recommendation on what time point in the cardiac cycle varying PVL size should be measured preferably. In our center we usually measure the third frame with visible PVL, unless this extent is clearly not representative as the average of the second to fifth frame with visible PVL (the first frame with visible PVL is always ignored because the jet is usually the smallest).

PVL jets at different locations may not only be seen in one beat but also in sequential phases of one beat or in different beats, as seen in a rocking prosthesis. This may

overestimate the true severity of PVL, although in the case of a rocking prosthesis PVL severity is likely to be severe and not overestimated [16].

In surgical prosthetic aortic valves there may be a relatively fixed relation between the circumferential extent of valve dehiscence and the actual leaking area (defined by circumferential and radial extent). Because of the different pathophysiology (surgical dehiscence versus TAVI malapposition) this relation will be less clear in TAVI patients. This may result in the patient with a paradoxically high VARC score but limited radial extent that may actually have less PVL compared to a patient with a smaller circumferential extent but truly (see discussion in previous sections on level of image acquisition) larger radial extent (Fig. 13).

A final reason for overestimation of PVL is the misinterpretation of a ventricular septal rupture after TAVI as PVL (Fig. 14) [17]. Careful colour and velocity Doppler imaging may easily differentiate between PVL and ventricular septal rupture.

Limitations of our observations

In this paper the focus was on PVL after TAVI. Evaluating the presence and severity of AR should obviously include an assessment of both valvular and paravalvular components, with finally a combined measurement of 'total' AR reflecting the total volume load imposed on the LV. At current follow-up duration significant valvular AR is rare; in our institute it is present in a small minority of patients, and constitutes usually only a trace, with more than mild AR seen in the presented series in only a few patients with a not well deployed stent. However, with longer follow-up duration valvular AR will undoubtedly make the assessment of AR severity even more complex.

We reported only on our experience with the CoreValve Revalving System©, because our Edwards SAPIEN™ cohort is too small to provide a meaningful analysis. To what extent the described problems may occur in the Edwards SAPIEN™ prosthesis or other, newer percutaneous aortic valves should be evaluated - and compared to the

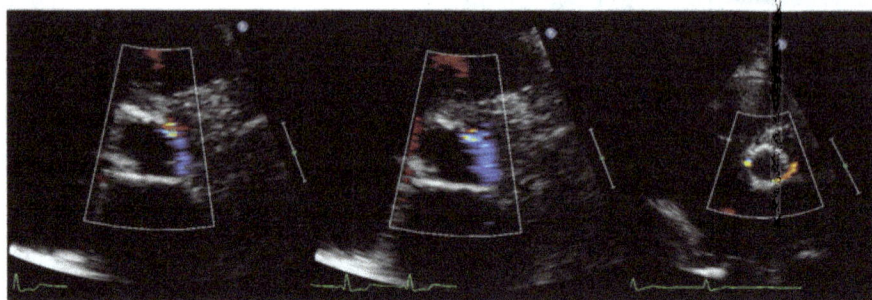

Fig. 10 Overestimation of circumferential extent because the jet seems to follow a (partly) circumferential course. Left two images showing partly mosaic coloured jet and partly blue coloured. The jet presumably runs a circumferential course and the blue parts should be not regarded as circumferential extent. Left image shows a jet flying away from the stent, similarly the red parts should not be measured

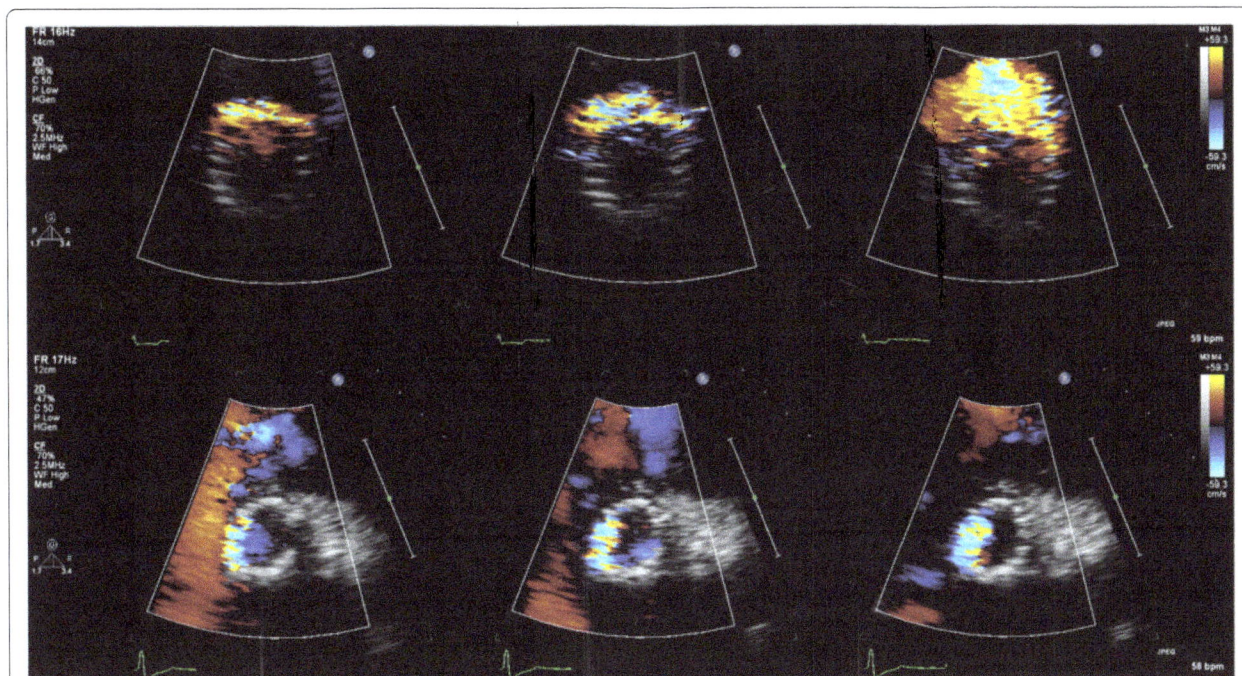

Fig. 11 The circumferential PVL extent on SAX imaging may be quite variable within one beat dependent on the longitudinal motion of the heart

CoreValve Revalving System© - in future studies. Some of the discussed limitations (acoustic shadowing, imaging level) may be generalizable, whereas others may be more specific for the CoreValve Revalving System©. Of note, comparative papers on PVL severity between different percutaneous valves should be interpreted with caution. Comparing results from centres implanting different prostheses are significantly influenced by operator dependent PVL recordings and measurements with unknown inter-observer and inter-institutional variability. Comparing the performance of two different prostheses in one single centre should take in consideration patient/prosthesis selection bias. In our center the Edwards Sapien prosthesis is used mainly in patients with known conduction abnormalities (pre-existing right bundle branch block) or a sigmoid interventricular septum, and the latter may be predisposing to a higher incidence of PVL [12].

Clinical implications and future perspectives

Studies that tried to predict the occurrence of PVL almost invariably divided PVL into less or more than mild. The methods to do so varied from abandoned echocardiographic methods to "according to VARC criteria". Even the last method is acknowledged by the VARC authors to be "not well-validated" [8] and is prone to important limitations as described in this paper and by Pibarot et al. [10]. The high variability in the incidence of more than mild PVL in CoreValve specific studies (15 % to 34 %) [12, 18] and the variable correlation with angiography and magnetic resonance imaging [19] may be in part explained by the limitations in PVL assessment. Similarly, studies that related PVL to mortality should therefore also be interpreted with caution [3].

In our opinion there are several ways to improve echocardiographic assessment of PVL severity. Most importantly,

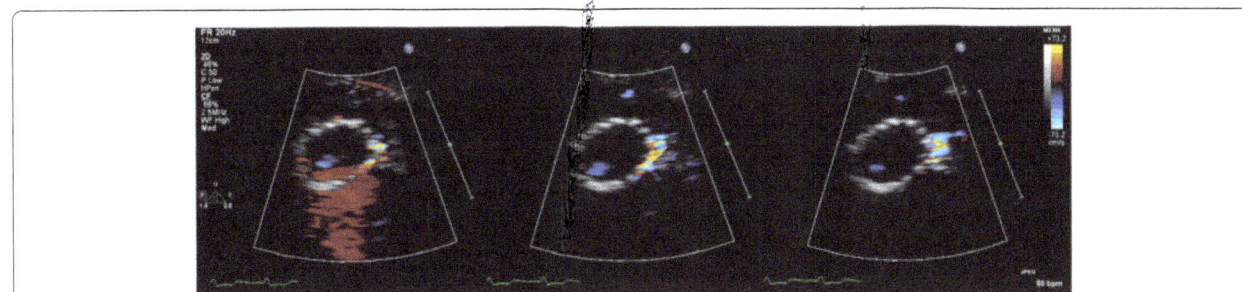

Fig. 12 Variable circumferential PVL extent within one beat independent on the longitudinal motion of the heart

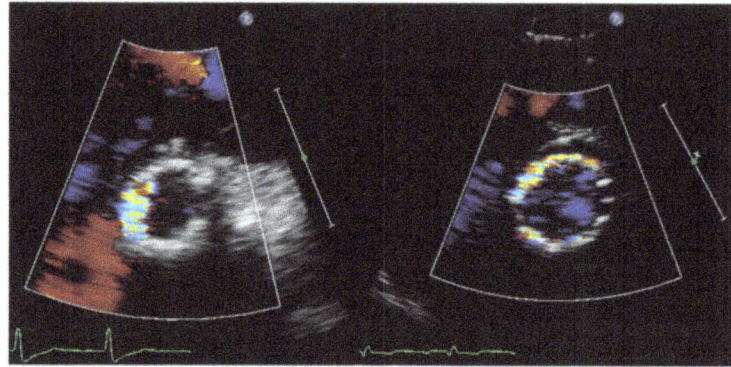

Fig. 13 Severity of PVL assessed by circumferential versus radial extent. Left image shows a VARC score of 24 % versus right image 45 %. In contrast, the "area" of leakage is 1,23 cm^2 versus 1,00 cm^2, respectively

sonographers and physicians should be aware of all the limitations of PVL assessment as described in this article and the final estimation of PVL severity should always integrate clinical data (symptoms and signs like the pulse-pressure and the Duroziez sign) with echocardiographic data (not only based on the circumferential extent but also on measures like the pressure half-time and backflow in the descending thoracic or abdominal aorta, although the value of these measurements in TAVI patients is not well established). In the future there are several ways to go:

- Use of a quantitative score model that incorporates apart from the SAX circumferential extent of PVL

also the radial extent and measurements from standard apical views. These latter views may provide additional information, and in the TAVI population apical views are usually of better quality. Of note, in the apical views the exit of the PVL is seen without interference of the stent, because the latter is positioned deeper in the scan sector. Such a score was recently proposed by Pibarot et al. [10] - The role of 2D transesophageal echocardiography (usually well tolerated by the elderly) should be explored further because of its superior quality compared to transthoracic echocardiography.

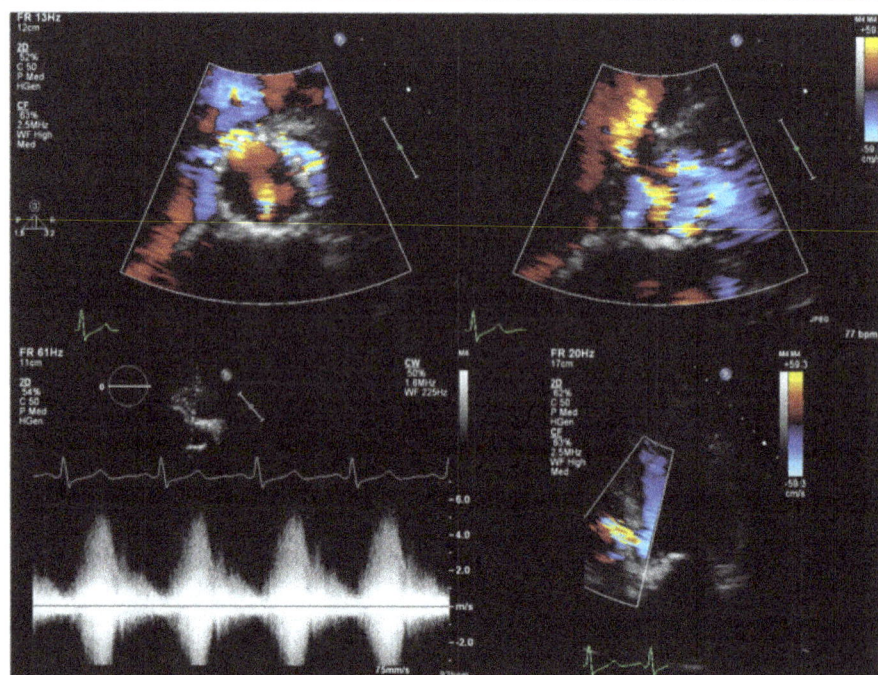

Fig. 14 Ventricular septal rupture after CoreValve implantation mimicking PVL

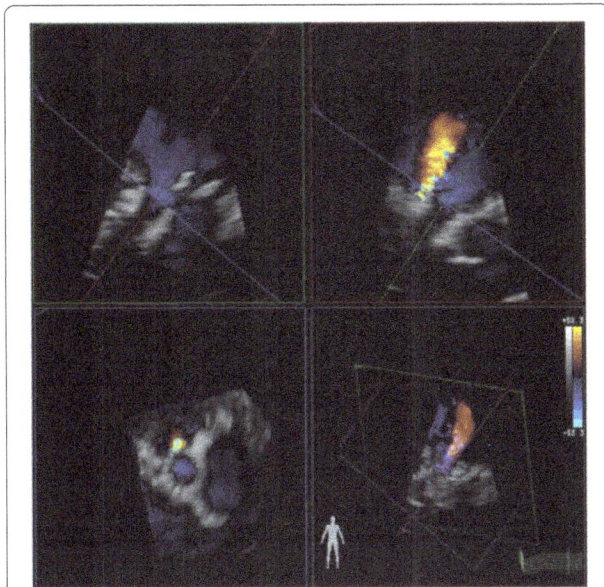

Fig. 15 Assessment of the neck of PVL with three dimensional echocardiography

– 3D colour flow imaging (Fig. 15) has by some been advocated as an accurate method to measure the vena contract of the PVL by imaging the SAX in a true perpendicular manner and imaging at the right level the "neck" of the PVL jet [20]. In our experience, the contribution of transthoracic 3D echocardiography to address the circumferential extent is rather low because of the lesser spatial (and temporal) resolution and the non-existence of a well-described neck in some patients. The role of 3D transesophageal echocardiography should be certainly explored further because of the better spatial resolution.

– Newly developed I-Rotate transducers do allow a full electronic rotation of 360° (adjustable by 5° steps) around the CoreValve prosthesis with excellent spatial and temporal resolution [21]. Similarly as studying the PVL extent of a mitral prosthesis with transesophageal echocardiography it may now be possible to study the PVL extent of a TAVI prosthesis by use of I-rotate colour Doppler in apical views, so avoiding interference with imaging of PVL jets by crushed native material or the stent (Fig. 16).

Conclusion

The transthoracic echocardiographic SAX analysis of PVL is prone to important limitations and difficulties that may result in overestimation or underestimation of PVL severity. Future guidelines should incorporate these limitations and provide clear advices how to deal with them, in particular in case of eccentric jets and variability in jet size.

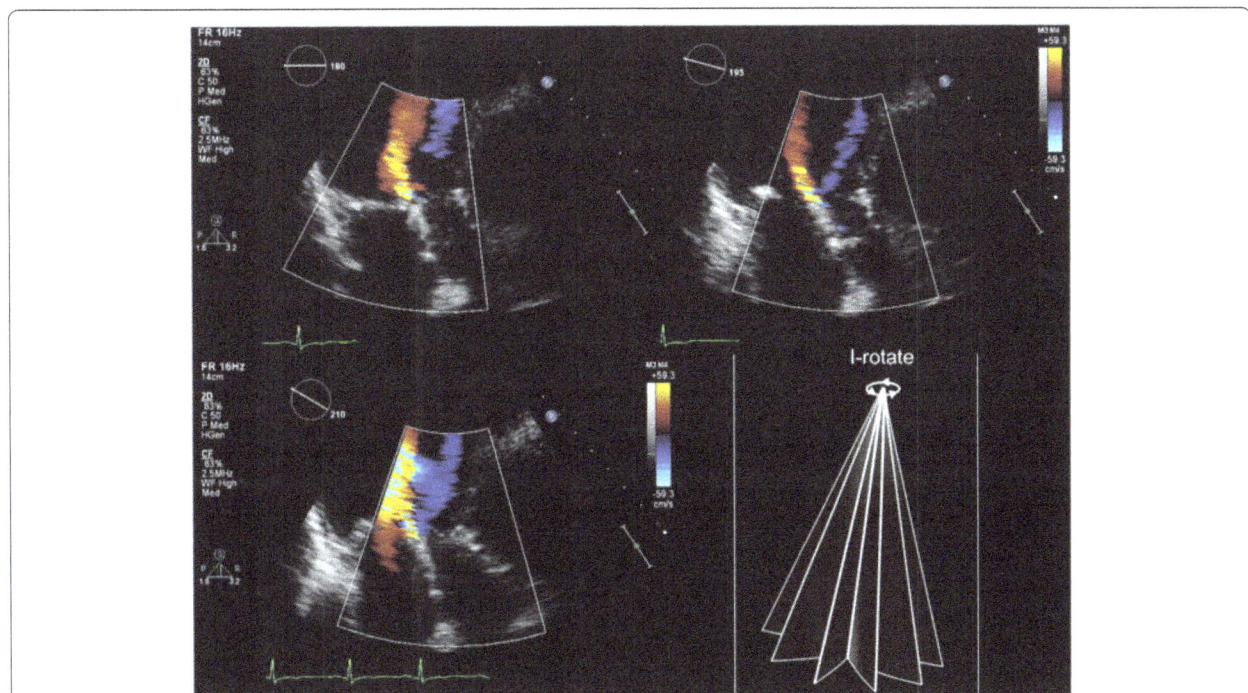

Fig. 16 I-Rotate imaging in an apical window of PVL seen in a CoreValve prosthesis. Colour Doppler images are acquired at 15 degrees intervals

Acknowledgements
None.

Funding
There are no sources of funding.

Authors' contributions
ML and OS conceived the study idea, performed data analysis and interpretation, and drafted the manuscript. All other authors reviewed and edited the manuscript. All authors read and approved the final manuscript.

Competing interests
The authors declare that they have no competing interests.

Author details
[1]From the department of Cardiology, Thoraxcenter, Erasmus University Medical Center, Thoraxcenter, Ba304, 's-Gravendijkwal 230, 3015, CE, Rotterdam, The Netherlands. [2]From the department of Cardiology, Ospedali Riuniti, Università degli Studi di Foggia, Foggia, Italy. [3]From the Cardialysis Cardiovascular Core Laboratory, Rotterdam, The Netherlands.

References

1. Leon MB, Smith CR, Mack M, Miller DC, Moses JW, Svensson LG, et al. Transcatheter aortic-valve implantation for aortic stenosis in patients who cannot undergo surgery. N Engl J Med. 2010;363:1597–607.
2. Smith CR, Leon MB, Mack MJ, Miller DC, Moses JW, Svensson LG, et al. Transcatheter versus surgical aortic-valve replacement in high-risk patients. N Engl J Med. 2011;364:2187–98.
3. Kodali SK, Williams MR, Smith CR, Svensson LG, Webb JG, Makkar RR, et al. Two-year outcomes after transcatheter or surgical aortic-valve replacement. N Engl J Med. 2012;366:1686–95.
4. Lancellotti P, Moura L, Pierard LA, Agricola E, Popescu BA, Tribouilloy C, et al. European Association of Echocardiography recommendations for the assessment of valvular regurgitation. Part 2: mitral and tricuspid regurgitation (native valve disease). Eur J Echocardiogr. 2010;11:307–32.
5. Zoghbi WA, Chambers JB, Dumesnil JG, Foster E, Gottdiener JS, Grayburn PA, et al. Recommendations for evaluation of prosthetic valves with echocardiography and doppler ultrasound: a report From the American Society of Echocardiography's Guidelines and Standards Committee and the Task Force on Prosthetic Valves, developed in conjunction with the American College of Cardiology Cardiovascular Imaging Committee, Cardiac Imaging Committee of the American Heart Association, the European Association of Echocardiography, a registered branch of the European Society of Cardiology, the Japanese Society of Echocardiography and the Canadian Society of Echocardiography, endorsed by the American College of Cardiology Foundation, American Heart Association, European Association of Echocardiography, a registered branch of the European Society of Cardiology, the Japanese Society of Echocardiography, and Canadian Society of Echocardiography. J Am Soc Echocardiogr. 2009;22:975–1014. quiz 82-4.
6. Zamorano JL, Badano LP, Bruce C, Chan KL, Goncalves A, Hahn RT, et al. EAE/ASE recommendations for the use of echocardiography in new transcatheter interventions for valvular heart disease. J Am Soc Echocardiogr. 2011;24:937–65.
7. Leon MB, Piazza N, Nikolsky E, Blackstone EH, Cutlip DE, Kappetein AP, et al. Standardized endpoint definitions for transcatheter aortic valve implantation clinical trials: a consensus report from the Valve Academic Research Consortium. Eur Heart J. 2011;32:205–17.
8. Kappetein AP, Head SJ, Genereux P, Piazza N, van Mieghem NM, Blackstone EH, et al. Updated standardized endpoint definitions for transcatheter aortic valve implantation: the Valve Academic Research Consortium-2 consensus document. Eur Heart J. 2012;33:2403–18.
9. Douglas PS, Waugh RA, Bloomfield G, Dunn G, Davis L, Hahn RT, et al. Implementation of echocardiography core laboratory best practices: a case study of the PARTNER I trial. J Am Soc Echocardiogr. 2013;26:348–58. e3.
10. Pibarot P, Hahn RT, Weissman NJ, Monaghan MJ. Assessment of paravalvular regurgitation following TAVR: a proposal of unifying grading scheme. JACC Cardiovasc Imaging. 2015;8:340–60.
11. Sherif MA, Abdel-Wahab M, Beurich HW, Stocker B, Zachow D, Geist V, et al. Haemodynamic evaluation of aortic regurgitation after transcatheter aortic valve implantation using cardiovascular magnetic resonance. EuroIntervention. 2011;7:57–63.
12. Sherif MA, Abdel-Wahab M, Stocker B, Geist V, Richardt D, Tolg R, et al. Anatomic and procedural predictors of paravalvular aortic regurgitation after implantation of the Medtronic CoreValve bioprosthesis. J Am Coll Cardiol. 2010;56:1623–9.
13. Schultz CJ, Tzikas A, Moelker A, Rossi A, Nuis RJ, Geleijnse MM, et al. Correlates on MSCT of paravalvular aortic regurgitation after transcatheter aortic valve implantation using the Medtronic CoreValve prosthesis. Catheter Cardiovasc Interv. 2011;78:446–55.
14. Ewe SH, Ng AC, Schuijf JD, van der Kley F, Colli A, Palmen M, et al. Location and severity of aortic valve calcium and implications for aortic regurgitation after transcatheter aortic valve implantation. Am J Cardiol. 2011;108:1470–7.
15. van Dalen BM, Bosch JG, Kauer F, Soliman OI, Vletter WB, ten Cate FJ, et al. Assessment of mitral annular velocities by speckle tracking echocardiography versus tissue Doppler imaging: validation, feasibility, and reproducibility. J Am Soc Echocardiogr. 2009;22:1302–8.
16. Jilaihawi H, Kashif M, Fontana G, Furugen A, Shiota T, Friede G, et al. Cross-sectional computed tomographic assessment improves accuracy of aortic annular sizing for transcatheter aortic valve replacement and reduces the incidence of paravalvular aortic regurgitation. J Am Coll Cardiol. 2012;59:1275–86.
17. Martinez MI, Garcia HG, Calvar JA. Interventricular septum rupture after transcatheter aortic valve replacement. Eur Heart J. 2012;33:190.
18. Sinning JM, Hammerstingl C, Vasa-Nicotera M, Adenauer V, Lema Cachiguango SJ, Scheer AC, et al. Aortic regurgitation index defines severity of peri-prosthetic regurgitation and predicts outcome in patients after transcatheter aortic valve implantation. J Am Coll Cardiol. 2012;59:1134–41.
19. Ribeiro HB, Orwat S, Hayek SS, Larose E, Babaliaros V, Dahou A, et al. Cardiovascular magnetic resonance to evaluate aortic regurgitation after transcatheter aortic valve replacement. J Am Coll Cardiol. 2016;68:577–85.
20. Goncalves A, Almeria C, Marcos-Alberca P, Feltes G, Hernandez-Antolin R, Rodriguez E, et al. Three-dimensional echocardiography in paravalvular aortic regurgitation assessment after transcatheter aortic valve implantation. J Am Soc Echocardiogr. 2012;25:47–55.
21. McGhie JS, Vletter WB, de Groot-de Laat LE, Ren B, Frowijn R, van den Bosch AE, et al. Contributions of simultaneous multiplane echocardiographic imaging in daily clinical practice. Echocardiography. 2014;31:245–54.

7

Investigation on left ventricular multi-directional deformation in patients of hypertension with different LVEF

Huimei Huang, Qinyun Ruan[*], Meiyan Lin, Lei Yan, Chunyan Huang and Liyun Fu

Abstract

Background: This study is aimed at investigating myocardial multi-directional systolic deformation in hypertensive with different left ventricular ejection fraction (LVEF), and exploring its contribution to LVEF.

Methods: One hundred and twenty-three patients with primary hypertension (HT) were divided into group A (LVEF ≥ 55%), group B (45% ≤ LVEF < 50%, or 50% ≤ LVEF < 55% + LVEDVI ≥ 97 ml/m^2), and group C (LVEF < 45%). Two-dimensional strain echocardiography (2DSE) including LV longitudinal strain (SL), radial strain (SR) and circumferential strain (SC) were measured.

Results: SL decreased gradually from group A, B to C (all $p < 0.05$) while SR and SC were reduced only in group B and C (all $p < 0.05$). All strain measurements correlated to LVEF, with the strongest correlation in SC ($r = -0.82$, $p < 0.01$) and the second in SL ($r = -0.76$). The diastolic E/e increased from group A, B to C.

Conclusions: Left ventricular multi-directional deformation correlated well to LVEF in hypertension and particularly SC, indicating that it was SC, not SL or SR, that makes the prominent contribution to left ventricular pump function.

Keywords: Hypertension, Heart failure, Myocardial contraction, Left ventricular ejection fraction, Strain, Echocardiography

Background

Heart failure with preserved ejection fraction (HFpEF) and heart failure with reduced EF (HFrEF) may be different stages of the identical disease [1]. Studies in patients of HFpEF revealed a general trend of a decrease in left ventricular ejection fraction (LVEF) although it remains in "normal range". In addition, there are abnormalities in other indices of left ventricular (LV) systolic function such as systolic mitral annulus velocity and displacement, LV myocardial strain and strain rate obtained by tissue doppler imaging (TDI) and 2-dimensional strain echocardiography (2DSE) [2–5]. Previous work including the one we conducted have shown a depressed LV longitudinal strain in the early stages of hypertensive LV remodeling (concentric remodeling and concentric hypertrophy) [6, 7]. Impaired LV longitudinal strain

occurs in some patients with hypertension and normal LVEF in the absence of heart failure [8]. However, with the progression of LV dysfunction, the characteristic of myocardial deformations in all directions is unknown. This study aimed to investigate myocardial multi-directional strain in hypertensive patients with normal, borderline and reduced left ventricular ejection fraction (LVEF), thus to explore the contribution of myocardial multi-directional deformation to LVEF.

Method

Study population

According to 2007 Guidelines for the management of arterial hypertension [9], hypertension was defined as systolic blood pressure ≥ 140 mmHg or diastolic blood pressure ≥ 90 mmHg. Inclusion criteria: One hundred and twenty-three patients (from October 2014 to October 2015) who had hypertension as defined above were enrolled in. Normal controls (NC) contains 40 age

* Correspondence: qyruan@126.com
Department of Ultrasound, the First Affiliated Hospital of Fujian Medical University, Fuzhou 350005, China

and sex matched volunteers who were free of cardiovascular or systemic diseases. Patients were excluded for the following reasons: poor image quality, atrial fibrillation, known coronary artery disease, regional wall motion abnormality in left ventricle, idiopathic cardiomyopathy, congenital heart disease, chest distress, exertional angina pectoris. According to LVEF, the subjects were divided into two groups: hypertension with normal LVEF (HT-NEF, LVEF $\geq$ 50%) and hypertension with reduced LVEF (HT-REF, LVEF < 50%). In order to investigate a "borderline" state, all the subjects were further divided into three sub-groups: group A, normal LVEF and LV end diastolic volume index (LVEF $\geq$ 55%, LVEDVI < 97 ml/m^2); group B, "borderline" LVEF and enlarged LV end diastolic volume index (45% $\leq$ LVEF < 50%, or 50% $\leq$ LVEF < 55% + LVEDVI $\geq$ 97 ml/m^2) and group C, reduced LVEF (LVEF < 45%).

Conventional Echocardiographic study

Echocardiography was performed in participants using GE VIVID E9 or GE VIVID E7 ultrasound scanner (GE Vingmed Ultrasound, Horten, Norway) with GE VIVID E9 or GE VIVID E7 probe (1.7-4.0 MHz). Conventional scans were acquired in standard left ventricular long axis, short axis and apical views. For parasternal short-axis views, three levels of LV were acquired, which were basal level, papillary muscle level and apical level. All echocardiographic measurements were averaged on three heart beats. Left ventricular ejection fraction (LVEF), left ventricular end-diastolic volume (LVEDV) and left atrial volume (LAV) were obtained by area-length method in standard apical views (biplane). Left ventricular internal dimension at end diastole and end systole (LVIDd, LVIDs), posterior wall thickness (LVPWT), septal thickness (IVST) and left atrial diameter (LAD) were acquired in parasternal long axis views. Left ventricular mass (LVM) was calculated based on the recently published guidelines [10]. LVEDV, LAV and LVM were indexed to body surface area (BSA). E/A ratio were measured from mitral inflow (measured at the tips of the mitral valve), peak early (E) and late (A) filling velocities. Tissue Doppler was applied at end-expiration in the pulsed-wave doppler mode at the level of the mitral annulus from an apical four-chamber view. Lateral and septal mitral annulus early diastolic velocities (e') were recorded and averaged to derive E/e' ratio. LV hypertrophy was defined as an LVMI $\geq$ 125 g/m^2 for men and LVMI $\geq$ 110 g/m^2 for women [9]. LV enlargement [10] was defined as an LVEDVI $\geq$ 97 ml/m^2.

LV systolic strain measurements by 2DSE

Myocardial strain measurements were performed using 2DSE [11–13]. The analysis was performed offline using commercial software (EchoPAC Software, version 113, General Electric Company, Horten, Norway). To optimize speckle tracking, 2D gray-scale harmonic images were obtained at a frame rate of >50 frames/s. In above software, myocardial deformation measurements were performed using tissue speckle tracking and the displacement of speckles of myocardium in each spot was analyzed and tracked frame by frame. After manual tracing of the endocardial border of the end-systolic frame and selecting the appropriate region of interest, i.e. the width of the region of interest was adjusted to fit the wall thickness as required, the software automatically determined six segments in each view. Each segmental strain curve was obtained by automatic frame-by-frame tracking of the acoustic markers in the myocardial tissue. The tracking quality was scored as either acceptable or unacceptable. For each subject, longitudinal strain values for all six LV myocardial segments in each of the apical four-chamber views were measured and averaged to derive the global LV longitudinal strain (SL). Circumferential and radial strain values were obtained in all 18 segments at the level of the three short-axis views. The average of peak systolic circumferential or radial strain values from the three short-axis views was calculated to derive global LV circumferential strain and radial strain (SC, SR). All the measurements were performed in triplicate and averaged from three regular heart beats. Segments with obvious bias tracking were excluded from the analysis.

Interobserver and Intraobserver variability

Ten patients were randomly-selected to assess interobserver and intraobserver variability in strain measurements. The interobserver variability was calculated as the SD of the difference between the measurements of two independent observers who were blinded to all other patient's data and expressed as a percent of the average value. The intraobserver variability was calculated as the SD of the difference between the first and second measurements by the same observer at 1-week interval and expressed as a percent of the average value.

Statistical analysis

Continuous data were presented as mean ± standard deviation (SD) or as percentages where appropriate. Comparisons among multiple groups was performed with one-way ANOVA if the data were normally distributed; otherwise, one-way ANOVA on ranks if the data distribution was not normal. Categorical variables were analyzed using χ^2 test, and Fisher's exact tests were used when appropriate. Pearson's correlation analysis was used to study the relation between two continuous variables. SPSS version 15 (IBM Corporation, Armonk, NY) was deployed to perform the majority of the statistical operations, where a p value less than 0.05 was considered statistically significant.

Results

Clinical characteristics and Echocardiographic measurements in HT

There was no difference in terms of age or sex among all patients groups and normal controls ($p > 0.05$), as shown in Table 1.

Besides reduced LVEF, patients in group HT-REF had lower annular systolic velocity and higher LAVI, LVIDd, LVMI, LVEDVI ($p < 0.05$); early diastolic e' velocity decreased and E/e' ratio increased progressively from NC to group HT-NEF and HT-REF (for each $p < 0.05$ in Table 1); there were no differences between group HT-NEF and NC in all strain measurements except that SL

decreased significantly, while all the strain measurements were significantly lower in group HT-REF compared to group HT-NEF ($p < 0.05$, Table 2).

Echocardiographic measurements in three HT sub-groups

Dilated LV and LA and increased LVMI appeared in all sub-groups with a progression from group A, B to C along with a diastolic in e' velocity and an increase in E/e' ratio. All the strain measurements except for apical SR showed a downward trend from group A, B to C, where SL was impaired in group A and was further impaired in group B and C. SC and SR were impaired in group B and C (all $p < 0.05$, Table 3, Fig. 1).

Table 1 Clinical characteristics and conventional echocardiographic measurements in hypertensive

	NC	HT-NEF (LVEF ≥ 50%)	HT-REF (LVEF < 50%)
	$n = 40$	$n = 81$	$n = 42$
Age(y)	53.75 ± 11.72	57.25 ± 11.70	57.55 ± 14.69
Gender(M/F)	26/14	60/21	36/6
LBBB/RBBB(n)	0	3	6
PAB(n)	0	3	1
PVB(n)	0	2	2
Abnormal blood lipid or DM(n)	0	2	10[△▲]
Renal dysfunction(n)	0	4	3
HR(beats/min)	67.60 ± 10.17	69.35 ± 11.90	78.33 ± 15.47[△▲]
SBP(mmHg)	122.48 ± 13.66	151.30 ± 19.91[△]	145.37 ± 25.80[△]
DBP(mmHg)	78.14 ± 10.44	88.48 ± 13.64[△]	89.11 ± 14.56[△]
LVIDd(cm)	4.70 ± 0.28	5.20 ± 0.56[△]	5.98 ± 0.86[△▲]
IVST (cm)	0.87 ± 0.12	1.19 ± 0.30[△]	1.22 ± 0.31[△]
LVPWT(cm)	0.76 ± 0.09	1.02 ± 0.21[△]	1.08 ± 0.24[△]
RWT	0.35 ± 0.04	0.43 ± 0.10[△]	0.40 ± 0.12
LVMI(g/m²)	76.41 ± 10.74	131.79 ± 44.35[△]	175.77 ± 49.84[△▲]
LAD(cm)	3.17 ± 0.59	3.97 ± 0.57[△]	4.39 ± 0.65[△▲]
LAVI(ml/ m²)	23.05 ± 8.69	31.72 ± 9.67[△]	40.01 ± 17.20[△▲]
FS(%)	34.29 ± 3.47	34.59 ± 4.25	18.43 ± 5.10[△▲]
LVEDVI(ml/ m²)	62.45 ± 8.60	76.14 ± 16.24[△]	109.06 ± 40.15[△▲]
LVEF(%)	62.56 ± 4.61	61.37 ± 5.20	37.30 ± 8.37[△▲]
PVA(m/s)	0.62 ± 0.20	0.77 ± 0.21[△]	0.70 ± 0.26
PVE(m/s)	0.64 ± 0.21	0.65 ± 0.21	0.73 ± 0.29
E/A	1.08 ± 0.39	0.96 ± 0.78	1.28 ± 0.90[▲]
E/e	7.53 ± 2.39	11.12 ± 4.16[△]	17.07 ± 11.20[△▲]
s(m/s)	0.07 ± 0.01	0.07 ± 0.03	0.05 ± 0.02[△▲]
a(m/s)	0.09 ± 0.02	0.09 ± 0.05	0.07 ± 0.08[▲]
e(m/s)	0.09 ± 0.03	0.07 ± 0.06[△]	0.05 ± 0.02[△▲]

Data are expressed as mean ± standard deviation (SD) or as number (ratio);

NC normal controls, *LVEF* left ventricular ejection fraction, *HT-NEF* hypertension with normal, *LVEF; HT-REF* hypertension with reduced LVEF, *HT* hypertension, *LBBB* left bundle branch block, *RBBB* right bundle branch block, *PAB* occasional premature atrial beats, *PVB* occasional premature ventricular beats, *DM* diabetes mellitus, *HR* heart rate, *SBP* systolic blood pressure, *DBP* diastolic blood pressure, *LVIDd* Left ventricular internal dimension in diastole, *IVST* Interventricular septal thickness, *LVPWT* Left ventricular posterior wall thickness, *RWT* Relative wall thickness, *LVM* Left ventricular mass, *LVMI* Left ventricular mass index, *LAD* Left atrial diameter, *LAVI* LA volume index, *FS* Fractional shortening, *LVEDVI* Left ventricular end-diastolic volume index, *LVEF* Left ventricular ejection fraction;

[△]:$p < 0.05$ vs NC group; [▲]:$p < 0.05$ vs group HT-NEF

Table 2 LV strain measurements in group HT-NEF and HT-REF

	NC	HT-NEF (LVEF ≥ 50%)	HT-REF (LVEF < 50%)
	$n = 40$	$n = 81$	$n = 42$
SL(%)	−20.16 ± 2.75	−18.27 ± 3.74$^\triangle$	−11.34 ± 3.85$^{\triangle\blacktriangle}$
SC-mv(%)	−18.31 ± 2.91	−17.54 ± 3.60	−10.54 ± 3.59$^{\triangle\blacktriangle}$
SC-pm(%)	−18.01 ± 2.79	−18.14 ± 3.02	−11.09 ± 4.12$^{\triangle\blacktriangle}$
SC-ap(%)	−21.37 ± 14.71	−23.01 ± 6.96	−15.01 ± 6.65$^{\triangle\blacktriangle}$
SR-mv(%)	43.99 ± 19.47	40.69 ± 14.48	20.42 ± 8.61$^{\triangle\blacktriangle}$
SR-pm(%)	42.75 ± 18.53	46.90 ± 16.95	22.83 ± 12.66$^{\triangle\blacktriangle}$
SR-ap(%)	22.84 ± 17.10	19.78 ± 17.22	11.94 ± 8.17$^{\triangle\blacktriangle}$

Data expressed as mean ± standard deviation (SD); *LV* left ventricular, *NC* normal controls, *LVEF* left ventricular ejection fraction, *HT-NEF* hypertension with normal LVEF, *HT-REF* hypertension with reduced LVEF, *SL* longitudinal strain, *SC* circumferential strain, *SR* radial strain; −mv, −pm, −ap indicates basal level, papillary and apical level;
$^\triangle p < 0.05$ vs NC; $^\blacktriangle p < 0.05$ vs group HT-NEF

Correlation analysis of strains with LVEF

We analyzed the correlations of systolic multi-directional strain with LVEF and found a good connection in all strains, where the correlation coefficients in SC, SL and SR were −0.82, −0.76 and 0.70 respectively in Fig. 2.

Discussion

In the present study, we compared the difference of LV multi-directional strain among patients in three different levels of LVEF, and investigated the correlation and

Table 3 Clinical characteristics and echocardiographic measurements of three sub-groups

	group A	group B	group C
	$n = 71$	$n = 13$	$n = 34$
Age(y)	57.99 ± 11.94	56.31 ± 14.07	57.62 ± 14.42
Gender(M/F)	53/18	11/2	28/6
HR(beats/min)	69.54 ± 11.97	66.92 ± 9.67	80.50 ± 15.81$^{\triangle\blacktriangle\star}$
LVIDd(cm)	5.17 ± 0.56$^\triangle$	5.61 ± 0.47$^{\triangle\blacktriangle}$	6.10 ± 0.88$^{\triangle\blacktriangle\star}$
RWT	0.44 ± 0.10$^\triangle$	0.41 ± 0.11	0.38 ± 0.12$^\blacktriangle$
LVEDVI(ml/ m^2)	74.61 ± 15.56$^\triangle$	91.14 ± 19.56$^{\triangle\blacktriangle}$	114.97 ± 41.34$^{\triangle\blacktriangle\star}$
LVMI(g/ m^2)	132.09 ± 44.70$^\triangle$	151.45 ± 42.37$^\triangle$	181.44 ± 51.20$^{\triangle\blacktriangle\star}$
LAD(cm)	3.99 ± 0.56$^\triangle$	4.11 ± 0.66$^\triangle$	4.45 ± 0.64$^{\triangle\blacktriangle\star}$
LAVI(ml/m^2)	31.33 ± 9.19$^\triangle$	31.91 ± 9.76$^\triangle$	42.69 ± 17.71$^{\triangle\blacktriangle\star}$
LVEF(%)	62.65 ± 4.14	49.45 ± 2.51$^{\triangle\blacktriangle}$	34.79 ± 7.24$^{\triangle\blacktriangle\star}$
s(m/s)	0.07 ± 0.03	0.06 ± 0.02	0.05 ± 0.02$^{\triangle\blacktriangle}$
E/e	11.13 ± 4.17$^\triangle$	11.19 ± 3.79	18.76 ± 11.78$^{\triangle\blacktriangle\star}$
e(m/s)	0.07 ± 0.06	0.06 ± 0.03$^\triangle$	0.05 ± 0.02$^{\triangle\blacktriangle}$

Data are expressed as mean ± standard deviation (SD) or as number (ratio); *HR* heart rate, *LVIDd* Left ventricular internal dimension in diastole, *RWT* Relative wall thickness, *LVEDVI* Left ventricular end-diastolic volume index, *LVMI* Left ventricular mass index, *LAD* Left atrial diameter, *LAVI* LA volume index, *LVEF* Left ventricular ejection fraction; the data of normal controls (NC) see Table one; group A, normal LVEF and LV end diastolic volume index, group B, "borderline" LVEF and enlarged LV end diastolic volume index, group C, reduced LVEF (LVEF < 45%). $^\triangle p < 0.05$ vs NC; $^\blacktriangle p < 0.05$ vs group A; $^\star p < 0.05$ group B

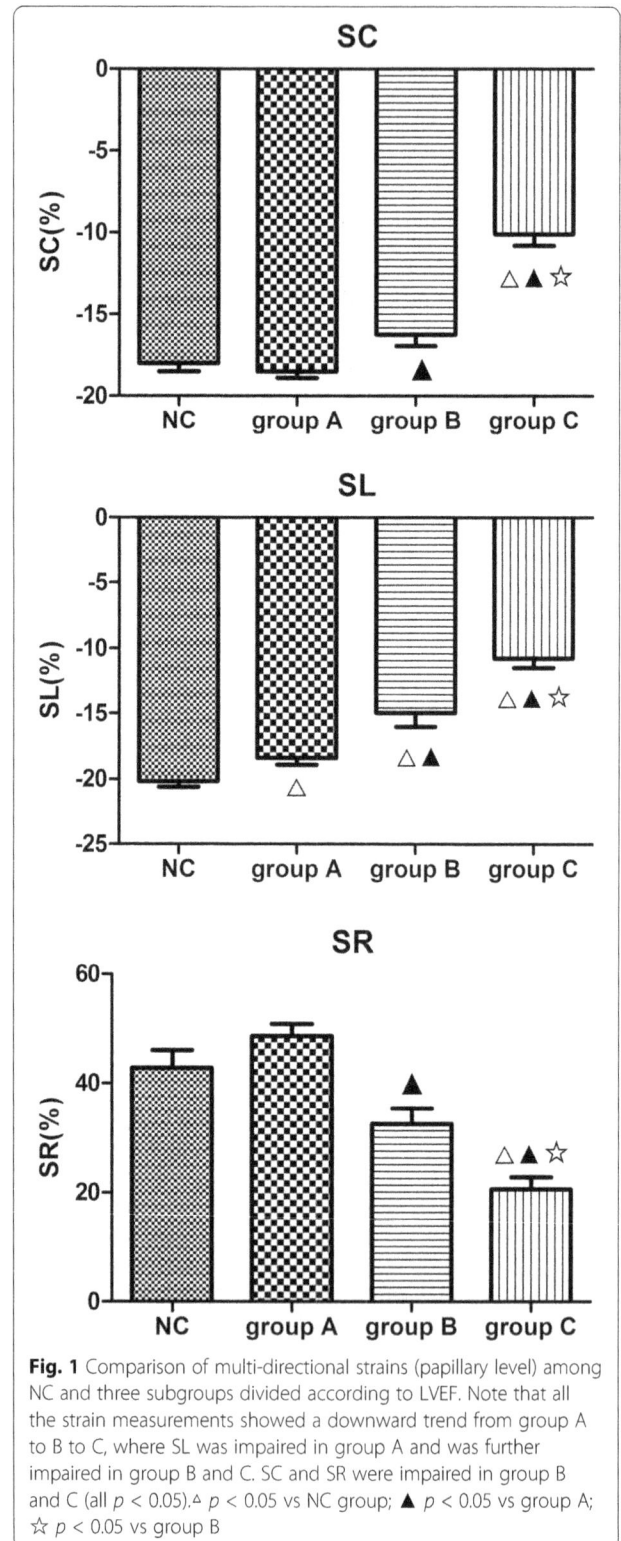

Fig. 1 Comparison of multi-directional strains (papillary level) among NC and three subgroups divided according to LVEF. Note that all the strain measurements showed a downward trend from group A to B to C, where SL was impaired in group A and was further impaired in group B and C. SC and SR were impaired in group B and C (all $p < 0.05$).$^\triangle$ $p < 0.05$ vs NC group; $^\blacktriangle$ $p < 0.05$ vs group A; * $p < 0.05$ vs group B

contribution of strain in each direction to global pump function, providing a continuous trend of LV performance in the progression of cardiac dysfunction in hypertension. The major findings were, (1) SL decreased early

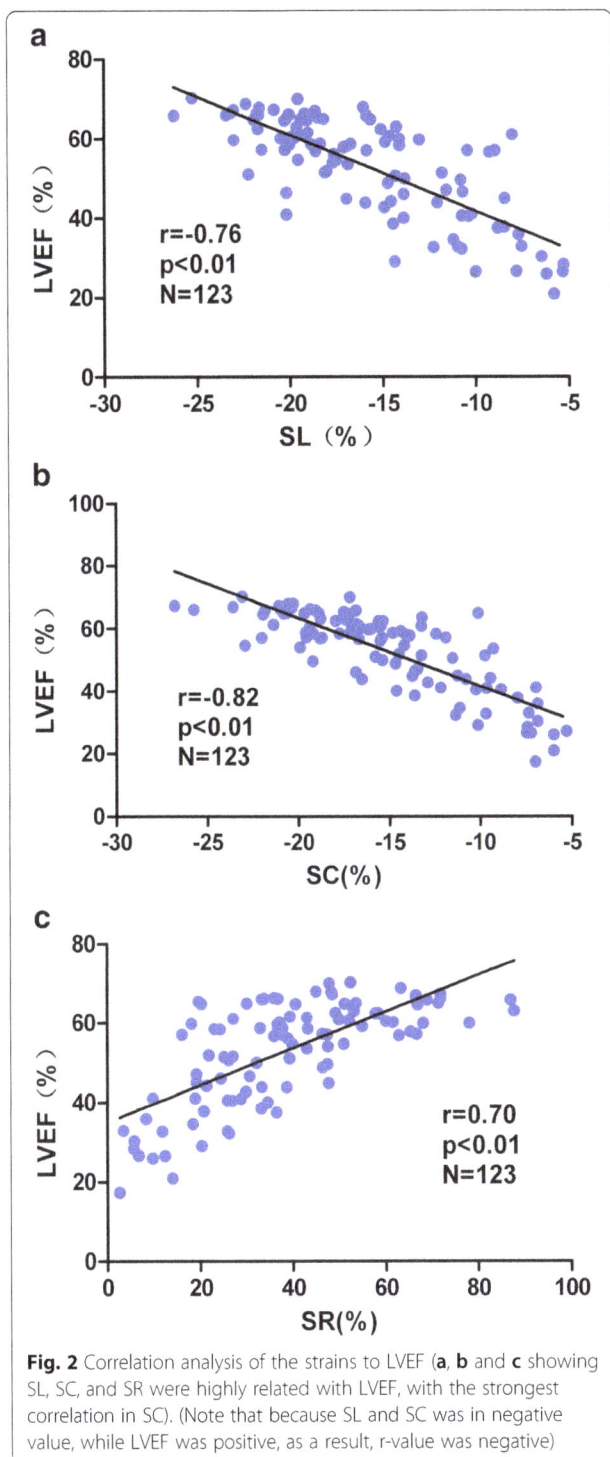

Fig. 2 Correlation analysis of the strains to LVEF (**a**, **b** and **c** showing SL, SC, and SR were highly related with LVEF, with the strongest correlation in SC). (Note that because SL and SC was in negative value, while LVEF was positive, as a result, r-value was negative)

Left ventricular remodeling and function in hypertension

LVMI, LVEDVI and LAVI increased from group A, B to C. With the decrease of LVEF, annular e' decreased together with s', and E/e' ratio increased. These results indicate that as the LV remodeling takes place, systolic performance is impaired together with diastolic dysfunction, which is in accordance with previous findings. In the progression from HFpEF to HFrEF, systolic dysfunction appeared while diastolic function deteriorated [3, 14]. HFpEF and HFrEF have similar pathophysiologic characteristics [14]. Biopsy of human myocardial tissue also showed HFpEF and HFrEF were injured to different degrees [15, 16], indicating that LV systolic and diastolic dysfunction are a continuous process, or two different stages in the progression of cardiac dysfunction [3].

Left ventricular myocardial multi-directional deformation in hypertension

Longitudinal strain (SL)

Similar to several former studies, we found SL decreased in the early stage of hypertensive heart failure. Kosmala et al. found SL firstly reduced in NYHA I-II, and became lower as the cardiac function deteriorated [17]. Reduced SC, SR appeared only in NYHA III-IV. Another study reported impaired SL and SR in HFpEF [12].

Radial strain (SR)

We found SR was preserved or even increased slightly in early stage of hypertensive heart disease with normal LVEF and decreased in later stages (borderline and reduced LVEF). In the early stage of remodeling (concentric remodeling), or before left ventricular function is significantly impaired, SR is preserved or increased in compensation for the decrease in SL [6, 17]. As observed in the present study, the increased SR may be considered as a compensation for the impaired SL in early stage of hypertension [6]. In addition, the radius of curvature of the circumferentially oriented myocardial fibers responsible for LV radial deformation is smaller than that of longitudinal ones, which might entail lower stress and consequently delayed functional impairment caused by pressure overload [17]. SR derived from speckle tracking from endocardial to epicardial layer was not purely originated from the contraction of midwall fiber but the whole heart muscle layers, and was decreased when all heart muscle layers was injured [17–19].

Circumferential strain (SC)

The present results of SC were in accord with previous studies [6, 12, 13]: SC was preserved or slightly increased as a compensation to maintain a normal LVEF, the reduction of which may lead to a decreased LVEF. Investigation by Wang et al. had revealed that there was no difference between HFpEF and normal control in SC,

in the stage of normal LVEF, while SC and SR began to decrease in patients with "borderline" LVEF (45%-55%) and deteriorated with LVEF reduced further. (2) Systolic strains in all directions highly correlated with LVEF, with the strongest correlation in SC ($r = -0.82$), indicating that it was SC, not SL or SR making the prominent contribution to left ventricular pump function.

while distinctly lowered SC only occurred in HFrEF [12]. Kouzu et al. found there was an increasing trend of SC in concentric remodeling, but a reduction in SC in patients with concentric hypertrophy and eccentric hypertrophy [6]. As mentioned above, mid-wall myocardial fibers were not affected in early stage and thus SC was preserved.

A recent study demonstrated that heart failure with normal LVEF had a poorer SC than normal subjects [8], where "normal LVEF" was defined as >45%, and the percentage of patients with abnormal SC was only 22% in patients of LVEF > 55%, lower than that with "borderline" LVEF (as described in our present study). In that study, patients in normal LVEF group mostly had a medical history of coronary disease or myocardial infarction which may indirectly lead to a decreased SC. In our present study, subjects with coronary artery disease or myocardial infarction were excluded, and we divided all the patients into 3 subgroups according to different LVEF, and we assessed LVEF using area-length method for better analysis of the correlation between LV multi-directional strain and global LV function.

The pathophysiological mechanisms

SL was impaired first in the early stage, and deteriorated together with decreased SR and SC with the progression of hypertensive remodeling. The pathological basis of these observations likely lies in hypertension-related fibrosis and myocyte hypertrophy progressing from subendocardial layer to the epicardium [20], and the subendocardial fibers primarily affect longitudinal strain [21]. Importantly, biopsy of human myocardium shows interstitial subendocardial fibrosis in patients with HFpEF [15, 16]. With progression of disease to the mid and outer myocardial layers, circumferential, and radial strain also decline as was seen in patients with depressed LVEF.

Correlations of strains to LVEF

The present study shows a significant correlation between longitudinal, circumferential, radial strain and LVEF. Impaired SL did not appear to impact LVEF because of the compensation of myocardial fibers in the mid and subepicardial layers. In the later stages of hypertension and with LV remodeling, other components of LV strain were also impaired [22]. In our study, SC related to LVEF best among all strains. Previous studies have also shown close correlation of SC or the time to peak of SC to LVEF [23, 24]. But some reports showed better correlation of SR with LVEF in patients of dilated cardiomyopathy in adolescents [25]. When LVEF is calculated from linear formula, where the only parameter used is from LV short axis dimension, SR was more strongly correlated with

LVEF. In our study, LVEF was evaluated by area-length method, where LV stroke volume originated from the whole LV endocardial displacements caused by longitudinal, radial and circumferential systolic deformation, thus all directions of strain measurements had significant correlation with LVEF, with SC contributing more to LVEF. Geometrically, systolic SC comes from the contraction of circumferential fibers, leading to both systolic wall thickening (systolic SR) and decrease in LV diameter and volume. The preserved SC and LV twist may contribute to the normal LVEF in patients with HFpEF, and an increasing SC may be a compensatory mechanism to maintain a normal LVEF in the early stage [11, 12], and accordingly, the decrease of multi-directional deformation especially SC and the deterioration of diastolic function may lead to reduced LVEF and HFrEF.

Limitations

We used 2DSE to reconstruct a 3D LV multi-directional strain, where images were obtained from different heart beats, and some detailed real myocardial dynamic information might be lost through heart motion in the chest in a cardiac cycle. Hence, the results might be less accurate than that of using a real time three dimensional strain. Since some LV short-axis views of apical level were challenging, we did not investigate LV twist, which would also contribute to preserved LVEF. We could not acquire detailed information of patients' managements and medication of hypertension, for most of them did not have a regular management or they were not able to provide reliable records.

Conclusions

Impaired left ventricular longitudinal strain and diastolic dysfunction happened early in patients with normal LVEF in hypertension, while circumferential and radial strains were preserved or increased slightly as a compensation for the decrease in local systolic function, and when all directions of strains were impaired, LVEF decreased together with a deteriorating LV diastolic function. Left ventricular multi-directional deformation correlated well to LVEF in hypertension, particularly SC, indicating that it was SC, not SL or SR making the prominent contribution to left ventricular pump function.

Acknowledgements
Not applicable.

Funding
This study was supported by National Natural Science Foundation of China (81171360).

Authors' contributions

QR designed the study; QR and HH performed the research, HH was a major contributor in writing the manuscript. ML, LY, CH and LF participated in the acquisition of echocardiographic images and given assistance in analysis of data. All authors read and approved the final manuscript.

Competing interests

The authors declare that they have no competing interests.

References

1. Paulus WJ, Tschope C, Sanderson JE, et al. How to diagnose diastolic heart failure: a consensus statement on the diagnosis of heart failure with normal left ventricular ejection fraction by the heart failure and echocardiography associations of the European Society of Cardiology. Eur Heart J. 2007;28:2539–50.
2. Yip G, Wang M, Zhang Y, Fung JW, Ho PY, Sanderson JE. Left ventricular long axis function in diastolic heart failure is reduced in both diastole and systole: time for a redefinition? Heart. 2002;87:121–5.
3. Yu CM, Lin H, Yang H, Kong SL, Zhang Q, Lee S. Progression of systolic abnormalities in patients with "isolated" diastolic heart failure. Circulation. 2002;105:1195–201.
4. Rosen BD, Edvardsen T, Lai S, et al. Left ventricular concentric remodeling is associated with decreased global and regional systolic function: the multi-ethnic study of atherosclerosis. Circulation. 2005;112:984–91.
5. Carluccio E, Biagioli P, Alunni G, et al. Advantages of deformation indices over systolic velocities in assessment of longitudinal systolic function in patients with heart failure and normal ejection fraction. Eur J Heart Fail. 2011;13:292–302.
6. Kouzu H, Yuda S, Muranaka A, et al. Left ventricular hypertrophy causes different changes in longitudinal, radial, and circumferential mechanics in patients with hypertension: a two-dimensional speckle tracking study. J Am Soc Echocardiogr. 2011;24:192–9.
7. Lin MY, Ruan QY, Gai YY, Zeng KQ, Xie LD. Investigation on myocardial systolic multi-dimensional deformation in hypertension patients with left ventricular remodeling by two-dimensional strain echocardiography. Chinese J Ultrasound Med. 2012;28(5):421–4.
8. Kraigher-Krainer E, Shah AM, Gupta DK, et al. Impaired systolic function by strain imaging in heart failure with preserved ejection fraction. J Am Coll Cardiol. 2014;63:447–56.
9. Mancia G, Backer GD, Dominiczak A, et al. 2007 guidelines for the management of arterial hypertension:the task force for the management of arterial hypertension of the European society of hypertension (ESH) and of the European society of cardiology (ESC). Eur Heart J. 2007;28:1462–536.
10. Lang RM, Badano LP, Mor-Avi V, et al. Recommendations for cardiac chamber quantification by echocardiography in adults: an update from the american society of echocardiography and the European association of cardiovascular imaging. J Am Soc Echocardiogr. 2015;28:1–39. e14
11. Phan TT, Shivu GN, Shivu GH, et al. Left ventricular torsion and strain patterns in heart failure with normal ejection fraction are similar to age-related changes. Eur J Echocardiogr. 2009;10:793–800.
12. Wang J, Khoury DS, Yue Y, Torre-Amione G, Nagueh SF. Preserved left ventricular twist and circumferential deformation, but depressed longitudinal and radial deformation in patients with diastolic heart failure. Eur Heart J. 2008;29:1283–9.
13. Mizuguchi Y, Oishi Y, Miyoshi H, Iuchi A, Nagase N, Oki T. The functional role of longitudinal, circumferential, and radial myocardial deformation for regulating the early impairment of left ventricular contraction and relaxation in patients with cardiovascular risk factors:a study with two-dimensional strain imaging. J Am Soc Echocardiogr. 2008;21:1138–44.
14. Kitzman DW, Little WC, Brubaker PH, et al. Pathophysiological characterization of isolated diastolic heart failure in comparison to systolic heart failure. JAMA. 2002;288:2144–50.
15. Heerebeek L, Borbely A, Niessen HW, et al. Myocardial structure and function differ in systolic and diastolic heart failure. Circulation. 2006;113:1966–73.
16. Borbely A, Velden J, Papp Z, et al. Cardiomyocyte stiffness in diastolic heart failure. Circulation. 2005;111:774–81.
17. Kosmala W, Plaksej R, Strotmann JM, et al. Progression of left ventricular functional abnormalities in hypertensive patients with heart failure: an ultrasonic two-dimensional speckle tracking study. J Am Soc Echocardiogr. 2008;21:1309–17.
18. Rademakers FE, Rogers WJ, Guier WH, et al. Relation of regional cross-fiber shortening to wall thickening in the intact heart: three dimensional strain analysis by NMR tagging. Circulation. 1994;89:1174–82.
19. Waldman LK, Nosan D, Villarreal F, Covell JW. Relation between transmural deformation and local myofiber direction in canine left ventricular. Circ Res. 1988;63:550–62.
20. Ishizu T, Seo Y, Kameda Y, et al. Left ventricular strain and transmural distribution of structural remodeling in hypertensive heart disease. Hypertension. 2014;63:500–6.
21. Cho GY, Marwick TH, Kim HS, et al. Global 2-dimensional strain as a new prognosticator in patients with heart failure. J Am Coll Cardiol. 2009;54:618–24.
22. Lewis RP, Sandler H. Relationship between changes in left ventricular dimensions and the ejection fraction in man. Circulation. 1971;104:548–57.
23. Carasso S, Cohen O, Mutlak D, et al. Relation of myocardial mechanics in severe aortic stenosis to left ventricular ejection fraction and response to aortic valve replacement. Am J Cardiol. 2011;107:1052–7.
24. Ortega M, Triedman JK, Geva T, Harrild DM. Relation of left ventricular dyssynchrony measured by cardiac magnetic resonance tissue tracking in repaired tetralogy of fallot to ventricular tachycardia and death. Am J Cardiol. 2011;107:1535–40.
25. Friedberg MK, Slorach C. Relation between left ventricular regional radial function and radial wall motion abnormalities using two-dimensional speckle tracking in children with idiopathic dilated cardiomyopathy. Am J Cardiol. 2008;102:335–9.

8

Definition of common carotid wall thickness affects risk classification in relation to degree of internal carotid artery stenosis: the Plaque At RISK (PARISK) study

J Steinbuch[1], AC van Dijk[2,3], FHBM Schreuder[4,5,6], MTB Truijman[4,5,6], J Hendrikse[7], PJ Nederkoorn[8], A van der Lugt[2], E Hermeling[4], APG Hoeks[1] and WH Mess[5*]

Abstract

Background: Mean or maximal intima-media thickness (IMT) is commonly used as surrogate endpoint in intervention studies. However, the effect of normalization by surrounding or median IMT or by diameter is unknown. In addition, it is unclear whether IMT inhomogeneity is a useful predictor beyond common wall parameters like maximal wall thickness, either absolute or normalized to IMT or lumen size. We investigated the interrelationship of common carotid artery (CCA) thickness parameters and their association with the ipsilateral internal carotid artery (ICA) stenosis degree.

Methods: CCA thickness parameters were extracted by edge detection applied to ultrasound B-mode recordings of 240 patients. Degree of ICA stenosis was determined from CT angiography.

Results: Normalization of maximal CCA wall thickness to median IMT leads to large variations. Higher CCA thickness parameter values are associated with a higher degree of ipsilateral ICA stenosis ($p < 0.001$), though IMT inhomogeneity does not provide extra information. When the ratio of wall thickness and diameter instead of absolute maximal wall thickness is used as risk marker for having moderate ipsilateral ICA stenosis (>50%), 55 arteries (15%) are reclassified to another risk category.

Conclusions: It is more reasonable to normalize maximal wall thickness to end-diastolic diameter rather than to IMT, affecting risk classification and suggesting modification of the Mannheim criteria.

Keywords: Atherosclerosis, Stenosis, Carotid IMT, Ultrasound, Carotid artery imaging

Background

An irregular intima-media thickness (IMT) of the common carotid artery (CCA) is indicative for atherosclerotic burden [1, 2] and hence, might be a useful predictor in risk assessment. In a vascular diseased patient population CCA-IMT irregularity is associated with nearby atherosclerosis [2]. Furthermore, in symptomatic patients high CCA-IMT irregularity is associated with a higher degree of stenosis of distal plaques [1] and is more prominent in symptomatic than in asymptomatic subjects [3].

However, as previously discussed by Bots et al. [4], it remains unclear whether IMT irregularity itself is a useful predictor in addition to maximal IMT. It has been shown that after adjustment for coronary risk factors the combined IMT irregularity of CCA, bulb and internal carotid artery (ICA) is a more accurate predictor for coronary artery disease than mean and maximum IMT [5]. But, for patients with cerebrovascular disease and ICA stenosis it is still unknown.

CCA-IMT progression is commonly used as surrogate endpoint for cardiovascular risk for evaluating drug therapy in interventional studies [6–9]. However, CCA-IMT is affected by the dynamic range and frequency bandwidth of the ultrasound system employed [10], while

* Correspondence: werner.mess@mumc.nl
[5]Clinical Neurophysiology, Maastricht University Medical Center, PO Box 58006202 Maastricht, AZ, The Netherlands
Full list of author information is available at the end of the article

for an elderly subject population image quality is generally poorer than for young healthy subjects. As a consequence the observed IMT distribution is subject to large relative errors. Moreover, CCA-IMT measures vary across studies [11], e.g., mean or maximal CCA-IMT with or without CCA plaque. According to the Mannheim consensus [12], plaques are defined as having a wall thickness 1) extending more than 500 μm into the lumen, 2) and higher than 50% of surrounding IMT and/or 3) higher than 1500 μm. Therefore, the Mannheim criteria use absolute maximal wall thickness (criterion 3) or wall thickness normalized to surrounding IMT (criterion 2) or a combination of both (criterion 1). Because IMT values are slightly higher than the ultrasound resolution (about 0.3 mm for commonly used ultrasound systems), normalization of maximum wall thickness with respect to the surrounding IMT (criterion 2) will introduce wide variations. Considering the interrelationship between wall thickness and artery diameter according to the Lamé's equation [13, 14] and the wider range in CCA diameter (6–9 mm) in a healthy population [15], it seems physiologically more reasonable to normalize absolute maximal wall thickness by diameter. Using local wall thickness normalized to either IMT (i.e., thickness-to-IMT ratio) or diameter (i.e., thickness-to-diameter ratio) instead of the CCA-IMT as surrogate endpoint may affect the interpretation of drug therapy results. In addition, normalized wall thickness may lead to reclassification of CCAs towards another risk category, e.g. risk of having more than 50% degree of ICA stenosis.

This study analyses the baseline results of a 2-year follow-up PARISK study in which the association between CCA wall parameters and risk of plaque rupture will be investigated [16]. As a first step, we will investigate the interrelationship of CCA-IMT parameters and their association with the degree of ipsilateral ICA stenosis. More specifically, we will investigate in a large group of symptomatic subjects 1) the relevance of absolute and normalized maximal wall thickness with or without CCA plaques, 2) their relation with CCA-IMT inhomogeneity and 3) the association between absolute wall thickness, thickness-to-diameter ratio, thickness-to-IMT ratio, CCA plaques and CCA-IMT inhomogeneity with the degree of ipsilateral ICA stenosis.

Methods
Study subjects
240 patients with mild-to-moderate ICA stenosis (<70% according to the NASCET criteria) and recent ischemic stroke, transient ischemic attack or amaurosis fugax, were included in the Plaque At RISK (PARISK) study (clinical trials.gov NCT01208025), an ongoing multicenter cohort study with 2-year follow-up. Details of the study were previously described [16]. The study was approved by the

Medical Ethics Committees of the participating centers and all patients gave written informed consent. Currently, only baseline observations are available.

Data acquisition
Longitudinal ultrasound B-mode recordings (40 mm width, 5 s, 37 fps) of both CCAs were acquired in duplicate of 233 patients at anterolateral and posterolateral angles with a Philips iU22 scanner (Philips Medical Systems, Bothell, USA) using different probes (17–5, 12–5 or 9–3 MHz) depending on the CCA depth. The distal end of the recorded CCA segment was located 1–2 cm proximal to the flow divider. During ultrasound recordings, patients lay in supine position with their head slightly tilted to the opposite side. Due to contra-indications (low renal clearance (<60 ml/min) or allergy to CT contrast media), only 201 patients were subjected to multidetector computed tomography angiography (MDCTA).

Echo edge detection
Wall thickness was extracted at end-diastole by edge detection of B-mode images with dedicated software developed by Maastricht University Medical Center (MUMC, Maastricht, The Netherlands) [17] by a trained observer blinded to the MDCTA results. The intra-subject precision of the adopted software for absolute IMT of an artery segment, i.e. the standard deviation of differences between duplicate recordings and their average, is on average 99 μm [1]. The maximum variation of IMT expected due to the ultrasound depth resolution is 150 μm [1]. For each B-mode frame, automatic wall detection of the media-adventitia transition at the anterior and posterior wall was performed for half-overlapping segments (width 3.7 mm) using a threshold of 65% (or half of the difference between this threshold and the maximum, i.e., 83%, in case of an echogenic lumen-intima boundary) of the maximal grey value of the adventitia segment [1]. The local diameter was defined as the local difference along the ultrasound beam between anterior and posterior media-adventitia transitions.

The diameter waveforms, as extracted by edge detection, were smoothed over time (0.2 s filter span) with a 2nd order zero-phase Savitsky-Golay filter. After discarding the end-segments, the mean diameter waveform was calculated and the end-diastolic frames identified. At those frames, the lumen-intima transition along the posterior wall was identified, based on the maximum of the first derivative of the echo amplitude, and corrected manually when necessary [1]. The spatial IMT distribution was obtained as the differences along the ultrasound beam between the posterior lumen-intima and media-adventitia transitions over the artery segment.

Absolute and normalized maximal wall thickness

For each end-diastolic image, the diameter and IMT were obtained as the spatial median while the maximal wall thickness as spatial maximum, and averaged (median) over all available heart beats (on average 5). Absolute maximal wall thickness was normalized to the median end-diastolic diameter, defined as thickness-to-diameter ratio, and to the median IMT, defined as thickness-to-IMT ratio. All parameters were averaged (median) over all ipsilateral recordings.

IMT inhomogeneity

Absolute IMT inhomogeneity was defined as the standard deviation of the IMT over the artery segment and averaged (median) over available heart beats and all ipsilateral recordings (anterolateral, posterolateral, duplicate). IMT inhomogeneity was also normalized to the local end-diastolic diameter, i.e., relative IMT inhomogeneity.

Degree of ICA stenosis

MDCTA images were analyzed with dedicated 3D analysis software (Leonardo and syngo.via; Siemens, Erlangen, Germany). Degree of stenosis in both carotid arteries (bifurcation or ICA), based on the European Carotid Surgery Trial criteria [18], was manually assessed perpendicularly to the central lumen line by a trained observer.

Statistical analysis

To compare the maximal wall thickness parameters, the parameters were transformed to a normal z-score distribution using the expression (value-mean)/SD. The mean and standard deviation (SD), used as reference in this equation, were derived for CCA arteries without plaques according to the Mannheim criteria. To compare maximal wall thickness parameters with IMT inhomogeneity, correlation coefficients were calculated.

Optimal cut-offs for absolute maximal wall thickness, thickness-to-diameter ratio and thickness-to-IMT ratio for the presence of a >50% ipsilateral stenosis were derived from ROC curves. The optimal cut-off follows from the shortest distance towards the upper left corner of the ROC curve. In addition, a Student t-test was used to assess the difference in degree of ICA stenosis for ipsilateral CCA arteries with low and high wall thickness parameters.

To establish the risk for having more than 50% degree of ipsilateral ICA stenosis, the CCAs were divided into low and high absolute maximal wall thickness, thickness-to-diameter ratio and thickness-to-IMT ratio according to the ROC defined cut-offs. Since the variation in IMT due to the ultrasound depth resolution (conservatively estimated at 300 μm) is about 150 μm, i.e. 2% for an end-diastolic diameter of 7.5 mm, the cut-off level for relative IMT inhomogeneity was tentatively set at 2% [1]. To investigate the effect of wall thickness parameters as risk markers on the defined risk categories, reclassification of arteries was defined as the number of CCAs that switched to another risk category, using either the maximal wall thickness parameters instead of the Mannheim criteria or thickness-to-diameter ratio instead of absolute maximal wall thickness. Values are quantified as mean ± SD. Significance level was set at $p < 0.05$.

Results

In total, 197 patients received an MDCTA as well as an ultrasound examination. Five patients were excluded due to insufficient quality of MDCTA ($N = 2$) or due to failure to have an ultrasound registration of both CCAs ($N = 3$). In addition, patients with an ICA occlusion or stent ($N = 3$) were excluded, leading to 189 included patients (371 CCAs; mean age 68 ± 9 years). Patient characteristics are shown in Table 1. Prior to the study we estimated the B-mode depth resolution both from the spatial speckle frequency (ensemble average power spectral density across image) and from the width at half-maximum of distinct lumen-intima echoes (average of 10 independent observations) at 264 and 267 um, respectively.

Absolute and normalized maximal wall thickness

Figure 1 contains a boxplot of absolute and normalized maximal wall thickness, expressed as normal z-scores. CCA arteries with plaques ($N = 140$) according to the Mannheim criteria clearly have a higher absolute maximal wall thickness, thickness-to-diameter ratio and thickness-to-IMT ratio than CCAs without plaques ($N = 231$; mean difference 5, 5 and 4, respectively, Student t-test p-value <0.001). The values of the thickness-to-IMT ratio of CCAs with plaques are spread over a wider range than the other wall thickness parameters (Fig. 1) due to resolution related

Table 1 Patient characteristics. Data are presented as mean ± SD (range or number of patients)

Number	189	-
Age	68 ± 9 (39–88)	years
Male	73 ($N = 138$)	%
BMI	27 ± 4 (17–43)	kg/m^2
Systolic blood pressure	140 ± 19 (97–210)	mmHg
Diastolic blood pressure	79 ± 9 (54–105)	mmHg
Pulse pressure	61 ± 16 (27–117)	mmHg
Stroke / TIA/ amaurosis fugax	46/42/12 ($N = 87/80/22$)	%
Current smoking	23 ($N = 43$)	%
Diabetes Mellitus	21 ($N = 41$)	%
Hypercholesterolemia	57 ($N = 107$)	%
Hypertension	59 ($N = 111$)	%

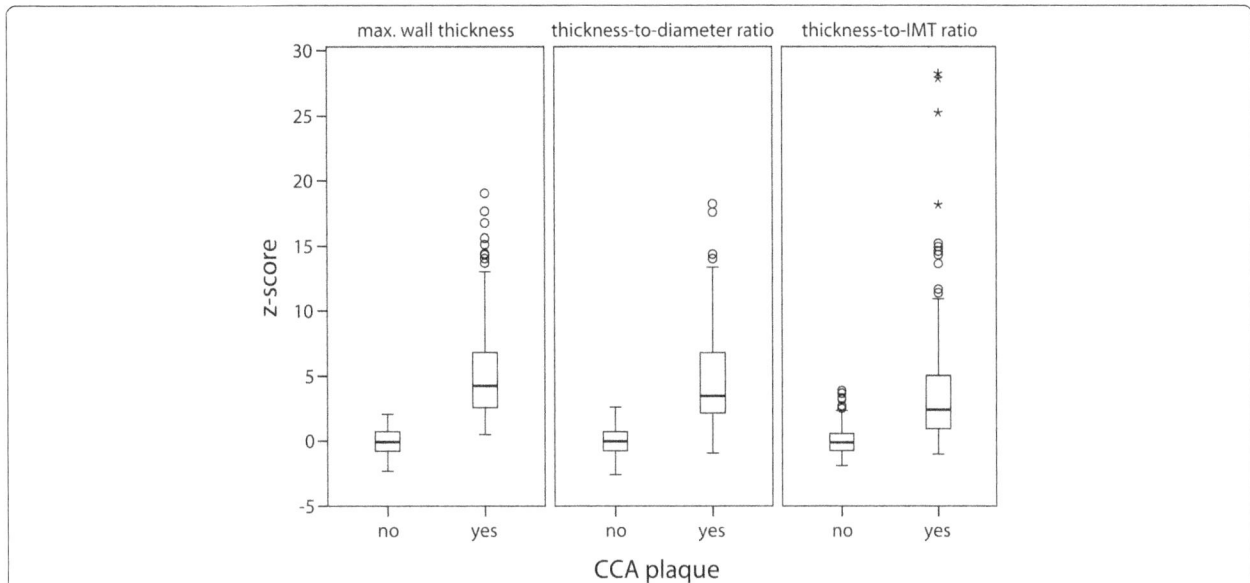

Fig. 1 Absolute maximal wall thickness, thickness-to-diameter ratio and thickness-to-IMT ratio of the CCA as function of the presence of CCA plaque. Values are presented as normal z-scores, based on the mean and SD of the thickness parameters for arteries without CCA plaques. Arteries with CCA plaques clearly have a significantly larger wall thickness. Normalized thickness-to-IMT has a wider distribution than maximal wall thickness and thickness-to-diameter ratio

variations. Therefore, thickness-to-IMT ratio is not considered for correlation with IMT inhomogeneity.

Maximal wall thickness and IMT inhomogeneity
Absolute maximal wall thickness is strongly correlated with absolute IMT inhomogeneity ($R = 0.76$, Fig. 2). In addition, maximal thickness-to-diameter ratio is also strongly associated with relative IMT inhomogeneity ($R = 0.73$, Fig. 2).

Maximal wall thickness and degree of ipsilateral ICA stenosis
ROC curves of absolute and normalized maximal wall thickness for detecting an ipsilateral ICA stenosis greater than 50% are shown in Fig. 3. Optimal cut-offs for absolute maximal wall thickness, thickness-to-diameter ratio and thickness-to-IMT ratio are 1277 µm, 17% and 129%, respectively. When only the side with the highest ICA plaque is considered, optimal cut-offs are 1191 µm, 16 and 124%, respectively.

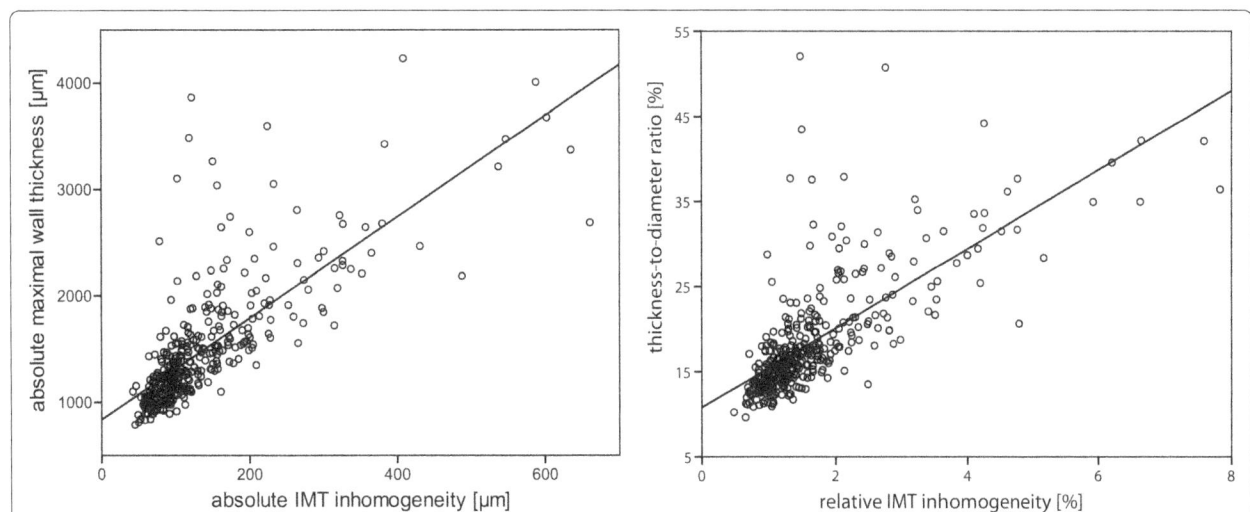

Fig. 2 Absolute maximal wall thickness as function of absolute IMT inhomogeneity (*left*) and thickness-to-diameter ratio as function of relative IMT inhomogeneity (*right*). A strong correlation exists between absolute maximal wall thickness and absolute IMT inhomogeneity ($R = 0.76$) and between thickness-to-diameter ratio and relative IMT inhomogeneity ($R = 0.73$)

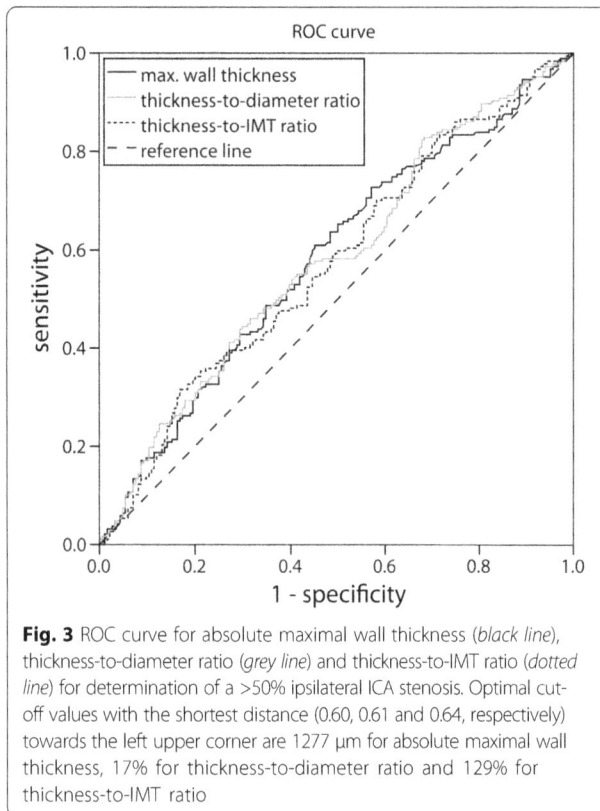

Fig. 3 ROC curve for absolute maximal wall thickness (*black line*), thickness-to-diameter ratio (*grey line*) and thickness-to-IMT ratio (*dotted line*) for determination of a >50% ipsilateral ICA stenosis. Optimal cut-off values with the shortest distance (0.60, 0.61 and 0.64, respectively) towards the left upper corner are 1277 μm for absolute maximal wall thickness, 17% for thickness-to-diameter ratio and 129% for thickness-to-IMT ratio

Risk stratification

Arteries were divided into two risk categories according to the ROC defined cut-offs for an ICA stenosis (see above). When thickness-to-IMT ratio instead of Mannheim criteria is used as risk marker, a large number of arteries (Table 2, $N = 95$, 26%) are reclassified to another risk category. Moreover, thickness-to-diameter ratio reclassifies 53 arteries (14%), whereas absolute maximal wall thickness reclassifies 56 arteries (15%). Since thickness-to-IMT ratio is more prone to resolution related variations (Fig. 1), only absolute maximal wall thickness and thickness-to-diameter ratio are considered for further analyses.

Patients with absolute maximal wall thickness below 1277 μm have a wide range of degree of ipsilateral ICA stenosis ($N = 174$), whereas patients with absolute wall thickness above 1277 μm ($N = 197$) exhibit a higher degree of ICA stenosis (Fig. 4). Both absolute maximal wall thickness and thickness-to-diameter ratio above cut-off values are associated with a higher ipsilateral stenosis degree (Tables 3 and 4, $52 \pm 15\%$ and $52 \pm 16\%$, respectively) than below the cut-off values (mean difference 8% and 7%, Student t-test p-value <0.001). This association remains borderline significant after excluding patients with CCA plaques (Tables 3 and 4, mean difference 7% and 5%, Student t-test p-value 0.02 and 0.15 respectively). Moreover, similar trends are seen when only the side with the highest ICA plaque is considered (Tables 3 and 4). In addition, CCAs with a plaque ($N = 140$) exhibit a stronger association with a higher distal stenosis degree than arteries without a plaque ($N = 231$; $52 \pm 15\%$ and $46 \pm 19\%$, respectively, mean difference 7%, Student t-test p-value < 0.001). When thickness-to-diameter ratio instead of absolute maximal wall thickness is used as risk marker for having more than ipsilateral 50% degree of ICA stenosis, 55 CCAs (15%) are reclassified towards the other risk category (of which $N = 20$ towards a higher category).

IMT inhomogeneity and degree of ipsilateral ICA stenosis

Arteries with a relative IMT inhomogeneity above 2% ($N = 81$) are associated with a higher degree of ipsilateral ICA stenosis ($53 \pm 11\%$) than arteries ($N = 290$) with a relative IMT inhomogeneity below 2% (mean difference 6%, Student t-test p-value <0.001).

Discussion

We evaluated the absolute and normalized maximal wall thickness and CCA-IMT inhomogeneity in patients with a recent cerebrovascular accident and mild-to-moderate ICA stenosis. Normalization by median IMT leads to large variations. Absolute maximal wall thickness and thickness-to-diameter ratio are strongly correlated with absolute and relative IMT inhomogeneity, respectively. IMT inhomogeneity does not provide extra information on top of absolute maximal wall thickness or thickness-to-IMT ratio in relation to the degree of ipsilateral ICA stenosis. Mainly CCA plaques are strongly associated with a higher degree of ipsilateral ICA stenosis. Although a similar trend is seen for both absolute

Table 2 Number of arteries with low or high maximal wall thickness parameters, stratified according to CCA plaque presence (Mannheim criteria). Using maximal wall thickness parameters as risk markers instead of Mannheim criteria results in reclassification of subjects towards another risk category. For example, the thickness-to-IMT ratio (right columns) reclassifies 70 and 25 subjects towards a higher and lower risk category, respectively, in total 26%

CCA plaque	Absolute maximal wall thickness		Thickness-to-diameter ratio		Thickness-to-IMT ratio	
	<1277 μm	>1277 μm	<17%	>17%	<129%	>129%
No	176	55	185	46	161	70
Yes	1	139	7	133	25	115
Total	177	194	192	179	186	185

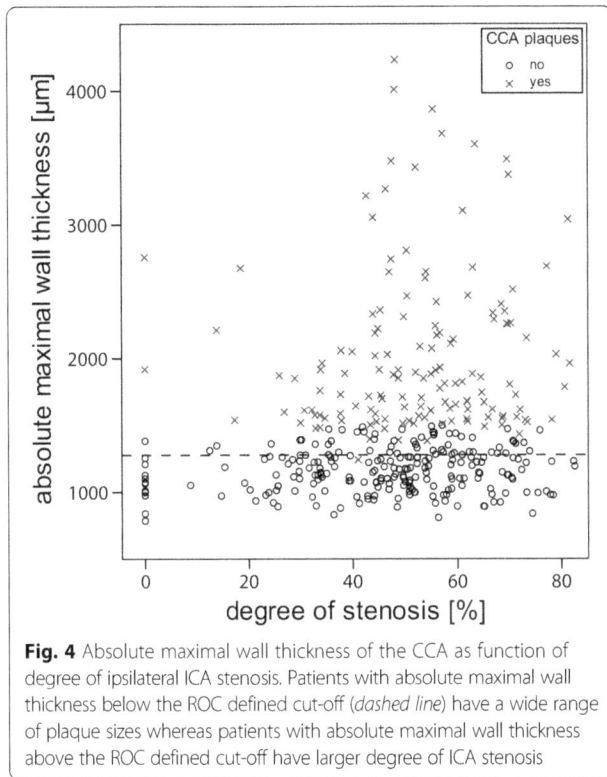

Fig. 4 Absolute maximal wall thickness of the CCA as function of degree of ipsilateral ICA stenosis. Patients with absolute maximal wall thickness below the ROC defined cut-off (*dashed line*) have a wide range of plaque sizes whereas patients with absolute maximal wall thickness above the ROC defined cut-off have larger degree of ICA stenosis

Table 4 ICA stenosis degree according to the ipsilateral thickness-to-diameter ratio cut-off for ICA stenosis at either side or for the largest ICA stenosis. Data are presented as mean ± SD. A high thickness-to-diameter ratio is indicative for a higher degree of ipsilateral ICA stenosis

ICA plaque	N ICAs	CCA plaque	Cut-off	ICA stenosis	p-value
Either side	192	yes/no	<17%	45 ± 19%	<0.001
	179		>17%	52 ± 16%	
	185	no	<17%	45 ± 19%	0.15
	46		>17%	50 ± 18%	
Largest	91	yes/no	<16%	56 ± 13%	0.03
	94		>16%	61 ± 12%	
	90	no	<16%	56 ± 13%	0.3
	23		>16%	58 ± 12%	

Risk stratification

Optimal cut-offs for absolute and normalized maximal wall thickness are derived from ROC curves for a >50% ipsilateral ICA stenosis (Fig. 3). We have chosen those plaques since the smaller plaques in the curved carotid bulb hardly induce hemodynamic changes [19, 20]. 96 CCAs (Table 2; 26%) are reclassified towards another risk category when thickness-to-IMT ratio rather than the Mannheim criteria are used as a risk marker for a >50% ipsilateral ICA stenosis. Since observed IMT values are generally noisy because they are slightly higher than the ultrasound depth resolution, normalization of maximum wall thickness with respect to median IMT will introduce wide variations. Therefore, it is questionable whether the Mannheim criterion [12], defining a plaque if the maximum thickness is 50% greater than the surrounding IMT, is consistent. Moreover, "surrounding IMT" is quite arbitrary (where does a plaque begin or end); that is why we decided to normalize the maximum thickness by the median IMT.

For the risk stratification of individual patients an optimal cut-off is needed. Although maximal wall thickness and thickness-to-diameter ratio show similar associations with the degree of ipsilateral ICA stenosis (Table 3 and 4), 55 arteries (15%) are reclassified when thickness-to-diameter ratio instead of absolute maximal wall thickness is used as risk marker for a >50% ipsilateral ICA stenosis. Alternately, an age dependent cut-off for absolute maximal wall thickness may be considered to correct for differences in CCA diameter [15, 21]. However, our population has a wide diameter distribution (8083 ± 1048 µm; range 5769–11702 µm), which cannot be explained by age differences only (68 ± 9 years; range 39–88 years). Since the vessel diameter depends on subject size, and diameter and wall thickness are interrelated via the Lamé's equation [13, 14], it seems more reasonable to use normalized rather than absolute maximal wall thickness values.

maximal wall thickness and thickness-to-diameter ratio, 15% of CCAs are reclassified when thickness-to-diameter ratio instead of absolute maximal wall thickness is used as risk marker for a >50% ipsilateral ICA stenosis.

Maximal wall thickness is normalized by the median end-diastolic diameter as well as the median IMT. As expected, patients with CCA plaques have a significantly higher absolute and normalized maximal wall thickness (p < 0.001). Normalization by the median IMT leads to similar values for arteries without CCA plaques, whereas a large variation is found for CCA arteries with large plaques (Fig. 1).

Table 3 ICA stenosis degree according to the ipsilateral absolute maximal wall thickness cut-off for ICA stenosis at either side or for the largest ICA stenosis. Data are presented as mean ± SD. A high absolute maximal wall thickness is indicative for a higher degree of ipsilateral ICA stenosis

ICA Plaque	N ICAs	CCA plaque	Cut-off	ICA stenosis	p-value
Either side	174	yes/no	<1277 µm	44 ± 20%	<0.001
	197		>1277 µm	52 ± 15%	
	173	no	<1277 µm	44 ± 20%	0.02
	58		>1277 µm	51 ± 16%	
Largest	64	yes/no	<1191 µm	55 ± 14%	0.006
	121		>1191 µm	60 ± 11%	
	64	no	<1191 µm	55 ± 14%	0.04
	54		>1191 µm	60 ± 12%	

Wall thickness parameters and ipsilateral stenosis degree

High relative IMT inhomogeneity and high thickness-to-diameter ratio are both associated with a higher degree of ICA stenosis (mean difference 6% and 7%, respectively, Student t-test p-value < 0.001). Since we look at local CCA features, the current p-value is lower than observed when the average relative IMT inhomogeneity of both CCAs is considered [1]. Because maximal wall thickness and thickness-to-diameter ratio are highly correlated with absolute and relative IMT inhomogeneity (Fig. 2) and similar trends are observed in relation to degree of stenosis, absolute or relative IMT inhomogeneity does not provide extra information on top of maximal wall thickness or thickness-to-diameter ratio. Mainly the presence of a CCA plaque dominates the association with a higher degree of ICA stenosis (mean difference 7%, Student t-test p-value < 0.001).

Plaques and wall thickness

Almost all CCAs with plaques according to the Mannheim consensus have a high maximal wall thickness and thickness-to-diameter ratio according to the cut-off derived with the ROC. Our population has a high incidence of CCA plaques (140 of 371 arteries; 38%). The presence of CCA plaques is rare in a healthy population, male 6% and female 3% [22], and is more prevalent (22%) in older subjects (>65 years) [23]. The relatively high incidence of CCA plaques in our population is attributable to the fact that subjects exhibited cerebrovascular symptoms and, therefore, belong to a diseased population.

It is questionable whether IMT and plaque formation are driven by the same process. IMT is strongly associated with hypertension and age [24] and is inheritable [25–27]. However, the heritability of plaque is less strong [27] and attributed to various genes [27–29]. Furthermore, since the intima thickness is approximately only 0.02 mm [30], IMT is mainly affected by hypertensive medial hypertrophy [31] whereas atherosclerosis is an inflammatory process where plaque formation starts with pathological intimal thickening and lesions containing lipid pools [32]. Therefore, IMT and plaque formation are likely different phenotypes [33–35]. Our study shows that the association between ICA stenosis and ipsilateral CCA plaques is highly significant (Table 3), which is in line with the concept of atherosclerosis as a more widespread instead of a focal disease, prompting a global rather than a focused vascular examination. Whether elevated CCA wall parameters are present before development of an ICA stenosis cannot be established in our study.

Conclusion

In conclusion, to evaluate wall thickness it is more reasonable to normalize maximal wall thickness by end-diastolic diameter rather than by IMT, suggesting a modification of the Mannheim criteria. Absolute or relative IMT inhomogeneity does not provide extra information on top of maximal wall thickness or thickness-to-diameter ratio. Mainly CCA plaques are strongly associated with a higher degree of ipsilateral ICA stenosis. Although a similar trend is seen for both absolute maximal wall thickness and thickness-to-diameter ratio, 55 arteries (15%) are reclassified when thickness-to-diameter ratio instead of absolute maximal wall thickness is used as risk marker for a >50% ICA stenosis. Whether this reclassification is clinically important and relative IMT inhomogeneity and thickness-to-diameter ratio have predictive value for plaque progression and cerebrovascular events will be evaluated in the follow-up phase of the PARISK study.

Abbreviations

CCA: Common carotid artery; CT: Computed tomography; ICA: Internal carotid artery; IMT: Intima-media thickness; MDCTA: Multidetector computed tomography angiography; MUMC: Maastricht University Medical Center; PARISK: Plaque At RISK; SD: Standard deviation

Acknowledgements

Not applicable.

Funding

This research was performed within the framework of the Center for Translational Molecular Medicine (www.ctmm.nl), project PARISK (Plaque At RISK; grant 01C-202) and supported by the Dutch Heart Foundation.

Authors' contributions

AD, FS, MT, JH, PN and AL made substantial contributions to patient inclusion, AH and JS to algorithm development, JS and AD to data analysis and JS, AH, EH and WM to data interpretation. All authors have contributed to the manuscript and have read and approved the submission of the manuscript.

Competing interests

The authors declare that they have no competing interests.

Author details

[1]Biomedical Engineering, Cardiovascular Research Institute Maastricht, Maastricht University, Maastricht, The Netherlands. [2]Radiology, Erasmus Medical Center, Rotterdam, The Netherlands. [3]Neurology, Erasmus Medical Center, Rotterdam, The Netherlands. [4]Radiology, Maastricht University Medical Center, Maastricht, The Netherlands. [5]Clinical Neurophysiology, Maastricht University Medical Center, PO Box 58006202 Maastricht, AZ, The Netherlands. [6]Neurology, Maastricht University Medical Center, Maastricht, The Netherlands. [7]Radiology, University Medical Center Utrecht, Utrecht, The Netherlands. [8]Neurology, Academic Medical Center, Amsterdam, The Netherlands.

References

1. Steinbuch J, van Dijk AC, Schreuder FH, Truijman MT, de Rotte AA, Nederkoorn PJ, van der Lugt A, Hermeling E, Hoeks AP, Mess WH. High Spatial Inhomogeneity in the Intima-Media Thickness of the Common Carotid Artery is Associated with a Larger Degree of Stenosis in the Internal Carotid Artery: The PARISK Study. Ultraschall in der Medizin 2016. doi:10.1055/s-0042-112220.

2. Graf IM, Schreuder FH, Hameleers JM, Mess WH, Reneman RS, Hoeks AP. Wall irregularity rather than intima-media thickness is associated with nearby atherosclerosis. Ultrasound Med Biol. 2009;35(6):955–61.

3. Saba L, Meiburger KM, Molinari F, Ledda G, Anzidei M, Acharya UR, Zeng G, Shafique S, Nicolaides A, Suri JS. Carotid IMT variability (IMTV) and its validation in symptomatic versus asymptomatic Italian population: can this be a useful index for studying symptomaticity? Echocardiography. 2012;29(9):1111–9.

4. Bots ML, den Ruijter HM. Variability in the intima-media thickness measurement as marker for cardiovascular risk? Not quite settled yet. Cardiovasc Diagn Ther. 2012;2(1):3–5.

5. Ishizu T, Ishimitsu T, Kamiya H, Seo Y, Moriyama N, Obara K, Watanabe S, Yamaguchi I. The correlation of irregularities in carotid arterial intima-media thickness with coronary artery disease. Heart Vessel. 2002;17(1):1–6.

6. Davidson MH, Rosenson RS, Maki KC, Nicholls SJ, Ballantyne CM, Mazzone T, Carlson DM, Williams LA, Kelly MT, Camp HS, et al. Effects of fenofibric acid on carotid intima-media thickness in patients with mixed dyslipidemia on atorvastatin therapy: randomized, placebo-controlled study (FIRST). Arterioscler Thromb Vasc Biol. 2014;34(6):1298–306.

7. Huang Y, Li W, Dong L, Li R, Wu Y. Effect of statin therapy on the progression of common carotid artery intima-media thickness: an updated systematic review and meta-analysis of randomized controlled trials. J Atheroscler Thromb. 2013;20(1):108–21.

8. Oyama J, Murohara T, Kitakaze M, Ishizu T, Sato Y, Kitagawa K, Kamiya H, Ajioka M, Ishihara M, Dai K, et al. The Effect of Sitagliptin on Carotid Artery Atherosclerosis in Type 2 Diabetes: The PROLOGUE Randomized Controlled Trial. PLoS Med. 2016;13(6):e1002051.

9. Ishigaki Y, Kono S, Katagiri H, Oka Y, Oikawa S. investigators N. Elevation of HDL-C in response to statin treatment is involved in the regression of carotid atherosclerosis. J Atheroscler Thromb. 2014;21(10):1055–65.

10. Gaarder M, Seierstad T. Measurements of carotid intima media thickness in non-invasive high-frequency ultrasound images: the effect of dynamic range setting. Cardiovasc Ultrasound. 2015;13:5.

11. Qu B, Qu T. Causes of changes in carotid intima-media thickness: a literature review. Cardiovasc Ultrasound. 2015;13:46.

12. Touboul PJ, Hennerici MG, Meairs S, Adams H, Amarenco P, Bornstein N, Csiba L, Desvarieux M, Ebrahim S, Hernandez Hernandez R, et al. Mannheim carotid intima-media thickness and plaque consensus (2004-2006-2011). An update on behalf of the advisory board of the 3rd, 4th and 5th watching the risk symposia, at the 13th, 15th and 20th European Stroke Conferences, Mannheim, Germany, 2004, Brussels, Belgium, 2006, and Hamburg, Germany, 2011. Cerebrovasc Dis. 2004;34(4):290–6.

13. Nichols WW, O'Rourke MF, Vlachopoulos C. McDonald's blood flow in arteries : theoretic, experimental, and clinical principles. 6th ed. London: Hodder Arnold; 2011.

14. Liang YL, Shiel LM, Teede H, Kotsopoulos D, McNeil J, Cameron JD, McGrath BP. Effects of Blood Pressure, Smoking, and Their Interaction on Carotid Artery Structure and Function. Hypertension. 2001;37(1):6–11.

15. Engelen L, Bossuyt J, Ferreira I, van Bortel LM, Reesink KD, Segers P, Stehouwer CD, Laurent S, Boutouyrie P. Reference values for local arterial stiffness. Part A. J Hypertens. 2015;33(10):1981–96.

16. Truijman MT, Kooi ME, van Dijk AC, de Rotte AA, van der Kolk AG, Liem MI, Schreuder FH, Boersma E, Mess WH, van Oostenbrugge RJ, et al. Plaque At RISK (PARISK): prospective multicenter study to improve diagnosis of high-risk carotid plaques. Int J Stroke. 2014;9(6):747–54.

17. Steinbuch J, Hoeks AP, Hermeling E, Truijman MT, Schreuder FH, Mess WH. Standard B-Mode Ultrasound Measures Local Carotid Artery Characteristics as Reliably as Radiofrequency Phase Tracking in Symptomatic Carotid Artery Patients. Ultrasound Med Biol. 2016;42(2):586–95.

18. European Carotid Surgery Trialists' Collaborative G. Randomised trial of endarterectomy for recently symptomatic carotid stenosis: final results of the MRC European Carotid Surgery Trial (ECST). Lancet. 1998;351(9113):1379–87.

19. Gijsen FJ, Palmen DE, van der Beek MH, van de Vosse FN, van Dongen ME, Janssen JD. Analysis of the axial flow field in stenosed carotid artery bifurcation models–LDA experiments. J Biomech. 1996;29(11):1483–9.

20. Ahmed SA, Giddens DP. Flow disturbance measurements through a constricted tube at moderate Reynolds numbers. J Biomech. 1983;16(12):955–63.

21. Engelen L, Ferreira I, Stehouwer CD, Boutouyrie P, Laurent S. Reference Values for Arterial Measurements C. Reference intervals for common carotid intima-media thickness measured with echotracking: relation with risk factors. Eur Heart J. 2013;34(30):2368–80.

22. Johnsen SH, Mathiesen EB, Joakimsen O, Stensland E, Wilsgaard T, Lochen ML, Njolstad I, Arnesen E. Carotid atherosclerosis is a stronger predictor of myocardial infarction in women than in men: a 6-year follow-up study of 6226 persons: the Tromso Study. Stroke. 2007;38(11):2873–80.

23. Scuteri A, Najjar SS, Orru M, Albai G, Strait J, Tarasov KV, Piras MG, Cao A, Schlessinger D, Uda M, et al. Age- and gender-specific awareness, treatment, and control of cardiovascular risk factors and subclinical vascular lesions in a founder population: the SardiNIA Study. Nutr Metab Cardiovasc Dis. 2009;19(8):532–41.

24. Al-Shali K, House AA, Hanley AJ, Khan HM, Harris SB, Mamakeesick M, Zinman B, Fenster A, Spence JD, Hegele RA. Differences between carotid wall morphological phenotypes measured by ultrasound in one, two and three dimensions. Atherosclerosis. 2005;178(2):319–25.

25. Fox CS, Polak JF, Chazaro I, Cupples A, Wolf PA, D'Agostino RA, O'Donnell CJ. Genetic and Environmental Contributions to Atherosclerosis Phenotypes in Men and Women: Heritability of Carotid Intima-Media Thickness in the Framingham Heart Study. Stroke. 2003;34(2):397–401.

26. Juo SH, Lin HF, Rundek T, Sabala EA, Boden-Albala B, Park N, Lan MY, Sacco RL. Genetic and environmental contributions to carotid intima-media thickness and obesity phenotypes in the Northern Manhattan Family Study. Stroke. 2004;35(10):2243–7.

27. Moskau S, Golla A, Grothe C, Boes M, Pohl C, Klockgether T. Heritability of carotid artery atherosclerotic lesions: an ultrasound study in 154 families. Stroke. 2005;36(1):5–8.

28. Pollex RL, Hegele R. Genetic determinants of carotid ultrasound traits. Curr Atheroscler Rep. 2006;8(3):206–15.

29. Al-Shali KZ, House AA, Hanley AJ, Khan HM, Harris SB, Zinman B, Mamakeesick M, Fenster A, Spence JD, Hegele RA. Genetic variation in PPARG encoding peroxisome proliferator-activated receptor gamma associated with carotid atherosclerosis. Stroke. 2004;35(9):2036–40.

30. Salonen JT, Salonen R. Ultrasound B-mode imaging in observational studies of atherosclerotic progression. Circulation. 1993;87(3 Suppl):II56–65.

31. Spence JD. Technology Insight: ultrasound measurement of carotid plaque–patient management, genetic research, and therapy evaluation. Nat Clin Pract Neurol. 2006;2(11):611–9.

32. Finn AV, Kolodgie FD, Virmani R. Correlation between carotid intimal/medial thickness and atherosclerosis: a point of view from pathology. Arterioscler Thromb Vasc Biol. 2010;30(2):177–81.

33. Spence JD, Hegele RA. Noninvasive phenotypes of atherosclerosis: similar windows but different views. Stroke. 2004;35(3):649–53.

34. Hegele RA, Al-Shali K, Khan HMR, Hanley AJG, Harris SB, Mamakeesick M, Zinman B, Fenster A, Spence JD, House AA. Carotid Ultrasound in One, Two and Three Dimensions. Vasc Dis Prev. 2005;2(1):87–91.

35. Spence JD. The importance of distinguishing between diffuse carotid intima-media thickening and focal plaque. Can J Cardiol. 2008;24:61C–4C.

9

Pilot study using 3D–longitudinal strain computation in a multi-parametric approach for best selecting responders to cardiac resynchronization therapy

Maxime Fournet[1,2], Anne Bernard[2,3], Sylvestre Marechaux[4], Elena Galli[1,2], Raphael Martins[1,2], Philippe Mabo[1,2], J. Claude Daubert[1,2], Christophe Leclercq[1,2], Alfredo Hernandez[2] and Erwan Donal[1,2,5*]

Abstract

Background: Almost all attempts to improve patient selection for cardiac resynchronization therapy (CRT) using echo-derived indices have failed so far. We sought to assess: the performance of homemade software for the automatic quantification of integral 3D regional longitudinal strain curves exploring left ventricular (LV) mechanics and the potential value of this tool to predict CRT response.

Methods: Forty-eight heart failure patients in sinus rhythm, referred for CRT-implantation (mean age: 65 years; LV-ejection fraction: 26%; QRS-duration: 160 milliseconds) were prospectively explored. Thirty-four patients (71%) had positive responses, defined as an LV end-systolic volume decrease ≥15% at 6-months. 3D–longitudinal strain curves were exported for analysis using custom-made algorithms. The integrals of the longitudinal strain signals ($I_{L,peak}$) were automatically measured and calculated for all 17 LV-segments.

Results: The standard deviation of longitudinal strain peak ($SDI_{L,peak}$) for all 17 LV-segments was greater in CRT responders than non-responders (1.18% s^{-1} [0.96; 1.35] versus 0.83% s^{-1} [0.55; 0.99], $p = 0.007$). The optimal cut-off value of $SDI_{L,peak}$ to predict response was 1.037%.s^{-1}. In the 18-patients without septal flash, $SDI_{L,peak}$ was significantly higher in the CRT-responders.

Conclusions: This new automatic software for analyzing 3D longitudinal strain curves is avoiding previous limitations of imaging techniques for assessing dyssynchrony and then its value will have to be tested in a large group of patients.

Keywords: Three-dimensional echocardiography, Heart failure, Cardiac resynchronization therapy, Dyssynchrony

Background

Cardiac resynchronization therapy (CRT) has emerged as a relevant therapeutic intervention for the treatment of chronic heart failure [1–5]. Based on current guidelines, patient selection for this costly therapy relies mainly on heart failure clinical status, ejection fraction (EF), and QRS characteristics (width and morphology). The proportion of non-responders remains relatively high, estimated at up to 30% [6, 7].

Several 2D echocardiographic indices of mechanical dyssynchrony have been proposed to better identify therapy responders, yet the lack of reproducibility and the non-optimal quantification of LV mechanical dyssynchrony (LVMD) achievable with these 2D echocardiographic indices in multicenter trials have cast some doubt on the techniques' clinical applicability [8–10].

In a further advancement, 3D speckle-tracking echocardiography (STE) has been proposed as an alternative and potentially more accurate method for quantifying LVMD and for identifying patients suitable for CRT [11–13].

These different approaches are typically based on analyzing differences in either myocardial velocity timing, by means of tissue Doppler imaging (TDI), or in

* Correspondence: erwan.donal@chu-rennes.fr
[1]Cardiologie et CIC-IT 1414, Centre Hospitalier Universitaire de Rennes, F-35000 Rennes, France
[2]LTSI, Université Rennes 1, INSERM, F-35000 Rennes, France
Full list of author information is available at the end of the article

myocardial deformation using 2D/3D STE. To describe the complexity of LV mechanics, we believe it is essential to perform a combined assessment of LV dyssynchrony and LV regional contractility using STE, particularly by means of longitudinal strain analysis.

We hypothesized that a new approach, based on automatic quantification of the integrals pertaining to 3D regional longitudinal strain signals, could provide valuable additional information about regional LV mechanics and function prior to any CRT procedure. The aims of this pilot study were to describe LV mechanics using 3D echocardiography integral-derived longitudinal strain parameters in patients eligible for CRT and to test the relevance of this new tool for predicting CRT response.

Methods

Study population

48 patients referred for CRT device implantation at two institutions, the Saint Philibert Catholic University Hospital (Lille, France) and the Rennes University Hospital (Rennes, France), were included in the study. Indications for CRT implantation were based on the 2010 ESC guidelines for CRT device use in heart failure [14]. The patients had no previous pacemaker or cardioverter-defibrillator implantation. Patients with a poor acoustic window were excluded ($n = 5$).

Ischemic etiology was defined by a history of previous myocardial infarction or prior coronary revascularization or if a > 75% stenosis was observed in ≥1 of the major epicardial coronary arteries [15]. The NYHA functional class reported was the highest reached by the patient. 12-lead surface electrocardiograms (ECGs) were recorded at 25 and 50 mm/s during intrinsic conduction before CRT-device implantation and then were analyzed by Rennes University's ECG Core Center. The morphology was classified as either LBBB or non-LBBB (non-specific intraventricular conduction delay) [16]. Only patients with a right bundle branch block were excluded.

The devices were implanted by a standard procedure. The electrophysiologist was blinded with respect to the localization of scar and the main aim during the implantation was to obtain the narrowest QRS at the end of the procedure.

All patients provided informed consent to participate in this study, which was performed in accordance with the principles outlined in the Declaration of Helsinki on research in human subjects (CNIL declaration no. 1620030 V. 0).

Two-dimensional echocardiography and speckle-tracking echocardiography

Baseline echocardiography was performed prior to CRT implantation (ViVid e9; GE Healthcare, Horten, Norway). Digital, routine, gray-scale, 2D Doppler TDI cineloops were obtained from three consecutive cardiac cycles, along with speckle tracking echocardiographic cineloops from one cardiac cycle, all from the apical view (gray-scale frame rate ≥ 50 Hz; color frame rate > 100 Hz; and 2-, 3-, 4-chamber apical views). Off-line analyses were performed on digitally stored images (BT12-EchoPAC PC; GE Healthcare).

The echocardiography examination was conducted according to the American Society of Echocardiography guidelines [17]. The LV volumes and LV ejection fraction (LVEF) were calculated using the biplane modified Simpson's rule. All of the measurements were averaged for three cardiac cycles. The LV pre-ejection interval and aortic valve closure values were determined using aortic Doppler profiles. LV global longitudinal strain (LVGLS) was measured off-line using automated functional imaging (AFI). After manual tracing of the endocardial LV border in the 4-, 2-, and 3-chamber views over one frame, the endocardial borders were automatically tracked throughout the cardiac cycle. LVGLS was averaged from all of the analyzable segments in all apical views.

Atrio-ventricular delay was calculated as the ratio between LV filling time and the RR interval. Atrio-ventricular dyssynchrony (AVD) was considered significant when the duration of LV filling time resulted <40% of the RR interval [18]. Interventricular dyssynchrony was defined as a left ventricular pre-ejection interval (LVPEI) >140 ms, with or without an interventricular mechanical delay (IVMD) >40 ms [18]. Intraventricular dyssynchrony was defined by the presence of one of the following: a septal to lateral wall delay by color TDI [19] ≥65 ms [20], or the presence of septal flash (SF). SF was defined as an early septal thickening or thinning within the isovolumetric contraction period, as detected both visually from the gray-scale short axis (SAX) and 4-chamber (4CH) views and from the parasternal long axis, SAX, and 4CH views obtained by M-mode [21].

Three-dimensional echocardiography and speckle-tracking echocardiography

Baseline 3D–echocardiography was performed in each patient prior to CRT implantation using a commercially available echocardiographic system (ViVid E9; GE Healthcare, Horten, Norway), equipped with a 4 V phased-array matrix transducer. Consecutive 6-beat ECG-gated subvolumes were acquired from the apical approach, using second-harmonic imaging during end-expiratory apnea, to generate the full-volume data set. We paid particular attention to encompassing the entire LV cavity within the data set, which was digitally stored in a raw-data format and was exported to a separate workstation equipped with the 4D–AutoLVQ package (EchoPAC V.110.1.3, GE Healthcare, Horten, Norway) for off-line analysis of STE LV myocardial longitudinal deformation.

The end-diastolic frames required for contour detection were automatically displayed in quad view. Manual alignment, achieved by pivoting and translating the four-chamber plane, was undertaken to align the three apical views so that the corresponding intersection line of all of the planes was placed in the middle of the LV cavity, crossing the LV apex and center of the mitral valve in each view. We subsequently used the semi-automated option to identify a fitting geometric model. Importantly, the software required only two single points to be input manually (one at the apex and the other at the tip of the mitral leaflet) on the end-diastolic and end-systolic frames of the four-chamber view slice. The software automatically detected the LV cavity endocardial border in 3D and provided the measured LV volumes. If the endocardial border detection was judged inadequate by the examiner, the LV endocardial borders were manually adjusted in multiplanar layout (three apical and three transverse planes) with a point-click method, immediately followed by secondary automated refinement of boundary detection according to the results. Following assessment of the LV volumes and ejection fraction, an automatic trace of the epicardial border was displayed to identify the region of interest required for LV mass and myocardial deformation measurements by means of 3D STE. This epicardial trace was manually adjusted in order to include the entire LV wall thickness using the same point-click method. The longitudinal deformation parameters were reported as global (both peak and end-systolic) and regional (only end-systolic) and were presented as color-coded polar maps and time-strain traces of an LV 17-segment model (Fig. 1). The time required for all this process is close to the time required to record the acquisitions and the export them on a computer where the computation will be performed automatically.

Automatic longitudinal strain integrals – new application

The 3D longitudinal strain signals were exported in text format to undergo dedicated analysis using custom-made methods and algorithms developed in Matlab software (Mathworks Inc., Natik, Massasuchetts, USA). This analysis included a regional characterization of the longitudinal strain integrals and extended to the 3D case of a set of methods initially developed by our group for 2D strain analysis [22]. The strain integrals represented the accumulated strain during different time intervals of the cardiac cycle. In this study, two particular markers were extracted for each of the 17 LV segments: 1) strain integrals from the beginning of the cardiac cycle (QRS onset) to the instant of the corresponding longitudinal strain peak ($I_{L,peak}$); and 2), strain integrals from the QRS onset to the instant of aortic valve closure ($I_{L,avc}$) (Fig. 2). All values exceeding -5% were considered to be noise (irrelevant information) and were thus not considered when calculating the integral.

We tested the integral-based indicators of the regional longitudinal strain signals, all of which were automatically calculated, revealing standard parameters such as "peak strain" (amplitude), "mean strain peak", and "$SD_{t,peak}$" (standard deviation of time to strain peak), along with novel measurements as detailed below.

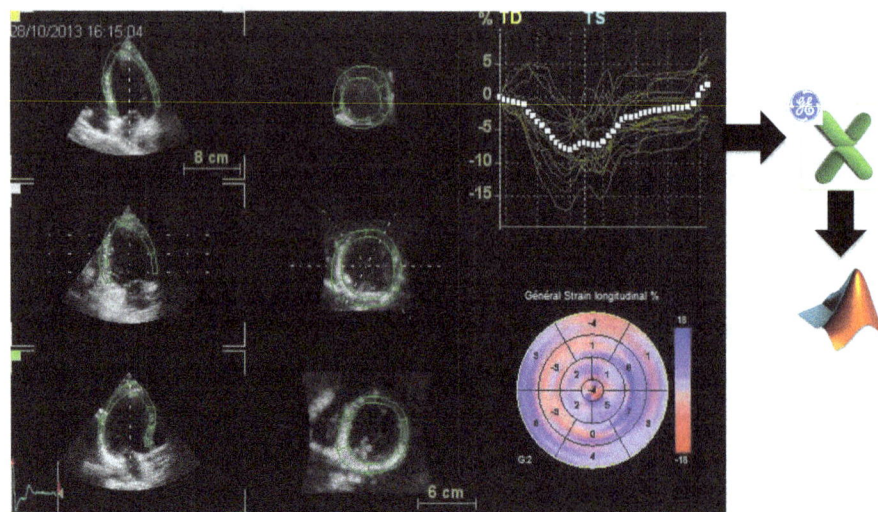

Fig. 1 LV dataset display with 3D speckle-tracking analysis of longitudinal myocardial deformation, using the 4D–AutoLVQ package (EchoPAC version 110.1.3, GE Healthcare, Horten, Norway). Microsoft Excel files of 3D longitudinal strain analyses were exported for dedicated analysis performed, with Matlab software (Mathworks Inc., USA)

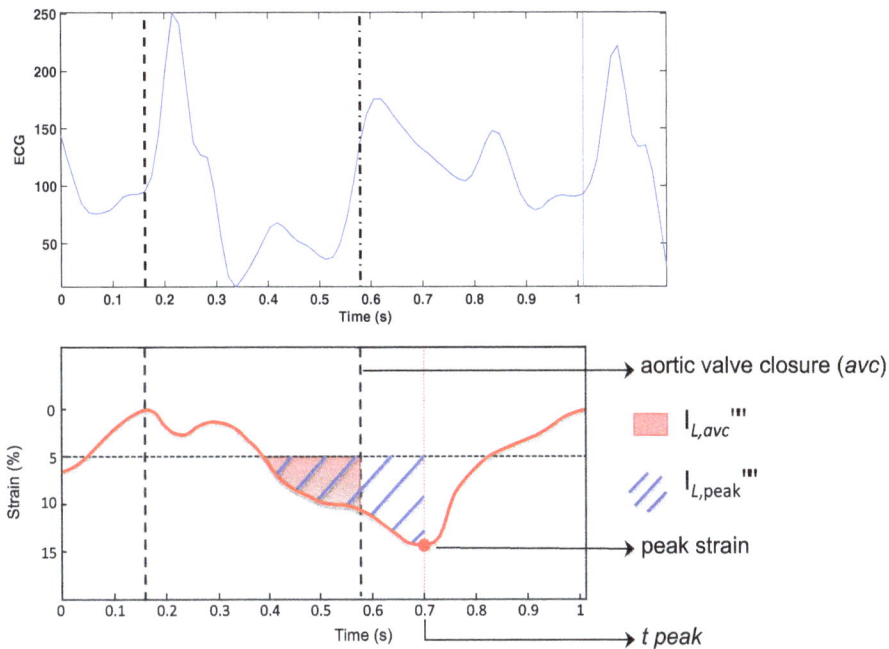

Fig. 2 Longitudinal strain curve of one LV segment, analyzed using custom-made algorithms. The *pink area* represents the integral of the longitudinal strain signal from the beginning of the cardiac cycle (QRS onset) to the instant of the aortic valve closure ($I_{L,avc}$). The *blue-shaded* area represents the integral of longitudinal strain signal from the beginning of the cardiac cycle to the instant of the corresponding longitudinal strain peak ($I_{L,peak}$). All values greater than −5% were considered noise and were thus not considered in calculating integrals. *t peak*: time to strain peak

- mean $I_{L,peak}$ and mean $I_{L,avc}$ represented the mean of $I_{L,peak}$ and $I_{L,avc}$ of all 17 LV segments, respectively.
- $SDI_{L,peak}$ and $SDI_{L,avc}$ were the standard deviation of the integrals of the strain signals $I_{L,peak}$ and $I_{L,avc}$ of all 17 segments, respectively. $SDI_{L,peak}$ and $SDI_{L,avc}$ corresponded to the energy dispersion for all 17 segments at the longitudinal strain peak and at the instant of aortic valve closure, respectively.
- DiffInt was calculated as the average of all 17 LV segments in terms of the difference between $I_{L,avc}$ and $I_{L,peak}$ for each segment. This value could be considered an indicator of the wasted energy developed by the ventricle after aortic valve closure.
- MSDI (maximal difference between strain peak instants) was calculated as the ratio of the time difference between the last and first strain peaks occurring during the cardiac cycle and the duration of the cardiac cycle.

Echocardiographic response

At 6-months post-implant, all of the patients were reassessed with 2D echocardiography. Response to CRT was defined as a ≥ 15% reduction in LV end-systolic volume, compared with baseline [23, 24].

Statistical analysis

All of the normally distributed data are displayed as the means and standard deviations, with non-normally distributed data expressed as medians and interquartile ranges (IQRs). Normality was evaluated by the Shapiro-Wilk test. Comparisons between the groups were performed using Student's t-test or the Welch two-sample t-test, with the Mann–Whitney U test applied for normally and non-abnormally distributed data. Categorical variables, expressed as counts and percentages, were compared using the chi-square test or Fisher's exact test, as appropriate. A *p*-value <0.05 was considered statistically significant. Sex, non-ischemic etiology, LBBB morphology, QRS ≥ 150 ms, GLS, atrioventricular dyssynchrony, IVMD >40 ms, LVPEI, DTI septo-lateral delay, septal flash, $SD_{t,peak}$, $SDI_{L,peak}$, DiffInt, and MSDI were covariates entered into the univariate model.

All variables showing a *p* < 0.1 were inserted in the multivariable logistic regression analysis (stepwise entry method). Variables with a *p*-value <0.1 in the multivariate model were considered possible contributors (according to the fact that this is a pilot study). For all of the variables in the multivariate model, the net odds ratio (OR) was reported, along with its 95% confidence interval (CI) and *p*-value. Receiver-operating characteristics curves were individually constructed for dyssynchrony parameters to determine the optimal threshold (closest to the top-left corner), sensitivity, specificity, positive and negative predictive values, and diagnostic accuracy. To explore the value in predicting response to CRT, of the tested 3D–strain parameters over the known variables (i.e.

QRS width, or septal flash) the ROC curves were traced and a comparison was done. In addition, and for assessing the complementarity or the concordance of the new potential 3D–strain tool vs the previously proposed predictive parameters, a Kappa test was performed. The analyses were performed using R software, version 3.0.3 (R Foundation for Statistical Computing, Vienna, Austria. URL: http://www.R-project.org/).

Results
Study population
A total of 48 heart-failure patients (mean age: 65 ± 10 years, 30 men) referred for CRT device implantation were included in this study. 15 patients (31%) had ischemic cardiomyopathy. The mean intrinsic QRS duration was 160 ms (IQR: 160–170), and a typical LBBB morphology was observed in 39 (79%) patients. The mean LVEF was 26 ± 6%.

At 6-months follow-up, 34 34 patients (71%) had a LV end-systolic volume reduction ≥15% (responders). Compared to non-responders, the responders were more often female (47 versus 14%, p = 0.033), had and had better LV performance at baseline as indicated by LVEF (28 ± 5% versus 23 ± 5%, p = 0.002), and GLS values (−9.8 ± 3.4% versus 6.5 ± 3.1%, p = 0.003). The main clinical and echocardiographic characteristics are shown in Table 1.

Classical dyssynchrony echocardiographic parameters
The classical dyssynchrony parameters were analyzed manually, with the results displayed in Table 2. No significant difference was observed in atrioventricular dyssynchrony between CRT-responders and non-responders. The prevalence of IVMD >40 msec and of septal flash were significantly higher in responders than in non-responders (91 versus 50%, p = 0.003 and 79 versus 21%, p = 0.001, respectively).

Automatic analyses and 3D integral-derived longitudinal strain parameters
In the overall population, the median strain peak was −10.2% (−11.6; −9.2), with no significant difference between CRT responders and non-responders (−10.6% [−11.7;-9.6] versus −9.7% [−11.3;-8.4], p = 0.302). The same relationship was observed for $SD_{t,peak}$ (101 ms [80; 123] versus 107 ms [66; 121], p = 0.626).

In the study population, mean $I_{L,avc}$ was lower than mean $I_{L,peak}$ (the mean of the differences: 0.97% s^{-1}, 95% CI: 0.82–1.13, p < 0.0001), and only Mean $I_{L,peak}$ was significantly higher in CRT responders than in non-responders (1.80 ± 0.62% s^{-1} versus 1.39 ± 0.41% s^{-1}, p = 0.029).

The $SDI_{L,peak}$ of all 17 LV segments differed significantly between CRT responders and non-responders (1.18% s^{-1} [0.96; 1.35] versus 0.83% s^{-1} [0.55; 0.99], p = 0.007). DiffInt and MSDI parameters were comparable between CRT responders and non-responders (Table 2).

Table 1 Baseline characteristics of patients

	All patients (n = 48)	CRT responders (n = 34, 71%)	CRT non-responders (n = 14, 29%)	P value
Age (years)	65 ± 10	64 ± 10	65 ± 11	0.893
Male, n (%)	30 (63%)	18 (53%)	12(86%)	0.033*
Ischemic etiology, n (%)	15(31%)	8 (24%)	7 (50%)	0.094
Heart rate (bpm)	69 ± 12	68 ± 12	71 ± 11	0.489
QRS duration (ms)	160 [160; 170]	160 [160; 170]	160 [153; 170]	0.649
QRS & 150 ms, n (%)	40 (83%)	29 (85%)	11 (79%)	0.676
LBBB morphology, n (%)	38 (79%)	27 (79%)	11 (79%)	1
ACE inhibitors or AR blockers, n (%)	46 (96%)	33 (97%)	13(93%)	0.503
β-blockers, n (%)	46 (96%)	33 (97%)	13(93%)	0.503
Diuretics, n (%)	28 (58%)	16 (47%)	12(86%)	0.014*
Antialdosterone, n (%)	18(38%)	14(41%)	4 (29%)	0.412
LVEF (%)	26 ± 6	28 ± 5	23 ± 5	0.002*
LVEDV (ml)	225 ± 85	209 ± 78	265 ± 89	0.037*
LVESV (ml)	169 ± 68	152 ± 57	207 ± 78	0.009*
Mitral regurgitation grade III-IV, n (%)	10(21%)	7(21%)	3(21%)	0.0767
TAPSE (mm)	21 + 4	21 ± 4	20 ± 5	0.78
GLS (%)	− 8.9 ± 3.6	− 9.8 ± 3.4	− 6.5 ± 3.1	0.003*

Data are presented as n (%), mean ± SD, median [IQR]. *ACE* angiotensin-converting enzyme inhibitor, *AR* angiotensin receptor, *GLS* global longitudinal strain, *LVEDV* left ventricular end-diastolic volume, *LVEF* left ventricular ejection fraction, *LVESV* left ventricular end-systolic volume, *TAPSE* tricuspid annular plane systolic excursion. * P value <0,05

Table 2 Classical dyssynchrony 2D–echocardiographic parameters and 3D- echocardiographic integral-based indicators of longitudinal strain

	All patients ($n = 48$)	CRT Responders ($n = 34$, 71%)	CRT Nonresponders ($n = 14$, 29%)	p Value
Atrioventricular dyssynchrony, n (%)	23 (48%)	16 (47%)	7 (50%)	0.853
IVMD >40 ms, n (%)	38 (79%)	31 (91%)	7 (50%)	0.003*
LVPEI (ms)	171 ± 27	175 ± 27	164 ± 28	0.189
DTI septo-lateral delay (ms)	110 [74;161]	114 [74;189]	93 [72;117]	0.162
Septal Flash, n (%)	30 (63%)	27 (79%)	3 (21%)	0.001*
Mean strain peak (%)	−10.2 [−11.6;-9.2]	−10.6 [−11.7;-9.6]	−9.7 [−11.3;-8.4]	0.302
$^{SD}t_{peak}$ (ms)	104 [80;123]	101 [80;123]	107 [66;121]	0.626
$^{Mean}I_{L,peak}$ (%.s-1)	1.68 ± 0.59	1.80 ± 0.62	1.39 ± 0.41	0.029*
Mean I^avc (%.s^{-1})	0.62 [0.34;0.90]	0.76 [0.44;0.92]	0.45 [0.24;0.77]	0.129
SDIL,peak (%.s^{-1})	1.09 [0.82;1.32]	1.18 [0.96;1.35]	0.83 [0.55;0.99]	0.007*
SDIL,avc (%.s-1)	0.85 ± 0.37	0.90 ± 0.35	0.72 ± 0.39	0.125
DiffInt (%.s-1)	0.57 ± 0.5	0.61 ± 0.47	0.47 ± 0.58	0.360
MSDI (ms)	0.35 ± 0.16	0.37 ± 0.16	0.29 ± 0.14	0.106

Data are presented as n (%), mean ± SD, median [IQR]. *DiffInt* average of 17 LV segments of the difference between $I_{L,avc}$ and $I_{L,peak}$ for each 17 LV segments, *DTI* doppler tissue imaging, *LVPEI* left ventricular pre-ejection interval, $I_{L,avc}$ integrals of longitudinal strain signals for each 17 LV segments from the beginning of the cardiac cycle (QRS onset) to the instant of aortic valve closure, $I_{L,peak}$ integrals of longitudinal strain signals for each 17 LV segments from the beginning of the cardiac cycle (QRS onset) to the instant of the corresponding longitudinal strain peak, *IVMD* interventricular mechanical delay, *MSDI* Maximal Difference between Strain peak Instants, *SD* standard deviation, $SDI_{L,peak}$ standard deviation of the integrals of strain signals $I_{L,peak}$ of 17 LV segments, $SDI_{L,avc}$ standard deviation of the integrals of strain signals $I_{L,avc}$ of 17 LV segments, t_{peak} time to strain peak. * p Value <0,05

Predictors of echocardiographic response

From all of the clinical, electrocardiographic, and echocardiographic variables entered into the model, the univariate regression analysis identified six variables with a p-value <0.1(Table 3). The multivariate regression analyses identified three variables as potentials predictors (Table 3): septal flash (OR: 14.1; 95% CI: 3.08−64.9, $p = 0.001$), $SDI_{L,peak}$ (OR: 12.1; 95% CI: 0.81−180, $p = 0.078$), and non-ischemic etiology (OR: 5.33; 95% CI: 0.92−31.1, $p = 0.063$). Among the 18 patients without

Table 3 Factors associated with good response to cardiac resynchronization therapy (univariate and multivariate regression analyses)

	Univariable OR (95% IC)	p Value	Multivariable OR (95% IC)	P value
Female	5.33 (1.03–27.5)	0.046*	1.64 (0.01–14.7)	0.657
Non-ischemic etiology	3.25 (0.87–12.1)	0.079*	5.33 (0.92–31.1)	0.063†
LBBB morphology	1.05 (0.23–4.83)	0.948		
QRS > 150 ms	1.58 (0.32–7.76)	0.572		
GLS	1.44 (1.11–1.89)	0.007*	1.22 (0.01–1.77)	0.223
Atrioventricular dyssynchrony	0.89 (0.26–3.09)	0.853		
IVMD >40 ms	10.3 (2.12–50.3)	0.004*	4.35 (0.53–36)	0.172
LVPEI	1.02 (0.99–1.04)	0.189		
DTI septo-lateral delay	1.01 (0.99–1.02)	0.1		
Septal Flash	14.1 (3.08–64.9)	0.001*	14.1 (3.08–64.9)	0.001†
$^{SD}t,peak$	49.1 (−)	0.604		
$^{SDI}L,peak$	18 (1.94–167)	0.011*	12.1 (0.81–180)	0.078†
DiffInt	0.55 (0.15–1.97)	0.354		
MSDI	41.8 (0.42–4200)	0.113		

DiffInt average of 17 LV segments of the difference between $I_{L,avc}$ and $I_{L,peak}$ for each 17 LV segments, *DTI* doppler tissue imaging, *GLS* global strain longitudinal, *IVMD* intraventricular mechanical delay, *LbBB* left bundle branch block morphology, *LVPEI* left ventricular pre-ejection interval, *MSDI* Maximal Difference between Strain peak Instants, *SD* standard deviation, $SDI_{L,peak}$ standard deviation of the integrals of strain signals $I_{L,peak}$ of 17 LV segments, t_{peak} time to strain peak. *All potential factors of positive response to CRT identified from the univariate analyses with a P value <0,1 were used in the multivariate logistic regression. † Variable with a P value <0,1 in the multivariate model were considered to be possible contributors of positive response of CRT septal flash, the $SDI_{L,peak}$ values were higher in CRT responders than in non-responders (1.12 ± 0.26% s^{-1}- versus 0.77 ± 0.34% s^{-1}, p = 0.03) (Table 4).

The receiver operator characteristic curve analysis for $SDI_{L,peak}$ values identified an optimal cut-off value of 1.037% s^{-1}, with a sensitivity (Se) of 70.6% and specificity (Sp) of 78.6% (Fig. 3). The positive predictive value (PPV), negative predictive value (NPV), and diagnostic accuracy for a cut-off of 1.037% s^{-1} were 89%, 52%, and 0.73, respectively (Table 5). For the septal flash, the Se, Sp, PPV, NPV, and diagnostic accuracy were 79%, 79%, 90%, 61%, and 0.79, respectively.

All of the multiparametric associations were tested, and they are displayed in Table 5. Better diagnostic accuracy was achieved with a combination of an $SDI_{L,peak}$ value >1.037% s^{-1} and interventricular dyssynchrony. The association of four parameters ($SDI_{L,peak}$ > 1.037% s^{-1}, atrioventricular dyssynchrony, interventricular dyssynchrony, and septal flash) increased the test specificity to 100%, although it decreased its sensitivity and NPV. The Kappa test testing the concordance between septal flash and $SDI_{L,peak}$ was 0.26 confirming that $SDI_{L,peak}$ is exploring another kind of mechanical dyssynchrony than septal flash. In addition combining the septal flash and the $SDI_{L,peak}$ > 1.037% s^{-1} lead to an area under the curve: AUC = 0.86.

Discussion

Our study investigated a new quantitative computation method for longitudinal strain curves. Integral-derived parameters were generated and described for the first time, and they were applied in heart failure patients eligible for CRT, producing the following primary findings: 1) automatic analysis of longitudinal strain curves provided new complementary data on LV mechanics by combining information on timing and LV regional performance; 2) the mean $I_{L,peak}$ and $SDI_{L,peak}$ of all 17 LV segments were higher in CRT responders than in non-responders; 3) While marginally significant in this study, $SDI_{L,peak}$ could have an independent value for predicting CRT response; and 4) combining a $SDI_{L,peak}$ value >1.037% s^{-1} and interventricular dyssynchrony appeared to be a promising multi-parametric approach for best predicting CRT response, and it was feasible and robust in patients with sufficient acoustic windows and a sinus rhythm. And perhaps the most important finding was that 3D strain-derived parameter could

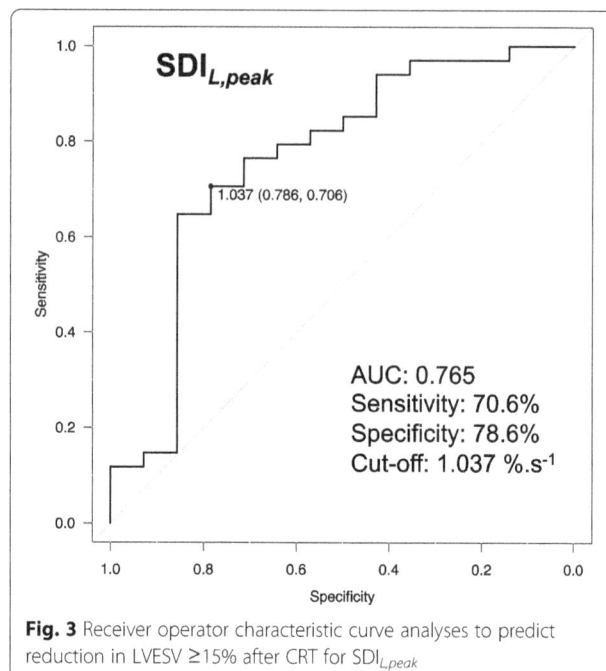

Fig. 3 Receiver operator characteristic curve analyses to predict reduction in LVESV ≥15% after CRT for $SDI_{L,peak}$

differentiate responders from non-responders among 18 patients without septal flash.

Automatic versus mechanical manual dyssynchrony analysis

Since the publication of the disappointing PROSPECT study results [8], several questions have remained unanswered regarding the real discriminatory value of mechanical dyssynchrony in CRT candidates.

The first source of error is undoubtedly related to the lack of standardized data-processing methods. Numerous parameters have been proposed [10]. After disappointing results and thanks to effort of scientists, it has been best understood how complex is cardiac mechanical, how complex is electromechanical coupling but also how valuable could be the imaging approach to best select patients for CRT [25–27]. It has been for instance, clearly shown that, patients with the same left-bundle branch block could exhibit completely different mechanical dyssynchrony patterns [28]. But, there are also, technical challenges to consider. The analysis of strain peaks can be difficult because there are different patterns of strain, which often have multiple peaks. Determining the relevant peak or peaks, along with the reproducibility of the timing of these peaks, remains a challenge. To overcome this

Table 4 3D–echocardiographic integral-based indicators of longitudinal strain in patients without Septal flash

	All patients without Septal flash (n = 18)	CRT responders without Septal flash (n = 7)	CRT non-responders without Septal flash (n = 11)	P value
$SDI_{L,peak}$ (%.s^{-1})	0.90 ± 0.35	1.12 ± 0.26	0.77 ± 0.34	0.03*
$SDI_{L,peak}$ > 1037%.s^{-1}	7 (39%)	5 (71%)	2 (18%)	0,049*

Data are presented as n (%), mean ± SD. $SDI_{L,peak}$ standard deviation of the integrals of strain signals $I_{L,peak}$ of 17 LV segments. * P value <0,05

Table 5 Sensitivity, specificity, positive predictive predictive value, negative predictive value, diagnostic accuracy in monoparametric and multiparametric analyses for reverse remodeling induced by cardiac resynchronization therapy

	Sensitivity	Specificity	Positive predictive value	Negative predictive value	Diagnostic accuracy
septal flash	79%	79%	90%	61%	0.79
SDI $_{L,peak}$ > 1.037%.s^{-1}	70.6%	7.6%	88.9%	52.4%	0.73
SDI $_{L,peak}$ > 1.037%.s^{-1} S Septal Flash	55.9%	92.9%	95%	46.4%	0.67
SDI $_{L,peak}$ > 1.037%.s^{-1} + AV	29.4%	92.9%	90.9%	35.1%	0.48
SDI $_{L,peak}$ > 1.037%.s^{-1} + IV	67.6%	92.9%	95.8%	54.2%	0.75
SDI $_{L,peak}$ > 1.037%.s^{-1} + AV + IV	29.4%	92.9%	90.9%	35.1%	0.48
SDI $_{L,peak}$ > 1.037%.s^{-1} + AV + IV + Septal Flash	23.5%	100%	100%	35%	0.46

AV atrioventricular dyssynchrony, *IV* interventricular dyssynchrony, *SDI L,peak* standard deviation of the integrals of strain signals

difficulty and also to consider not only peaks and dyssynchrony but regional myocardial function as well, a number of authors have proposed novel operator-independent methods that automatically assess function and dyssynchrony, using predefined algorithms [28–31]. In our study, heart failure patients with dilated or ischemic cardiomyopathy were considered eligible for CRT. All of the patients presented with severe LV dysfunction, an altered LVGLS as detectable on 2D echocardiography, an altered mean strain peak with a very low amplitude of strain curves, and significant dispersion of time to strain peak ($SD_{t,peak}$). We thus proposed a new 3D automatic assessment of regional LV mechanics, avoiding as much as possible potential human error.

Toward a new step by step approach for assessing left ventricular dyssynchrony assessment and for CRT response prediction

Mechanical dyssynchrony assessment could have 2 steps. As the first step, septal flash should be searched for using a simple visual and/or M-mode approach. If septal flash (and/or apical rocking) is not found, 3D echo should be performed in the next step as an attempt to detect a novel predictor of volumetric response. In the present study, we confirmed such results but also that the septal flash is highly relevant [21]. That is emphasizing the potential value of multiparametric scores like the L2ANDS2 score [32]. However, septal flash was found in 79% of CRT responders and in only approximately 60% of all of the patients, regardless of cardiomyopathy etiology. In patients without any septal flash, $SDI_{L,peak}$ was significantly higher in CRT responders, suggesting that this new predictor could provide additional information for the optimal selection of CRT patients. After the performing of a multiparametric evaluation of mechanical dyssynchrony that considers the three levels of dyssynchrony (atrioventricular, interventricular, and intra-ventricular), it appeared rather clear that this imaging approach could be of additive value to ECG [33]. A combination of very simple dyssynchrony parameters, such as atrioventricular, interventricular and septal flash, which are easy to

measure and are reproducible, with automated strain-derived parameters, should probably be tested in larger groups of patients based on the current, first validation. The combination of an $SDI_{L,peak}$ > 1.037% s^{-1} and interventricular dyssynchrony appeared to be an interesting multiparametric approach for predicting a good CRT response.

This "second step" three-dimensional STE appeared promising for several reasons [34]: (I) all 17 segments of the LV were evaluated in their 3D motion, along with the relationships among them, thus avoiding the 'out-of-plane' phenomenon inherent to 2D imaging; (II) the full LV volume was assessed during a 6-beat acquisition, allowing for a rapid evaluation of the global and regional all-directional contractions; and (III) all of the 3D echocardiographic strain markers (longitudinal, radial, and circumferential area) exhibited good reproducibility [35]. In our study, the feasibility rate of 3D STE was 83%, with the scientific literature reporting feasibility rates ranging from 63 to 83% [36]. This feasibility rate is likely to increase further with the advent of new transducer technologies. Until now, the principal 3D echocardiography parameter has been the standard deviation of time to minimal systolic volume [11]. This parameter has proved a feasible and reliable parameter of LV mechanical dyssynchrony, which might even provide additional value compared to the current selection criteria for accurate CRT response prediction [11]. This approach is only looking at the analysis of the differences in timings. The assessment of remaining LV regional contractility is lacking [11]. In a small study, 3D strain dyssynchrony index, (area tracking approach using the average difference between peak and end-systolic area strain, derived from 16 LV segments), was proposed for predicting CRT-response [13]. An integrative approach of dyssynchrony and function, using a new longitudinal strain integral-derived method, has appeared more relevant [29, 37]. This approach is likely to be of particular interest in ischemic diseases for distinguishing the passive movement of scarred tissue segments [38]. The mean $I_{L,avc}$ was lower than the mean $I_{L,peak}$ in our patients, indicating that most segments reached their maximal deformation after aortic valve closure. $SDI_{L,peak}$, corresponding to the energy dispersion for all 17 segments at the longitudinal strain peak, appeared to be promising for the assessment of LV dyssynchrony and the prediction of LV reverse remodeling following CRT.

Study limitations

That is a first pilot study, using one kind of echo-machine in a limited number of patients but in two centers. The goal was to 'validate' a tool that was planned to be use in largest population. Since a large intervendor variability has been demonstrated in 3D strain systems, the cut-off values identified are valid only for GE technology [39]. Only the integral-derived longitudinal strain parameters were measured in this study [40]. One limitation to the image acquisition for 3D speckle-tracking was the relatively slow volume rate of 32 ± 7 volumes/s. The volume rate and the image definition will improved in next generation of 3D–probes, it will improve the value of our automatic approach that will be applicable in atrial fibrillation patients thanks to the single beat capabilities.

Another limitation is related to fact that it is a pilot study with the use of an endpoint that is questionable. LV-remodeling is not a perfect surrogate marker of the hardest clinical endpoints. The Endpoint proposed by Packer will have to be considered [41].

Conclusion

This new automatic analysis of 3D longitudinal strain curves, using integral-derived parameters, provided original information on LV mechanics by combining timings and LV regional contractility data. This approach could be of value for improving patient selection for CRT.

Abbreviation

3D: Three-dimensional; 4CH: Four-chamber; AFI: Automated function imaging; CRT: Cardiac resynchronization therapy; DiffInt: The average of 17 LV segments of the difference between $I_{L,avc}$ and $I_{L,peak}$ for each segment; $I_{L,avc}$: The integrals of longitudinal strain signals for all 17 LV segments from the beginning of the cardiac cycle (QRS onset) to the moment of the aortic valve closure; $I_{L,peak}$: The integrals of longitudinal strain signals for all 17 LV segments from the beginning of the cardiac cycle (QRS onset) to the moment of the corresponding longitudinal strain peak; IQR: Interquartile range; IVMD: Interventricular mechanical delay; LBBB: Left bundle branch block; LV: Left ventricular; LVEF: Left ventricular ejection fraction; LVGLS: Left ventricular global longitudinal strain; LVPEI: Left ventricular pre-ejection interval; MSDI: Maximal difference between strain peak instants; NYHA: New York Heart Association; PPV: Positive predictive value; $SD_{t,peak}$: Standard deviation of time to strain peak; STE: Speckle-tracking echocardiography; TDI: Tissue doppler imaging

Acknowledgements

To the whole team and especially the research nurses at the CIC-IT 1414

Funding

For performing the study, we receive a grant from the 'fondation de l'Avenir' (Fondation de France). Grant ET2–654.

Authors' contributions

All the authors validated and provided correction to the manuscript. The concept was imagined by Alfredo Hernandez, Maxime Fournet, Anne Bernard and Erwan Donal. Elena Galli provided a substantial help. Christophe Leclercq helps as well and implanted all the patients. Sylvestre Marechaux provided patients and data. Philippe Mabo lead the research lab and agreed and reviewed the work as well as Jean-Claude Daubert and Raphael Martins. All authors read and approved the final manuscript.

Competing interests

The authors declare that they have no competing interests.

Author details

[1]Cardiologie et CIC-IT 1414, Centre Hospitalier Universitaire de Rennes, F-35000 Rennes, France. [2]LTSI, Université Rennes 1, INSERM, F-35000 Rennes, France. [3]Service de Cardiologie, CHU Tours, F-37000 Tours, France. [4]Service de Cardiologie, Saint Philibert Catholic University Hospital, Lille, France. [5]Service de Cardiologie, Hôpital Pontchaillou, CHU Rennes, F-35033 Rennes, France.

References

1. Cazeau S, Leclercq C, Lavergne T, Walker S, Varma C, Linde C, et al. Effects of multisite biventricular pacing in patients with heart failure and intraventricular conduction delay. N Engl J Med. 2001;344(12):873–80.
2. Cleland JG, Daubert JC, Erdmann E, Freemantle N, Gras D, Kappenberger L, et al. The effect of cardiac resynchronization on morbidity and mortality in heart failure. N Engl J Med. 2005;352(15):1539–49.
3. Linde C, Abraham WT, Gold MR, Daubert C, Group RS. Cardiac resynchronization therapy in asymptomatic or mildly symptomatic heart failure patients in relation to etiology: results from the REVERSE (REsynchronization reVErses Remodeling in systolic left vEntricular dysfunction) study. J Am Coll Cardiol. 2010;56(22):1826–31.
4. Moss AJ, Hall WJ, Cannom DS, Klein H, Brown MW, Daubert JP, et al. Cardiac-resynchronization therapy for the prevention of heart-failure events. N Engl J Med. 2009;361(14):1329–38.
5. Tang AS, Wells GA, Talajic M, Arnold MO, Sheldon R, Connolly S, et al. Cardiac-resynchronization therapy for mild-to-moderate heart failure. N Engl J Med. 2010;363(25):2385–95.
6. European Heart Rhythm A, European Society of C, Heart Rhythm S, Heart Failure Society of A, American Society of E, American Heart A, et al. 2012 EHRA/HRS expert consensus statement on cardiac resynchronization therapy in heart failure: implant and follow-up recommendations and management. Heart Rhythm. 2012;9(9):1524–76.
7. European Society of C, European Heart Rhythm A, Brignole M, Auricchio A, Baron-Esquivias G, Bordachar P, et al. 2013 ESC guidelines on cardiac pacing and cardiac resynchronization therapy: the task force on cardiac pacing and resynchronization therapy of the European Society of Cardiology (ESC). Developed in collaboration with the European heart rhythm association (EHRA). Europace. 2013;15(8):1070–118.
8. Chung ES, Leon AR, Tavazzi L, Sun JP, Nihoyannopoulos P, Merlino J, et al. Results of the predictors of response to CRT (PROSPECT) trial. Circulation. 2008;117(20):2608–16.
9. Ruschitzka F, Abraham WT, Singh JP, Bax JJ, Borer JS, Brugada J, et al. Cardiac-resynchronization therapy in heart failure with a narrow QRS complex. N Engl J Med. 2013;369(15):1395–405.
10. Gorcsan J 3rd, Abraham T, Agler DA, Bax JJ, Derumeaux G, Grimm RA, et al. Echocardiography for cardiac resynchronization therapy: recommendations for performance and reporting–a report from the American Society of Echocardiography Dyssynchrony writing group endorsed by the Heart Rhythm Society. J Am Soc Echocardiogr. 2008;21(3):191–213.
11. Kapetanakis S, Kearney MT, Siva A, Gall N, Cooklin M, Monaghan MJ. Real-time three-dimensional echocardiography: a novel technique to quantify global left ventricular mechanical dyssynchrony. Circulation. 2005;112(7):992–1000.
12. Thebault C, Donal E, Bernard A, Moreau O, Schnell F, Mabo P, et al. Real-time three-dimensional speckle tracking echocardiography: a novel technique to quantify global left ventricular mechanical dyssynchrony. Eur J Echocardiogr. 2011;12(1):26–32.

13. Tatsumi K, Tanaka H, Matsumoto K, Hiraishi M, Miyoshi T, Tsuji T, et al. Mechanical left ventricular dyssynchrony in heart failure patients with narrow QRS duration as assessed by three-dimensional speckle area tracking strain. Am J Cardiol. 2011;108(6):867–72.

14. Dickstein K, Vardas PE, Auricchio A, Daubert JC, Linde C, McMurray J, et al. 2010 focused update of ESC guidelines on device therapy in heart failure: an update of the 2008 ESC guidelines for the diagnosis and treatment of acute and chronic heart failure and the 2007 ESC guidelines for cardiac and resynchronization therapy. Developed with the special contribution of the heart failure association and the European heart rhythm association. Eur Heart J. 2010;31(21):2677–87.

15. Felker GM, Shaw LK, O'Connor CM. A standardized definition of ischemic cardiomyopathy for use in clinical research. J Am Coll Cardiol. 2002;39(2):210–8.

16. Zareba W, Klein H, Cygankiewicz I, Hall WJ, McNitt S, Brown M, et al. Effectiveness of cardiac resynchronization therapy by QRS morphology in the multicenter automatic defibrillator implantation trial-cardiac resynchronization therapy (MADIT-CRT). Circulation. 2011;123(10):1061–72.

17. Lang RM, Badano LP, Mor-Avi V, Afilalo J, Armstrong A, Ernande L, et al. Recommendations for cardiac chamber quantification by echocardiography in adults: an update from the american society of echocardiography and the European association of cardiovascular imaging. Eur Heart J Cardiovasc Imaging. 2015;16(3):233–71.

18. Cazeau S, Bordachar P, Jauvert G, Lazarus A, Alonso C, Vandrell MC, et al. Echocardiographic modeling of cardiac dyssynchrony before and during multisite stimulation: a prospective study. Pacing Clin Electrophysiol. 2003;26(1 Pt 2):137–43.

19. Sogaard P, Egeblad H, Kim WY, Jensen HK, Pedersen AK, Kristensen BO, et al. Tissue Doppler imaging predicts improved systolic performance and reversed left ventricular remodeling during long-term cardiac resynchronization therapy. J Am Coll Cardiol. 2002;40(4):723–30.

20. Bax JJ, Bleeker GB, Marwick TH, Molhoek SG, Boersma E, Steendijk P, et al. Left ventricular dyssynchrony predicts response and prognosis after cardiac resynchronization therapy. J Am Coll Cardiol. 2004;44(9):1834–40.

21. Parsai C, Bijnens B, Sutherland GR, Baltabaeva A, Claus P, Marciniak M, et al. Toward understanding response to cardiac resynchronization therapy: left ventricular dyssynchrony is only one of multiple mechanisms. Eur Heart J. 2009;30(8):940–9.

22. Bernard A, Donal E, Leclercq C, Schnell F, Fournet M, Reynaud A, et al. Impact of Cardiac Resynchronization Therapy on Left Ventricular Mechanics: Understanding the Response through a New Quantitative Approach Based on Longitudinal Strain Integrals. J Am Soc Echocardiogr. 2015;28(6):700–708.

23. Yu CM, Fung WH, Lin H, Zhang Q, Sanderson JE, Lau CP. Predictors of left ventricular reverse remodeling after cardiac resynchronization therapy for heart failure secondary to idiopathic dilated or ischemic cardiomyopathy. Am J Cardiol. 2003;91(6):684–8.

24. Bertini M, Hoke U, van Bommel RJ, Ng AC, Shanks M, Nucifora G, et al. Impact of clinical and echocardiographic response to cardiac resynchronization therapy on long-term survival. Eur Heart J Cardiovasc Imaging. 2013;14(8):774–81.

25. Galli E, Leclercq C, Donal E. Mechanical dyssynchrony in heart failure: still a valid concept for optimizing treatment? Arch Cardiovasc Dis. 2017;110(1):60–8.

26. Bernard A, Donal E, Leclercq C, Schnell F, Fournet M, Reynaud A, et al. Impact of cardiac resynchronization therapy on left ventricular mechanics: understanding the response through a new quantitative approach based on longitudinal strain integrals. J Am Soc Echocardiogr. 2015;28(6):700–8.

27. Brunet-Bernard A, Leclercq C, Donal E. Defining patients at-risk of non-response to cardiac resynchronization therapy. Value of rest and exercise echocardiography. Int J Cardiol. 2014;171(2):279–81.

28. Leenders GE, Lumens J, Cramer MJ, De Boeck BW, Doevendans PA, Delhaas T, et al. Septal deformation patterns delineate mechanical dyssynchrony and regional differences in contractility: analysis of patient data using a computer model. Circ Heart Fail. 2012;5(1):87–96.

29. Prinzen FW, Vernooy K, De Boeck BW, Delhaas T. Mechano-energetics of the asynchronous and resynchronized heart. Heart Fail Rev. 2011;16(3):215–24.

30. Russell K, Eriksen M, Aaberge L, Wilhelmsen N, Skulstad H, Gjesdal O, et al. Assessment of wasted myocardial work: a novel method to quantify energy loss due to uncoordinated left ventricular contractions. Am J Physiol Heart Circ Physiol. 2013;305(7):H996–1003.

31. Szulik M, Tillekaerts M, Vangeel V, Ganame J, Willems R, Lenarczyk R, et al. Assessment of apical rocking: a new, integrative approach for selection of candidates for cardiac resynchronization therapy. Eur J Echocardiogr. 2010;11(10):863–9.

32. Brunet-Bernard A, Marechaux S, Fauchier L, Guiot A, Fournet M, Reynaud A, et al. Combined score using clinical, electrocardiographic, and echocardiographic parameters to predict left ventricular remodeling in patients having had cardiac resynchronization therapy six months earlier. Am J Cardiol. 2014;113(12):2045–51.

33. Lafitte S, Reant P, Zaroui A, Donal E, Mignot A, Bougted H, et al. Validation of an echocardiographic multiparametric strategy to increase responders patients after cardiac resynchronization: a multicentre study. Eur Heart J. 2009;30(23):2880–7.

34. Tanaka H, Hara H, Saba S, Gorcsan J 3rd. Usefulness of three-dimensional speckle tracking strain to quantify dyssynchrony and the site of latest mechanical activation. Am J Cardiol. 2010;105(2):235–42.

35. Reant P, Barbot L, Touche C, Dijos M, Arsac F, Pillois X, et al. Evaluation of global left ventricular systolic function using three-dimensional echocardiography speckle-tracking strain parameters. J Am Soc Echocardiogr. 2012;25(1):68–79.

36. Jasaityte R, Heyde B, D'Hooge J. Current state of three-dimensional myocardial strain estimation using echocardiography. J Am Soc Echocardiogr. 2013;26(1):15–28.

37. Lim P, Donal E, Lafitte S, Derumeaux G, Habib G, Reant P, et al. Multicentre study using strain delay index for predicting response to cardiac resynchronization therapy (MUSIC study). Eur J Heart Fail. 2011;13(9):984–91.

38. Lim P, Pasquet A, Gerber B, D'Hondt AM, Vancraeynest D, Gueret P, et al. Is postsystolic shortening a marker of viability in chronic left ventricular ischemic dysfunction? Comparison with late enhancement contrast magnetic resonance imaging. J Am Soc Echocardiogr. 2008;21(5):452–7.

39. Badano LP, Cucchini U, Muraru D, Al Nono O, Sarais C, Iliceto S. Use of three-dimensional speckle tracking to assess left ventricular myocardial mechanics: inter-vendor consistency and reproducibility of strain measurements. Eur Heart J Cardiovasc Imaging. 2013;14(3):285–93.

40. Mor-Avi V, Lang RM, Badano LP, Belohlavek M, Cardim NM, Derumeaux G, et al. Current and evolving echocardiographic techniques for the quantitative evaluation of cardiac mechanics: ASE/EAE consensus statement on methodology and indications endorsed by the Japanese Society of Echocardiography. Eur J Echocardiogr. 2011;12(3):167–205.

41. Packer M. Development and evolution of a hierarchical clinical composite end point for the evaluation of drugs and devices for acute and chronic heart failure: a 20-years perspective. Packer M Circulation. 2016;134(21):1664–78.

10

Accuracy of echocardiographic area-length method in chronic myocardial infarction: comparison with cardiac CT in pigs

Haitham Ballo[1,2]* , Miikka Tarkia[1], Matti Haavisto[1], Christoffer Stark[2,3], Marjatta Strandberg[2], Tommi Vähäsilta[2,3], Virva Saunavaara[1], Tuula Tolvanen[1], Mika Teräs[1], Ville-Veikko Hynninen[4], Timo Savunen[3], Anne Roivainen[1,5], Juhani Knuuti[1] and Antti Saraste[1,2,6]

Abstract

Background: We evaluated echocardiographic area-length methods to measure left ventricle (LV) volumes and ejection fraction (EF) in parasternal short axis views in comparison with cardiac computed tomography (CT) in pigs with chronic myocardial infarction (MI).

Methods: Male farm pigs with surgical occlusion of the left anterior descending coronary artery ($n = 9$) or sham operation ($n = 5$) had transthoracic echocardiography and cardiac-CT 3 months after surgery. We measured length of the LV in parasternal long axis view, and both systolic and diastolic LV areas in parasternal short axis views at the level of mitral valve, papillary muscles and apex. Volumes and EF of the LV were calculated using Simpson's method of discs (tri-plane area) or Cylinder-hemiellipsoid method (single plane area).

Results: The pigs with coronary occlusion had anterior MI scars and reduced EF (average EF $42 \pm 10\%$) by CT. Measurements of LV volumes and EF were reproducible by echocardiography. Compared with CT, end-diastolic volume (EDV) measured by echocardiography showed good correlation and agreement using either Simpson's method ($r = 0.90$; mean difference -2, 95% CI -47 to 43 mL) or Cylinder-hemiellipsoid method ($r = 0.94$; mean difference 3, 95% CI -44 to 49 mL). Furthermore, End-systolic volume (ESV) measured by echocardiography showed also good correlation and agreement using either Simpson's method ($r = 0.94$; mean difference 12 ml, 95% CI: -16 to 40) or Cylinder-hemiellipsoid method ($r = 0.97$; mean difference:13 ml, 95% CI: -8 to 33). EF was underestimated using either Simpson's method ($r = 0.78$; mean difference -6, 95% CI -11 to 1%) or Cylinder-hemiellipsoid method ($r = 0.74$; mean difference -4, 95% CI-10 to 2%).

Conclusion: Our results indicate that measurement of LV volumes may be accurate, but EF is underestimated using either three or single parasternal short axis planes by echocardiography in a large animal model of chronic MI.

Keywords: Ejection fraction, Transthoracic echocardiography, Cardiac CT

Background

The biplane method of disks (modified Simpson's rule) is the currently recommended 2D method to assess left ventricle (LV) volumes and ejection fraction (EF) [1]. Accordingly, LV volumes should be measured from the apical four- and two chamber views. When apical views are not technically feasible or poor apical endocardial definition precludes accurate tracing, an alternative method to calculate LV volumes is the area-length method, in which the LV is assumed to be hemiellipsoid or bullet shaped [1]. The LV cross-sectional area is computed by planimetry in the parasternal short-axis view or views and the length of the ventricle measured from the midpoint of the mitral valve annular plane to the apex. Variations of the method include the use of different mathematical models and LV cross-sectional

---
* Correspondence: Haitham.Ballo@utu.fi
[1]Turku PET Centre, University of Turku and Turku University Hospital, Kiinamyllynkatu 4-8, Turku 20520, Finland
[2]Heart Center, Turku University Hospital and University of Turku, Turku, Finland
Full list of author information is available at the end of the article

area in the mid-ventricle only or mid-ventricle, basal and apical levels [2–6].

Area-length methods have been validated ex vivo after formalin fixation or in vivo with x-ray cineangiography or radionuclide techniques in normal hearts and in various pathological conditions [3–8]. However, there is limited data validating the use of area-length method for measurement of LV volumes and EF in the presence of regional wall motion abnormalities caused by chronic myocardial infarction (MI) [2]. Furthermore, the quality of 2D images has improved over time. We hypothesized that area-length method would enable accurate LV volume quantification in parasternal short axis images and that computation of LV cross-sectional area at three levels (modified Simpson's method) of the LV would be preferable to one level only (Cylinder-hemiellipsoid method) in the presence of MI scar.

The purpose of this study was to validate echocardiographic area-length methods to quantify LV volumes and EF in parasternal short axis and long axis images using dynamic cardiac computed tomography (CT) as a reference in the presence of regional dysfunction caused by chronic MI in a pig model. Furthermore, we compared Simpson's method of discs and Cylinder-hemiellipsoid methods, which are based on LV area measurements at the level of mitral valve, papillary muscles and apex or at the level of papillary muscles only, respectively.

Methods

Experimental animals and general study protocol

Male Finnish Landrace pigs [age 3 months, weight 28 ± 4 kg (range 19–43 kg)] had either a sham operation (control group) or a concurrent 2-step occlusion of the left anterior descending (LAD) coronary artery with distal ligation for the preconditioning of the heart and subsequent implantation of a proximal ameroid constrictor (chronic MI group) as described recently. The ameroid constrictor will occlude resulting in large MI [9]. After a 3-month follow-up, echocardiography, CT and positron emission tomography (PET) were performed in the same imaging session.

All pigs were housed and fed in individual pens under a 12-h light/12-h dark cycle. Animals were fed with normal farm pig diet (Pekoni 90, Hankkija-Maatalous Oy, Hyvinkää, Finland). Water was provided ad libitum. Animal health was monitored on a daily basis. All animal experiments were made according to European Community Guidelines for the use of experimental animals and approved by Finnish National Animal Experiment Board.

There were 21 pigs in the chronic MI group that survived the 3-month follow-up until the imaging studies. Detailed procedural and long-term survival in this model has been reported previously [9]. Six pigs were excluded due to inability to obtain echo images because of logistic reasons or inadequate imaging windows related to the surgery scar. Another 6 were excluded due to inability to perform cardiac CT due to logistic reasons. Ten animals had a sham operation. One sham-operated animal was sacrificed due to oesophageal obstruction. Three were excluded due to missing or incomplete echocardiographic images. One was excluded due to inability to perform cardiac CT due to logistic reasons. Thus, the final study group consisted of 9 pigs with MI and 5 sham-operated controls.

Anaesthesia and hemodynamic monitoring

Prior to the surgical operation or imaging studies, animals were anaesthetized with intramuscular (i.m.) administration of midazolam 1 mg/kg (Midazolam Hameln, Hameln Pharmaceuticals GmbH, Hameln, Germany) and xylazine 4 mg/kg (Rompun vet, Bayer Animal Health GmbH, Leverkusen, Germany) and connected to a respirator and ventilated mechanically (tidal volume 8–10 mL/kg, frequency 14–18 min^{-1}, Dräger Oxylog 3000, Drägerwerk AG, Lübeck, Germany). An ear vein was cannulated using a 22G venous catheter and anesthesia was maintained with intravenous (i.v.) infusion of propofol 10–50 mg/kg/h (Propofol Lipuro, B. Braun Melsungen AG, Melsungen, Germany) combined with fentanyl 4–8 µg/kg/h i.v. (Fentanyl-Hameln, Hameln Pharmaceuticals GmbH, Hameln, Germany). Femoral artery was cannulated for hemodynamic monitoring during the imaging studies. Diastolic, systolic and mean arterial pressure and heart rate were recorded using a pressure transducer (TruWave, Edwards Lifesciences Corp., Irvine, CA, USA) connected to an anesthesia monitor (Datex Ohmeda S5, GE Healthcare Finland Oy, Helsinki, Finland).

Surgical operation and medication

Animals were operated on as previously described [9]. A short left anterior thoracotomy was performed to allow a direct view of the LAD. The pericardium was opened and tented and a complete ligation of the distal LAD was made immediately after the second diagonal branch using a 5-0 monofilament polypropylene suture (Prolene, Ethicon, and Norderstedt, Germany). Approximately 15 min later, the proximal LAD was prepared free and an ameroid constrictor (2.50 mm or 2.75 mm, model MRI-2.50-TI and MRI-2.75-TI; Research Instruments SW, Escondido, CA, USA) was placed around the LAD. Ameroid size was selected on the basis of the diameter of the LAD. In the control group, a sham operation including thoracotomy and pericardial dissection without the LAD occlusion or implantation of the ameroid was performed.

For analgesia, fentanyl 4–8 µg/kg i.v. was administered intraoperatively and fentanyl 2–4 µg/kg/h (Matrifen transdermal patch, Takeda Pharma A/S, Roskilde, Denmark) postoperatively for 3–7 days. Bupivacain 25 mg i.m. (Bicain, Orion Pharma, and Espoo, Finland) was administered locally to anesthetize the thoracotomy wound at the end of the operation. A single dose of cefuroxime 30 mg/kg i.v. (Cefuroxime, Orion Pharma, and Espoo, Finland) was administered preoperatively for antibiotic prophylaxis. In order to prevent ventricular arrhythmias, amiodarone (Cordarone, Sanofi-Synthelabo Ltd, Newcastle upon Tyne, UK) was administered 8 mg/kg perorally (p.o.) daily for 1 week before and for 2 weeks after the surgery. Amiodarone 6 mg/kg i.v, metoprolol 0.2 mg/kg i.v. (Seloken, Genexi, Fontenaysous Bois, France) and magnesium sulphate (MgSO$_4$) 25 mg/kg i.v. (Addex-magnesiumsulfaatti, Fresenius Kabi AB, Uppsala, Sweden) were administered intraoperatively. Clopidogrel 3 mg/kg p.o. (Plavix, Sanofi Winthrop Industrie S.A., Ambarès et Lagrave, France) was administered daily 1 day before and daily for 2 weeks after the surgery to prevent premature thrombosis of the LAD.

Transthoracic echocardiography
Echocardiographic studies were performed by a portable Vivid Q device and MS5 transducer (GE, Hjorten, Norway). The anesthesized animals were studied in supine position. Left or right parasternal views were used to visualize the LV. 2D parasternal long axis view including the apex and short-axis views obtained at the level of the mitral valve (basal LV level), papillary muscles (papillary level), and apex (apical level). All images were stored in DICOM format, and analysed off-line using Echo PAC PC 113 software (GE, Hjorten, Norway).

Echocardiography image analysis
Area of the LV cavity was measured planimetrically by manually tracing the endocardial borders in short axis views at the level of mitral valve, papillary muscles and apex. Papillary muscles and trabeculations were included within the cavity. End-diastole was identified at the beginning of the QRS complex of the simultaneously recorded electrocardiography (ECG) and the systolic frame was selected as the one with smallest LV cavity. LV length was measured in parasternal long axis view from the apex to the level of the mitral valve annulus. Each measurement was repeated 2 times and mean of them recorded.

Reproducibility of the measurements was tested by repeated analysis of images of 5 pigs by the same or two independent observers and coefficient of variation (CV) was calculated.

The end-diastolic volume (EDV), end-systolic volume (ESV) and EF were calculated using two different methods:

The modified Simpson's method [3–6]: The volume of the two basal thirds of LV is determined using the Simpson's rule, but volume of apex is estimated separately as the volume of an ellipsoid volume segment using formula:

$$Volume = (A_1 + A_2)(L/3) + (A_3/2)(L/3) + (\pi/6)(L/3)^3.$$

Where A$_1$, A$_2$, and A$_3$ are LV areas at the level of mitral valve, papillary muscles and apex; and L is the maximum length of ventricle

Cylinder-hemiellipsoid [3–5]: Is a combined figure model in which the LV is divided into cylinder and hemiellipsoid. The volume is calculated from the formula.

$$Volume = 5/6AL.$$

Where A is LV cavity area at the level of papillary muscles and L length of the LV.

The LV EF was then calculated according to formula:

$$\frac{\text{End-diastolic volume–End-systolic volume}}{\text{End-diastolic volume}} \times 100$$

Dynamic cardiac CT
End-diastolic and end-systolic volumes (EDV, ESV) and ejection fraction (EF) were evaluated by helical computed tomography angiography (CTA, GE Discovery VCT, General Electric Medical Systems, Wankesha, WI, USA) with iodinated contrast agent (Omnipaque 350 mg I/mL, Amersham Health AS, Nydalen, Oslo, Norway). Contrast agent (100 mL) was administered at 4 mL/s via the ear vein and flushed with 100 mL of physiological saline. CTA scanning was performed during breath-hold and started immediately when contrast agent appeared into the LV. A 3-lead ECG was used for cardiac triggering and CTA images were reconstructed with retrospective gating at 0–90% at 10% interval relative to the cardiac cycle. Left ventricular EDV and ESV were calculated by tracing the endocardial borders with semi-automated analysis software (CardIQ Function Xpress) and ADW 4.5 work station (GE Medical Systems, Milwaukee, WI, USA).

[^{11}C]acetate PET
Size of the MI was defined by PET perfusion imaging with [^{11}C]acetate as described [9]. [^{11}C]acetate [782 ± 65 MBq (range 689–874 MBq)] was injected i.v. via the

ear vein as a slow bolus. The acquisition frames were as follows: 10 × 10 s, 1 × 60 s, 5 × 100 s, 5 × 120 s, 5 × 240 s (total duration 41 min). The acquired PET data was reconstructed with an iterative VUE Point algorithm. There were 2 iterations and 24 subsets in reconstruction. The whole transaxial field of view (70 cm) was reconstructed in 128 × 128 matrix yielding pixel size of 5.47 mm × 5.47 mm. The measurements were corrected for scatter, random counts and dead time. The device produces 47 axial planes with a slice thickness of 3.27 mm. Images were analysed using cardiac image analysis Carimas 2 software (Turku PET Centre, Turku, Finland; http://www.turkupetcentre.fi/carimas), polar maps of myocardial blood flow were generated, and MI was defined as the area of the LV (%) with resting perfusion <60% of the maximum.

Tissue samples
Immediately after the imaging studies, the animals were sacrificed by i.v. injection of potassium chloride. Heart was excised and sliced horizontally to four slices from base to apex.

In order to confirm the presence of MI, samples were incubated for 15 min in 1% 2,3,5-triphenyltetrazolium chloride (TTC) (Sigma-Aldrich, Saint Louis, MO, USA) diluted in phosphate-buffered saline (pH 7.4) at 37 °C. Stained myocardial samples were photographed from both sides.

Statistical analysis
All data were expressed as mean ± SD. Linear regression analysis and Pearson's correlation were used to compare CT and two-dimensional echocardiography. The degree of agreement was analyzed by using Bland-Altman method. Student's t-test for non-paired data was used to compare means of two groups. p value > 0.05 was considered as significant.

Results
Basic characteristics of animals
The final study group consisted of 9 pigs with coronary ligation and 5 sham-operated controls. Mean weight was 104 ± 16 kg (range 84–130 kg). The hemodynamic parameters measured at the time of imaging are shown in Table 1.

Table 1 Hemodynamic characteristics of pigs with myocardial infarction (MI) and controls

Cardiovascular index	Control (n = 5)	MI (n = 9)	All (n = 14)	p
Heart rate (bpm)	110 ± 18	86 ± 18	95 ± 21	0.16
Systolic blood pressure (mmHg)	142 ± 18	120 ± 18	128 ± 20	0.19
Diastolic blood pressure (mmHg)	96 ± 6	78 ± 15	84 ± 15	0.12

None of the sham-operated pigs had MI, whereas an area of MI was detected in the apical and/or mid-ventricular slices of the anterior septum and anterior wall in 8 animals with an ameroid constrictor implanted based on TTC staining of myocardial slices. In these pigs, the MI size varied from 3 to 57% of the LV and the average size was 23 ± 19% as shown by PET perfusion imaging.

Measurement of LV volumes and EF
Representative echocardiographic and CT images used for delineation of the LV cavity are shown in Fig. 1. LV diastolic volume, systolic volume and EF by cardiac CT and echocardiography using either Simpson's method or Cylinder-hemiellipsoid method are shown in Table 2. In pigs with MI, average LV volumes or EF measured by echocardiography did not differ significantly from those measured by CT (Table 2). Although LV diastolic volumes were similar in pigs with MI and controls, systolic volumes were larger and EF was lower in pigs with MI than controls.

Reproducibility of repeated measurements by the same or two observers are shown in Table 3. CV was always lower than 11% indicating good reproducibility.

Agreement between echocardiography and cardiac CT
The correlations between LV volumes and EF measured by echocardiography and dynamic cardiac CT are shown in Fig. 2. There were good correlations between LV diastolic volumes measured with CT and either the Simpson's (r = 0.90, p = 0. 001) or Cylinder-hemiellipsoid (r = 0.94, p = 0. 0002) methods. good correlations were also found between LV systolic volumes measured with CT and the Simpson's (r = 0.94, p = 0. 0003) or Cylinder-hemiellipsoid (r = 0.97, p < 0.0001) methods. There was a relatively good correlation between EF measured by CT and Simpson's method (r = 0.78, p = 0. 01) or Cylinder-hemiellipsoid method (r = 0.74, p = 0. 02).

Bland-Altman plots between LV volumes and EF measured by CT or echocardiography are shown in Fig. 3. There was a good agreement between LV diastolic volumes measured by CT and either Simpson's method (mean difference: −2 ml, 95% CI: −47 to 43) or Cylinder-hemiellipsoid method (mean difference: 3 ml, 95% CI: −44 to 49). Compared with CT, LV systolic volumes were overestimated by the Simpson's method (mean difference: 12 ml, 95% CI: −16 to 40) and by Cylinder-hemiellipsoid method (mean difference: 13 ml, 95% CI: −8 to 33). Compared with CT, both Simpson's method and Cylinder-hemiellipsoid method underestimated the LV EF (mean difference: −6%, 95% CI: −11% to 1%and −4%, 95% CI: −10% to 2%, respectively).

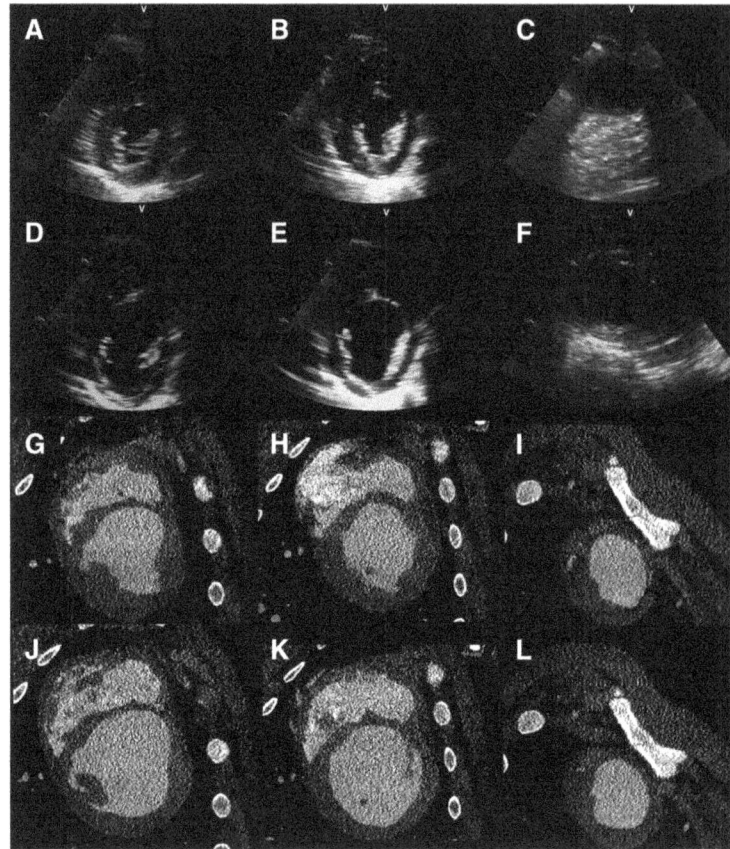

Fig. 1 Echocardiographic parasternal short-axis views of the left ventricle (LV) at the level of mitral valve (**a** and **d**), papillary muscles (**b** and **e**) and apex (**c** and **f**) at systole (**a**, **b** and **c**) and end-diastole (**d**, **e** and **f**). Short axis cardiac CT views of the LV of the same pig at the level of mitral valve (**g** and **j**), papillary muscles (**h** and **k**) and apex (**i** and **l**) at systole (**g**, **h** and **i**) and end-diastole (**j**, **k** and **l**). The pig had myocardial infarction involving of45% of the LV

Table 2 Left ventricle volumes at diastole (EDV) and systole (ESV) and ejection fraction (EF) measured by cardiac CT or echocardiography and either Simpson's, or Cylinder-hemiellipsoid methods in pigs with chronic myocardial infarction (MI) and controls

	Control ($n = 5$)	MI ($n = 9$)	All ($n = 14$)	p
EDV (mL)				
Cardiac CT	140 ± 19	227 ± 96	196 ± 88	0.07
Modified Simpson's	124 ± 18	225 ± 126 [a]	189 ± 111	0.1
Cylinder hemiellipsoid	112 ± 22	230 ± 140 [b]	188 ± 125	0.09
ESV (mL)				
Cardiac CT	49 ± 2	137 ± 79	106 ± 76	0.03
Modified Simpson's	59 ± 14	149 ± 98 [c]	117 ± 89	0.07
Cylinder hemiellipsoid	47 ± 14	150 ± 94 [d]	113 ± 90	0.03
EF (%)				
Cardiac CT	64 ± 4	42 ± 10	50 ± 14	<0.001
Modified Simpson's	53 ± 5	37 ± 8 [e]	42 ± 11	0.0015
Cylinder hemiellipsoid	59 ± 7	38 ± 6 [f]	46 ± 12	<0.001

[a] $P = 0.86$ vs. Cardiac CT, [b] $P = 0.85$ vs. Cardiac CT, [c] $P = 0.72$ vs. Cardiac CT, [d] $P = 0.82$ vs. Cardiac CT, [e] $P = 0.1$ vs. Cardiac CT, [f] $P = 0.3$ vs. Cardiac CT

Table 3 Coefficients of variation (CV) between repeated measurements by the same (Intra-observer) and two (Inter-observer) observers in 5 pigs

Echocardiographic index	Intra-observer CV (%)	Inter-observer CV (%)
Modified Simpson's		
Ejection fraction	8.2	10.4
End-diastolic volume	2.5	6.4
End-systolic volume	4.7	10.9
Cylinder hemiellipsoid		
Ejection fraction	9.3	10.4
End-diastolic volume	1.9	10.3
End-systolic volume	2.5	6.4

Discussion

These results suggest that area-length methods obtained using parasternal short axis projections are valid alternatives for the assessment of LV volume, although EF was appears to be underestimated in the presence of chronic MI when apical views are not technically feasible.

We found that LV volumes and can be measured relatively accurately, but EF is underestimated using echocardiography and area-length methods in the presence of regional wall motion abnormality due to chronic MI. Comparable estimates can be obtained with hemiellipsoid method and modified Simpson's methods when CT was used as a reference. We used a novel pig model of chronic MI. In this model, ameroid constrictor gradually occludes the LAD resulting in large MI. Two-step occlusion improves survival of animals and enables long-term follow-up studies. The technique resulted in variable MI size and none of the pigs showed signs of overt heart failure. Although systemic hemodynamic were variable, there was a tendency towards lower heart rate and blood pressure in pigs with MI that may be related to enhanced cardioinhibitory response to the anaesthetic agents in the presence of cardiac dysfunction. As in many other animal models, apical echocardiographic windows are not possible to obtain in pig due to chest anatomy that necessitates the use of parasternal views only. Therefore, our findings have implications for translational studies using pig models of MI and ischemic heart failure.

Area-length methods have been previously validated in ex vivo formalin fixed hearts and in patients using X-ray cineangiography or radionuclide ventriculography as a gold standard [3–8]. The patient series included total number of approximately 50 patients with different pathologies, including as ischemic heart disease, cardiomyopathy, valvular heart disease, constrictive pericarditis or hypertrophy [6–8]. Regional wall motion abnormalities were reported to be present in many patients. One experimental study has been performed after acute (1 h) occlusion of the LAD in dog. In these studies, reasonably good correlations were obtained between area-length echocardiography and the reference standard using either Simpsons's technique or the hemiellipsoid method. In the presence of LAD occlusion, both Simpson's technique and the hemiellipsoid technique provided good correlations when short axis image from the papillary muscle level including the region with wall motion abnormality was included [8]. Our study adds to the previous studies by systematically comparing area-length method with cardiac CT in the presence of LV dysfunction caused by chronic MI that is a common cause of heart failure. Quantification of LV volume and EF by CT is based on delineation of actual chamber volumes that has been shown to be accurate when compared with magnetic resonance imaging (MRI) [10]. However, cardiac MRI is considered as the gold standard for this purpose [11, 12].

As in previous studies we found that volumes were accurately measured by the area-length method. In this study, we measured the longest length of the LV from the apical long axis view. This is in line with a previous study recommending the use of the apical long-axis view due to low risk of foreshortening of the image, and providing an additional endocardial reference position in the aorta [13]. In pig, it was feasible to visualize the entire length of the LV except a small tip in the apex in some animals from parasternal long axis view.

Simpson's method and the cylinder hemiellipsoid methods were used in the present study since they have shown good accuracy in previous studies. We also tested cylinder truncated cone and cylinder cone-cone models (data not shown), but their performance in measuring LV volumes was inferior to Simpson's or cylinder hemiellipsoid methods.

Study limitations

Although reproducibility of measurements was good, high operative mortality resulted in small sample size that can affect comparisons of small differences between methods [9]. Therefore, the results should be confirmed in a larger series. In general, the accuracy of estimation of left ventricular volumes and EF on 2D echocardiography is limited by geometrical assumptions, standardized image positions with respect to LV long axis, and accurate tracing of LV endocardial boundaries [5, 7, 14]. In addition, measurement of long axis length may be affected, because the cardiac apex not always visualized in the long axis view.

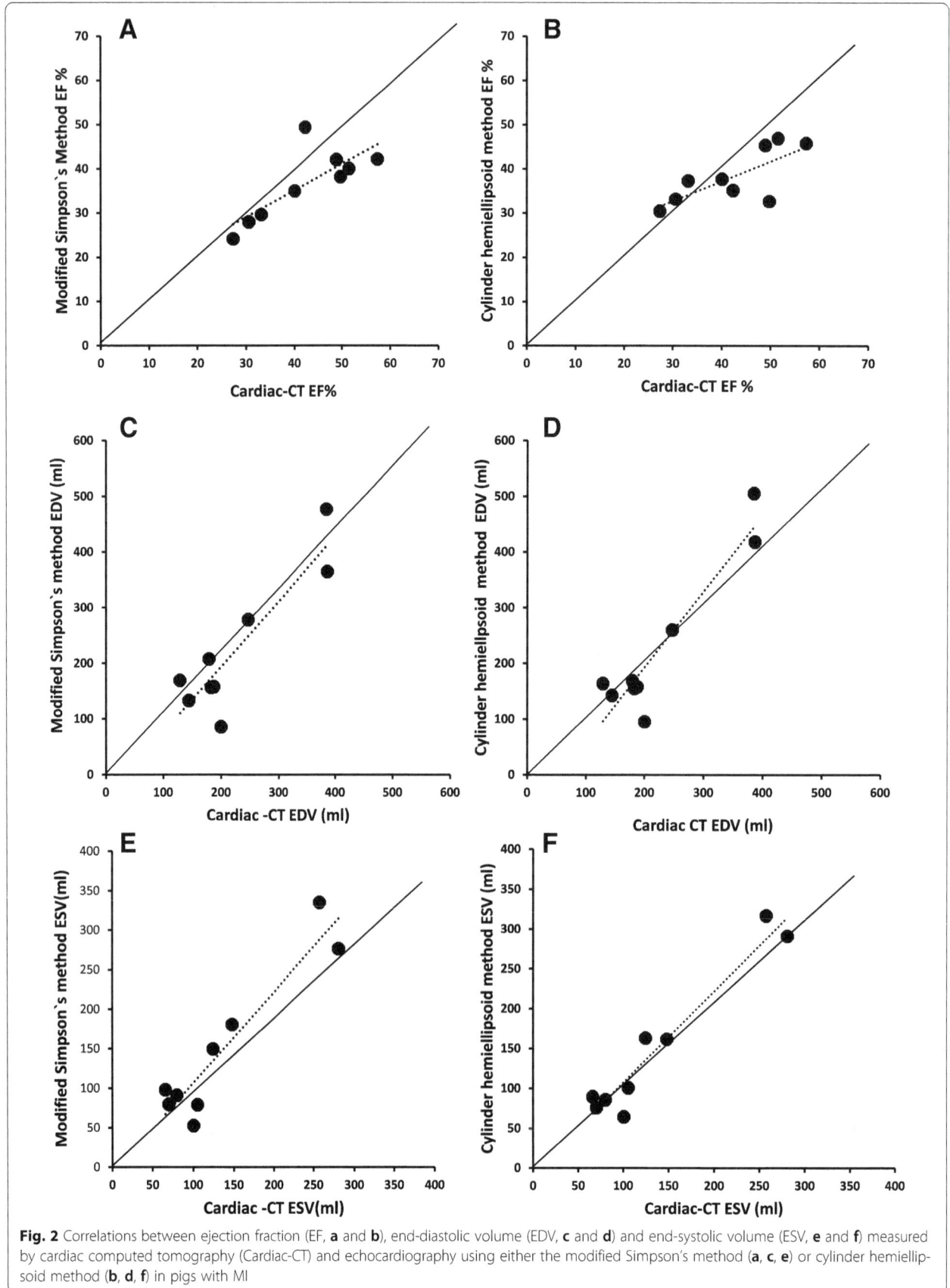

Fig. 2 Correlations between ejection fraction (EF, **a** and **b**), end-diastolic volume (EDV, **c** and **d**) and end-systolic volume (ESV, **e** and **f**) measured by cardiac computed tomography (Cardiac-CT) and echocardiography using either the modified Simpson's method (**a**, **c**, **e**) or cylinder hemiellipsoid method (**b**, **d**, **f**) in pigs with MI

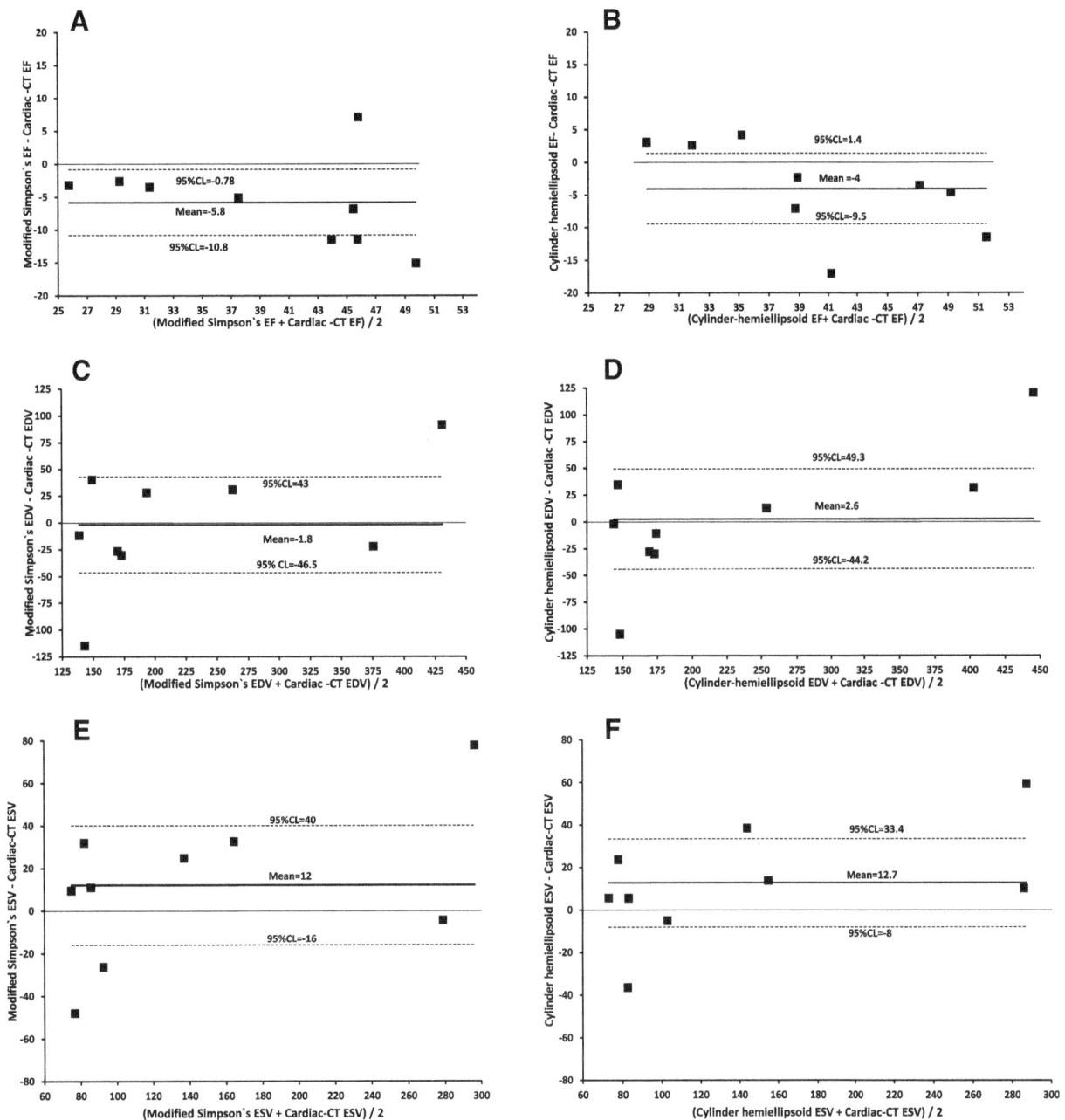

Fig. 3 Bland-Altman analysis for agreement between ejection fraction (EF, **a** and **b**), end-diastolic volume (EDV, **c** and **d**) and end-systolic volume (ESV, **e** and **f**) measured by cardiac computed tomography (Cardiac-CT) and echocardiography using either the modified Simpson's method (**a**, **c**, **e**) or cylinder hemiellipsoid method (**b**, **d**, **f**) in pigs with MI

Conclusions

Our results indicate that measurement of LV volumes may be accurate, but EF is underestimated in parasternal short axis images using transthoracic echocardiography in a large animal model of chronic MI.

Abbreviations

CT: Computed tomography; CTA: Computed tomography angiography; CV: Coefficient of variation; ECG: Electrocardiography; EDV: End-diastolic volume; EF: Ejection fraction; ESV: End-systolic volume; LAD: Left anterior descending coronary artery; LV: Left ventricle; MI: Myocardial infarction; MRI: Magnetic resonance imaging; PET: Positron emission tomography; TTC: 2,3,5-triphenyltetrazolium chloride; TTE: Transthoracic echocardiogram

Acknowledgements

Not applicable.

Funding

This work was supported by Tekes—the Finnish Funding Agency for Technology Innovation; the Finnish Cultural Foundation and Finnish Foundation for Cardiovascular Research. It was conducted in the Finnish

Centre of Excellence in Cardiovascular and Metabolic Diseases supported by the Academy of Finland, University of Turku, Turku University Hospital, and Åbo Akademi University.

Authors' contributions
MT, TS, AR, JK, AS the designers of the study, HB, MT, MH, CS, MS, TV, VS, TT, MT, VVH, TS, JK, AS Carried out the experiments and analysed the data, all authors were writing and drafting the manuscript. All authors read and approved the final manuscript.

Authors' information
Haitham Ballo is a PhD student supported by the Clinical Investigation Doctoral Programme of the University of Turku Graduate School.

Competing interests
The authors declare that they have no competing interests.

Author details
[1]Turku PET Centre, University of Turku and Turku University Hospital, Kiinamyllynkatu 4-8, Turku 20520, Finland. [2]Heart Center, Turku University Hospital and University of Turku, Turku, Finland. [3]Research Centre of Applied and Preventive Cardiovascular Medicine, University of Turku, Turku, Finland. [4]Department of Anesthesiology, Intensive Care, Emergency Care and Pain Medicine, Turku University Hospital, Turku, Finland. [5]Turku Center for Disease Modeling, University of Turku, Turku, Finland. [6]Institute of Clinical Medicine, University of Turku, Turku, Finland.

References
1. Lang RM, Badano LP, Mor-Avi V, Afilalo J, Armstrong A, Ernande L, Flachskampf FA, Foster E, Goldstein SA, Kuznetsova T, Lancellotti P, Muraru D, Picard MH, Rietzschel ER, Rudski L, Spencer KT, Tsang W, Voigt JU. Recommendations for cardiac chamber quantification by echocardiography in adults: an update from the American Society of Echocardiography and the European Association of Cardiovascular Imaging. Eur Heart J Cardiovasc Imaging. 2015;16:233-70.
2. Picard MH, Popp RL, Weyman AE. Assessment of Left Ventricular Function by Echocardiography: A Technique in Evolution. J Am Soc Echocardiogr. 2008;21:14-21.
3. Wyatt HL, Heng MK, Meerbaum S, Hestenes JD, Cobo JM, Davidson RM, Corday E. Cross-sectional echocardiography. I. Analysis of mathematic models for quantifying mass of the left ventricle in dogs. Circulation. 1979;60:1104-13.
4. Wyatt HL, Meerbaum S, Heng MK, Gueret P, Corday E. Cross-sectional echocardiography. II. Analysis of mathematic models for quantifying volume of the formalin-fixed left ventricle. Circulation. 1980;61:1119-25.
5. Wyatt HL, Meerbaum S, Heng MK, Gueret P, Corday E. Cross-sectional echocardiography: III. Analysis of mathematic models for quantifying volume of symmetric and asymmetric left ventricles. Am Heart J. 1980;100:821-8.
6. Folland ED, Parisi AF, Moynihan PF, Jones DR, Feldman CL, Tow DE. Assessment of left ventricular ejection fraction and volumes by real-time, two-dimensional echocardiography. A comparison of cineangiographic and radionuclide techniques. Circulation. 1979;60:760-6.
7. Helak JW, Reichek N. Quantitation of human left ventricular mass and volume by two-dimensional echocardiography: in vitro anatomic validation. Circulation. 1981;63:1398-407.
8. Gueret P, Meerbaum S, Wyatt HL, Uchiyama T, Lang TW, Corday E. Two-dimensional Echocardiographic Quantitation of Left Ventricular Volumes and Ejection Fraction Importance of Accounting for Dyssynergy in Short-axis Reconstruction Models. Circulation. 1980;62:1308-18.
9. Tarkia M, Stark C, Haavisto M, Kentala R, Vähäsilta T, Savunen T, Strandberg M, Hynninen VV, Saunavaara V, Tolvanen T, Teräs M, Rokka J, Pietilä M, Saukko P, Roivainen A, Saraste A, Knuuti J. Cardiac remodeling in a new pig model of chronic heart failure: Assessment of left ventricular functional, metabolic, and structural changes using PET, CT, and echocardiography. J Nucl Cardiol. 2015;22:655-65.
10. Greupner J, Zimmermann E, Grohmann A, Dübel HP, Althoff TF, Borges AC, Rutsch W, Schlattmann P, Hamm B, Dewey M. Head-to-head comparison of left ventricular function assessment with 64-row computed tomography, biplane left cineventriculography, and both 2- and 3-dimensional transthoracic echocardiography: comparison with magnetic resonance imaging as the reference standard. J Am Coll Cardiol. 2012;59:1897-907.
11. Gardner BI, Bingham SE, Allen MR, Blatter DD, Anderson JL. Cardiac magnetic resonance versus transthoracic echocardiography for the assessment of cardiac volumes and regional function after myocardial infarction: an intrasubject comparison using simultaneous intrasubject recordings. Cardiovasc Ultrasound. 2009;7:38.
12. Bellenger NG, Burgess MI, Ray SG, Lahiri A, Coats AJ, Cleland JG, Pennell DJ. Comparison of left ventricular ejection fraction and volumes in heart failure by echocardiography, radionuclide ventriculography and cardiovascular magnetic resonance; are they interchangeable? Eur Heart J. 2000;21:1387-96.
13. Nosir YF, Vletter WB, Boersma E, Frowijn R, Ten Cate FJ, Fioretti FM, Roelandt JR. The apical long-axis rather than the two-chamber view should be used in combination with the four-chamber view for accurate assessment of left ventricular volumes and function. Eur Heart J. 1997;18:1175-85.
14. Chukwu EO, Barasch E, Mihalatos DG, Katz A, Lachmann J, Han J, Reichek N, Gopal AS. Relative Importance of Errors in Left Ventricular Quantitation by Two-Dimensional Echocardiography: Insights from Three-Dimensional Echocardiography and Cardiac Magnetic Resonance Imaging. J Am Soc Echocardiogr. 2008;21:990-7.

11

Rotational method simplifies 3-dimensional measurement of left atrial appendage dimensions during transesophageal echocardiography

Chaim Yosefy[1,3]*, Yulia Azhibekov[2], Boris Brodkin[1], Vladimir Khalameizer[1], Amos Katz[1] and Avishag Laish-Farkash[1]

Abstract

Background: Not all echo laboratories have the capability of measuring direct online 3D images, but do have the capability of turning 3D images into 2D ones "online" for bedside measurements. Thus, we hypothesized that a simple and rapid rotation of the sagittal view (green box, x-plane) that shows all needed left atrial appendage (LAA) number of lobes, orifice area, maximal and minimal diameters and depth parameters on the 3D transesophageal echocardiography (3DTEE) image and LAA measurements after turning the images into 2D (Rotational 3DTEE/"Yosefy Rotation") is as accurate as the direct measurement on real-time-3D image (RT3DTEE).

Methods: We prospectively studied 41 consecutive patients who underwent a routine TEE exam, using QLAB 10 Application on EPIQ7 and IE33 3D-Echo machine (BORTHEL Phillips) between 01/2013 and 12/2015. All patients underwent 64-slice CT before pulmonary vein isolation or for workup of pulmonary embolism. LAA measurements were compared between RT3DTEE and Rotational 3DTEE versus CT.

Results: Rotational 3DTEE measurements of LAA were not statistically different from RT3DTEE and from CT regarding: number of lobes (1.6 ± 0.7, 1.6 ± 0.6, and 1.4 ± 0.6, respectively, p = NS for all); internal area of orifice (3.1 ± 0.6, 3.0 ± 0.7, and 3.3 ± 1.5 cm^2, respectively, p = NS for all); maximal LAA diameter (24.8 ± 4.5, 24.6 ± 5.0, and 24.9 ± 5.8 mm, respectively, p = NS for all); minimal LAA diameter (16.4 ± 3.4, 16.7 ± 3.3, and 17.0 ± 4.4 mm, respectively, p = NS for all), and LAA depth (20.0 ± 2.1, 19.8 ± 2.2, and 21.7 ± 6.9 mm, respectively, p = NS for all).

Conclusion: Rotational 3DTEE method for assessing LAA is a simple, rapid and feasible method that has accuracy similar to that of RT3DTEE and CT. Thus, rotational 3DTEE ("Yosefy rotation") may facilitate LAA closure procedure by choosing the appropriate device size.

Keywords: 3-dimensional transesophageal echocardiography, Left atrial appendage, Imaging, Computed tomography, Rotation

Abbreviations: "Yosefy rotation", Rotational 3DTEE; 2DTEE, 2D transesophageal echocardiography; 3DTEE, 3D transesophageal echocardiography; AA, Atrial fibrillation; BSA, Body surface area; CT, Computed tomography; IVS-D, Inter-ventricular septum diameter; LAA, Left atrial appendage; LPW-D, Left posterior ventricular wall diameter; LVEDD, Left ventricular end diastolic diameter; LVEF, Left ventricular ejection fraction; LVESD, Left ventricular end systolic diameter; MPR, Multiplanar reconstruction; MRI, Magnetic resonance imaging; MS, Mitral stenosis; OAC, Oral anticoagulation; PE, Pulmonary embolism; PVI, Pulmonary vein isolation; RT3DTEE, Real-time-3D image; TEE, Transesophageal echocardiography; TTE, Transthoracic echocardiography

* Correspondence: yosefy@barzi.health.gov.il
[1]Department of Cardiology, Barzilai Medical Center, Ben-Gurion University of the Negev, Ashkelon, Israel
[3]Noninvasive Cardiology Unit, Barzilai Medical Center, Ashkelon 78306, Israel
Full list of author information is available at the end of the article

Background

Ninety percent of clots in patients with non-valvular atrial fibrillation (AF) occur in the left atrial appendage (LAA). The shape and location of LAA allow for stasis of blood in AF, mitral stenosis (MS), and other low cardiac output conditions. Clots may remain hidden because of the three-dimensional (3D) complexity of the LAA [1, 2]. Complex LAA morphology characterized by an increased number of LAA lobes (≥3) was associated with the presence of LAA thrombus independently of clinical risk and blood stasis [1].

Over the last years, minimally invasive epicardial techniques and catheter-based transseptal techniques have been developed for occlusion of the LAA orifice to reduce stroke risk [3–5]. These devices and procedures may provide an alternative to oral anticoagulation (OAC) for AF patients at high risk for stroke but with contraindications for chronic OAC [6–8].

Accurate knowledge of LAA anatomy and dimensions has become a key guiding stage before introducing LAA closure devices [7, 9, 10]. LAA assessment should be done prior to procedure [7, 11–13]. Currently, 2D transesophageal echocardiography (2DTEE) at a cut plane angulation of 135° is the recommended method to size maximal LAA orifice diameter before introducing a percutaneous LAA closure device [9, 10, 14, 15]. However, 2DTEE does not adequately allow complete spatial visualization of the LAA [11–13, 16]. Thus, three-dimensional imaging modalities [11–13] such as cardiac magnetic resonance imaging (MRI), computed tomography (CT), and Real-Time-3-Dimensional Transesophageal Echocardiography (RT3DTEE) may be more accurate [15, 17–19].

Recent trials show better performance of RT3DTEE for the assessment of LAA anatomy compared with 2DTEE regarding LAA orifice area, LAA ejection fraction calculation, and LAA volume [15, 20–22]. Our group showed that bedside direct online RT3DTEE measurements of LAA maximal orifice diameter are more accurate than 2DTEE measurements and are as accurate as CT as gold standard [16]. Thus, direct RT3DTEE measurements may facilitate LAA closure procedure by choosing the appropriate device size. However, not all echo laboratories have the capability of using this method that directly measures the 3D images (RT3DTEE) but yet have the capability to online turn 3D images into 2D ones for bedside measurements.

We analyzed LAA measurements using a simpler and faster 3D method: after conversion of the 3D image into three 2D planes (X,Y,Z), the operator uses a 360° rotation of the sagittal plane (green box, x-plane), that enables him to rapidly choose the image which shows all the LAA parameters needed for the introduction of the invasive procedure in one single "stop shop" image (Rotational 3DTEE/"Yosefy Rotation"). Our aim was to validate the accuracy of Rotational 3DTEE versus the former direct online RT3DTEE method for LAA assessment.

Methods

Study population

A total of 41 consecutive patients who underwent a routine indicated 3DTEE and 64-slice CT, either before pulmonary vein isolation (PVI) ablation (n = 34) for precise definition of LA and pulmonary veins anatomy, or for workup of pulmonary embolism (PE) (n = 7) (Table 1). In this group of patients, 64-slice CT was used as reference technique to test the accuracy of 3DTEE-derived measurements of LAA parameters. We compared Rotational 3DTEE LAA measurements versus RT3DTEE.

Echocardiography

Forty-one consecutive patients (out of 43 patients) who underwent the routine echocardiography exam using EPIQ7 and iE33 echo machine (Philips Medical Systems, Andover, MA) between January 2013 and December 2015 and had a good echogenic window, were included in the study. All images were digitally stored for offline analysis (QLAB 10.0 cardiac 3DQ, Philips Medical Systems).

Table 1 Baseline demographics and echocardiographic characteristics of the study population

	Study population (n = 41)
Age (years)	62.9 ± 12.7
Male	21 (51 %)
BSA (m^2)	1.9 ± 0.2
Height (meters)	1.7 ± 0.1
Weight (kg)	84.1 ± 15.9
Indication of CT	Before PVI – 34
	PE workup – 7
Echocardiographic measurements (RT3DTEE)	
LVEF (est. %)	59.9 ± 6.9
LPW-D (mm)	10.1 ± 0.2
IVS-D (mm)	10.8 ± 2.4
LVESD (mm)	31.3 ± 3.7
LVEDD (mm)	48.8 ± 4.5
Pulmonary pressure (mmHg)	33.0 ± 14.0
RA area (cm^2)	17.6 ± 4.5
LA area (cm^2)	22.7 ± 5.3
LA diameter (ap) (mm)	39.8 ± 6.8
Ascending aorta diameter (mm)	32.4 ± 3.4
Aortic root diameter (mm)	30.4 ± 3.2

BSA body surface area, *CT* computed tomography, *est* estimated, *IVS-D* inter-ventricular septum diameter, *LPW-D* left posterior ventricular wall diameter, *LVEDD* left ventricular end diastolic diameter, *LVEF* left ventricular ejection fraction, *LVESD* left ventricular end systolic diameter, *PE* pulmonary embolism, *PVI* pulmonary vein isolation, *RT3DTEE* real-time 3-dimensional transesophageal echocardiography

Internal area of LAA orifice, LAA depth, maximal LAA diameter, minimal LAA diameter, and number of LAA lobes were compared between Rotational 3DTEE and RT3DTEE and to the CT as the gold standard method. All echocardiographic data have been reviewed by a single operator (CY) who was blinded to CT results done by a single operator (YA).

Transesophageal echocardiography

Transesophageal echocardiography (TEE) was performed using a commercially available fully sampled matrix-array TEE transducer and ultrasound system (X7–2 t Live 3D TEE transducer).

Real-Time-3-Dimensional Transesophageal Echocardiography (RT3DTEE)

RT3DTEE imaging was performed acquiring the usual pyramidal data set large enough to include the entire LAA. The zoom mode was used to improve visualization of LAA.

The internal area of the LAA orifice, as well as the minimal and maximal diameters of the LAA orifice (D_{max} and D_{min}, respectively), were measured directly from the original 3D views, along a plane connecting the origin of the left Circumflex artery to the roof of the LAA, below the ligament of Marshall, as previously shown by our group [16]. These measurements were assessed online using the EPIQ 7 echo machine (Philips Medical Systems, Andover, MA), since they could not be measured off-line on QLAB 10.0 software. The LAA depth (i.e., the longest distance from LAA orifice at the Circumflex artery level to the tip of the LAA) was measured off-line from the long-axes views, using dedicated software (QLAB 10.0). On these datasets we tried to measure LAA 3D volume using the same tracking method that we used for LA volume measurement, as previously described [23].

Rotational 3DTEE

Our 3D protocol for LAA dimensions measurements was as follows: Data acquisition included all the LAA in 3D zoom mode. We chose the 3DQ (and not 3DQadv) application and found the ECG guided end systole (i.e., end of T-wave) for the maximal LAA dimensions. We magnified multiplanar reconstruction (MPR) 2D images, then adjusted and cropped the lines to the optimal alignment. After optimizing the blue line to the circumflex artery level and decreasing the gain in the volume mode, we took the sagittal plane (green box, x-plane) and screened a 360° rotation. This 360° rotation ("Yosefy rotation"), is simpler and faster 3D method: it uses a rotation of the sagittal plane (in the green box, x-plane) that enables the operator to rapidly choose the image which gives him all the LAA parameters needed to introduce the invasive procedure in one single "stop shop" image (including: number of lobes - during the rotation; orifice area; maximal and minimal diameters - in the axial blue box; and depth - in the green box). In contrast to the usual time consuming MPR methods, in which each of the above parameters is taken at different angles (0°, 45°, 90°, 135°) and frames, using our rotation, we easily find the "stop shop" image point where all the above LAA parameters are measured (Fig. 1).

All 3D measurements of LAA were performed at ventricular end-systole. All the patients included in our study were in sinus rhythm during the echocardiographic studies. Nevertheless, in patients who are in

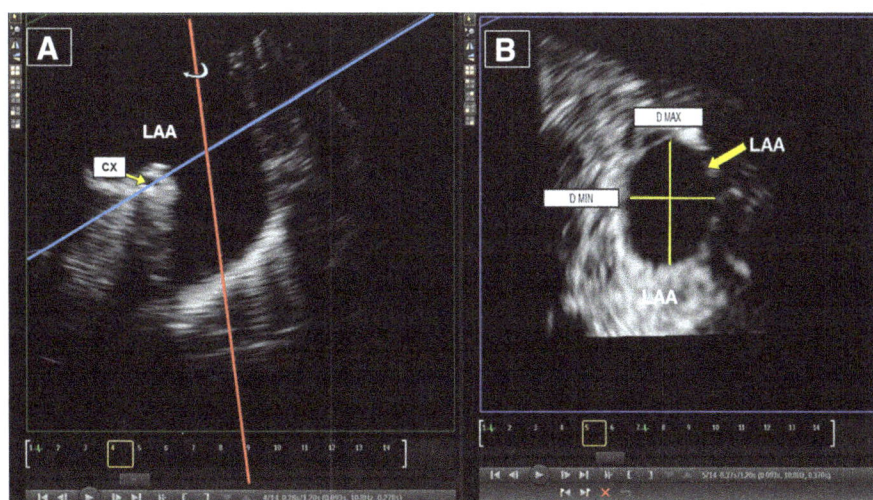

Fig. 1 Three dimensional transesophageal echocardiography (3DTEE) measurements of left atrial appendage (LAA) using 360°, Rotational 3DTEE method (see text and panel **a**); and measurement of maximal (Dmax) and minimal (Dmin) diameters at the level of the circumflex (Cx) artery (panel **b** Video clip is attached)

atrial fibrillation at the time of transesophageal echocardiography (TEE), we usually average measurements from ≥3 cardiac cycles.

Sixty-four-slice computed tomography

All forty-one patients underwent clinically indicated 64-slice CT (Philips Brilliance CT 64 Power-Philips Medical Systems, Eindhoven, The Netherlands) within one week of transthoracic and transesophageal echocardiography. All patients were in sinus rhythm during the CT scan. A retrospective ECG-gating protocol was used. Scanning parameters were the following: detector collimation of 0.625 mm, total z-axis coverage of 40 mm per rotation, gantry rotation speed of 0.35 s, tube voltage of 120 kV, pitch of 0.16 to 0.24, and ECG modulated tube current ranging from 400 to 800 mA. The bolus tracking technique was used to trigger the acquisition, with a four-cavity view as the region of interest. A total of 70–100 mL of iodinated, nonionic contrast agent (Iomeron 350, Bracco Imaging S.p.A.) was injected continuously into the antecubital vein (100–120 mL at 5.0 mL/s). Scanning was initiated during a single breath hold for an acquisition time of 5 to 7 s. All images were reconstructed with an effective slice thickness of 0.625 mm. ECG-gating protocol reconstruction of the image data was performed starting from early systole (10 % of R-R interval) and ending at end-diastole (90 % of R-R interval) using 10 % steps. Reconstructed image data were transferred to a remote workstation (IntelliSpace Portal, Philips) for post-processing. For the purpose of the current study, image data sets reconstructed at end-systole (40 % of R-R interval) were used for analysis. Using MPR, measurements of the area of the LAA orifice were performed from the short-axis view as well as the maximum (D_{max}) and minimum (D_{min}) diameters (Fig. 2), and the maximum depth of LAA was measured as the longest distance from LAA orifice to the tip of LAA. All the patients included in our study were in sinus rhythm during the imaging studies. Nevertheless, in patients who are in atrial fibrillation at the time of CT scanning, we usually average measurements from ≥3 cardiac cycles.

Statistical analysis

Continuous variables are presented as percentages and means ± standard deviation. Categorical data are presented as absolute numbers and percentages. Continuous variables were compared using independent Student t-test; categorical variables were compared using chi-square test or Fisher's exact test. A 2-sided p-value $< .05$ was considered to indicate statistical significance for all tests. Analyses were carried out using SPSS version 21.0 statistical package (SPSS IBM. Inc.).

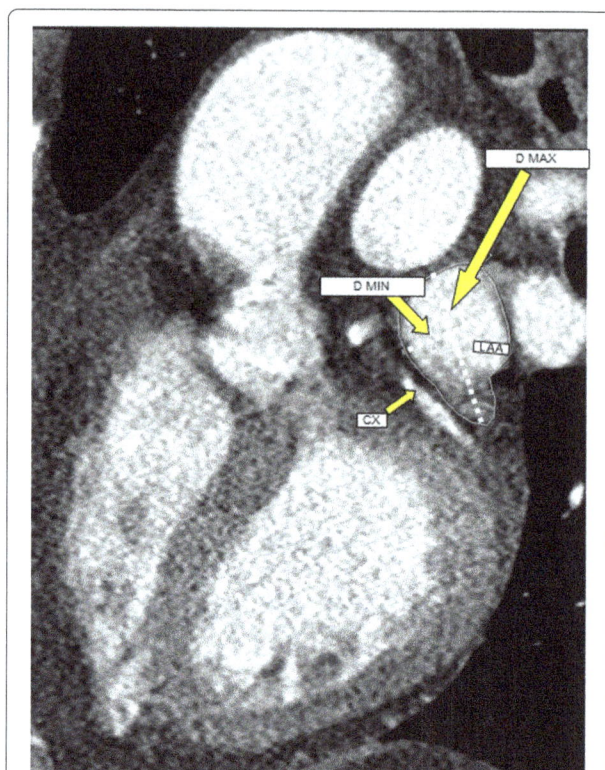

Fig. 2 CT images of LAA orifice maximal diameter and area at the level of circumflex (Cx) artery (arrow). (D_{max} = largest diameter, D_{min} = minimal diameter)

The intra-observer reproducibility of Rotational 3DTEE method for the measurement of all LAA parameters was demonstrated by performing the measurements of Rotational 3DTEE and CT in 10 randomized patients from our study by the same operator (CY for the TEE and YA for the CT), to assure they were not significantly different by paired t test. The measurements of LAA orifice area, maximal and minimal diameters and depth were calculated to obtain their SD and test the mean value versus 0.

Inter-observer variability was assessed between two observers in 10 patients selected randomly from our study patients. The measurements using Rotational 3DTEE and CT methods were obtained independently by two expert operators for each modality (CY and Doodit Mimon for the TEE and YA and Victor Lapis for the CT) blinded to the results of each other. Inter-observer variability was defined as the SD of the differences between observers and expressed as a percentage of the means.

Results

Baseline characteristics

Baseline characteristics of the study population ($n = 41$) are shown in Table 1. All patients had full readable

Rotational 3DTEE and RT3DTEE images. Thus, there was 100 % feasibility of LAA assessment.

Comparison between Rotational 3DTEE and RT3DTEE

Rotational 3DTEE measurements of LAA were not statistically different from RT3DTEE regarding: number of lobes (1.6 ± 0.7 and 1.6 ± 0.6, respectively, $p = NS$); area of orifice (3.1 ± 0.6 and 3.0 ± 0.7 cm^2, respectively, $p = NS$); maximal LAA diameter (24.8 ± 4.5, 24.6 ± 5.0 mm, respectively, $p = NS$) (Fig. 3); minimal LAA diameter (16.4 ± 3.4, 16.7 ± 3.3 mm, respectively, $p = NS$) (Fig. 4); and LAA depth (20.0 ± 2.1 and 19.8 ± 2.2 mm, respectively, $p = NS$) (Fig. 5).

As in our previous study [16], LAA volume could not be measured directly using RT3DTEE due to inability of the technology to track the lobe borders.

Comparison between Rotational 3DTEE and CT

Rotational 3DTEE measurements were not different from CT measurements regarding: number of LAA lobes (1.6 ± 0.7 and 1.4 ± 0.6, respectively, $p = NS$); area of orifice (3.1 ± 0.6 and 3.3 ± 1.5 cm^2, respectively, $p = NS$); maximal LAA diameter (24.8 ± 4.5, 24.9 ± 5.8 mm, respectively, $p = NS$) (Fig. 3); minimal LAA diameter (16.4 ± 3.4, 17.0 ± 4.4 mm, respectively, $p = NS$) (Fig. 4); and LAA depth (20.0 ± 2.1 and 21.7 ± 6.9 mm, respectively, $p = NS$) (Fig. 5).

The Bland-Altman analysis shows good correlation and low variability between LAA orifice area, maximal and minimal diameters and depth measured by Rotational 3DTEE and by CT scanning (Fig. 6a-d).

Inter-observer variability of LAA orifice area, maximal and minimal diameters and depth measured by Rotational 3DTEE and by CT scan methods was calculated and compared between the two observers. The variability of the mean values was 3.9, 4.1, 2.9 and 3.1 %, respectively, for the Rotational 3DTEE, and 3.2, 3.6, 2.7 and 3.8 %, respectively, for the CT. The observers concordance was with good agreement ($r = 0.97$, 0.95, 0.95 and 0.97, respectively) between the two methods.

Intra-observer variability of calculated LAA orifice area, maximal and minimal diameters and depth measurements for the Rotational 3DTEE were 3.9, 2.8, 4.3 and 3.5 %, respectively, and for the CT scan method: 3.7, 2.3, 3.9 and 2.7 %, respectively, indicating a reasonable range of variability for this technique. The same observer concordance of different measurements was with good agreement ($r = 0.95$, 0.94, 0.95 and 0.97, respectively) for the Rotational 3DTEE and $r = 0.95$, 0.94, 0.99, 0.95, respectively, for the CT scan method.

Discussion

Precise knowledge of LAA anatomy and dimensions has become a key guiding stage before implanting LAA closure devices [7, 9–13, 24]. Bedside RT3DTEE measurements of LAA maximal orifice diameter were shown to be more accurate than 2DTEE and are as accurate as CT as the gold standard [16]. However, not all echo laboratories have the capability of measuring direct online 3D images, but do have the capability of turning 3D images into 2D ones "online" for bedside measurements.

In this study we introduced a simpler and faster 3D method: it uses a rotation of the sagittal plane (green box, x-plane), that enables the operator to rapidly choose the image which gives him all the LAA parameters needed for the invasive procedure in one single "stop shop" image. This includes number of lobes, orifice

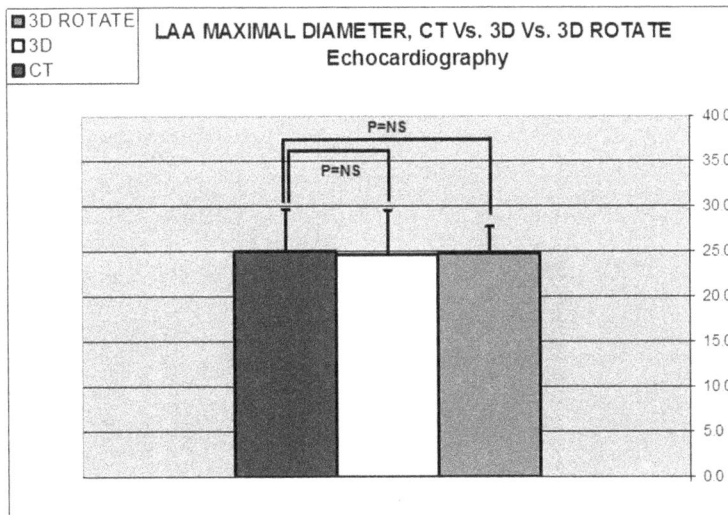

Fig. 3 Histogram comparing LAA maximal diameter using different imaging methods ($n = 41$). Comparison between computed tomography (CT) (24.9 ± 5.8 mm), direct Real-Time 3-Dimensional Transesophageal Echocardiography (3D) (24.6 ± 5.0 mm), and Rotational 3DTEE (3D Rotate) (24.8 ± 4.5 mm), ($p = NS$ for all)

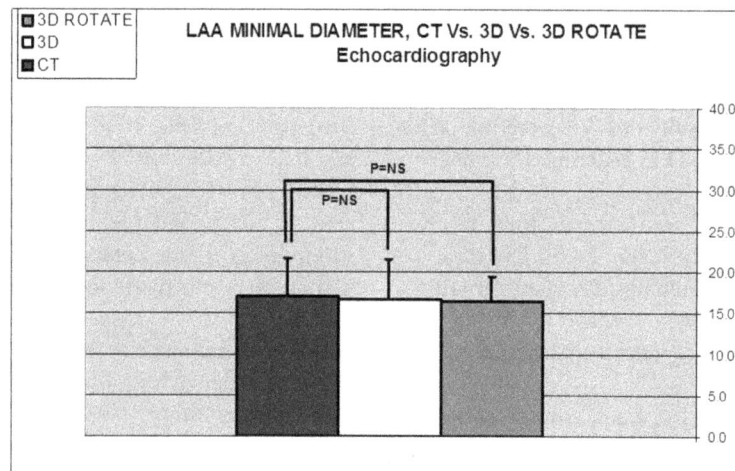

Fig. 4 Histogram comparing LAA minimal diameter using different imaging methods ($n = 41$). Comparison between computed tomography (CT) (17.0 ± 4.4 mm), direct Real-Time 3-Dimensional Transesophageal Echocardiography (3D) (16.7 ± 3.3 mm), and Rotational 3DTEE (3D Rotate) (16.4 ± 3.4 mm), ($p =$ NS for all)

area, maximal and minimal diameters and LAA depth. In contrast to the usual time consuming MPR methods, in which each of the above parameters are taken in different angles ($0°$, $45°$, $90°$, $135°$) and frames, using our rotation, we could easily find the "stop shop" image point where all LAA parameters are measured (Fig. 1).

Thus, rotational 3DTEE (Yosefy rotation) may facilitate percutaneous LAA closure procedure for stroke prophylaxis in patients with non-valvular AF by choosing the appropriate LAA closure-device size. As it is simple and fast it can be repeated as many times needed before and during the procedure to ensure device size and proper implantation and LAA closure. Its accuracy

is emphasized by the Bland-Altman analysis that shows good correlation and low variability between LAA orifice area, maximal and minimal diameters and depth measured by Rotational 3DTEE (3D Rotate) and by CT scanning (Fig. 6a-d). Also, the calculated differences between LAA orifice area, maximal and minimal diameters and depth were concordant ($r =$ around 0.95), indicating a reasonable range of variability for this technique.

Recent evolving data show better performance of RT3DTEE for the assessment of LAA anatomy compared with 2DTEE [13, 15, 16, 20–22]. Nucifora et al. [20] have published a study showing that RT3DTEE is more accurate than 2DTEE for assessment of LAA

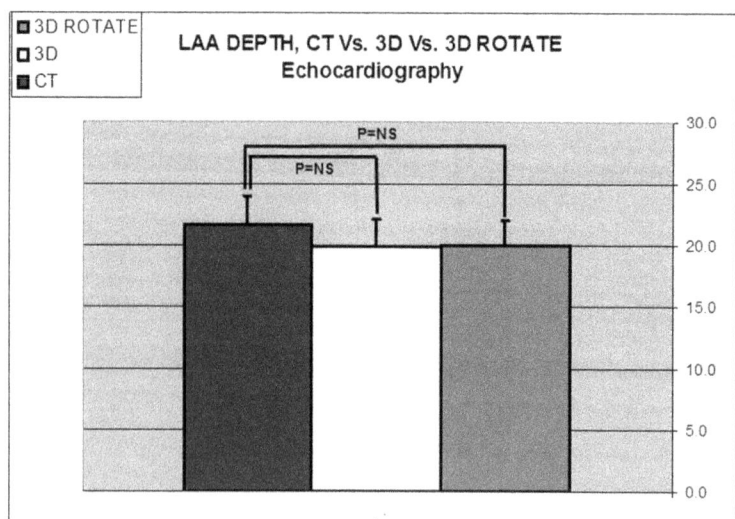

Fig. 5 Histogram comparing LAA depth using different imaging methods ($n = 41$). Comparison between computed tomography (CT) (21.7 ± 6.9 mm), direct Real-Time 3-Dimensional Transesophageal Echocardiography (3D) (19.8 ± 2.2 mm), and Rotational 3DTEE (3D Rotate) (20.0 ± 2.1 mm), ($p =$ NS for all)

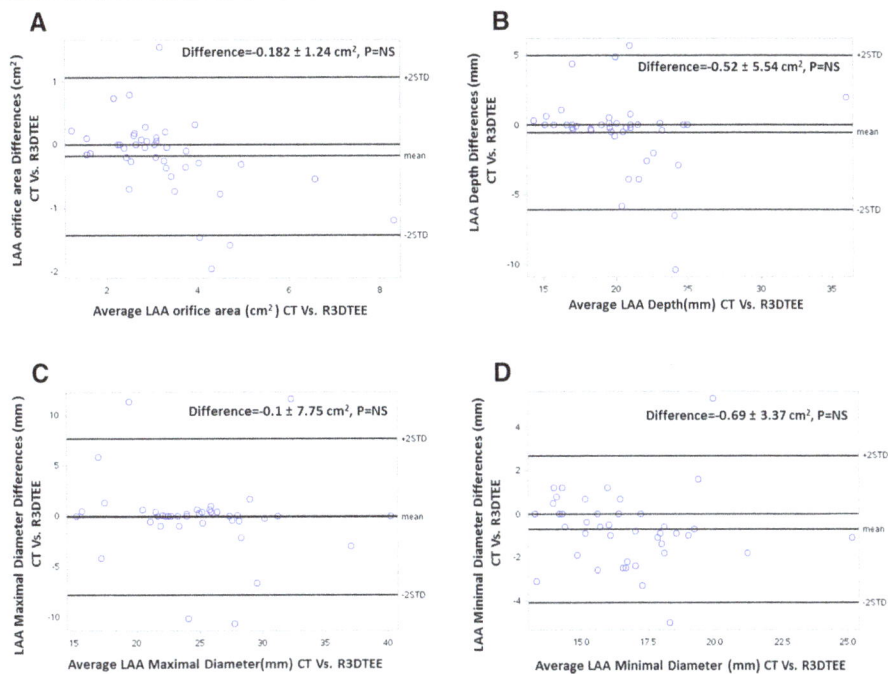

Fig. 6 Bland-Altman analysis of differences between left atrial appendage (LAA) orifice area (**a**), depth (**b**), maximal (**c**), and minimal (**d**), diameters by CT scanning Vs. Rotational 3DTEE

orifice area: 137 patients (99 of them had AF) underwent 2DTEE and RT3DTEE, with CT used as a reference in 46 of them. RT3DTEE showed higher correlation with CT for the assessment of LAA orifice area, compared with 2DTEE. Our group showed in a previous study [16] that although no difference was found between LAA depth measurements using RT3DTEE and 2DTEE, compared to measurements with the direct RT3DTEE method, in 23.3 % of patients the commonly "recommended" 135° 2DTEE was not the cut plane angulation with maximal orifice diameter, thus underestimating this diameter and potentially complicating proper implantation of the device. In contrast, bedside RT3DTEE LAA measurements were not statistically different from those with CT.

Our method to size the LAA is different from the three methods that are already being used. The three methods include: the standard 2D methods using four angles (0°, 45°, 90°, 135°) [7], the 3D multiplane reconstruction (MPR) method using the three orthogonal planes from the three original pyramid 3D volume dataset [20], and the 3D TEE with on-image caliper measurement, as described in our previous work [16]. The main difference in our current technique is that we do not use different MPR orthogonal planes to find each of the LAA parameters, but we use a "stop shop" image point where all LAA parameters are measured. Thus, this technique enhances the time and simplifies LAA measurements, as shown in the attached video clip and in Fig. 1.

Thus, RT3DTEE is slowly evolving as a first-line method for sizing LAA due to its accuracy and its real-time and inherent bedside capabilities [16, 25, 26]. Compared to CT and MRI, it is faster, cheaper, and more comfortable to access; and as opposed to CT it is not associated with radiation exposure and contrast administration, while providing high quality images [27]. It may lower the cost of LAA closure procedure by also avoiding the need to exchange unsuitable devices and may reduce the risk of complications by lowering the number of failed attempts due to inappropriate device size [28, 29]. These advantages are in addition to its excellent capabilities in ruling out LA thrombus prior to the procedure [30].

The closure device is available in various sizes to accommodate individual variations on LAA anatomy. Proper positioning and sizing are essential for safety and efficacy (ref). Undersizing of the device has the potential risk of device migration or embolization and may favor peri-device leakage. Oversizing of the device should also be avoided because this may cause cardiac perforation, pericardial effusion, and cardiac tamponade.

Important aspects for LAA occlusion include the correct sizing of the landing zone diameters for the selected device and the measurement of the depth and orientation of the main anchoring lobe and the number and origin of additional lobes. Because of the substantial variations in LAA anatomy that impact device selection and efficacy, an accurate assessment of anatomic LAA characteristics is crucial before an LAA closure procedure [24].

The choice of an appropriate occlusion device depends on accurate measurements of the landing zone diameters. To achieve a secure and stable device position, the size of the occlusion device is usually selected to be a few millimeters larger in diameter than the measurements of the landing zone. The maximum length of the anchoring lobe has to be measured in addition (in the expected axis of the device) to ensure that this lobe has enough space to accommodate the selected device. Different device types require different measurements because the different occluder systems vary slightly. The angle between the ostium, the neck, and the main anchoring lobe should be evaluated because it can influence the choice of the puncture site and/or the curve of the delivery sheath. The number and origin of additional LAA lobes also needs to be assessed. Some LAA morphologies are more challenging for device closure than others; thus, LAA anatomy should be defined before any planned closure-device procedure [24].

Previous works [1, 20] used MPR for measurements on the 3D images and only as a second stage analysis do they measure LAA size by using the cut planes of each lobule at the X,Y,Z axes. Our group described a new method that measures LAA size directly on the 3D image [16]. The advantages of this method are its efficiency and speed. The measurements are given immediately, bedside, without the need for further analysis of the image.

Many echo laboratories have the capability of turning 3D images into 2D ones "online" for bedside measurements but some of them do not have the capability of measuring direct online 3D images (i.e., RT3DTEE) as we have shown before [16]. Thus, we tried to use a simpler, practical method for measuring LAA size that combines the accuracy and real time capabilities of 3D echo on one hand, and the simplicity and bedside availability of 2D echo on the other hand.

We showed that a fast and simple rotation of the introducer that demonstrates maximal diameter of LAA orifice on the 3D image (Yosefy rotation) and LAA measurements after turning the images into 2D (Rotational 3DTEE) has a similar accuracy to that of the former direct measurement on 3D image (RT3DTEE) and to CT. Our 3D protocol for LAA dimensions measurements was described in detail. We showed that rotational 3DTEE measurements of LAA were not statistically different from RT3DTEE and from CT regarding number of lobes, internal area of LAA orifice, maximal LAA diameter, and LAA depth. We believe that either RT3DTEE or Rotational 3DTEE should replace CT scan before and during implantation of percutaneous LAA occlusion devices.

Limitations

Whenever there is a need for volume measurement by 3D echocardiography, MPR can be applied (by using cut planes of each lobule at the X,Y,Z axes, calculating the volume and adding to the volume of the other lobes). However, this method is not practical, is slow and inefficient, and thus was not used in our 3DTEE studies.

Conclusions

Rotational 3DTEE method is a fast, simple and feasible method that has similar accuracy as RT3DTEE and CT in assessing LAA anatomy. Thus, bedside rotational 3DTEE may facilitate LAA closure procedure by choosing the appropriate device size.

Funding
This research was not supported by any company.

Authors' contributions
CY and BB performed the echocardiography; AL-F, VK, and AK performed the PVI; YA performed the CT scans; AL-F, YA, and CY wrote the article and the others reviewed it. All authors read and approved the final manuscript.

Competing interests
The authors declare that they have no competing interests.

Author details
[1]Department of Cardiology, Barzilai Medical Center, Ben-Gurion University of the Negev, Ashkelon, Israel. [2]Department of Imaging, Barzilai Medical Center, Ben-Gurion University of the Negev, Ashkelon, Israel. [3]Noninvasive Cardiology Unit, Barzilai Medical Center, Ashkelon 78306, Israel.

References
1. Yamamoto M, Seo Y, Kawamatsu N, et al. Complex LAA morphology and LAA thrombus formation in patients with AF. Circ Cardiovasc Imaging. 2014; 7:337–43.
2. Donal E, Yamada H, Leclercq C, Herpin D. The left atrial appendage, a small, blind-ended structure: a review of its echocardiographic evaluation and its clinical role. Chest. 2005;128:1853–62.
3. Bayard YL, Omran H, Neuzil P, et al. PLAATO (Percutaneous Left Atrial Appendage Transcatheter Occlusion) for prevention of cardioembolic stroke in non-anticoagulation eligible atrial fibrillation patients: results from the European PLAATO study. EuroIntervention. 2010;6:220–6.
4. Park JW, Bethencourt A, Sievert H, et al. Left atrial appendage closure with Amplatzer cardiac plug in atrial fibrillation: initial European experience. Catheter Cardiovasc Interv. 2011;77:700–6.
5. Holmes DR, Reddy VY, Turi ZG, et al. PROTECT AF Investigators, Percutaneous closure of the left atrial appendage versus warfarin therapy for prevention of stroke in patients with atrial fibrillation: a randomized non-inferiority trial. Lancet. 2009;374:534–42.
6. Camm AJ, Lip GY, De Caterina R, et al. ESC Committee for Practice Guidelines (CPG), 2012 focused update of the ESC Guidelines for the management of atrial fibrillation. Eur Heart J. 2012;33:2719–47.
7. Meier B, Blaauw Y, Khattab A, et al. EHRA/EAPCI expert consensus statement on catheter-based left atrial appendage occlusion. Europace. 2014;16:1397–416.
8. Price MJ, Valderrábano M. Left atrial appendage closure to prevent stroke in patients with atrial fibrillation. Circulation. 2014;130:202–12.
9. Cruz-Gonzalez I, Yan BP, Lam YY. Left atrial appendage exclusion: state-of-the-art. Catheter Cardiovasc Interv. 2010;75:806–13.
10. Chue CD, de Giovanni J, Steeds RP. The role of echocardiography in percutaneous left atrial appendage occlusion. Eur J Echocardiogr. 2011;12:i3–10.

11. Karakus G, Kodali V, Inamdar V, et al. Comparative assessment of left atrial appendage by transesophageal and combined two- and three-dimensional transthoracic echocardiography. Echocardiography. 2008;25(8):918–24.

12. Kumar V, Nanda NC. Is it time to move on from two-dimensional transesophageal to three-dimensional transthoracic echocardiography for assessment of left atrial appendage? Review of existing literature. Echocardiography. 2012;29:112–6.

13. Gorani D, Dilic M, Kulic M, et al. Comparison of two and three dimensional transthoracic versus transesophageal echocardiography in evaluation of anatomy and pathology of left atrial appendage. Med Arch. 2013;67:318–21.

14. Lacomis JM, Goitein O, Deible C, et al. Dynamic multidimensional imaging of the human left atrial appendage. Europace. 2007;9:1134–40.

15. Valocik G, Kamp O, Mihciokur M, et al. Assessment of the left atrial appendage mechanical function by three-dimensional echocardiography. Eur J Echocardiogr. 2002;3:207–13.

16. Yosefy C, Laish-Farkash A, Azhibekov Y, et al. A new method for direct three-dimensional measurement of left atrial appendage dimensions during transesophageal echocardiography. Echocardiography. 2016;33(1):69–76.

17. Budge LP, Shaffer KM, Moorman JR, et al. Analysis of in vivo left atrial appendage morphology in patients with atrial fibrillation: a direct comparison of transesophageal echocardiography, planar cardiac CT, and segmental three-dimensional cardiac CT. J Interv Card Electrophysiol. 2008; 23:87–93.

18. Heist EK, Refaat M, Danik SB, et al. Analysis of the left atrial appendage by magnetic resonance angiography in patients with atrial fibrillation. Heart Rhythm. 2006;3:1313–8.

19. Wang Y, Di Biase L, Horton RP, et al. Left atrial appendage studied by computed tomography to help planning for appendage closure device placement. J Cardiovasc Electrophysiol. 2010;21:973–82.

20. Nucifora G, Faletra FF, Regoli F, et al. Evaluation of the left atrial appendage with real-time 3-dimensional transesophageal echocardiography. Implications for catheter-based left atrial appendage closure. Circ Cardiovasc Imaging. 2011;4:514–23.

21. Shah SJ, Bardo DM, Sugeng L, et al. Real-time three-dimensional transesophageal echocardiography of the left atrial appendage: initial experience in the clinical setting. J Am Soc Echocardiogr. 2008;21:1362–8.

22. Nakajima H, Seo Y, Ishizu T, et al. Analysis of the left atrial appendage by three-dimensional transesophageal echocardiography. Am J Cardiol. 2010; 106:885–92.

23. Yosefy C, Shenhav S, Feldman V, et al. Left atrial function during pregnancy: a three-dimensional echocardiographic study. Echocardiography. 2012;29(9): 1096–101.

24. Wunderlich NC, Beigel R, Swaans MJ, Ho SY, Siegel RJ. Percutaneous interventions for left atrial appendage exclusion: options, assessment, and imaging using 2D and 3D echocardiography. JACC Cardiovasc Imaging. 2015;8(4):472–88.

25. Bai W, Chen Z, Wang H, Wei X, Rao L: GW25-e0158 Assessment of the Left Atrial Appendage using Real-time Three Dimensional Transesophageal Echocardiography. J Am Coll Cardiol 2014;64(16_S). doi:10.1016/j.jacc.2014.06.1060

26. Sommer M, Roehrich A, Boenner F, et al. Value of 3D TEE for LAA Morphology. JACC: Cardiovasc Imaging. 2015;8(9):1107–10.

27. Brinkman V, Kalbfleisch S, Auseon A, Pu M. Real time three-dimensional transesophageal echocardiography-guided placement of left atrial appendage occlusion device. Echocardiography. 2009;26:855–8.

28. Reddy VY, Holmes D, Doshi SK, Neuzil P, Kar S. Safety of percutaneous left atrial appendage closure: results from the Watchman left atrial appendage system for embolic protection in patients with AF (Protect AF) clinical trial and the continued access registry. Circulation. 2011;123:417–24.

29. Stollberger C, Schneider B, Finsterer J. Serious complications from dislocation of a watchman left atrial appendage occluder. J Cardiovasc Electrophysiol. 2007;18:880–1.

30. Latcu DG, Rinaldi JP, Saoudi N. Real-time three-dimensional transoesophageal echocardiography for diagnosis of left atrial appendage thrombus. Eur J Echocardiogr. 2009;10:711–2.

12

Equivocal tests after contrast stress-echocardiography compared with invasive coronary angiography or with CT angiography: CT calcium score in mildly positive tests may spare unnecessary coronary angiograms

Nicola Gaibazzi[*] ⓘ, Guido Pastorini, Andrea Biagi, Francesco Tafuni, Claudia Buffa, Silvia Garibaldi, Francesca Boffetti and Giorgio Benatti

Abstract

Background: Imaging stress tests are not ideally accurate to predict anatomically obstructive CAD, leading to a non-trivial rate of unnecessary iCA. This may depend on the threshold used to indicate iCA, and maybe CTA or, one step earlier, CT calcium score could spare most unnecessary iCA in only mildly positive cSE. We assessed the diagnostic accuracy of contrast stress-echocardiography (cSE) in comparison with invasive coronary angiography (iCA), and CT angiography (CTA) only in case of equivocal tests, to find hints helping reduce falsely positive cSE in the suspicion of coronary artery disease (CAD).

Methods: Patients who were indicated cSE for suspected CAD between 2012 and 2016, who also underwent iCA were selected and diagnostic results compared. A second group, specifically with equivocal cSE who underwent CTA was also analyzed.

Results: 137 subjects with equivocal cSE and CTA and 314 with cSE (any result) and iCA were selected. In the CTA-equivocal cSE group, an Agatston score < 105 and a coronary flow reserve (CFR-LAD) <1.7 had very high negative predictive value (99%, 92% respectively) to exclude obstructive CAD. The Agatston score was the most significant incremental predictor of CAD beyond clinical variables (chi square 31 to 47, $p < 0.001$). In the iCA group a more-than-mild reversible wall motion abnormality (WMA) demonstrated high positive predictive value for CAD (89%), while CFR-LAD appeared less useful. More-than-mild reversible WMA was the most significant predictor of CAD beyond clinical variables (chi square 37.5 to 56, $p < 0.001$).

Conclusions: Our data suggest iCA should be indicated only for more-than-mild reversible WMA at cSE, due to the very high positive predictive value for CAD of this finding, while mildly positive tests should be shifted to non-invasive CT, with CTA performed only for coronary calcium Agatston score > 100, since lower scores demonstrated very high negative predictive value for CAD, not justifying proceeding to CTA and even less to iCA.

Keywords: Stress-echocardiography, Computed tomography angiography, Coronary artery disease, Equivocal tests

* Correspondence: ngaibazzi@gmail.com
Department of Cardiology, Parma University Hospital, Via Gramsci 14, 43123 Parma, Italy

Background

Recent stress-echocardiography studies have been mostly focused on prognostic stratification [1]; however, the diagnostic gatekeeping role to invasive tests more directly impacts on patients clinical management, aiming to avoid financial and biological downstream costs of unnecessary invasive coronary angiograms (iCA). The recent NICE guidelines [2] suggest the "anatomical" multislice CT coronary angiography (CTA) approach to be preferred over functional stress-testing in the suspicion of coronary artery disease (CAD), emphasizing the general disappointment regarding the suboptimal diagnostic performance of functional tests. In fact, functional tests still over-predict obstructive CAD in 1/3 to ½ of patients who are then indicated iCA [3, 4], and, more surprisingly, this has not improved since 1977, when Erikssen et al. first reported that coronary angiograms of patients selected for suspected CAD showed "..a ratio of 2 true positives to 1 false positive" [5]. Diagnostic tests are usually forced into a binary classification, positive or negative, and imaging functional tests for suspected CAD make no exception. This simplistic classification does not fit for all patients. In today's low-pretest probability practice [6], negative tests represent the vast majority of stress-echocardiograms, positive tests represent a minority, and a third class, not so rare, is represented by "equivocal" tests, which is impossible to classify. In our lab we suggest iCA for patients testing positive for reversible ischemia, while CTA is proposed specifically for patients with equivocal tests, in line with existing recommendations on CTA appropriateness. A wealth of variables can be collected from our routine vasodilator contrast stress-echocardiography (cSE) protocol, comprising wall motion (WM), Doppler coronary flow reserve of the left anterior descending coronary artery (CFR-LAD), myocardial perfusion, ECG abnormalities, and anginal symptoms. We assessed diagnostic accuracy data of cSE in the iCA and CTA groups, to find hints helping modify our practice and minimize false positive cSE sent to iCA. Our lab's routine practice to assess multiple variables and indicate iCA not only on the basis of WM, but also on myocardial perfusion, CFR-LAD data or clinical suspicion, makes WM accuracy data only partially affected by referral bias.

Methods

Patients

From our cSE database we retrospectively selected patients who were indicated cSE for suspected CAD between 2012 and 2016. We selected patients who were either indicated a) iCA after cSE (<90 days) for any clinical reason, whatever the cSE result, or b) multislice CTA specifically after equivocal cSE, defined as mild reversible WM abnormalities, or normal WM but abnormal findings among the other parameters assessed

during cSE. Figure 1 shows the flow diagram of patients selection. Patients who underwent iCA within 90 days (either because of a positive cSE or any other clinical reason, comprising the results of other stress-tests) were selected and cSE and iCA data compared. In the second group, equivocal cSE who were indicated and underwent CTA within 90 days were also selected and results analyzed; in this CTA group we also applied the exclusion criteria of prior coronary revascularization or myocardial infarction, not applied to the iCA group, to exclude patients with possible stent-related artifacts, a known diagnostic limitation of CTA.

Diabetes mellitus was defined as a fasting plasma glucose level > 125 mg/dL or the need for insulin or oral hypoglycemic agents. Hypercholesterolemia was defined as total cholesterol >200 mg/dL or treatment with lipid lowering medications. Hypertension was defined as blood pressure > 140/90 mmHg or use of antihypertensive medication.

The study was approved by the Institutional Review Board of the Parma Medical Center and all patients gave informed consent.

Contrast stress-echocardiography

Our protocol for accelerated high-dose dipyridamole contrast stress-echocardiography has been described elsewhere [7]; briefly, it consists in rest and peak vasodilation assessments of the following three imaging parameters: WM, myocardial perfusion and Doppler CFR-LAD for peak diastolic velocity stress/rest ratio, after small boluses of 0.5 ml SonoVue microbubble ultrasound contrast. Stress acquisition is performed after dipyridamole administration of 0.84 mg/kg infused in 6 min. Wall motion analysis is the only assessment strictly required for the protocol, perfusion imaging and CFR-LAD being assessed only when feasible, mostly depending on the specific operator preferences and technical skills. The left ventricle is divided in 17 segments according to the recommendations of the American and European Societies of Echocardiography [8]. Myocardial perfusion is visually assessed, normal myocardial perfusion after dipyridamole was assigned if myocardium was fully replenished 1.5–2 s after the end of the flash impulse, normal myocardial replenishment at rest was defined as complete replenishment within 4 s after the flash impulse. Segmental wall motion was graded as follows: normal = 1; hypokinetic = 2; akinetic = 3; and dyskinetic = 4. Reversible ischemia was defined as the occurrence of a stress-induced new dyssynergy or worsening of rest hypokinesia in ≥1 segment.

Definition of equivocal or positive cSE test

Following our lab guidelines, CTA was indicated only after an equivocal cSE, which was strictly defined based

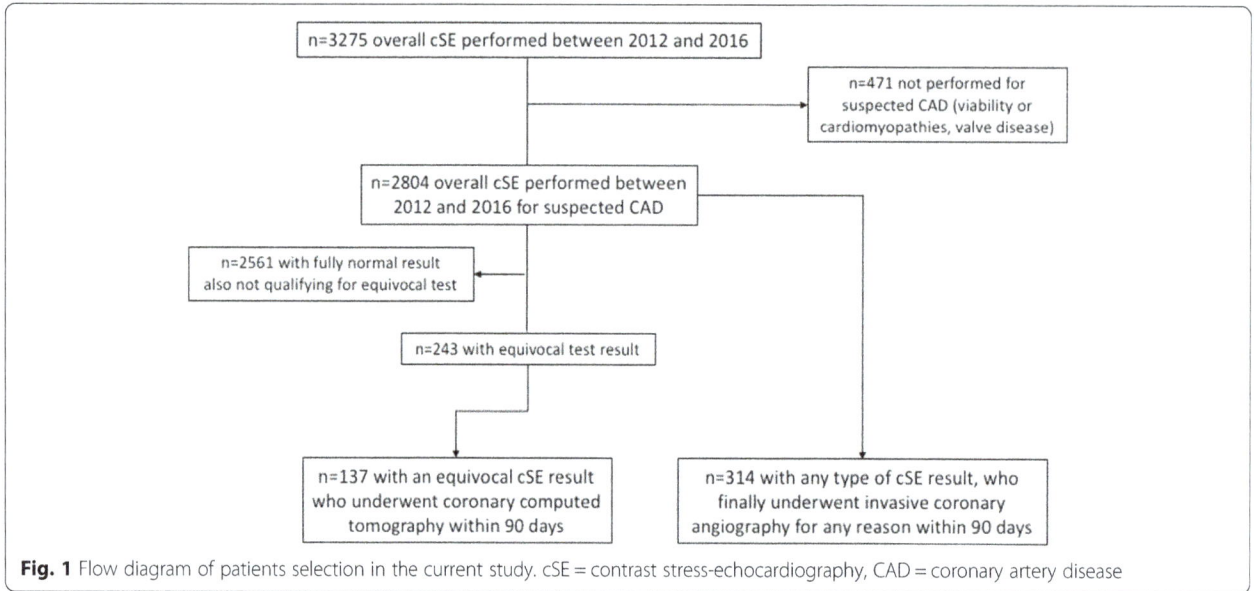

Fig. 1 Flow diagram of patients selection in the current study. cSE = contrast stress-echocardiography, CAD = coronary artery disease

either on only mildly abnormal wall motion score index (WMSI) delta between rest and stress (≤0.06) as a standalone criterion or, alternatively, normal WM behavior (WMSI delta = 0) but 2 "minor" abnormal findings among the following: a) mild reversible perfusion defects (affecting ≤2 segments), b) abnormal but not extremely reduced CFR-LAD (between 1.5 and 1.99), c) reversible downsloping or horizontal ST deviation of >1 mm in at least 2 ECG leads, d) anginal symptoms at peak

vasodilation. The definition of a frankly positive cSE, encompassed either a more severe WMSI delta (>0.06) as a standalone criterion or, alternatively, WMSI delta ≤0.06 but associated with >2 other ancillary abnormal variables or only 2 of such variables, but showing extremely abnormal values, limited to myocardial perfusion or CFR-LAD. Figure 2 clarifies stress-echocardiography criteria used to define equivocal cSE or positive tests in our echolab.

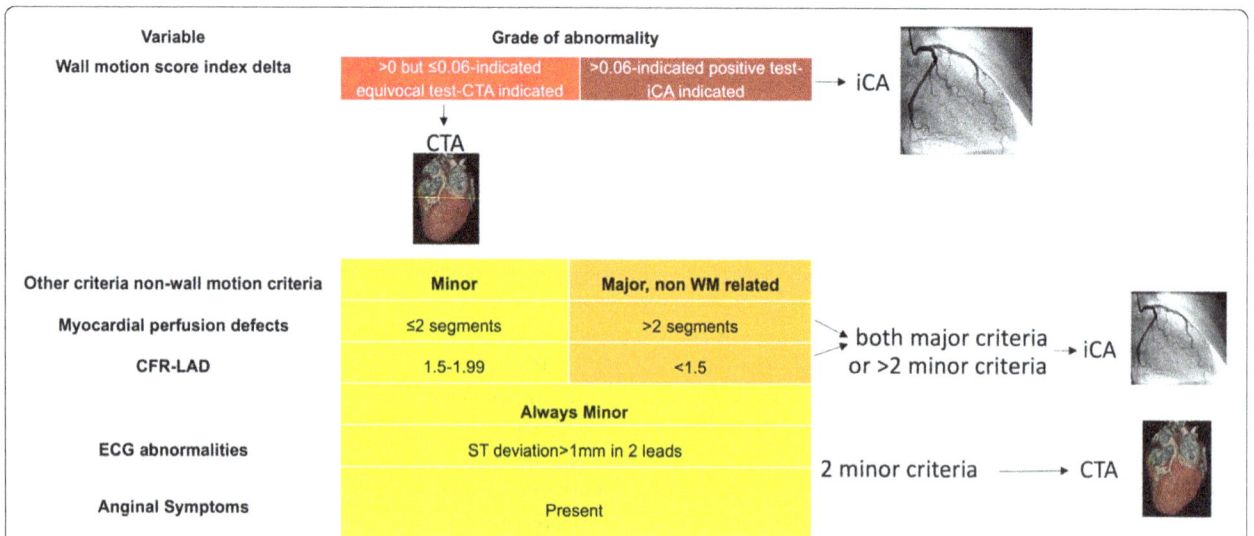

Fig. 2 Pre-specified criteria suggested in our lab to define equivocal contrast stress-echocardiograms (who are indicated CTA) based on wall motion and the other available variables. Additionally to the standalone wall motion score index delta criterion, patients with 2 minor criteria were also defined equivocal tests and indicated CTA, while more than 2 minor or two major were also defined positive tests and indicated iCA. Yellow colour represents minor criteria, orange means major criteria, but unrelated to wall motion assessment. CTA = CT angiography, iCA = invasive coronary angiography, CFR-LAD = coronary flow reserve of the left anterior descending coronary artery. Yellow boxes identify minor criteria, Orange are major non-WM criteria, while light red and dark red indicate WM mild and more-than-mild ischemia

Coronary Calcium and CTA

The study was performed with a Definition Flash system (Siemens, Forchheim, Germany). Gantry rotation time was 280 ms, which provides a temporal resolution of 75 ms using a heart rate independent single-segment reconstruction and high pitch up to 3.4. Detector collimation is $2 \times 64 \times 0.6$ mm. A z-axis flying focal spot is applied which results in an acquisition of 2×128 slices per rotation. Two scans were performed in all patients: one to visualize coronary artery calcium and one angiography scan. First patients underwent non-enhanced prospective electrocardiography (ECG)-gated sequential scan to measure coronary calcium score. The corresponding images for calcium scoring were reconstructed with a slice width of 2.5–3 mm and slice spacing of 1.25–1.5 mm and the tube voltage was 120 kVp. A region of interest was drawn over the areas of calcification and the Agatston score was automatically calculated by the software. A cutoff value above 130 Hounsfield units defined calcification and lesion area was multiplied by a density factor derived from the maximal Hounsfield units. Scans for coronary CTA were performed with breath held in inspiration. CTA was performed with adaptive electrocardiographic pulsing. A prospective ECG-triggering high-pitch spiral mode or retrospective ECG gating spiral mode were used. All images were reviewed on a workstation (Leonardo Siemens) equipped with a dedicated software tool for calcium scoring (Calcium Scoring CT, Siemens).

Invasive Coronary Angiography

Angiograms were performed by standard technique via radial or femoral approach. Obstructive CAD was primarily defined as stenosis >50% in any major epicardial coronary artery, but the alternative stenosis cutoff of >70% was also assessed. Left main trunk with at least 50% stenosis was always considered as >70% CAD. Invasive coronary angiography wad graded by visual inspection of the cath-lab physician performing the diagnostic procedure.

Statistics

This was an observational retrospective study of data collected in clinical practice. All data were expressed as mean (±standard deviation) or median (and interquartile range—IQR) or number (percentage), as appropriate. Comparisons between patients with at least one significant coronary stenosis and patients with unaffected coronaries (or <50% stenosis) were made by unpaired t-test or the Wilcoxon rank sum test and test for proportions, as appropriate. We created receiver operating characteristic (ROC) curves of considered parameters, and we calculated area under the curve (AUC) to estimate their predictive power for the presence of CAD. Accuracy

data were reported using common definitions of sensitivity, specificity, positive and negative predictive values. Logistic regression models were used to evaluate how demographics, clinical risk factors or imaging parameters predicted the presence of CAD and the potential incremental value using change in models chi square. Coronary artery disease was by default defined as the presence of at least one >50% visually-assessed coronary artery stenosis; when the alternative definition of more severe >70% coronary artery stenosis was used and assessed, this was expressly specified in the manuscript. A p value <0.05 was considered statistically significant. StatsDirect 3 statistical software (StatsDirect Ltd. http://www.statsdirect.com) was used.

Results

Out of overall 3275 cSE performed between 2012 and 2016, we found 137 subjects satisfying the definition for equivocal cSE who underwent CTA after cSE and within 90 days, who had no history of prior myocardial infarction or revascularization (specific exclusion criteria for the CTA group), and 314 who underwent iCA within 90 days after cSE.

Equivocal cSE and CTA data

In the 137 patients, CTA demonstrated no or <50% coronary stenosis in 96 patients (70%) (no CAD group), while in 41 (30%) demonstrated at least one >50% coronary artery stenosis (CAD group); among such 41 patients, 14 had at least one coronary artery stenosis >70% or left main disease >50%. Only 26 subjects out of the overall 41 patients in whom CTA reported at least >50% stenosis subsequently underwent iCA, which confirmed CTA findings in 22 (85%) with 4 patients (15%) being over-diagnosed by CTA with >50% stenosis, downgraded to <50% at iCA.

Baseline risk factors, cSE and CTA data are shown in Table 1, which highlights few significant differences between the CAD and no CAD groups: age was significantly higher in the group with CAD (Median 65 vs 57 y/o, $p < 0.0001$), as it was the prevalence of hypertension, active smoking and hypercholesterolemia ($p < 0.05$ for all).

The only cSE imaging variable significantly differing between the 2 groups was CFR-LAD, which was lower in the CAD group (median 1.9 vs 2.0, $p < 0.005$), while the CT-derived coronary calcium, measured as the Agatston score, was significantly higher in the CAD group (median 269 vs 2, $p < 0.001$).

Figure 3 shows the ROC curves, on the left using the calculated best cutoff of >150 for the Agatston score to predict >50% CAD at CTA, demonstrating an area under the curve (AUC) = 0.843 (95% CI 0,765 to 0,920), a negative predictive value of 87,5% (95% CI 79% to

Table 1 Baseline demographics, clinical variables, stress-echocardiography and computed tomography angiograms data in the entire population and in the subgroups with or without obstructive coronary artery disease > 50%

	Entire population($n = 137$)	CAD > 50% ($n = 41$)	No CAD > 50% ($n = 96$)	p
Age, median (IQR)	59 (11)	65 (10)	57 (11)	<0.0001
Male Gender (%)	79 (58%) (57%)	28 (68%)	51 (53%)	0.1
Hypertension (%)	83 (60%)	30 (73%)	53 (55%)	0.048
Family history of CAD (%)	37 (27%)	11 (27%)	26 (27%)	0.9
Smoking (%)	26 (19%)	14 (34%)	12(13%)	0.003
Hypercolesterolemia (%)	62 (45%)	25 (61%)	37 (39%)	0.015
Diabetes mellitus (%)	16 (12%)	7 (17%)	9 (9%)	0.2
Coronary Calcium Agatston score, Median (IQR)	25 (175)	269 (917)	2 (42)	<0.0001
Coronary stenosis >50% but <70%	27 (20%)	27 (66%)	–	–
At least one stenosis more than 70%	14 (10%)	14 (34%)	–	–
Bridge, tortuous course or coronary anomaly, sum, (%)	21, 24, 17 = 62 (45%)	9, 6, 7 = 22 (54%)	12, 18, 10 = 40 (42%)	0.2
Any reversible WM abnormality	18 (13%)	5 (12%)	13 (13%)	0.9
Reversible myocardial perfusion abnormality	78 (56%)	21 (51%)	57 (60%)	0.37
CFR-LAD Median (IQR)	2,0 (0.2)	1,9 (0.3)	2 (0.2)	0.003

CAD coronary artery disease, *IQR* interquartile range, *WM* wall motion, *CFR-LAD* coronary flow reserve of the left anterior descending coronary artery

93%) and a positive predictive value of 75% (95% CI 58% to 88%); on the right the ROC curve for the prediction of more severe >70% CAD, using the specific best cutoff of >105, showing superimposable AUC value (0.843, 95% CI 0,713 to 0,973), but an increased negative predictive value of 99% (95% CI 94% to 100%) and a decreased positive predictive value, of only 27,5% (95% CI 15% to 44%).

From the ROC curve for CFR-LAD to predict >50% CAD at CTA, the best cutoff was <1.8, demonstrating a suboptimal AUC = 0.339 (95% CI 0,234 to 0,443), a negative predictive value of 78% (95% CI 68% to 86%) and a positive predictive value of 58% (95% CI 39% to 75%), while the ROC curve recalculated for the prediction of more severe >70% CAD showed an AUC of 0.370 (95% CI 0,195 to 0,546) using the calculated best cutoff of <1.7, an increased negative predictive value of 92% (95% CI 85% to 97%) and a positive predictive value of only 28,5% (95% CI 11% to 52%).

Full accuracy data in this CTA group of patients with equivocal cSE are shown in Fig. 4, highlighting the very high negative predictive value of an Agatston score < 105

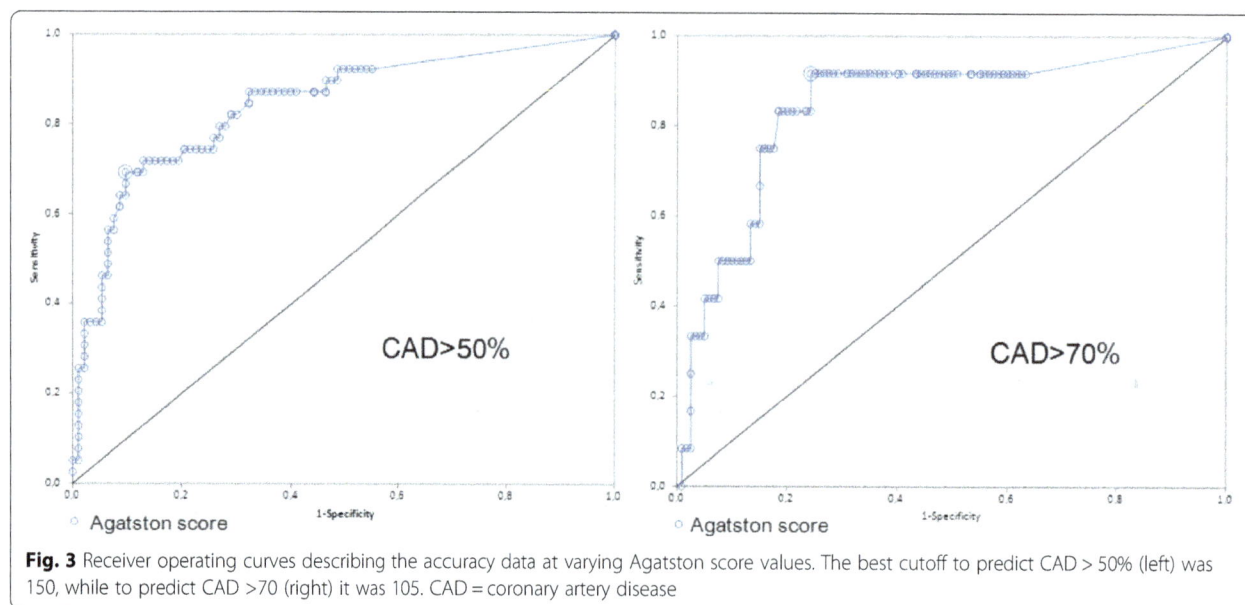

Fig. 3 Receiver operating curves describing the accuracy data at varying Agatston score values. The best cutoff to predict CAD > 50% (left) was 150, while to predict CAD >70 (right) it was 105. CAD = coronary artery disease

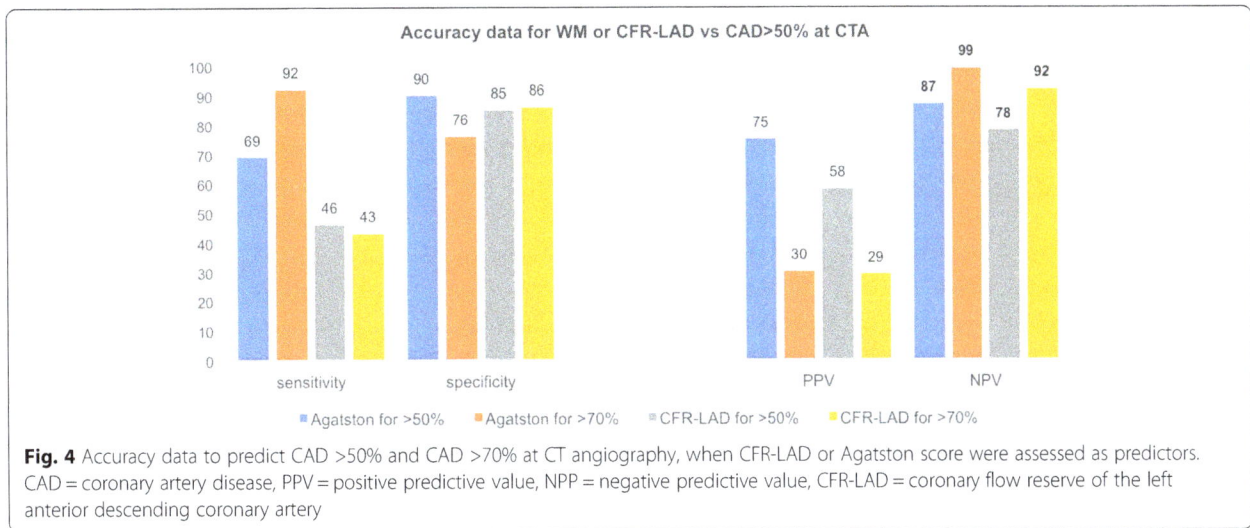

Fig. 4 Accuracy data to predict CAD >50% and CAD >70% at CT angiography, when CFR-LAD or Agatston score were assessed as predictors. CAD = coronary artery disease, PPV = positive predictive value, NPP = negative predictive value, CFR-LAD = coronary flow reserve of the left anterior descending coronary artery

(and also of a CFR < 1.7) to exclude the presence of CAD > 70%.

Figure 5 graphically demonstrates the incremental diagnostic benefit of adding CFR-LAD data (chi square increases from 30.89 to 41.04, $p < 0.005$) or the Agatston score (chi square increases from 30.89 to 47.28, $p < 0.001$) over baseline demographics + clinical risk factors.

Contrast Stress-echocardiography and iCA data

In the 314 patients with available iCA, 73 (23%) demonstrated no or <50% coronary stenosis in (no CAD group), while 241 (77%) demonstrated at least one >50% coronary artery stenosis (CAD group); among such 241 patients, most ($n = 222$, 92%) had also at least one coronary artery stenosis >70% or left main trunk disease >50%. Reversible wall motion abnormalities of any degree (delta WMSI > 0) were found in 206 (66%) patients, while only 164 (52%) demonstrated a reversible more-than-mild wall motion abnormality (WMSI > 0.06),

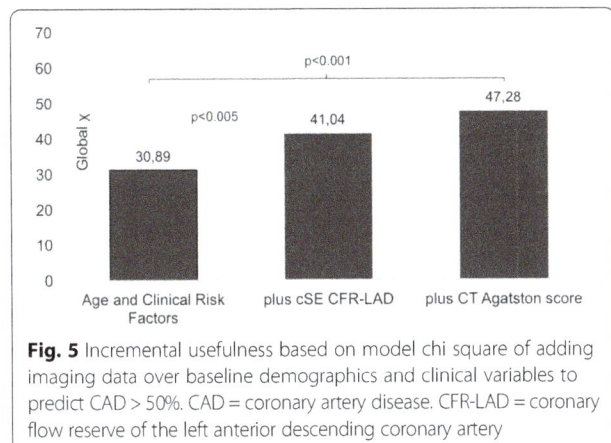

Fig. 5 Incremental usefulness based on model chi square of adding imaging data over baseline demographics and clinical variables to predict CAD > 50%. CAD = coronary artery disease. CFR-LAD = coronary flow reserve of the left anterior descending coronary artery

highlighting that half of patients who underwent iCA did so not mainly driven by cSE wall motion results, but other cSE variables, other functional tests or clinical variables. CFR-LAD data were available only for 208 (66%) and myocardial perfusion data in 176 (56%) in this real-world cohort of 314 patients, highlighting the less than optimal feasibility of such two imaging parameters compared with standard WM when cSE data are prospectively collected in routine clinical practice, not selecting operators based on their advanced technical skills. Accuracy to predict CAD for such only partly available variables was calculated limited to patients in which they were measurable.

Baseline risk factors, cSE and iCA data are shown in Table 2, which highlights few significant differences between the CAD and no CAD groups: age was significantly higher in the group with CAD (median 67 vs 53, $p = 0.005$), as it was the prevalence of male gender, hypertension, dyslipidemia and diabetes mellitus ($p < 0.05$ for all), while smoking habit and prior myocardial infarction were apparently more frequent, but only of borderline statistical significance ($p = 0.05$).

The presence of any degree of reversible WM abnormality during cSE was more frequent in the CAD (71%) vs no CAD (48%) groups ($p < 0.001$) but also present in almost half of patients with no stenosis < 50% at iCA, while when considering positive for ischemia only more-than-mild reversible WM abnormalities (WMSI delta > 0.06) such false positive rate of WM abnormalities fell to 29%. The only other cSE imaging variable differing between the 2 groups was a reduced CFR-LAD < 2 (best cutoff calculated from ROC curve in this iCA group was 1.96 and we decided to use the literature standard 2.0), which was significantly more frequent in the CAD group vs no CAD group (58% vs 40%, $p = 0.026$).

Table 2 Baseline demographics and clinical variables, stress-echocardiography and invasive coronary angiograms data in the entire population and in the subgroups with or without obstructive coronary artery disease > 50%

	Entire population (n = 314)	CAD > 50% (n = 241)	No CAD > 50% (n = 73)	p
Age, median (IQR)	66 (17)	67 (15)	63 (16)	0.005
Male Gender (%)	229 (73%) (57%)	186 (77%)	43 (59%)	0.002
Hypertension (%)	227 (72%)	183 (76%)	44 (60%)	0.008
Family history of CAD (%)	93 (30%)	72 (30%)	21 (29%)	0.855
Smoking (%)	120 (38%)	99 (41%)	21(29%)	0.057
Hypercolesterolemia (%)	188 (60%)	152 (63%)	36 (49%)	0.035
Diabetes mellitus (%)	71 (23%)	63 (26%)	8 (11%)	0.006
Prior Miocardial infarction	73 (23%)	62 (26%)	11 (15%)	0.059
Coronary stenosis >50%	241 (77%)	241 (100%)	0	–
At least one stenosis more than 70%	222 (71%)	222 (92%)	0	–
Any reversible WM abnormality	206 (66%)	172 (71%)	35 (48%)	0.0002
More than mild reversible WM abnormality (>0.06)	164 (52%)	146 (61%)	18 (25%)	<0.0001
Reversible myocardial perfusion abnormality	136/176 (77%)[a]	105/130 (81%)[a]	31/46 (67%)[a]	0.063
CFR-LAD < 2	110/208 (53%)[a]	87/151 (58%)[a]	23/57 (40%)[a]	0.026
Normal WM + normal or unavailable myocardial perfusion and CFR-LAD	59 (19%)	44 (18%)	15 (20%)	0.66

CAD coronary artery disease, *IQR* interquartile range, *WM* wall motion, *CFR-LAD* coronary flow reserve of the left anterior descending coronary artery
[a]Myocardial perfusion and CFR-LAD percentages are related to the total number of patients in whom such variables could actually be technically measured

Figure 6 shows the ROC curves for reversible WM abnormalities based on WMSI delta to predict CAD, for CAD > 50% demonstrating an AUC = 0.696 (95% CI 0.636 to 0.756), a negative predictive value of 63,3% (95% CI 55% to 71%) and a positive predictive value of 90% (95% CI 84% to 94%), and for CAD > 70% an AUC = 0.658, 95% CI 0.596 to 0.720), but a negative predictive value of 57% (95% CI 48% to 65%) with a positive predictive value of 83.5% (95% CI 77% to 89%).

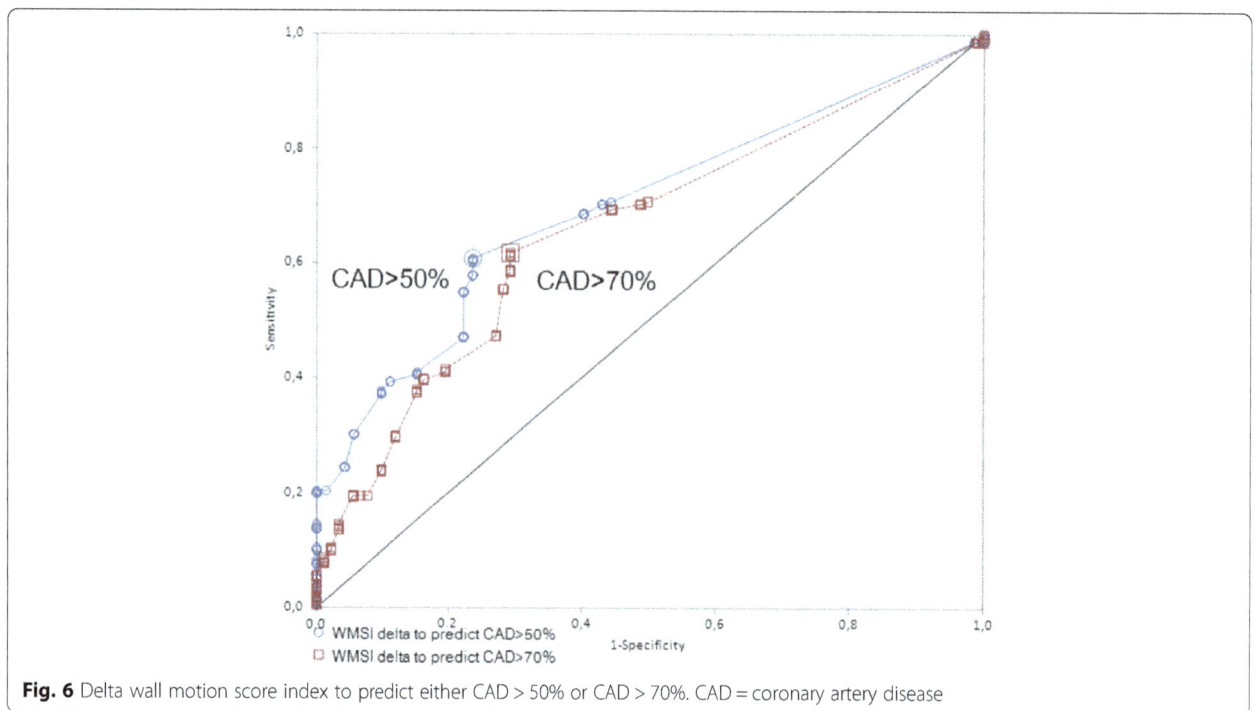

Fig. 6 Delta wall motion score index to predict either CAD > 50% or CAD > 70%. CAD = coronary artery disease

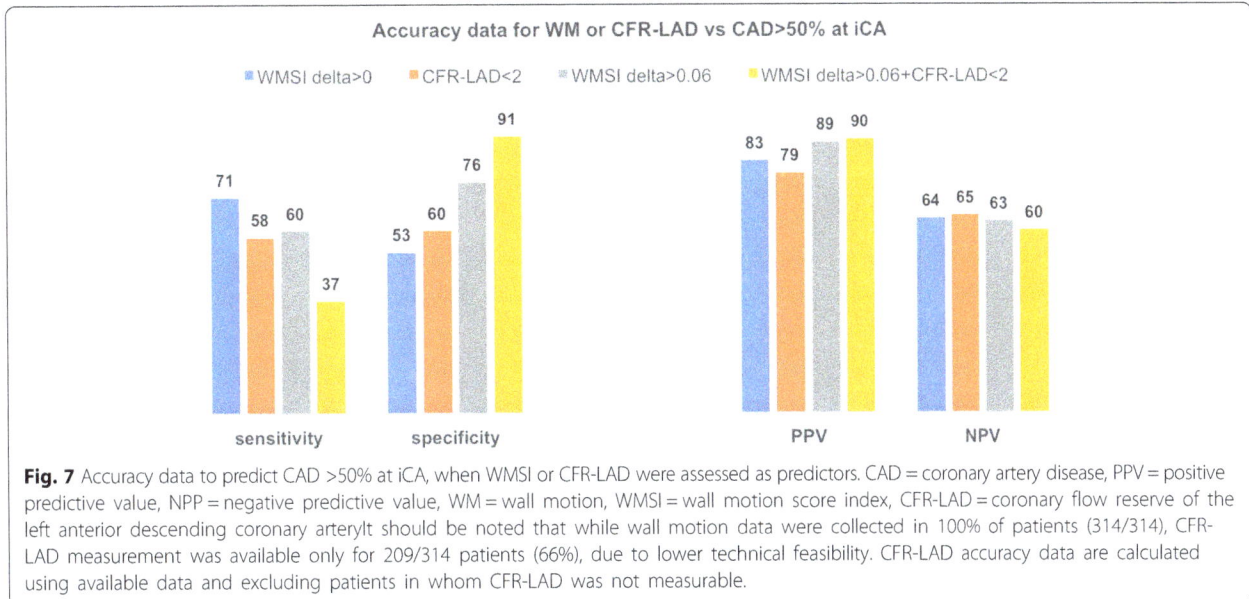

Fig. 7 Accuracy data to predict CAD >50% at iCA, when WMSI or CFR-LAD were assessed as predictors. CAD = coronary artery disease, PPV = positive predictive value, NPP = negative predictive value, WM = wall motion, WMSI = wall motion score index, CFR-LAD = coronary flow reserve of the left anterior descending coronary arteryIt should be noted that while wall motion data were collected in 100% of patients (314/314), CFR-LAD measurement was available only for 209/314 patients (66%), due to lower technical feasibility. CFR-LAD accuracy data are calculated using available data and excluding patients in whom CFR-LAD was not measurable.

Full accuracy data in this iCA group are shown in Fig. 7, which highlights the high positive predictive value of cSE data, in particular of a more than mild reversible WM abnormality (WMSI delta >0.06) to predict CAD; CFR-LAD appeared less useful and also the combination of the two parameters did not increase significantly the predictive value of simple WMSI delta >0.06. On the other hand, all tested variables demonstrated a low negative predictive value for CAD.

Figure 8 graphically demonstrates that WMSI data (delta >0.06) add to baseline demographics and risk factors for the prediction of CAD >50% (chi square increases from 37.5 to 56.4, $p < 0.001$) while adding CFR-LAD data did not (chi square increase from 37.5 to 39.3, p = ns).

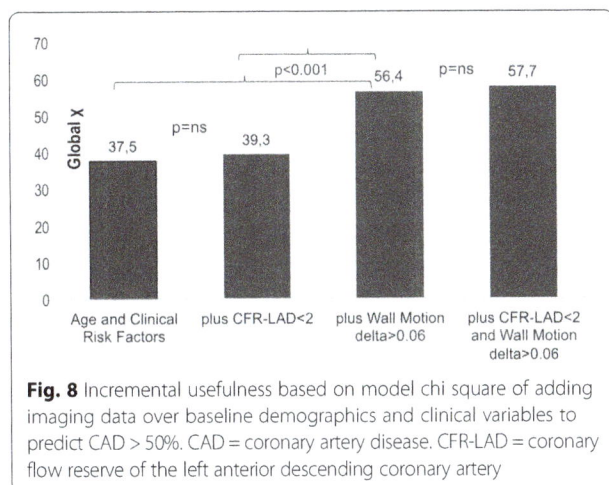

Fig. 8 Incremental usefulness based on model chi square of adding imaging data over baseline demographics and clinical variables to predict CAD > 50%. CAD = coronary artery disease. CFR-LAD = coronary flow reserve of the left anterior descending coronary artery

Discussion

Our data confirm the common sense that once a functional imaging test for suspect CAD is performed, only patients showing more than mild degree of ischemia, in this case reversible WM abnormality, should be indicated iCA, by so doing possibly decreasing to trivial or "one-digit" percentage the subsequent "normal" findings of non-obstructive CAD at iCA.

This was never specifically confirmed for stress-echocardiography and it is not a trivial issue, since many (if not most) positive stress-echocardiograms performed in the low CAD prevalence population, which nowadays undergoes functional testing, demonstrate limited WMSI delta; the physician is consequently left with a clinical dilemma regarding what to do next in these cases.

Patients with equivocal results or only mildly positive WM behavior are not immune to CAD, but they may be rather indicated non-invasive CTA; further, coronary calcium score could be used first in this case, as a gatekeeper, to decide whether to proceed or not to full contrast CTA, based on an Agatston score threshold of 100 (an easy cutoff to memorize), since a lower score in our cohort demonstrated a very high (99%) negative predictive value for CAD > 70%, which would not justify routinely proceeding to CTA. Non-contrast CT calcium scoring is cheaper and biologically safer than CTA (even more if compared with iCA) for both being non-invasive and implying only trivial radiation.

The implementation of this hypothetical flow-chart (Fig. 9) derived from our dataset to optimize the diagnostic process after cSE would possibly reduce the number of equivocal cSE finally proceeding to iCA, but also

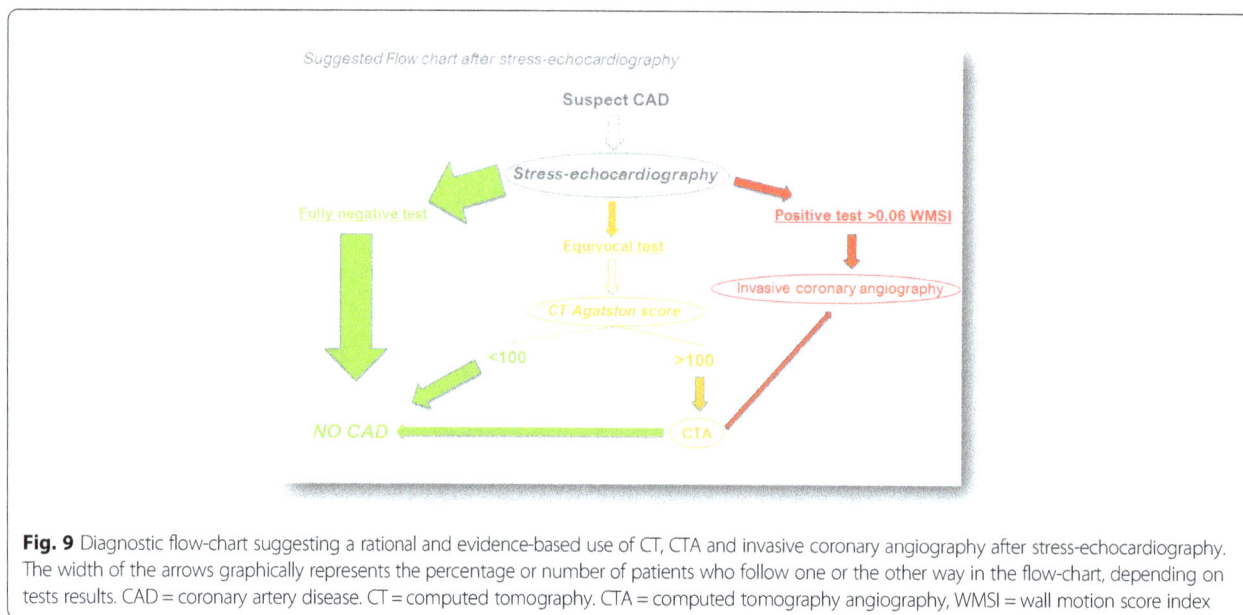

Fig. 9 Diagnostic flow-chart suggesting a rational and evidence-based use of CT, CTA and invasive coronary angiography after stress-echocardiography. The width of the arrows graphically represents the percentage or number of patients who follow one or the other way in the flow-chart, depending on tests results. CAD = coronary artery disease. CT = computed tomography. CTA = computed tomography angiography, WMSI = wall motion score index

to full CTA, simply using a 0–100 Agatston score to skip subsequent CTA, and still identifying the same overall number of patients with CAD. This strategy is retrospectively derived by our data, and should definitely be confirmed in a prospective validation cohort.

CFR-LAD less than 1.7 in cSE equivocal tests also demonstrated a high negative predictive value, almost as good as the CT Agatston score, but suboptimal feasibility of this measurement may be perceived as an issue for less experienced operators.

Although most patients with an equivocal cSE were finally reassured by CTA regarding the absence of anatomically severely obstructive CAD, this group with equivocal cSE tests hides a non-trivial percentage of patients with CAD who should not be overlooked or simply reassured.

Why not "go functional" if accuracy could be similar?

While the Recent NICE guidelines [2] suggest that CTA should be preferred over functional imaging stress-testing in the suspicion of CAD, and we mostly agree due to the limited diagnostic accuracy of both ECG or imaging stress-tests when used as gatekeepers to iCA [9, 10], CTA could instead more realistically play the role of the missing link between functional tests and iCA. This would result particularly effective for the "grey zone" of patients with equivocal tests showing no or mildly abnormal WM behavior, who could be more confidently indicated iCA, maximizing the percentage who are finally diagnosed with obstructive CAD, and minimizing false-positive cSE undergoing iCA.

Starting from a functional test, instead of an anatomical one, has the main advantage that semi-quantitative

inducible ischemia data are still today the mainstay (together with invasive coronary fractional flow measurements) to indicate subsequent coronary revascularization in stable CAD. Consequently, diagnostic, prognostic and therapeutic indications may all be assessed within a single test, in the specific case of cSE with a very low biological and economic cost, compared with a "CTA-for-all" strategy. CTA also has non-zero false positive rate compared with iCA, as it is apparently also confirmed in our study, which would be amplified if used indiscriminately.

Limitations

This is a retrospective and single-center study and the strategy suggested needs to be further tested in a prospective and multicenter validation cohort.

Contrast stress-echocardiograms were routinely performed by 4 different operators and cSE interpretation is to some degree subjective, although it has been demonstrated that using contrast for endocardial border enhancement, as it was in our study in 100% of studies, the variability of interpretation is very significantly reduced [11, 12].

Myocardial perfusion and CFR-LAD data were not available for all patients, mostly due to the multiple operators involved in the clinical routine of our echolab, which is the setting of this study, not all being specifically trained or skilled in myocardial perfusion imaging and CFR-LAD, but WM remains the mainstay and the most widely used marker during stress-echocardiography to indicate iCA, and our diagnostic strategy in fact focused on WM behavior. The finding of myocardial perfusion data resulting almost useless to predict the presence of obstructive CAD (the prevalence of reversible perfusion defects was not significantly different between CAD and no CAD groups) may derive from cSE being performed by several different operators after 2012 in our lab, only rarely skilled in this complicated imaging method and interpretation, differently from prior studies published from our lab, when myocardial perfusion assessments were conducted and interpreted mostly by a single and experienced operator.

Conclusions

Our data suggest that iCA should be indicated only for more than mild reversible ischemia by WM assessment at cSE, due to the very high positive predictive value of this variable for CAD, while mildly positive tests may rather be shifted to non-invasive CTA. Further, coronary calcium score could be assessed, as a gatekeeper, to proceed only in case of an Agatston score > 100 to CTA, since a lower score in our cohort demonstrated such a high negative predictive value for CAD that it would not justify proceeding to CTA. A significant percentage of patients with mildly positive cSE today usually sent to iCA would be more efficiently managed shifting them to non-contrast CT calcium scoring first, which is cheap and biologically safer for both being non-invasive and implying only trivial radiation.

Abbreviations
AUC: Area under the curve; CAD: Coronary artery disease; CFR-LAD: Coronary flow reserve of the left anterior descending coronary artery; cSE: Contrast stress-echocardiography; CT: Computed tomography; CTA: CT angiography; ECG: Electrocardiogram; iCA: Invasive coronary angiography; ROC: Receiver operating characteristic; WM: Wall motion; WMSI: Wall motion score index

Acknowledgements
Not applicable.

Funding
No external funding declared.

Authors' contributions
NG (first author, corresponding author) analyzed and interpreted the patient data, drafting/revising the manuscript, control and guarantee that all aspects of the work was investigated and resolved. GP, AB, FT, CB, SG, GB acquisition of data, analysis and interpretation of data, revising the manuscript, control and guarantee that all aspects of the work was investigated and resolved. All authors read and approved the final manuscript.

Competing interests
All other authors declare that they have no conflict of interests.

References

1. Cortigiani L, Borelli L, Raciti M, Bonvenzi F, Picano E, Molinaro S, Sicari R. Prediction of mortality by stress echocardiography in 2835 diabetic and 11 305 nondiabetic patients. Circ Cardiovasc Imaging. 2015;8(5). https://doi.org/10.1161/CIRCIMAGING.114.002757.
2. National Institute for Health and Clinical Excellence. Chest pain of recent onset: assessment and diagnosis of recent onset chest pain or discomfort of suspected cardiac origin (update). CG95. London: National Institute for Health and Clinical Excellence; 2016.
3. Erikssen J, Rasmussen K, Forfang K, Storstein O. Exercise ECG and Case history in the diagnosis of latent coronary heart disease among presumably healthy middle-aged men. Eur J Cardiol. 1977;5:463–76.
4. Patel MR, Dai D, Hernandez AF, et al. Prevalence and predictors of nonobstructive coronary artery disease identified with coronary angiography in contemporary clinical practice. Am Heart J. 2014;167:846–52.e2.
5. Patel MR, Peterson ED, Dai D, et al. Low diagnostic yield of elective coronary angiography. N Engl J Med. 2010;362:886–95. doi: https://doi.org/10.1056/NEJMoa0907272. Erratum in: N Engl J Med 2010; 363:498.
6. Carpeggiani C, Landi P, Michelassi C, Sicari R, Picano E. The declining frequency of inducible myocardial ischemia during stress echocardiography over 27 consecutive years (1983-2009). Int J Cardiol. 2016;224:57–61.
7. Gaibazzi N, Rigo F, Lorenzoni V, et al. Comparative prediction of cardiac events by wall motion, wall motion plus coronary flow reserve, or myocardial perfusion analysis: a multicenter study of contrast stress echocardiography. J Am Coll Cardiol Img. 2013;6:1–12.
8. Lang RM, Badano LP, Mor-Avi V, et al. Recommendations for cardiac chamber quantification by echocardiography in adults: an update from the American Society of Echocardiography and the European Association of Cardiovascular Imaging. Eur Heart J Cardiovasc Imaging. 2015;16:233–70.
9. Ladapo JA, Blecker S, Elashoff MR, et al. Clinical implications of referral bias in the diagnostic performance of exercise testing for coronary artery disease. J Am Heart Assoc. 2013;2:e000505.
10. Neglia D, Rovai D, Caselli C, et al, EVINCI Study Investigators. Detection of significant coronary artery disease by noninvasive anatomical and functional imaging. Circ Cardiovasc Imaging. 2015;8. pii: e002179. doi: https://doi.org/10.1161/CIRCIMAGING.114.002179.
11. Hoffmann R, von Bardeleben S, Kasprzak JD, Borges AC, ten Cate F, Firschke C, Lafitte S, Al-Saadi N, Kuntz-Hehner S, Horstick G, Greis C, Engelhardt M, Vanoverschelde JL, Becher H. Analysis of regional left ventricular function by cineventriculography, cardiac magnetic resonance imaging, and unenhanced and contrast-enhanced echocardiography: a multicenter comparison of methods. J Am Coll Cardiol. 2006;47:121–8.
12. Plana JC, Mikati IA, Dokainish H, et al. A randomized cross-over study for evaluation of the effect of image optimization with contrast on the diagnostic accuracy of dobutamine echocardiography in coronary artery disease the OPTIMIZE trial. J Am Coll Cardiol Img. 2008;1:145–52.

13

Identification of the main determinants of abdominal aorta size: a screening by Pocket Size Imaging Device

Roberta Esposito[1], Federica Ilardi[1], Vincenzo Schiano Lomoriello[1], Regina Sorrentino[1], Vincenzo Sellitto[1], Giuseppe Giugliano[1], Giovanni Esposito[1], Bruno Trimarco[1] and Maurizio Galderisi[1,2*]

Abstract

Background: Ultrasound exam as a screening test for abdominal aorta (AA) can visualize the aorta in 99% of patients and has a sensitivity and specificity approaching 100% in screening settings for aortic aneurysm. Pocket Size Imaging Device (PSID) has a potential value as a screening tool, because of its possible use in several clinical settings. Our aim was to assess the impact of demographics and cardiovascular (CV) risk factors on AA size by using PSID in an outpatient screening.

Methods: Consecutive patients, referring for a CV assessment in a 6 months period, were screened. AA was visualized by subcostal view in longitudinal and transverse plans in order to determine the greatest anterior-posterior diameter. After excluding 5 patients with AA aneurysm, 508 outpatients were enrolled. All patients underwent a sequential assessment including clinical history with collection of CV risk factors, physical examination, PSID exam and standard Doppler echoc exam using a 2.5 transducer with harmonic capability, both by expert ultrasound operators, during the same morning. Standard echocardiography operators were blinded on PSID exam and viceversa.

Results: Diagnostic accuracy of AA size by PSID was tested successfully with standard echo machine in a subgroup ($n = 102$) (rho $= 0.966$, $p < 0.0001$). AA diameter was larger in men than in women and in ≥50 -years old subjects than in those <50 -years old (both $p < 0.0001$). AA was larger in patients with coronary artery disease (CAD) ($p < 0.0001$). By a multivariate model, male sex ($p < 0.0001$), age and body mass index (both $p < 0.0001$), CAD ($p < 0.01$) and heart rate ($p = 0.018$) were independent predictors of AA size (cumulative $R^2 = 0.184$, $p < 0.0001$).

Conclusion: PSID is a reliable tool for the screening of determinants of AA size. AA diameter is greater in men and strongly influenced by aging and overweight. CAD may be also associated to increased AA diameter.

Keywords: Abdominal aorta, Pocket size imaging device, Ultrasound, Aging, Cardiovascular risk factors, Coronary artery disease

Background

Abdominal aortic aneurysm (AAA) is a localized abnormal dilatation of the aorta defined as a diameter ≥30 mm or a >50% increase of the aortic diameter at the diaphragm [1]. Incidence of AAA is increasing [2] due mainly to life prolongation in the current era. The incidence of AAAs in the general population is about 1.0 to 1.5% [3]. This incidence is particularly high in presence of male gender, advanced age, arterial systemic hypertension, family history of AAA, peripheral artery disease or coronary artery disease (CAD), and/or cerebrovascular disease [4–6]. The most feared complication is rupture, which relates directly to size and is especially frequent in patients with AAA >5.5 cm [7]. AAA rupture entails 85–90% overall mortality, 60% pre-hospital and from 40 to 70% in-hospital (following emergency interventions) [8]. AAAs usually do not produce symptoms and ruptured aneurysms often occur without warning. This comprehensive information highlights the need for an early detection of abdominal aorta

* Correspondence: mgalderi@unina.it
[1]Department of Advanced Biomedical Sciences, Division of Cardiology, Federico II University Hospital, Naples, Italy
[2]Interdepartimental Laboratory of Cardiac Imaging, Federico II University Hospital, Via S. Pansini 5,bld 1, 80131 Naples, Italy

(AA) dilatation, together with identification of high-risk patients that could benefit from a screening program.

Ultrasound exam as a screening test for AAA is able to visualize the aorta in 99% of patients and has a sensitivity and specificity approaching 100% in screening settings for AAA [9, 10]. In addition, ultrasound test is non invasive, fast, relatively inexpensive, and without biological risk of radiation. The feasibility of population-based ultrasound screening of AAA has been established through large randomized screening trials [11, 12]. Pocket Size Imaging Device (PSID) is an ultrasound machine not classifiable as a standard echocardiographic machine because of impossibility of calculating chamber volumes and quantifying valvular flow by pulsed or continuous Doppler. It has a potential value as a screening tool [13, 14], because of its possible use in several clinical settings.

The present study was designed to identify the influence of demographic variables and cardiovascular (CV) risk factors on AA size in a screening of outpatient population using PSID and to validate it in comparison to standard transthoracic echo-Doppler exam.

Methods

Five hundred thirteen consecutive patients, referring to Echo-lab of Federico II University hospital for a CV assessment in a 6 months period, were screened. All subjects gave written informed consent and the study was approved by the Institutional Ethical Committee. During the screening, 5 patients with AAA (diameter ≥ 3.0 cm in maximum antero-posterior or latero-lateral dimensions) were identified and excluded from subsequent analysis. The final study population included 508 outpatients (M/F = 305/203). All the patients underwent a sequential assessment including: 1. clinical history with collection of CV risk factors; 2. physical examination; 3. PSID exam (Vscan, GE, Horten, Norway) and 4. standard Doppler echocardiographic exam (Vivid E9 ultrasound scanner, GE, Horten, Norway) using a 2.5 transducer with harmonic capability, both by expert ultrasound operators, during the same morning. Standard echocardiography operators were blinded on PSID exam and viceversa.

Arterial systemic hypertension was diagnosed if systolic blood pressure (BP) exceeded 140 mmHg and/or diastolic BP exceeded 90 mmHg, or if the patient was taking antihypertensive drugs [15]. Hypercholesterolemia was defined as plasma total cholesterol >200 mg/dL, plasma low-density lipoprotein cholesterol >130 mg/dL, or when the patient used lipid-lowering medications [16]. Diabetes mellitus was diagnosed if plasma fasting glucose exceeded 126 mg/dL or if the patient used hypoglycaemic drugs [17]. A history of CAD was documented by hospital records, it including acute coronary syndromes, angina pectoris, previous coronary

revascularization procedures and positive inducible ischemia test.

AA ultrasound exam was performed using a PSID (unit + probe = 390 g) which provides 2-D, black and white and colour flow images (fixed pulse-repetition frequency and colour-box size), and is connected to a broad-bandwith, phased array probe (1.7–3.8 MHz). The flow sector represents blood flow within an angle of 30°. Videos (automatic autocycle without ECG need) and images can be produced and stored in separate folders, recalled via a gallery function and transferred to hardware by an intermediate docking station. In the present study we utilized an abdominal setting whereas the alternative cardiac/thoracic setting was not applied. AA was visualized using subcostal and abdominal views, with the patient lying supine. No abdominal preparation was required. The entire AA was first visualized in longitudinal and transverse plans from the diaphragm to the aorta bifurcation in order to determine the greatest aortic diameter, which was considered for statistical analyses. Antero-posterior and latero-lateral outer diameters were measured in the transverse plane, at the largest portion of infrarenal aorta [18, 19] (Fig. 1). In a subgroup of 102 patients the diagnostic accuracy of AA size measurements obtained by PSID was tested in comparison with the same measurements taken by a standard echocardiographic machine.

Statistical analyses

Statistical analyses were performed by SPSS package, release 12 (SPSS Inc, Chicago, Illinois, USA). Data are presented as mean value ± SD. Descriptive statistics were done by one-factor ANOVA (Bonferroni post-hoc test). Intra-class correlation analysis was used to assess agreement of AA size between PSID and standard echo. The null hypothesis was rejected at $p \leq 0.05$.

Results

The feasibility of AA measurements by both PSID and standard echo machine was 100%.

Figure 2 shows the univariate relation between AA size measured by PSID and that taken by standard echocardiography. The agreement between the two instrumentations was also excellent (rho = 0.966, 95% CI = 0.956–0.974, $p < 0.0001$).

Demographic characteristics and CV risk factors of the study population are listed in Table 1. Of note, hypertensive patients were 64.9% of the study population, the majority being under anti-hypertensive therapy.

AA diameter was larger in men (1.84 ± 0.35 cm) than in women (1.65 ± 0.29 cm) ($p < 0.0001$) and in patients with > 50 years (1.80 ± 0.36 cm), compared with patients >50 years old (1.64 ± 0.25 cm) ($p < 0.0001$). Of note, smokers had larger AA diameter in comparison with

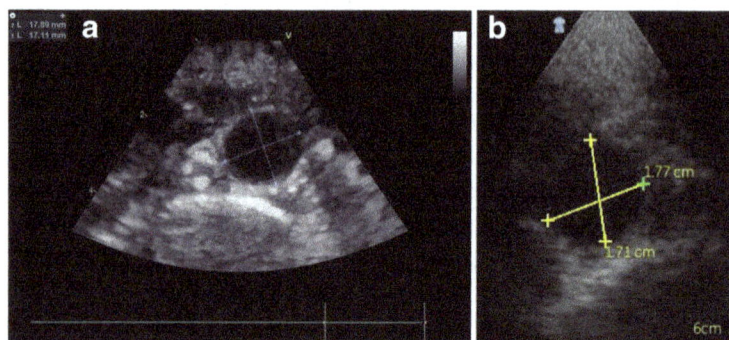

Fig. 1 AA visualized in longitudinal and transverse plans from the diaphragm to the bifurcation of the aorta. Antero-posterior and latero-lateral outer diameters were measured in the transverse plane, at the largest portion of infrarenal aorta. The figure shows the good concordance of the two measured diameters between standard echocardiography (panel **a**) and PSID (panel **b**): 17.89 mm versus 1.77 cm and 17.11 mm versus 1.71 cm

non smokers ($p = 0.007$) as well as hypercholesterolemic ($p < 0.01$) versus non hypercholesterolemic. Conversely, the presence of both arterial hypertension and diabetes mellitus did not differentiate larger AA diameters. AA was larger also in patients with CAD (1.93 ± 0.43 cm) than in those without (1.72 ± 0.31 cm) ($p < 0.0001$).

In the pooled population, AA diameter was positively related to age ($p < 0.0001$) (Fig. 3), systolic BP ($p < 0.005$) (Fig. 4), mean BP and pulse pressure (both $r = 0.11$, $p < 0.01$), weight, height and body mass index (BMI) (all $p < 0.0001$) (Fig. 5). Diastolic BP and heart rate were not significantly related with AA size.

In a multiple linear regression analysis performed in the pooled population, after adjusting for several confounders, male sex, age and BMI (all $p < 0.0001$), and, with a lesser extent, CAD ($p < 0.01$) and heart rate ($p = 0.018$) were independent predictors of AA size whereas cigarette

smoking and hypercholesterolemia did not enter the model (cumulative $R^2 = 0.184$, SEE $= 0.31$ cm, $p < 0.0001$) (Table 2).

Discussion

The present study demonstrates (1) PSID's excellent feasibility and accuracy in assessing AA size in comparison to standard echocardiography and that (2) by using this tool, male sex, age, body mass index are major independent determinants of AA size, whereas the presence of CAD and increased heart rate should not be underestimated.

PSID is a latest generation, portable device that allows to acquire real-time 2D and colour Doppler images, giving the chance to obtain linear and area measurements of cardiac and vascular structures. Its additional diagnostic value to the simple physical examination has been shown [20–22], particularly in conditions such as evaluation of left ventricular size and function [21–23], right ventricular heart failure [21, 24], mitral valve prolapse [25] and pleural or pericardial effusions [26]. Being a very small unit it offers the potential possibility of an easy and practical use and effectiveness for population screening [13]. The screening for AAA using PSID by experienced physicians has been already proposed as a valuable extension of routine physical examination in

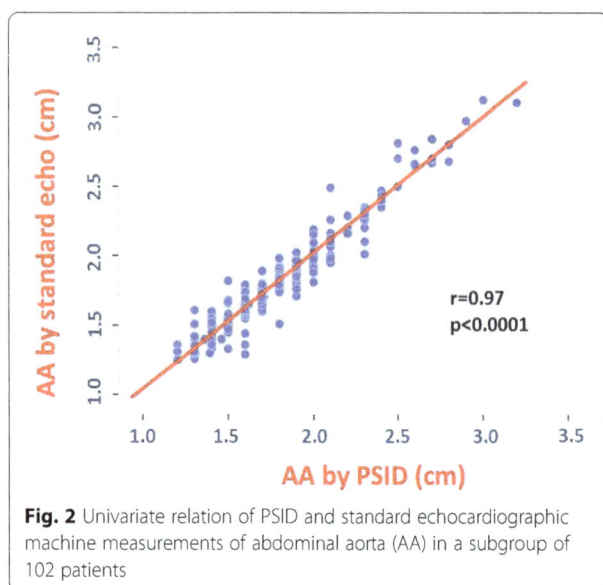

Fig. 2 Univariate relation of PSID and standard echocardiographic machine measurements of abdominal aorta (AA) in a subgroup of 102 patients

Table 1 Characteristics of Study Population

Variable	Patients ($n = 508$)
Sex (M/F)	305/203
Age (years)	57.0 ± 15.5
Arterial Hypertension, n (%)	330 (64.9%)
Hypercholesterolemia, n (%)	228 (44.8%)
Type II diabetes mellitus, n (%)	77 (15.1%)
Cigarette smoking, n (%)	115 (22.6%)
Coronary artery disease, n (%)	90 (17.7%)
Anti-hypertensive therapy, n (%)	290 (57.1%)

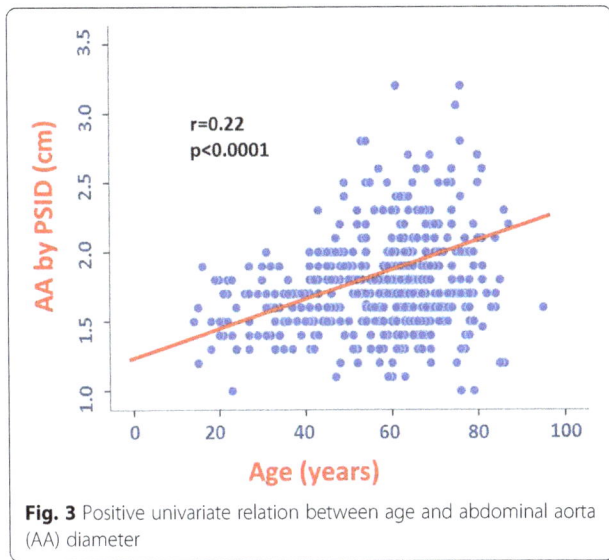

Fig. 3 Positive univariate relation between age and abdominal aorta (AA) diameter

vascular patients. It appeared to have a 100% of agreement with a standard ultrasound machine in diagnosing aneurysms in 204 patients hospitalized in a cardiology institute [27]. Another study showed a good diagnostic accuracy in measuring AA size in comparison with standard ultrasound exam in patients referring for acute myocardial infarction in coronary care unit [28]. The present study is in agreement with these findings since we found an excellent concordance between measurements of AA taken by PSID and those obtained by a standard ultrasound machine. Accordingly, PSID can be judged as a valuable tool for detecting AA dilation.

AAA represents still nowadays an important cause of mortality in the western countries [29]. To date, in expert hands, ultrasound exam represents a consolidated tool for AA assessment [30]. Therefore, an effective screening plan

could be valuable to prevent extreme AA dilation and rupture and appropriately address high risk patients towards surgery. The importance of an early detection of AA dilatation has been indirectly proven by the observation that AAA and AA rupture can be reasonably excluded in old patients with abdominal pain admitted in emergency department if they had a normal AA size on a previously performed computed tomography or ultrasound exam [31]. A recent study has also shown that a systematic and targeted approach based on CV risk assessment could be very useful to identify undiagnosed cases [32]. The cost-effectiveness of AAA screening programs has been demonstrated in men with >65 years [33]. Even women should be involved in these programs, because, in spite of the lower prevalence, AAA in woman has a higher risk of rupture [34].

By using standard ultrasound machines, determinants of AAA have been more extensively investigated than factors influencing AA size itself. In an unselected population of 742 patients, Bekkers et al. observed that AAA prevalence increased with age, especially in men [35]. In the very large sample size of Tromso study, the prevalence of AAA increased with age, additional factors being represented by smoke, low serum high density lipoprotein cholesterol and antihypertensive therapy [36]. In a meta-analysis of 15 cross-sectional studies, male sex was strongly associated with AAA (OR 5.69), while cigarette smoking (OR 2.41), history of myocardial infarction (OR 2.28) or peripheral vascular disease (OR 2.50) showed moderate associations and arterial hypertension was only weakly associated with AAA (OR 1.33) [37]. The association of obesity with AAA is controversial. Body mass index was not associated with AAA presence and growth in the experiences of Tagaki et al. [38, 39]. However, in a large cohort of 12.203 men who had an ultrasound examination of their AA and filled out a questionnaire including demographic, behavioural and medical variables, AAA was significantly associated with a waist/hip ratio greater than 0.9 [35].

In our study population, we extended the screening to outpatients without overt AAA. By this assessment. male sex, age and BMI were all major independent determinants of AA size, whereas the association of higher heart rate and AA was marginal but significant. Although this latter finding is in disagreement with a cross sectional study showing a negative correlation between heart rate and AA diameter [40], it is conceivable that tachycardia could exert a detrimental effect on AA size [41]. Systolic BP showed a positive univariate relation with AA diameter in our study population but this association disappeared in the multivariate model. Conversely, in a recent study diastolic BP was a risk factor of AAA expansion [42]. The undergoing anti-hypertensive therapy of the majority of our patients (57%, see Table 1) could have

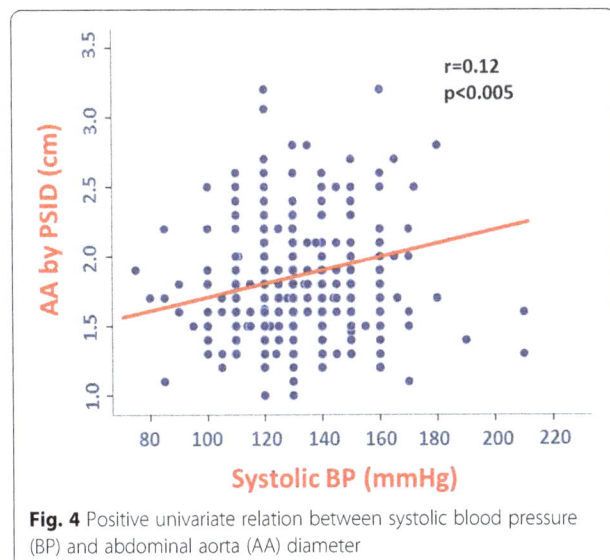

Fig. 4 Positive univariate relation between systolic blood pressure (BP) and abdominal aorta (AA) diameter

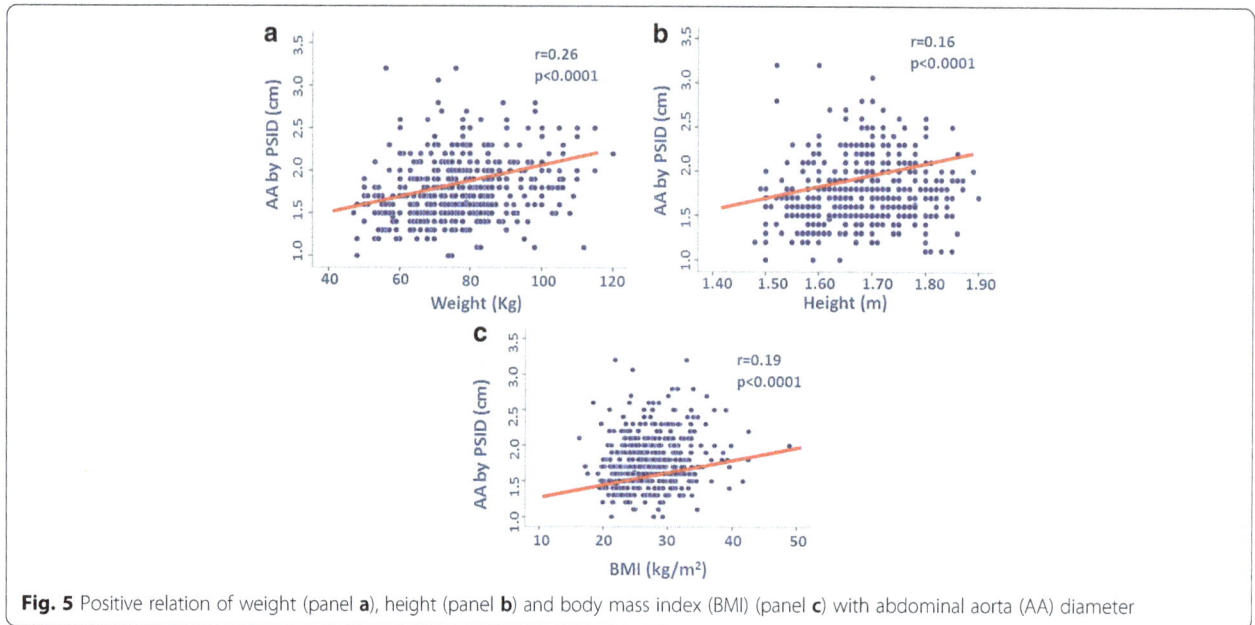

Fig. 5 Positive relation of weight (panel **a**), height (panel **b**) and body mass index (BMI) (panel **c**) with abdominal aorta (AA) diameter

blunted the association between increased afterload due to hypertension and AA size of the present study. The independent association of CAD with AA size is consistent with the data of Bekkers et al., who found a significant association of AAA with established coronary and peripheral arterial disease [35] and also with a meta-analysis of 15 cross-sectional studies [37]. Cigarette smoking and hypercholesterolemia were not independently associated with increased AA size, findings which are in disagreement with some previous studies assessing determinants of AAA [36, 37]. It has however to be taken into account that the rate of smoking in our population sample was relatively low and that the present study investigated determinants of AA diameter in earlier stages than that explored in these previous observations on AAA.

Table 2 Independent predictors of AA Size by multiple linear regression analysis

Dependent variable	Predictor	Standardized β coefficient	P value
AA size	Male sex	0.279	<0.0001
	Age	0.174	<0.0001
	BMI	0.170	<0.0001
	HR	0.099	=0.018
	Systolic BP	0.018	0.671
	Cigarette smoking	0.019	0.654
	Hypercholesterolemia	0.040	0.352
	Coronary artery disease	0.106	<0.01

Cumulative $R^2 = 0.184$, SEE = 0.31 cm, $p < 0.0001$
AA abdominal aorta, *BP* blood pressure, *BMI* body mass index, *HR* heart rate

Study limitations

The main limitation of the present study is represented by the fact that we demonstrated the diagnostic capability of PSID in measuring AA and not AAA. However, looking at our correlation between AA data assessed by PSID and standard echo we can suppose that PSID-derived measurements of AAA could be also consistent with those taken by standard echo machine. Another limitation could be considered our lack of correlation data between AA and ascending aorta, an association previously reported by Agricola et al. in patients with known AAA [42]. Finally, PSID derived AA size in the present study was measured by experts in cardiac ultrasound whereas it could be even more important to collect measurements taken by non expert operators.

Conclusion

The physical examination does not always allow diagnosis of AAA in patients without a very large AA diameter [43]. The findings of the present study demonstrate that the use of a miniaturized and portable device such as PSID could allow to widen the spectrum of patients susceptible of screening, allowing AA visualization also during a routine medical examination. Thus, the physician has the opportunity to complete the evaluation of patients, especially those at higher CV risk, to precociously detect patients with abnormalities of AA size and possibly treat cardiovascular risk factors more aggressively.

Abbreviations
AA: Abdominal aorta; AAA: Abdominal aorta aneurysm; CAD: Coronary artery disease; CV: Cardiovascular; PSID: Pocket size imaging device

Funding
No funding.

Authors' contributions
RE and FI designed the study and drafted the manuscript, VSL, RS and VS participated in the design of the study and performed the statistical analyses, GG participated in the study design and coordination and helped to draft the manuscript, GE, BT and MG conceived the study and its designed and revised critically the final manuscript All authors read and approved the final manuscript.

Competing interests
The authors declare that they have no competing interest.

References

1. Braunwald E, Fauci AS, Kasper DL, Hauser S, Longo DL, Jameson JL. Harrison's principles of internal medicine. 15th ed. New York: McGraw-Hill; 2001.

2. Spittell PC, Ehrsam JE, Anderson L, Seward JB. Screening for abdominal aortic aneurysm during transthoracic echocardiography in a hypertensive patient population. J Am Soc Echocardiogr. 1997;10:722–7.

3. Salo JA, Soisalon-Soininen S, Bondestam S, Mattila PS. Familial occurrence of abdominal aortic aneurysm. Ann Intern Med. 1999;130:637–42.

4. Karanjia PN, Madden KP, Lobner S. Coexistence of abdominal aortic aneurysm in patients with carotid stenosis. Stroke. 1994;25:627–30.

5. Folsom AR, Yao L, Alonso A, Lutsey PL, Missov E, Lederle FA, Ballantyne CM, Tang W. Circulating biomarkers and abdominal aortic aneurysm incidence: The Atherosclerosis Risk in Communities (ARIC) Study. Circulation. 2015;132:578–85.

6. Giugliano G, Perrino C, Schiano V, Brevetti L, Sannino A, Schiattarella GG, Gargiulo G, Serino F, Ferrone M, Scudiero F, Carbone A, Bruno A, Amato B, Trimarco B, Esposito G. Endovascular treatment of lower extremity arteries is associated with an improved outcome in diabetic patients affected by intermittent claudication. BMC Surg. 2012;12 Suppl 1:S19.

7. Lederle FA, Johnson GR, Wilson SE, Ballard DJ, Jordan Jr WD, Blebea J, Littooy FN, Freischlag JA, Bandyk D, Rapp JH, Salam AA, Veterans Affairs Cooperative Study #417 Investigators. Rupture rate of large abdominal aortic aneurysms in patients refusing or unfit for elective repair. JAMA. 2002;287:2968–72.

8. Health Quality Ontario. Ultrasound screening for abdominal aortic aneurysm: an evidence-based analysis. Ont Health Technol Assess Ser. 2006;6:1–67.

9. Quill DS, Colgan MP, Sumner DS. Ultrasonic screening for the detection of abdominal aortic aneurysms. Surg Clin North Am. 1989;69:713–20.

10. Eisenberg MJ, Geraci SJ, Schiller NB. Screening for abdominal aortic aneurysms during transthoracic echocardiography. Am Heart J. 1995;130:109–15.

11. Ashton HA, Buxton MJ, Day NE, Kim LG, Marteau TM, Scott RA, Thompson SG, Walker NM, Multicentre Aneurysm Screening Study Group. The Multicentre Aneurysm Screening Study (MASS) into the effect of abdominal aortic aneurysm screening on mortality in men: a randomised controlled trial. Lancet. 2002;360:1531–9.

12. Seelig MH, Malouf YL, Klingler PJ, Oldenburg WA, Atkinson EJ. Clinical utility of routine screening for abdominal aortic aneurysm during echocardiography. Vasa. 2000;29:265–8.

13. Sicari R, Galderisi M, Voigt JU, Habib G, Zamorano JL, Lancellotti P, Badano LP. The use of pocket sixe imaging device: a position statement of the European Association of Echocardiography. Eur J Echocardiogr. 2011;12:85–7.

14. Galderisi M, Santoro A, Versiero M, Lomoriello VS, Esposito R, Raia R, Farina F, Schiattarella PL, Bonito M, Olibet M, de Simone G. Improved cardiovascular diagnostic accuracy by pocket size imaging device in non-cardiologic outpatients: the NaUSiCa (Naples Ultrasound Stethoscope in Cardiology) study. Cardiovasc Ultrasound. 2010;8:51.

15. Mancia G, Fagard R, Narkiewicz K, Redon J, Zanchetti A, Böhm M, Christiaens T, Cifkova R, De Backer G, Dominiczak A, Galderisi M, Grobbee DE, Jaarsma T, Kirchhof P, Kjeldsen SE, Laurent S, Manolis AJ, Nilsson PM, Ruilope LM, Schmieder RE, Sirnes PA, Sleight P, Viigimaa M, Waeber B, Zannad F, Redon J, Dominiczak A, Narkiewicz K, Nilsson PM, Burnier M, Viigimaa M, Ambrosioni E, Caufield M, Coca A, Olsen MH, Schmieder RE, Tsioufis C, van de Borne P, Zamorano JL, Achenbach S, Baumgartner H, Bax JJ, Bueno H, Dean V, Deaton C, Erol C, Fagard R, Ferrari R, Hasdai D, Hoes AW, Kirchhof P, Knuuti J, Kolh P, Lancellotti P, Linhart A, Nihoyannopoulos P, Piepoli MF, Ponikowski P, Sirnes PA, Tamargo JL, Tendera M, Torbicki A, Wijns W, Windecker S, Clement DL, Coca A, Gillebert TC, Tendera M, Rosei EA, Ambrosioni E, Anker SD, Bauersachs J, Hitij JB, Caulfield M, De Buyzere M, De Geest S, Derumeaux GA, Erdine S, Farsang C, Funck-Brentano C, Gerc V, Germano G, Gielen S, Haller H, Hoes AW, Jordan J, Kahan T, Komajda M, Lovic D, Mahrholdt H, Olsen MH, Ostergren J, Parati G, Perk J, Polonia J, Popescu BA, Reiner Z, Rydén L, Sirenko Y, Stanton A, Struijker-Boudier H, Tsioufis C, van de Borne P, Vlachopoulos C, Volpe M, Wood DA. 2013 ESH/ESC Practice guidelines for the management of arterial hypertension. Eur Heart J. 2013;34:2159–219.

16. Reiner Z, Catapano AL, De Backer G, Graham I, Taskinen MR, Wiklund O, Agewall S, Alegria E, Chapman MJ, Durrington P, Erdine S, Halcox J, Hobbs R, Kjekshus J, Filardi PP, Riccardi G, Storey RF, Wood D, ESC Committee for Practice Guidelines (CPG) 2008–2010 and 2010–2012 Committees, European Association for Cardiovascular Prevention & Rehabilitation. ESC/EAS Guidelines for the management of dyslipidaemias: the Task Force for the management of dyslipidaemias of the European Society of Cardiology (ESC) and the European Atherosclerosis Society (EAS). Eur Heart J. 2011;32:1769–818.

17. Rydén L, Grant PJ, Anker SD, Berne C, Cosentino F, Danchin N, Deaton C, Escaned J, Hammes HP, Huikuri H, Marre M, Marx N, Mellbin L, Ostergren J, Patrono C, Seferovic P, Uva MS, Taskinen MR, Tendera M, Tuomilehto J, Valensi P, Zamorano JL, ESC Committee for Practice Guidelines (CPG), Zamorano JL, Achenbach S, Baumgartner H, Bax JJ, Bueno H, Dean V, Deaton C, Erol C, Fagard R, Ferrari R, Hasdai D, Hoes AW, Kirchhof P, Knuuti J, Kolh P, Lancellotti P, Linhart A, Nihoyannopoulos P, Piepoli MF, Ponikowski P, Sirnes PA, Tamargo JL, Tendera M, Torbicki A, Wijns W, Windecker S. ESC Guidelines on diabetes, pre-diabetes, and cardiovascular diseases developed in collaboration with the EASD: the Task Force on diabetes, pre-diabetes, and cardiovascular diseases of the European Society of Cardiology (ESC) and developed in collaboration with the European Association for the Study of Diabetes (EASD). Eur Heart J. 2013;34:3035–87.

18. Johnston KW, Rutherford RB, Tilson MD, Shah DM, Hollier L, Stanley JC. Suggested standards for reporting on arterial aneurysms: Subcommittee on reporting standards for arterial aneurysms, ad hoc Committee on reporting standards, Society for Vascular Surgery and North American Chapter, International Society for Cardiovascular Surgery. J Vas Surg. 1991;13:452–8.

19. Erbel R, Aboyans V, Boileau C, Bossone E, Bartolomeo RD, Eggebrecht H, Evangelista A, Falk V, Frank H, Gaemperli O, Grabenwöger M, Haverich A, Iung B, Manolis AJ, Meijboom F, Nienaber CA, Roffi M, Rousseau H, Sechtem U, Sirnes PA, Allmen RS, Vrints CJ, ESC Committee for Practice Guidelines. 2014 ESC Guidelines on the diagnosis and treatment of aortic diseases: Document covering acute and chronic aortic diseases of the thoracic and abdominal aorta of the adult. The Task Force for the Diagnosis and Treatment of Aortic Diseases of the European Society of Cardiology (ESC). Eur Heart J. 2014;35:2873–926.

20. Cardim N, Fernandez Golfin C, Aubele A, Aubele A, Toste J, Cobos MA, Carmelo V, Nunes I, Oliveira AG, Zamorano J. Usefulness of a new miniaturized echocardiographic system in outpatient cardiology consultations as an extension of physical examination. J Am Soc Echocardiogr. 2011;24:117–24.

21. Prinz C, Dohrmann J, van Buuren F, Bitter T, Bogunovic N, Horstkotte D, Faber L. Diagnostic performance of hand-held echocardiography for the assessment of basic cardiac morphology and function: a validation study in routine cardiac patients. Echocardiography. 2012;29:887–94.

22. Michalski B, Kasprzak JD, Szymczyk E, Lipiec P. Diagnostic utility and clinical usefulness of the pocket echocardiographic device. Echocardiography. 2012;29:1–6.

23. Gianstefani S, Catibog N, Whittaker AR, et al. Pocket-size imaging device: effectiveness for ward-based transthoracic studies. Eur Heart J Cardiovasc Imaging. 2013;14:1132–9.

24. Schiano-Lomoriello V, Esposito R, Santoro C, de Simone G, Galderisi M. Early markers of right heart involvement in regular smokers by Pocket Size Imaging Device. Cardiovasc Ultrasound. 2015;13:33.

25. Kimura BJ, Scott R, De Maria AN. Accuracy and cost-effectiveness of single-view echocardiographic screening for suspected mitral valve prolapse. Am J Med. 2000;108:331–3.

26. Lisi M, Cameli M, Mondillo S, Luzzi L, Zacà V, Cameli P, Gotti G, Galderisi M. Incremental value of pocket size imaging device for bedside diagnosis of unilateral pleural effusions and ultrasound-guided thoracentesis. Interact Cardiovasc Thorac Surg. 2012;15:596–601.

27. Cueff C, Keenan NG, Krapf L, Steg PG, Cimadevilla C, Ducrocq G, Michel JB, Vahanian A, Messika-Zeitoun D. Screening for abdominal aortic aneurysm in

coronary care unit patients with acute myocardial infarction using portable transthoracic echocardiography. Eur Heart J Cardiovasc Imaging. 2012;13:574–8.

28. Prance SE, Wilson YG, Cosgrove CM, Walker AJ, Wilkins DC, Ashley S. Ruptured abdominal aortic aneurysms: selecting patients for surgery. Eur J Vasc Endovasc Surg. 1999;17:129–32.

29. Kostun ZW, Malik RK. Screening for abdominal aortic aneurysms. Clin Imaging. 2016;40:321–4.

30. Hahn B, Bonhomme K, Finnie J, Adwar S, Lesser M, Hirschorn D. Does a normal screening ultrasound of the abdominal aorta reduce the likelihood of rupture in emergency department patients? Clin Imaging. 2016;3:398–401.

31. Jones GT, Hill BG, Curtis N, Kabir TD, Wong LE, Tilyard MW, Williams MJ, van Rij AM. Comparison of three targeted approaches to screening for abdominal aortic aneurysm based on cardiovascular risk. Br J Surg. 2016;103:1139–46.

32. Bergqvist D, Bjorck M, Wanhainen A. Abdominal aortic aneurysm–to screen or not to screen. Eur J Vasc Endovasc Surg. 2008;35:13–8.

33. Wanhainen A, Lundkvist J, Bergqvist D, Björck M. Cost-effectiveness of screening women for abdominal aortic aneurysm. J Vasc Surg. 2006;43:908–14.

34. Jamrozik K, Norman PE, Spencer CA, Parsons RW, Tuohy R, Lawrence-Brown MM, Dickinson JA. Screening for abdominal aortic aneurysm: lessons from a population-based study. Med J Aust. 2000;173:345–50.

35. Bekkers SC, Habets JH, Cheriex EC, Palmans A, Pinto Y, Hofstra L, Crijns HJ. Abdominal aortic aneurysm screening during transthoracic echocardiography in an unselected population. J Am Soc Echocardiogr. 2005;18:389–93.

36. Singh K, Bonaa KH, Jacobsen BK, Bjork L, Solberg S. Prevalence of and risk factors for abdominal aortic aneurysms in a population-based study: The Tromso Study. Am J Epidemiol. 2001;154:236–44.

37. Cornuz J, Sidoti Pinto C, Tevaearai H, Egger M. Risk factors for asymptomatic abdominal aortic aneurysm: systematic review and meta-analysis of population-based screening studies. Eur J Public Health. 2004;14:343–9.

38. Takagi H, Umemoto T. A meta-analysis of the association of obesity with abdominal aortic aneurysm presence. Int Angiol. 2015;34:383–91.

39. Takagi H, Umemoto T. The association between body mass index and abdominal aortic aneurysm growth: a systematic review. Vasa. 2016;45:119–24.

40. Wei R, Liu LS, Wang LW, Zhang T, Liu J, Zuo SW, Jia SH, Song YX, Wu ZY, Duan C, Ge YY, Li HB, Xiong J, Jia X, Wang X, Kong W, Xu XP, Guo W, Huo Y. Association of resting heart rate with infrarenal aortic diameter: A cross-sectional study in chinese hypertensive adults. Eur J Vasc Endovasc Surg. 2015;50:714–21.

41. Bhak RH, Wininger M, Johnson GR, Lederle FA, Messina LM, Ballard DJ, Wilson SE, Aneurysm Detection and Management (ADAM) Study Group. Factors associated with small abdominal aortic aneurysm expansion rate. JAMA Surg. 2015;150:44–50.

42. Agricola E, Slavich M, Tufaro V, Fisicaro A, Oppizzi M, Melissano G, Bertoglio L, Marone E, Civilini E, Margonato A, Chiesa R. Prevalence of thoracic ascending aortic aneurysm in adult patients with known abdominal aortic aneurysm: an echocardiographic study. Int J Cardiol. 2013;168:3147–8.

43. Fink HA, Lederle FA, Roth CS, Bowles CA, Nelson DB, Haas MA. The accuracy of physical examination to detect abdominal aortic aneurysm. Arch Intern Med. 2000;160:833–6.

14

Noninvasive assessment of pulmonary arterial capacitance by pulmonary annular motion velocity in children with ventricular septal defect

Yasunobu Hayabuchi*⊕, Akemi Ono, Yukako Homma and Shoji Kagami

Abstract

Background: We hypothesized that longitudinal pulmonary arterial deformation during the cardiac cycle reflects pulmonary arterial capacitance. To examine this hypothesis, we assessed whether tissue Doppler-derived pulmonary annular motion could serve as a novel way to evaluate pulmonary arterial capacitance in pediatric patients with ventricular septal defect (VSD).

Methods: In this prospective study, pulmonary annular velocity was measured in children (age, 6 months–5 years) with a preoperative VSD (VSD group, $n = 35$) and age-matched healthy children (Control group, $n = 23$). Pulmonary artery capacitance was calculated by two methods. Systolic pulmonary arterial capacitance (sPAC) was expressed as the stroke volume/pulmonary arterial pulse pressure. Diastolic pulmonary arterial capacitance (dPAC) was determined according to a two-element windkessel model of the pulmonary arterial diastolic pressure profile.

Results: Pulmonary annular velocity waveforms comprised systolic bimodal (s1′ and s2′) and diastolic e′ and a′ waves in all participants. The peak velocities of s1′, s2′, and e′ were significantly lower in the VSD group than in the Control group. On multiple regression analysis, sPAC was an independent variable affecting the peak velocities of the s1′, s2′, and e′ waves ($\beta = 0.41$, 0.62, and 0.35, respectively). The dPAC affected the s1′ wave peak velocity ($\beta = 0.34$). The time durations of the s1′ and e′ waves were independently determined by the sPAC ($\beta = 0.49$ and 0.27).

Conclusion: Pulmonary annular motion velocity evaluated using tissue Doppler is a promising method of assessing pulmonary arterial capacitance in children with VSD.

Keywords: Tissue Doppler imaging, Pulmonary annular motion, Pulmonary arterial compliance, Children

Abbreviations: BSA, Body surface area; dPAC, Diastolic pulmonary arterial capacitance; DPAP, Diastolic pulmonary arterial pressure; HR, Heart rate; ICT, Isovolumic contraction time; IRT, Isovolumic relaxation time; LVEDD, Left ventricular end-diastolic dimension; LVEF, Left ventricular ejection fraction; LVFS, Left ventricular fractional shortening; MPAP, Mean pulmonary arterial pressure; PA, Pulmonary artery; PAH, Pulmonary arterial hypertension; PAPP, Pulmonary arterial pulse pressure; PASV, Pulmonary artery stroke volume; PVRi, Pulmonary vascular resistance indexed for body surface area; Qp/Qs, Pulmonary to systemic blood flow ratio; RV, Right ventricle; RVEDP, Right ventricular end-diastolic pressure; RVEF, Right ventricular ejection fraction; RVOT, Right ventricular outflow tract; RVSP, Right ventricular systolic pressure; sPAC, Systolic pulmonary arterial capacitance; SPAP, Systolic pulmonary arterial pressure; TDI, Tissue Doppler imaging; VSD, Ventricular septal defect

* Correspondence: hayabuchi@tokushima-u.ac.jp
Department of Pediatrics, Tokushima University, Kuramoto-cho-3, Tokushima
770-8305, Japan

Background

Pulmonary vascular hemodynamic assessment has traditionally evaluated pulmonary vascular resistance (PVR) [1–3]. However, PVR primarily reflects small vessel status and the static component of the pulmonary circulation [4], and it does not reflect the properties of the large and medium pulmonary vessels or account for pulsatile elements of the pulmonary circulation. Pulmonary artery (PA) capacitance reflects the dynamic component of the pulmonary circulation and is thought to be determined largely by the properties of the large proximal capacitance vessels [5]. Because it is the immediate environment encountered by the right ventricle (RV), PA capacitance is a major determinant of RV work [5]. It has recently been shown that lower PA capacitance is strongly associated with worse survival in patients with pulmonary arterial hypertension (PAH) [5–7]. Furthermore, PA capacitance is also reported to be a strong prognostic indicator in patients with left ventricular dysfunction, even in patients with normal PVR [8]. Consequently, accurate determination and serial follow-up of PA capacitance are important in the management of patients with various cardiac diseases with congestive heart failure. However, despite its potential importance for RV performance and clinical outcomes, PA capacitance is not routinely measured. Noninvasive quantitative assessment of PA capacitance remains challenging.

We have previously reported that the pulmonary annular motion velocity waveform obtained using tissue Doppler imaging (TDI) reflects right ventricular outflow tract (RVOT) performance [9]. In the present study, we hypothesized that the pulmonary annular motion would be affected not only by RVOT function, but also by PA capacitance because the pulmonary annulus is located adjacent to the RVOT and PA. In large arteries, deformation of the arterial wall during systole and diastole occurs in the radial and longitudinal directions (Additional file 1). The present study attempted to assess the relationship between the longitudinal pulmonary arterial deformation and capacitance.

The aim of this study, therefore, was to determine whether tissue Doppler-derived pulmonary annular motion velocity can be used as a noninvasive assessment of PA capacitance in children with ventricular septal defect (VSD).

Methods

Study population

The prospective study group comprised consecutive 35 pediatric patients with a preoperative VSD (VSD group; mean age, 2.3 ± 1.5 years; range, 0.6–5.0 years). These patients were scheduled for surgical closure. Twenty-three age-matched healthy children without electrocardiographic or echocardiographic abnormalities (Control group; age, 2.5 ± 1.6 years; range, 0.6–5.0 years) were also enrolled. The patients underwent cardiac catheterization within 3 days of assessment by echocardiography. Data collected between December 2012 and December 2015 were analyzed. All protocols were approved by the Institutional Review Board of the Tokushima University Hospital and conformed to the ethical guidelines of the Declaration of Helsinki (1975). The parents of all subjects provided their written, informed consent for their children to participate in the study.

Echocardiographic study

Standard and pulsed Doppler tissue echocardiography proceeded using a Preirus digital ultrasound system (Hitachi-Aloka Medical Co., Tokyo, Japan) equipped with 1–5 and 3–7 MHz sector transducers. All Doppler data were acquired from patients in the left lateral decubitus position during shallow respiration or end-expiratory apnea. Pulmonary annular motion velocity was measured using TDI in the long-axis view of the RVOT and PA. Guided by the two-dimensional images, a sample volume with a fixed length of 5.0 mm was placed on the pulmonary annulus of the RV free wall side, as indicated by the yellow arrow [9]. Figures 1a and b show a representative example of the color TDI and profile of the pulmonary annular velocity in a healthy child. Furthermore, tricuspid annular motion was recorded in the four-chamber view for the sake of comparison (Fig. 1c). The ultrasound beam was positioned parallel to the direction of the pulmonary and tricuspid annular motions. All tissue Doppler parameters were measured during three consecutive heart cycles by a single physician who was blinded to patient condition, and mean values were calculated.

In addition to pulsed TDI, participants were assessed by conventional, two-dimensional, M-mode, pulsed, continuous, and color Doppler echocardiography. The left ventricular ejection fraction (LVEF) was calculated from apical two-chamber and four-chamber images using the biplane Simpson's technique. All parameters were measured over three cardiac cycles and then averaged.

Cardiac catheterization

All VSD patients underwent cardiac catheterization within 3 days of echocardiography. Catheterization and angiography using an Integris Allura 9 Biplane (Phillips Medical Systems, Best, The Netherlands) proceeded using 4–6 Fr catheters. All patients were intubated and examined by biplane anteroposterior and lateral projection angiography. Ventricular volume was assessed by means of ventriculography and calculated using Simpson's rule by quantitative CAW2000 cardiac analysis software (ELK Corporation, Osaka, Japan). During cardiac catheterization, the main PA pressure was measured

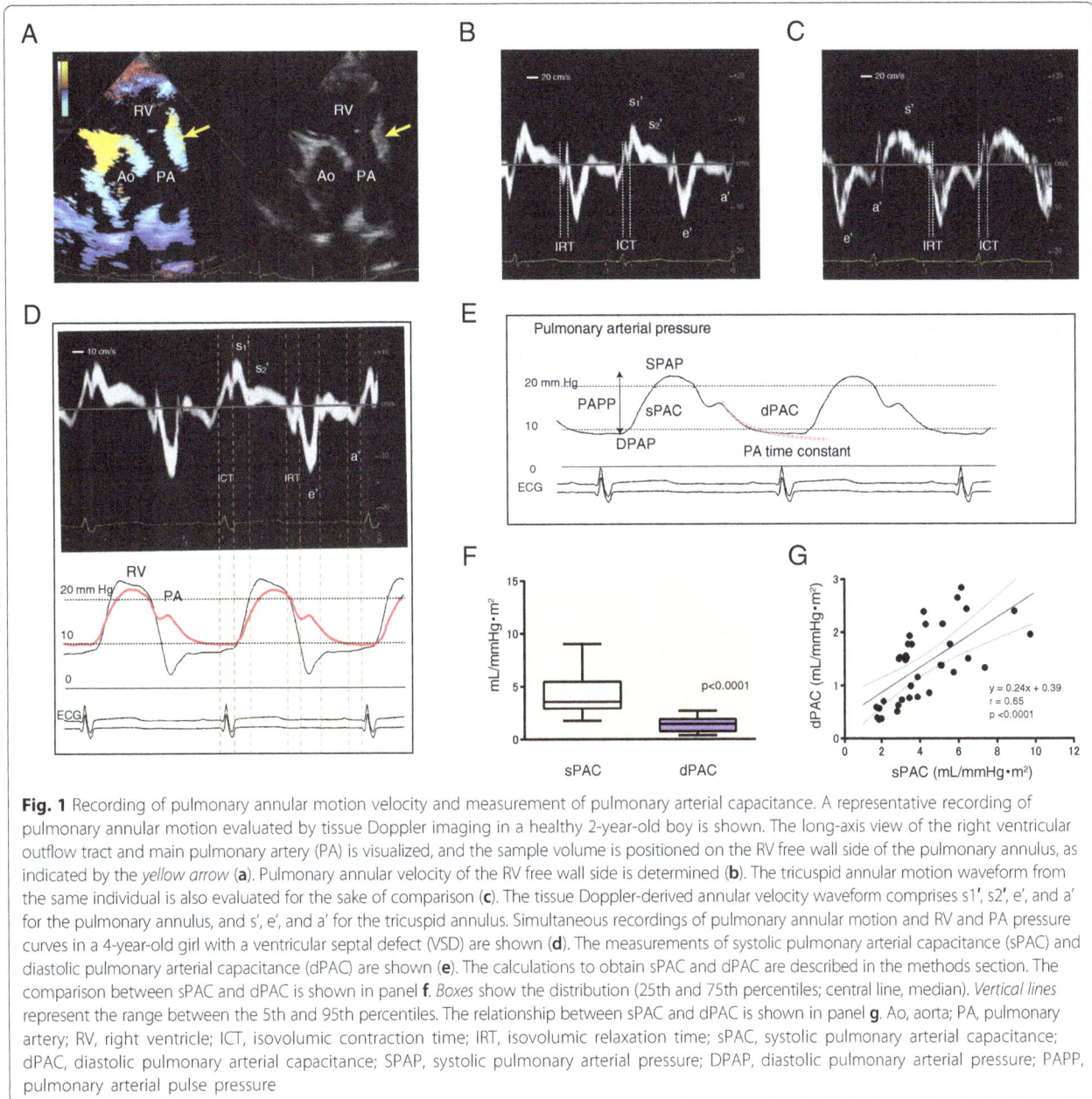

Fig. 1 Recording of pulmonary annular motion velocity and measurement of pulmonary arterial capacitance. A representative recording of pulmonary annular motion evaluated by tissue Doppler imaging in a healthy 2-year-old boy is shown. The long-axis view of the right ventricular outflow tract and main pulmonary artery (PA) is visualized, and the sample volume is positioned on the RV free wall side of the pulmonary annulus, as indicated by the *yellow arrow* (**a**). Pulmonary annular velocity of the RV free wall side is determined (**b**). The tricuspid annular motion waveform from the same individual is also evaluated for the sake of comparison (**c**). The tissue Doppler-derived annular velocity waveform comprises s1', s2', e', and a' for the pulmonary annulus, and s', e', and a' for the tricuspid annulus. Simultaneous recordings of pulmonary annular motion and RV and PA pressure curves in a 4-year-old girl with a ventricular septal defect (VSD) are shown (**d**). The measurements of systolic pulmonary arterial capacitance (sPAC) and diastolic pulmonary arterial capacitance (dPAC) are shown (**e**). The calculations to obtain sPAC and dPAC are described in the methods section. The comparison between sPAC and dPAC is shown in panel **f**. *Boxes* show the distribution (25th and 75th percentiles; central line, median). *Vertical lines* represent the range between the 5th and 95th percentiles. The relationship between sPAC and dPAC is shown in panel **g**. Ao, aorta; PA, pulmonary artery; RV, right ventricle; ICT, isovolumic contraction time; IRT, isovolumic relaxation time; sPAC, systolic pulmonary arterial capacitance; dPAC, diastolic pulmonary arterial capacitance; SPAP, systolic pulmonary arterial pressure; DPAP, diastolic pulmonary arterial pressure; PAPP, pulmonary arterial pulse pressure

using a high-fidelity manometer-tipped 0.014-inch pressure wire (PressureWire Aeris; St Jude Medical, Inc., St. Paul, MN, USA) to compare with pulmonary annular motion velocity (Fig. 1d). Pulmonary blood flow was calculated using the Fick principle. Stroke volume indexed to body surface area (BSA) was calculated from the pulmonary blood flow in 1 min divided by the heart rate (HR), expressed in mL/m^2. PVR was calculated using the standard formula; that is, PVR was calculated as the mean PAP minus PA wedge pressure/pulmonary blood flow (PVR; expressed in Wood units·m^2).

PA capacitance was calculated by two methods. One was designated systolic PA capacitance (sPAC), which

can be determined from measures of pulse pressure and stroke volume indexed to BSA. The sPAC was expressed as the stroke volume/pulse pressure (sPAC; mL/mmHg · m^2) [6–8]. Furthermore, PA capacitance was also estimated in a different way. Diastolic PA capacitance (dPAC) was approximated according to a two-element windkessel model that assumes that compliance and hemodynamic resistance are constant during the measurement [10–12]. Previous studies reported that PA capacitance can be calculated from the PA pressure profile during diastole. The time constant (tau) of the exponentially decaying curve can be obtained from the fitting curve calculated from diastolic PA pressure. The dPAC

$(mL/mmHg \cdot m^2)$ was calculated from PVR and the PA time constant (tau) (Fig. 1e).

Statistical analysis

All data are expressed as means ± standard deviation (S.D.) or as medians with the 5th–95th percentiles. Statistical significance was determined using the Mann-Whitney U-test or Student's t-test, as appropriate. Linear regression analyses were performed for correlations between the pulmonary annular motion velocity and hemodynamic parameters, and Pearson's or Spearman's correlation coefficients were calculated, as appropriate. Variables with $p < 0.10$ on univariate analysis were "candidates" for a backwards stepwise (inclusion criteria/exclusion criteria: $p < 0.05/p > 0.1$, respectively) multivariate analysis, and those with $p < 0.05$ were "retained" in the model. Multiple regression analysis was used to identify hemodynamic variables affecting the pulmonary annular motion waveform. All statistical data were calculated using Prism version 6.0 (GraphPad Software, San Diego, CA, USA) and JMP 11 (SAS Institute, Inc., Cary, NC, USA) installed on a desktop computer. A value of $p < 0.05$ was considered significant. Intra-observer and inter-observer reproducibilities of TDI measurements were assessed using Bland-Altman analysis in a blinded manner. Data were recorded and assessed at 5-minute intervals by observers 1 and 2 from 20 randomly selected participants (VSD, $n = 10$; Controls, $n = 10$). For intra-observer variability, data were analyzed twice, 8 weeks apart. Inter-observer variability was assessed by analyzing data from two separate observers blinded to each other's results.

Results

No subjects were excluded from the subsequent analyses due to suboptimal recording from poor echocardiographic imaging. Accordingly, the study group included 23 healthy children (2.5 ± 1.6 years; range, 0.6–5.0 years) and 35 VSD patients (mean age, 2.3 ± 1.5 years; range, 0.6–5.0 years). Table 1 shows the clinical, echocardiographic, and hemodynamic data of the participants. Age, height, and HR did not differ significantly between the VSD group and the Control group, whereas body weight and BSA were significantly lower in the VSD group than in the Control group. Left ventricular end-diastolic dimension (LVEDD), left ventricular fractional shortening (LVFS), and LVEF were significantly higher in the VSD group than in the Control group.

Figure 1b shows the pulmonary annular velocity curve. The tricuspid annular motion is shown in Fig. 1c for comparison with the pulmonary annular velocity waveform. The systolic wave was monomodal (s') for the tricuspid annular velocity and bimodal (s1' and s2') for the pulmonary annular motion velocity. The systolic

waveform peaked earlier in pulmonary annular motion than in the tricuspid annular velocity curve. The shapes of the e' and a' waves in diastole were similar. Simultaneous recordings of pulmonary annular motion, RV pressure, and PA pressure in a patient with VSD are shown (Fig. 1d). The pulmonary s1' wave corresponds to the steep RV pressure elevation during early systole. The s2' wave coincides with mid to late systolic phase around the peak RV and PA pressure. Measurements of the sPAC and the dPAC are shown with the PA pressure profile (Fig. 1e). The comparison between the sPAC and dPAC obtained from the VSD group is demonstrated in Fig. 1f. The sPAC was significantly higher than the dPAC ($4.2 ± 1.9$ vs. $1.4 ± 0.7$ $mL/mmHg \cdot m^2$, $p < 0.0001$). There was a significant correlation between these parameters (Fig. 1g; $r = 0.65$, $p < 0.0001$).

Pulmonary annular motion was compared between the Control and VSD groups (Fig. 2). The peak velocities of the s1', s2', and e' waves were significantly lower in the VSD group than in the Control group ($9.9 ± 1.9$ vs. $11.5 ± 2.2$ cm/s, $p = 0.0070$; $3.4 ± 0.7$ vs. $4.1 ± 1.1$ cm/s, $p = 0.0107$; $8.8 ± 2.3$ vs. $13.0 ± 2.7$ cm/s, $p < 0.0001$, respectively). The s1' duration, s2' duration, e' duration, and a' duration were significantly shorter in the VSD group ($p = 0.0008$, <0.0001, 0.0392, and 0.0008, respectively), whereas isovolumic contraction time (ICT) and isovolumic relaxation time (IRT) were not significantly different between the two groups.

Next, the relationships between the parameters obtained from TDI-derived pulmonary and tricuspid annular motion and right heart performance were examined in the VSD group. Table 2 summarizes the univariate regression analysis. TDI-derived parameters were significantly correlated with and determined by RV and PA function. Figure 3 shows the relationship between the sPAC and the pulmonary annular motion waveform. The peak velocity of the pulmonary annular s1' wave was significantly correlated with the sPAC ($r = 0.58$, $p = 0.0002$). The s2' and e' velocity also showed significant correlations with the sPAC ($r = 0.62$, $p < 0.0001$; $r = 0.66$, $p < 0.0001$; respectively). ICT and IRT measured using TDI and the time duration of each wave were also assessed in terms of their correlations with the sPAC. The sPAC had significant correlations with s1' and e' and a' wave duration ($r = 0.49$, $p = 0.0029$; $r = 0.48$, $p = 0.0034$; $r = 0.44$, $p = 0.0088$; respectively), whereas there were no significant correlations with ICT, IRT, and s2' wave duration. Figure 4 shows the relationship between dPAC and TDI-derived pulmonary annular motion. The peak velocities of pulmonary annular s1', s2', and e' wave were significantly correlated with the dPAC ($r = 0.60$, $p = 0.0002$; $r = 0.46$, $p = 0.0051$; $r = 0.55$, $p = 0.0006$; respectively). In regard to the timing issue, the e' wave duration was significantly correlated with the dPAC ($r = 0.53$, $p = 0.0011$).

Table 1 Clinical characteristics of the subjects

		Control ($n = 23$)	VSD ($n = 35$)	p values
Sex (male/female)		11/12	20/15	n.s.
Age (y)		2.5 ± 1.6	2.3 ± 1.5	n.s.
Weight (kg)		13.8 ± 3.3	11.4 ± 4.1	0.0224
Height (cm)		91.1 ± 7.1	88.7 ± 8.1	n.s.
Body surface area (m^2)		0.58 ± 0.07	0.53 ± 0.08	0.0177
Heart rate (bpm)		90 ± 12	92 ± 17	n.s.
QRS duration (msec)		87 ± 6	89 ± 13	n.s.
Systolic blood pressure (mmHg)		80 ± 7	77 ± 6	n.s.
Diastolic blood pressure (mmHg)		46 ± 6	45 ± 6	n.s.
LVEDD (mm)		25.8 ± 3.1	29.2 ± 4.4	0.0022
LVFS (%)		32.6 ± 5.9	38.7 ± 6.1	0.0004
LVEF (%)		63.4 ± 5.6	69.3 ± 6.2	0.0005
Qp/Qs		-	2.04 ± 0.92	-
RVSP (mmHg)		-	35.4 ± 13.0	-
RVEDP (mmHg)		-	7.6 ± 2.1	-
RVEF (%)		-	53.0 ± 9.1	-
SPAP (mmHg)		-	29.0 ± 9.9	-
DPAP (mmHg)		-	11.5 ± 3.3	-
MPAP (mmHg)		-	19.7 ± 6.2	-
PAPP (mmHg)		-	17.5 ± 8.0	-
PVRi (Wood U m^2)		-	1.44 ± 0.8	-
PASV (ml/m^2)		-	62.7 ± 20.7	-
Transmitral flow (m/sec)	E	1.05 ± 0.17	1.11 ± 0.19	n.s.
	A	0.41 ± 0.07	0.51 ± 0.17	0.0099
Transtricuspid flow (m/sec)	E	0.64 ± 0.12	0.49 ± 0.18	0.0009
	A	0.29 ± 0.09	0.31 ± 0.13	n.s.
Mitral annular motion (cm/sec)	s'	8.4 ± 1.6	9.5 ± 2.7	0.0292
	e'	14.6 ± 2.8	15.7 ± 2.9	n.s.
	a'	5.0 ± 2.3	6.1 ± 2.4	n.s.
Tricuspid annular motion (cm/sec)	s'	12.5 ± 2.2	13.6 ± 1.8	0.0418
	e'	14.2 ± 2.3	12.7 ± 3.2	n.s.
	a'	6.6 ± 2.3	6.5 ± 2.1	n.s.

LVEDD left ventricular end-diastolic dimension, *LVFS* left ventricular fractional shortening, *LVEF* left ventricular ejection fraction, *Qp/Qs* pulmonary to systemic blood flow ratio, *RVSP* right ventricular systolic pressure, *RVEDP* right ventricular end-diastolic pressure, *RVEF* right ventricular ejection fraction, *SPAP* systolic pulmonary arterial pressure, *DPAP* diastolic pulmonary arterial pressure, *MPAP* mean pulmonary arterial pressure, *PAPP* pulmonary arterial pulse pressure, *PVRi* pulmonary vascular resistance indexed for body surface area, *PASV* pulmonary artery stroke volume, *n.s.* not significant

Next, multiple regression analysis for predictors of the pulmonary annular motion waveform was performed (Table 3). The analysis showed that the sPAC had an effect on the peak velocities of s1′, s2′, and the e′ wave and the time duration of the s1′ and a′ waves ($\beta = 0.41$, $p = 0.0131$; $\beta = 0.62$, $p < 0.0001$; $\beta = 0.35$, $p = 0.0314$; $\beta = 0.49$, $p = 0.0029$; and $\beta = 0.27$, $p = 0.0488$, respectively). The dPAC affected the s1′ wave peak velocity ($\beta = 0.34$, $p = 0.0354$). The other right heart performance parameters, including RVEDP, RVSP, and Qp/Qs, also had an

impact on pulmonary annular motion. Importantly, although RVEF had been assumed to determine pulmonary annular motion, no significant relationship was demonstrated with pulmonary annular motion in the VSD group.

Reproducibility

The inter- and intra-observer reproducibilities of the TDI analysis of pulmonary annular motion were determined from Bland-Altman analysis of 20 randomly

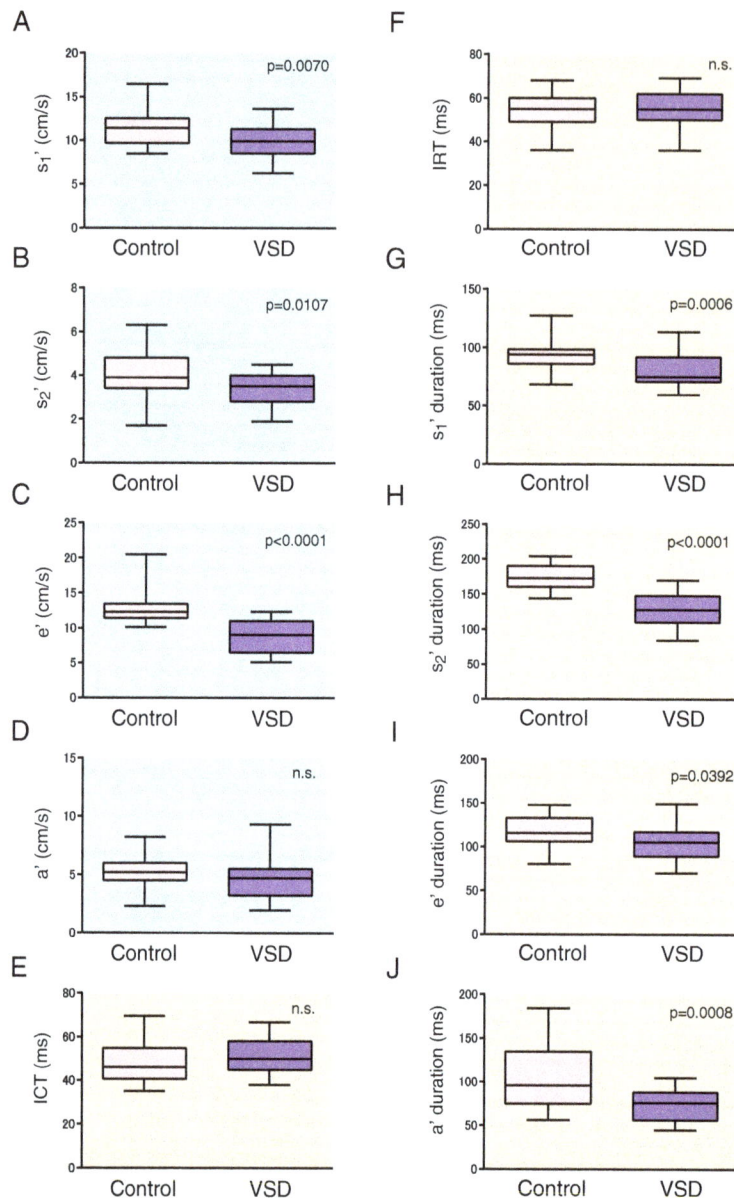

Fig. 2 Comparison of pulmonary annular and tricuspid annular motion velocities between the Control group and the VSD group. The comparison is shown in terms of peak velocity (**a–d**) and time duration (**e–j**). *Boxes* show the distribution of peak velocity (25th and 75th percentiles; central line, median). *Vertical lines* represent the range between the 5th and 95th percentiles. ICT, isovolumic contraction time; IRT, isovolumic relaxation time

selected participants (VSD group, $n = 10$; Control group, $n = 10$). Table 4 shows the inter- and intra-observer reproducibilities obtained from the Bland-Altman plots (bias $\pm$ 2SDs [95 % limit of agreement]). They showed minimal bias and substantial agreement for reproducibility.

Discussion

The present results showed that the pulmonary annular motion waveform is mainly determined by PA capacitance. Assessment of pulmonary annular motion is useful for estimating PA capacitance in children with VSD.

Pulmonary annular TDI was found to be a simple, rapid, reproducible, and highly distinctive method for evaluating PA capacitance.

Recent reports demonstrated that PA capacitance has great impact on the prognosis in various cardiac diseases [5–8]. Patients require lifelong follow-up that includes serial assessment of PA capacitance. Therefore, noninvasive assessment of PA capacitance is considered quite important. However, its assessment is challenging due to the difficulty of measurement and poor reproducibility. Therefore, an invasive method is necessary to accurately

Table 2 Correlations between tissue Doppler parameters and pulmonary hemodynamics

	sPAC	dPAC	SPAP	DPAP	MPAP	PAPP	RVSP	RVEDP	PVRi	PASV	Qp/Qs	RVEF
Pulmonary annulus motion												
s1' (cm/sec)	$r=0.58$ $p=0.0002$	$r=0.60$ $p=0.0002$	$r=-0.39$ $p=0.0209$	n.s.	$r=-0.45$ $p=0.0072$	$r=-0.35$ $p=0.0386$	$r=-0.41$ $p=0.0138$	$r=-0.34$ $p=0.0431$	$r=-0.59$ $p=0.0002$	n.s.	n.s.	$r=0.35$ $p=0.0362$
s2' (cm/sec)	$r=0.62$ $p<0.0001$	$r=0.46$ $p=0.0051$	$r=-0.50$ $p=0.0022$	n.s.	$r=-0.41$ $p=0.0141$	$r=-0.50$ $p=0.0022$	$r=-0.45$ $p=0.0071$	n.s.	$r=-0.43$ $p=0.0104$	n.s.	n.s.	n.s.
e' (cm/sec)	$r=0.66$ $p<0.0001$	$r=0.55$ $p=0.0006$	$r=-0.59$ $p=0.0002$	n.s.	$r=-0.44$ $p=0.0078$	$r=-0.65$ $p<0.0001$	$r=-0.57$ $p=0.0004$	$r=0.44$ $p=0.0079$	$r=-0.55$ $p=0.0006$	n.s.	$r=-0.50$ $p=0.0023$	n.s.
a' (cm/sec)	n.s.	n.s.	n.s.	n.s.	n.s.	n.s.	n.s.	n.s.	n.s.	n.s.	n.s.	n.s.
ICT (msec)	n.s.	n.s.	n.s.	n.s.	n.s.	n.s.	n.s.	n.s.	n.s.	n.s.	n.s.	n.s.
IRT (msec)	n.s.	n.s.	n.s.	n.s.	n.s.	n.s.	n.s.	n.s.	n.s.	n.s.	n.s.	n.s.
s1' duration (msec)	$r=0.49$ $p=0.0029$	n.s.	n.s.	n.s.	n.s.	n.s.	n.s.	n.s.	n.s.	n.s.	n.s.	n.s.
s2' duration (msec)	n.s.	n.s.	$r=-0.42$ $p=0.0128$	n.s.	$r=-0.35$ $p=0.0378$	$r=-0.41$ $p=0.0136$	$r=-0.35$ $p=0.0394$	n.s.	n.s.	n.s.	$r=-0.47$ $p=0.0047$	n.s.
e' duration (msec)	$r=0.48$ $p=0.0034$	$r=0.53$ $p=0.0011$	$r=-0.67$ $p<0.0001$	$r=-0.38$ $p=0.0251$	$r=-0.58$ $p=0.0003$	$r=-0.67$ $p<0.0001$	$r=-0.58$ $p=0.0003$	$r=0.38$ $p=0.0235$	$r=-0.46$ $p=0.0056$	n.s.	$r=-0.63$ $p<0.0001$	n.s.
a' duration	$r=0.44$ $p=0.0086$	n.s.	$r=-0.53$ $p=0.0011$	n.s.	$r=-0.47$ $p=0.0046$	$r=-0.53$ $p=0.0011$	$r=-0.47$ $p=0.0044$	$r=0.48$ $p=0.0037$	n.s.	n.s.	$r=-0.64$ $p<0.0001$	n.s.
Tricuspid annulus motion												
s' (cm/sec)	$r=0.36$ $p=0.0332$	$r=0.43$ $p=0.0107$	$r=-0.47$ $p=0.0043$	n.s.	$r=-0.39$ $p=0.0193$	$r=-0.54$ $p=0.0008$	$r=-0.35$ $p=0.0418$	n.s.	$r=-0.38$ $p=0.0260$	n.s.	$r=-0.53$ $p=0.0011$	$r=0.39$ $p=0.0310$
e' (cm/sec)	n.s.	n.s.	$r=-0.45$ $p=0.0062$	n.s.	n.s.	$r=-0.41$ $p=0.0136$	$r=-0.39$ $p=0.0209$	$r=-0.34$ $p=0.0451$	n.s.	n.s.	$r=-0.35$ $p=0.0407$	n.s.
a' (cm/sec)	n.s.	n.s.	$r=0.53$ $p=0.0011$	$r=0.42$ $p=0.0126$	$r=0.49$ $p=0.0028$	$r=0.49$ $p=0.0030$	$r=0.49$ $p=0.0024$	n.s.	n.s.	n.s.	$r=0.55$ $p=0.0006$	n.s.
ICT (msec)	n.s.	n.s.	n.s.	n.s.	n.s.	n.s.	n.s.	n.s.	n.s.	n.s.	n.s.	n.s.
IRT (msec)	n.s.	n.s.	n.s.	n.s.	n.s.	n.s.	n.s.	n.s.	n.s.	n.s.	n.s.	n.s.
s' duration (msec)	n.s.	n.s.	$r=-0.41$ $p=0.0118$	n.s.	$r=-0.39$ $p=0.0228$	$r=-0.46$ $p=0.0051$	$r=-0.43$ $p=0.0021$	n.s.	n.s.	n.s.	$r=-0.36$ $p=0.0138$	n.s.
e' duration (msec)	$r=0.35$ $p=0.0232$	n.s.	n.s.	n.s.	n.s.	n.s.	n.s.	n.s.	n.s.	n.s.	n.s.	n.s.
a' duration (msec)	n.s.	n.s.	n.s.	n.s.	n.s.	n.s.	n.s.	n.s.	n.s.	n.s.	n.s.	n.s.

sPAC systolic pulmonary arterial capacitance, dPAC diastolic pulmonary arterial capacitance, SPAP systolic pulmonary arterial pressure, DPAP diastolic pulmonary arterial pressure, MPAP mean pulmonary arterial pressure, PAPP pulmonary arterial pulse pressure, RVSP right ventricular systolic pressure, RVEDP right ventricular end-diastolic pressure, PVRi pulmonary vascular resistance indexed for body surface area, PASV stroke volume to pulmonary artery, Qp/Qs pulmonary to systemic blood flow ratio, RVEF right ventricular ejection fraction

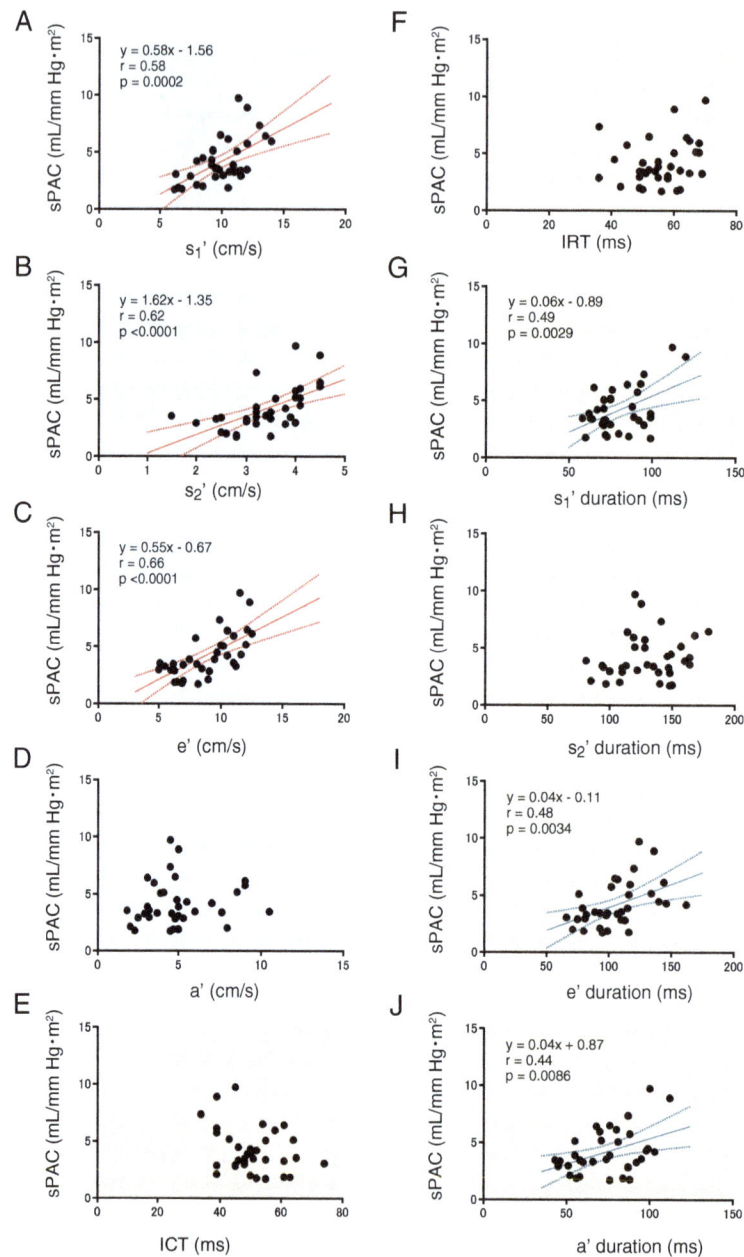

Fig. 3 The relationship between the pulmonary annular motion waveform and systolic pulmonary arterial capacitance (sPAC) in the VSD group. The relationship was evaluated in terms of peak velocity (**a–d**) and time duration (**e–j**) in each wave. There are significant correlations between the peak velocities of pulmonary s1′, s2′, e′, and sPAC (**a–c**). The pulmonary s1′, e′, and a′ wave durations are significantly correlated with sPAC (**g**, **i**, and **j**, respectively). Linear regression lines with 95 % confidence interval (*dashed lines*) are indicated. sPAC, systolic pulmonary arterial capacitance; ICT, isovolumic contraction time; IRT, isovolumic relaxation time

assess PA capacitance in clinical practice. Several studies have been conducted to identify noninvasive ways for estimating PA capacitance using echocardiographic parameters [13, 14]. These studies attempted echocardiographic estimation of PA capacitance from the PA pulse pressure and RV stroke volume. Systolic PA pressure was estimated from the tricuspid regurgitation velocity by the modified Bernoulli equation. RV stroke volume was calculated using

the pulmonary valve diameter measured in the parasternal short-axis view and the velocity-time integral of the PA Doppler flow [13]. In other reports, the right pulmonary arterial diameter change during the cardiac cycle was used to calculate PA capacitance [14]. However, these methods are complex and time-consuming, errors can easily occur, and they have low reproducibility. Previous reports that attempted echocardiographic estimation of PA

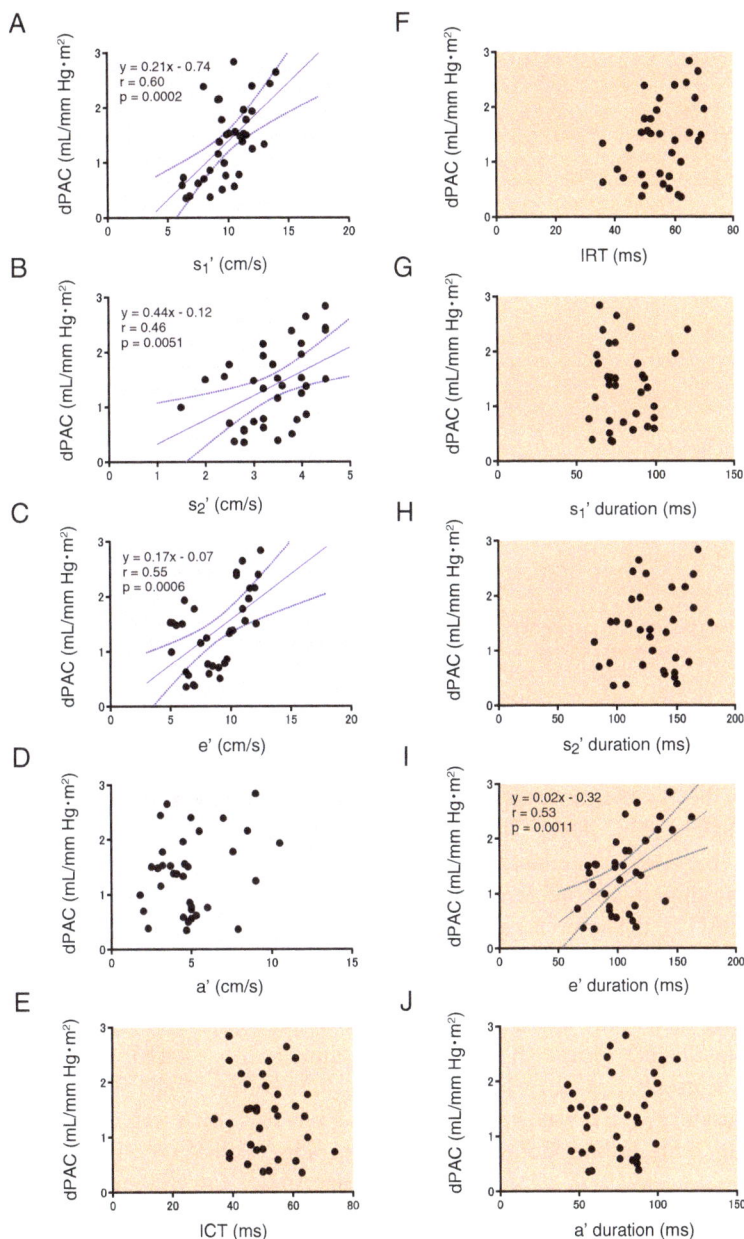

Fig. 4 The relationship between the pulmonary annular motion waveform and diastolic pulmonary arterial capacitance (dPAC) in the VSD group. The relationship was evaluated in terms of peak velocity (**a–d**) and time duration (**e–j**) in each wave. There are significant correlations between the peak velocities of pulmonary s1', s2', e' and dPAC (**a–c**). The e' wave duration is significantly correlated with dPAC (I). Linear regression lines with 95 % confidence interval (*dashed lines*) are indicated. dPAC, diastolic pulmonary arterial capacitance; ICT, isovolumic contraction time; IRT, isovolumic relaxation time

capacitance all had limitations due to poor reproducibility and difficulty, because accurate quantitative assessment by two-dimensional echocardiography is hampered by the complex geometry and difficult depiction. Pulmonary arterial wall strain evaluated by speckle tacking method can be a candidate for evaluating PA distensibility and capacitance. However, in our preliminary experimental study, the tracking was insufficient and the reproducibility was quite low. Therefore, nongeometric methods to assess PA

compliance and PA deformation should be explored. One such method, TDI, allows the quantitative assessment of longitudinal PA deformation.

To the best of our knowledge, this is the first application of pulmonary annular motion velocity obtained by TDI as a tool for PA capacitance assessment. We postulated that the PA longitudinal deformation reflects stroke volume, and that the pulmonary annular motion waveform shows PA capacitance.

Table 3 Results of stepwise multiple regression analysis for variables predicting accuracy of pulmonary annular motion parameters

Objective variable	Explanatory variables	B	SE	β	p values	VIF
s1′ (cm/sec)	sPAC	0.41	0.16	0.41	0.0131	1.76
	dPAC	0.95	0.43	0.34	0.0354	1.74
	RVEDP	−0.37	0.11	−0.39	0.0021	1.02
s2′ (cm/sec)	sPAC	0.24	0.05	0.62	<0.0001	1.00
e′ (cm/sec)	sPAC	0.37	0.19	0.35	0.0314	2.08
	RVSP	−0.05	0.02	−0.28	0.0432	1.71
	RVEDP	0.46	0.12	0.42	0.0005	1.04
a′ (cm/sec)	n.a.	-	-	-	-	-
ICT (msec)	n.a.	-	-	-	-	-
IRT (msec)	n.a.	-	-	-	-	-
s1′ duration (msec)	sPAC	3.76	1.17	0.49	0.0029	1.00
s2′ duration (msec)	Qp/Qs	−12.71	4.19	−0.47	0.0047	1.00
e′ duration (msec)	n.a.	-	-	-	-	-
a′ duration (msec)	sPAC	2.66	1.30	0.27	0.0488	1.11
	Qp/Qs	−9.19	3.18	−0.44	0.0070	1.48

B unstandardized coefficient, *SE* standard error, *β* standardized partial regression coefficient, *VIF* variance inflation factor, *sPAC* systolic pulmonary arterial capacitance, *dPAC* diastolic pulmonary arterial capacitance, *SPAP* systolic pulmonary arterial pressure, *RVSP* right ventricular systolic pressure, *RVEDP* right ventricular end-diastolic pressure, *Qp/Qs* pulmonary to systemic blood flow ratio, *n.a.* not available

In the present study, PA capacitance was represented by two parameters: sPAC and dPAC. There was a significant correlation between the two parameters, although sPAC was significantly higher than dPAC. The significant difference between the two parameters was assumed to be caused by the time phase difference during the cardiac cycle. The sPAC is the arterial capacitance from end-diastole to systole, whereas the dPAC is the capacitance from end-systole to diastole.

The peak velocities of the pulmonary annular s1′, s2′, e′, and a′ waves were significantly lower in the VSD group than in the Control group (Fig. 2), whereas the peak velocity of the tricuspid s′ wave was significantly higher in the VSD group than in the Control group

Table 4 Inter- and intra-observer reproducibility

Parameter variability	Inter-observer variability	Intra-observer
Peak velocity of s1′	0.15 ± 2.12 cm/s	−0.14 ± 2.14 cm/s
Peak velocity of s2′	−0.04 ± 1.25 cm/s	−0.05 ± 1.36 cm/s
Peak velocity of e′	0.27 ± 1.72 cm/s	0.29 ± 1.46 cm/s
Peak velocity pf a′	0.19 ± 1.43 cm/s	0.18 ± 2.41 cm/s
ICT	−5.34 ± 15.14 ms	−4.31 ± 10.22 ms
IRT	2.21 ± 10.03 ms	−1.31 ± 9.33 ms
s1′ duration	3.64 ± 10.31 ms	1.92 ± 8.13 ms
s2′ duration	−0.33 ± 18.75 ms	−0.29 ± 16.85 ms
e′ duration	0.88 ± 13.54 ms	−0.72 ± 11.14 ms
a′ duration	5.22 ± 9.36 ms	3.98 ± 6.38 ms

Inter- and intra-observer variabilities (bias ± 2 SD [95 % limit of agreement]) are shown

(Table 1). This discrepancy between pulmonary and tricuspid annular motions might have resulted from the different RV contractility properties between RV inflow and outflow regional properties that originate from the RV geometry, including myocardial fiber orientation [15, 16]. Furthermore, we assumed that PA motion velocity might be affected by PA properties, including PA capacitance. The annular motions are presumed to be affected by RV performance and the adjacent structures [9]. The pulmonary annulus and tricuspid annulus are located adjacent to the PA and right atrium, respectively. Tricuspid annular motion would be affected by right atrial stiffness, contraction, and pressure. Pulmonary annular motion is assumed to be affected by PA properties, including arterial pressure, compliance, and stiffness. These conditions might contribute to the opposite results for the peak velocities of pulmonary and tricuspid annular motions in the VSD group.

The present data demonstrated that pulmonary annular motion parameters can be used to represent PA capacitance. On multiple regression analysis, PA capacitance independently affected the pulmonary annular motion waveform and parameters. Importantly, RVEF was not an independent variable that determined pulmonary annular motion. This is likely due to the fact that PA stroke volume is not correlated with RVEF because VSD shunt flow is directly expelled to the PA during systole in the VSD group. The present data indicate that pulmonary annular motion is determined not by RV contraction, but by PA deformation in children with VSD. Nevertheless, the present study demonstrated the significant negative correlation between the pulmonary annular s1′ wave and RVEDP in the VSD group. Furthermore, RVSP and RVEDP affect the peak velocity of the e′ wave. It would be useful to investigate the relationship between pulmonary annular motion velocity and RV performance or RV overload. Further studies are necessary to determine the various factors affecting pulmonary annular motion.

Limitations

The sample cohort was relatively small, but TDI parameters were compared between patients and age-matched healthy individuals, and distinctive waveforms were found in the patient group. We postulated that PA expansion by the stroke volume and distensibility is similar in the radial and longitudinal directions. However, a directional difference might be present, which might generate systematic measurement error. The detailed characteristics of stiffness and elasticity in the PA radial and longitudinal directions should be elucidated in the future. Next, some degree of angulation between the Doppler beam and the true direction of longitudinal PA elasticity might exist. The long-axis view of the RVOT and PA was obtained, and the ultrasound beam was parallel to the direction of the pulmonary annular motions. We considered that this is the most appropriate cross-sectional view to observe the expansion and contraction of the PA.

A significant correlation between the s1′ wave and RVEDP was found. Furthermore, RVSP and RVEDP had effects on the peak velocity of the e′ wave in the VSD group. These indicate that RV performance also affects pulmonary annular motion. It is necessary to note that PA capacitance is not the only factor determining pulmonary annular motion. From another point of view, it would be meaningful to investigate the relationship between pulmonary annular motion velocity and RV performance or RV overload. Further studies are needed to determine the utility of pulmonary annular motion.

Lastly, although it was demonstrated that TDI-derived pulmonary annular motion parameters reflect PA capacitance, no attempt was made to determine the most useful parameter and derive the prediction formula to evaluate PA capacitance in the present study. The correlations found between pulmonary annular motion parameter and PA capacitance are relatively weak. Further studies of larger patient populations are needed to determine the most valuable parameter and the normal range of pulmonary annular motion for the evaluation of PA capacitance. Moreover, a further study with other disease populations would be necessary to establish the importance of the TDI-derived pulmonary annular motion waveform for the estimation of PA capacitance.

Conclusions

Pulmonary annular TDI is a promising echocardiographic tool for evaluating PA capacitance in children with VSD. It can be a simple, rapid, reproducible, and highly distinctive method for evaluating PA capacitance.

Acknowledgements
Not applicable.

Funding
This research received no grant from any funding agency in the public, commercial, or not-for-profit sectors.

Authors' contributions
Yasunobu Hayabuchi was responsible for idea formation, study designing, performing echocardiography and reviewing the article. Akemi Ono contributed in idea formation, study designing, performig echocardiography, drafting and reviewing the article. Yukako Homma and Akemi Ono were responsible for data gathering and helped in analysis and drafting the article. Shoji Kagami was responsible for critical review and editing the manuscript. All authors read and approved the final manuscript.

Competing interests
The authors declare that they have no competing interests.

References
1. Rosenzweig EB, Widlitz AC, Barst RJ. Pulmonary arterial hypertension in children. Pediatr Pulmonol. 2004;38:2–22.
2. Raymond RJ, Hinderliter AL, Willis PW, Ralph D, Caldwell EJ, Williams W, et al. Echocardiographic predictors of adverse outcomes in primary pulmonary hypertension. J Am Coll Cardiol. 2002;39:1214–9.
3. Abman SH, Hansmann G, Archer SL, Ivy DD, Adatia I, Chung WK, et al. Pediatric Pulmonary Hypertension: Guidelines From the American Heart Association and American Thoracic Society. Circulation. 2015;132:2037–99.
4. McGregor M, Sniderman A. On pulmonary vascular resistance: the need for more precise definition. Am J Cardiol. 1985;55:217–21.
5. Mahapatra S, Nishimura RA, Sorajja P, Cha S, McGoon MD. Relationship of pulmonary arterial capacitance and mortality in idiopathic pulmonary arterial hypertension. J Am Coll Cardiol. 2006;47:799–803.
6. Mahapatra S, Nishimura RA, Oh JK, McGoon MD. The prognostic value of pulmonary vascular capacitance determined by Doppler echocardiography in patients with pulmonary arterial hypertension. J Am Soc Echocardiogr. 2006;19:1045–50.
7. Sajan I, Manlhiot C, Reyes J, McCrindle BW, Humpl T, Friedberg MK. Pulmonary arterial capacitance in children with idiopathic pulmonary arterial hypertension and pulmonary arterial hypertension associated with congenital heart disease: relation to pulmonary vascular resistance, exercise capacity, and survival. Am Heart J. 2011;162:562–8.
8. Pellegrini P, Rossi A, Pasotti M, Raineri C, Cicoira M, Bonapace S, et al. Prognostic relevance of pulmonary arterial compliance in patients with chronic heart failure. Chest. 2014;145:1064–70.
9. Hayabuchi Y, Ono A, Kagami S. Pulmonary annular motion velocity assessed using Doppler tissue imaging - Novel echocardiographic evaluation of right ventricular outflow tract function. Circ J. 2016;80:168–75.
10. Reuben SR. Compliance of the human pulmonary arterial system in disease. Circ Res. 1971;29:40–50.
11. Stergiopulos N, Meister JJ, Westerhof N. Evaluation of methods for estimation of total arterial compliance. Am J Physiol Heart Circ Physiol. 1995;268:H1540–8.
12. Henriksen JH, Fuglsang S, Bendtsen F, Christensen E, Møller S. Arterial compliance in patients with cirrhosis: stroke volume-pulse pressure ratio as simplified index. Am J Physiol Gastrointest Liver Physiol. 2001;80:G584–94.
13. Friedberg MK, Feinstein JA, Rosenthal DN. Noninvasive assessment of pulmonary arterial capacitance by echocardiography. J Am Soc Echocardiogr. 2007;20:186–90.

15

Cardiac shock-wave therapy in the treatment of coronary artery disease: systematic review and meta-analysis

Greta Burneikaitė[1,2,7]*, Evgeny Shkolnik[3,4], Jelena Čelutkienė[1,2]*, Gitana Zuozienė[1,2], Irena Butkuvienė[1,2], Birutė Petrauskienė[1,2], Pranas Šerpytis[1,2], Aleksandras Laucevičius[1,5] and Amir Lerman[6]

Abstract

Aim: To systematically review currently available cardiac shock-wave therapy (CSWT) studies in humans and perform meta-analysis regarding anti-anginal efficacy of CSWT.

Methods: The Cochrane Controlled Trials Register, Medline, Medscape, Research Gate, Science Direct, and Web of Science databases were explored. In total 39 studies evaluating the efficacy of CSWT in patients with stable angina were identified including single arm, non- and randomized trials. Information on study design, subject's characteristics, clinical data and endpoints were obtained. Assessment of publication risk of bias was performed and heterogeneity across the studies was calculated by using random effects model.

Results: Totally, 1189 patients were included in 39 reviewed studies, with 1006 patients treated with CSWT. The largest patient sample of single arm study consisted of 111 patients. All selected studies demonstrated significant improvement in subjective measures of angina symptoms and/or quality of life, in the majority of studies left ventricular function and myocardial perfusion improved. In 12 controlled studies with 483 patients included (183 controls) angina class, Seattle Angina Questionnaire (SAQ) score, nitrates consumption were significantly improved after the treatment.
In 593 participants across 22 studies the exercise capacity was significantly improved after CSWT, as compared with the baseline values (in meta-analysis standardized mean difference SMD = −0.74; 95% CI, −0.97 to −0.5; $p < 0.001$).

Conclusions: Systematic review of CSWT studies in stable coronary artery disease (CAD) demonstrated consistent improvement of clinical variables. Meta-analysis showed a moderate improvement of exercise capacity.
Overall, CSWT is a promising non-invasive option for patients with end-stage CAD, but evidence is limited to small sample single-center studies. Multi-center adequately powered randomised double blind studies are warranted.

Keywords: Cardiac shock wave therapy, coronary artery disease, stable angina pectoris, refractory angina

Background

A substantial number of patients suffer from disabling angina despite having undergone invasive treatment methods and continuation on optimal medical treatment (OMT) [1]. Such condition is defined as a refractory angina (RFA) [2]. In many cases, stable coronary artery disease (CAD) becomes too diffuse and extensive to be treated by traditional revascularization methods. The

annual mortality rate of RFA in recent studies is in the range of 3–4% [3, 4].

Several new alternative treatment methods of RFA are being investigated. A number of studies showed that transmyocardial [5] and percutaneous myocardial laser revascularization [6, 7], spinal cord stimulation [8] and stem cell therapy [9–11] may reduce angina symptoms and improve exercise capacity, myocardial perfusion and function. Nevertheless, these treatment modalities are invasive, quite expensive or still at a preclinical stage.

Enhanced external counter-pulsation is a non-invasive option suggested for CAD patients. However, the recent studies were inconclusive and found no or small differences

---
* Correspondence: gburneikaite@gmail.com; jelena.celutkiene@santa.lt
[1]Clinic of Cardiac and Vascular Diseases, Faculty of Medicine, Vilnius University, Vilnius, Lithuania
Full list of author information is available at the end of the article

between test and control groups with respect to change in angina or exercise duration [12, 13].

Ultrasound-guided cardiac shock wave (SW) therapy is another promising non-invasive modality in patients with stable CAD. Experimental studies showed that SW might induce shear stress to endothelial cells and produce complex cascade of short- and long-term reactions leading to angiogenesis [14, 15]. The observed immediate increase in blood flow due to local vasodilation and the formation of new capillaries in the treated tissue [16–18] has led to its application in cardiovascular medicine. Since 1999 [19], cardiac shock-wave therapy (CSWT) as a tool for the management of RFA has been investigated in a considerable number of clinical studies.

Our aim was to systematically review and analyse currently available data from CSWT studies in humans and perform meta-analysis regarding efficacy of CSWT on exercise capacity.

Materials and methods
Inclusion criteria, search strategy, methods of data collection and analysis were elaborated in a protocol.

Data sources
We searched for articles evaluating the efficacy of CSWT in CAD patients from the following medical bibliographic databases: Cochrane Controlled Trials Register, Medline, Medscape, Research Gate, Science Direct, Web of Science (from 1999 to April of 2016), and Google Web. Publications were selected by predefined criteria and reviewed by two authors (GB, ES) following PRISMA statement [20]. Disagreements were discussed with other author (JC). The search terms included coronary artery disease, ischemic heart disease, refractory angina treatment, stable angina treatment combined with extracorporeal cardiac shock wave therapy, myocardial shock wave therapy, extracorporeal myocardial revascularisation. We also searched for references in review articles and abstracts.

Study selection criteria
In order to be included, trials had to assess the treatment with CSWT of CAD patients, written in English. Selected studies included patients with stable CAD proven by coronary angiography or computed tomography angiography, not amenable to revascularization, angina class II-IV (Canadian Cardiology Society, CCS), despite OMT, and

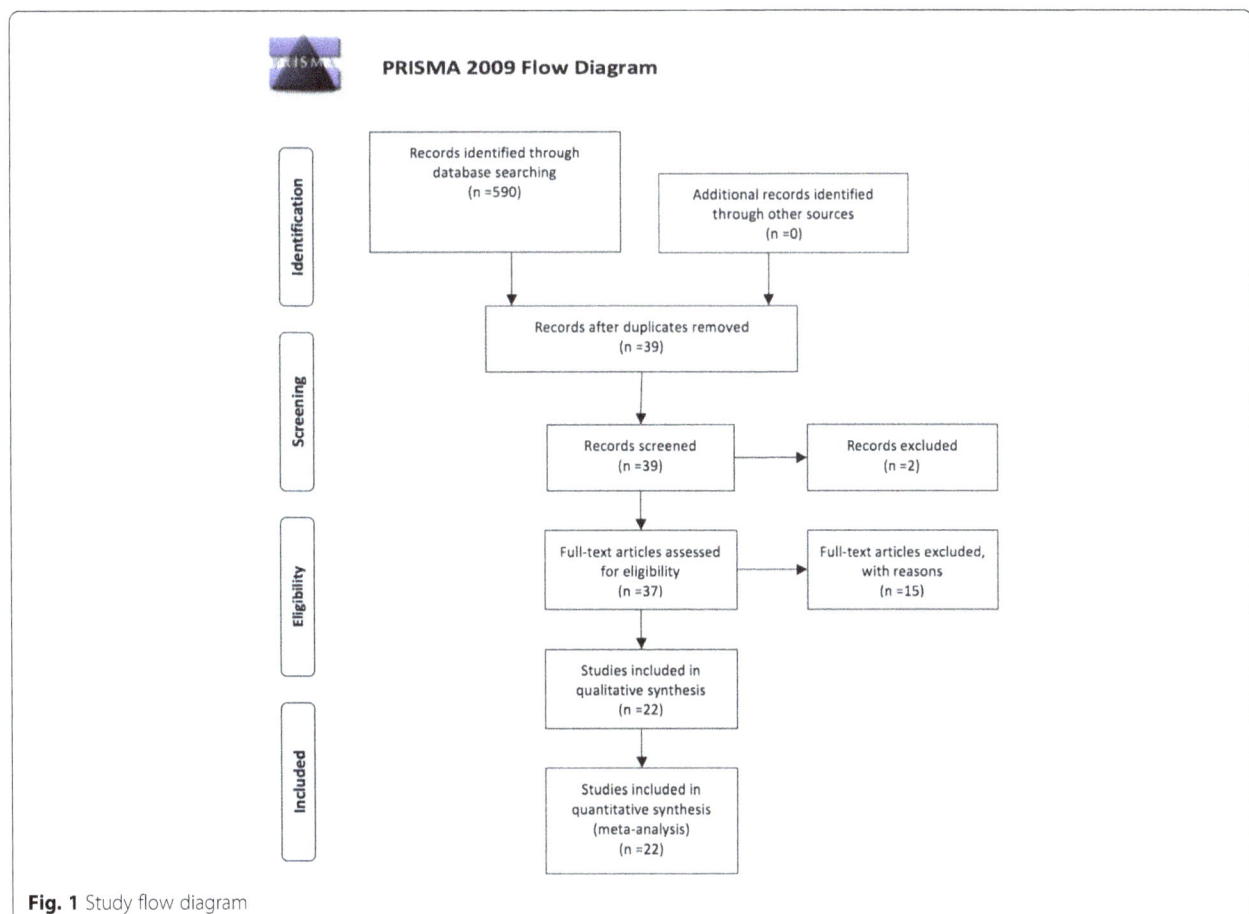

Fig. 1 Study flow diagram

documented stress induced myocardial ischemia. Trials investigating combination of CSWT with stem cell therapy were not included.

Data extraction

Information on 1) study design (including study type, method of randomization and blinding of patients, study personnel and outcome assessors), 2) sample size and patients characteristics (including age, sex), 3) intervention strategies (including treatments schedule, follow up duration), 4) outcome measures (including (short-acting nitrates consumption per week, CCS angina class and New York Heart Association [NYHA] functional class, Seattle Angina Questionnaire (SAQ) scores, and parameters

of the functional tests as exercise duration, workload, global and regional left ventricular [LV] function, myocardial perfusion) were extracted into Microsoft Excel (Microsoft, Seattle, Wash., USA) spread sheets.

Statistical analysis

Variables were presented as mean value ± standard deviation (SD) for continuous data with normal distribution and as median with interquartile range (IQR: Q1, Q3) for data not normally distributed, whereas categorical variables were expressed as number (%).

Assessment of risk of bias randomized trials was performed in accordance with the Cochrane Collaboration tool [21] and was based on information on concealment

Table 1 PRISMA checklist

Section/topic	Number	Checklist item	Reported on page #
TITLE			
Title	1	Identify the report as a systematic review, meta-analysis, or both.	1
ABSTRACT			
Structured summary	2	Provide a structured summary including, as applicable: background; objectives; data sources; study eligibility criteria, participants, and interventions; study appraisal and synthesis methods; results; limitations; conclusions and implications of key findings; systematic review registration number.	2
INTROCUTION			
Rationale	3	Describe the rationale for the review in the context of what is already known.	3
Objectives	4	Provide an explicit statement of questions being addressed with reference to participants, interventions, comparisons, outcomes, and study design (PICOS).	3
METHODS			
Protocol and registration	5	Indicate if a review protocol exists, if and where it can be accessed (e.g., Web address), and, if available, provide registration information including registration number.	3
Eligibility criteria	6	Specify study characteristics (e.g., PICOS, length of follow-up) and report characteristics (e.g., years considered, language, publication status) used as criteria for eligibility, giving rationale.	4
Information sources	7	Describe all information sources (e.g., databases with dates of coverage, contact with study authors to identify additional studies) in the search and date last searched.	4
Search	8	Present full electronic search strategy for at least one database, including any limits used, such that it could be repeated.	4
Study selection	9	State the process for selecting studies (i.e., screening, eligibility, included in systematic review, and, if applicable, included in the meta-analysis).	4
Data collection process	10	Describe method of data extraction from reports (e.g., piloted forms, independently, in duplicate) and any processes for obtaining and confirming data from investigators.	4
Data items	11	List and define all variables for which data were sought (e.g., PICOS, funding sources) and any assumptions and simplifications made.	4
Risk of bias in individual studies	12	Describe methods used for assessing risk of bias of individual studies (including specification of whether this was done at the study or outcome level), and how this information is to be used in any data synthesis.	4–5
Summary measures	13	State the principal summary measures (e.g., risk ratio, difference in means).	Table 2, 4–5
Synthesis of results	14	Describe the methods of handling data and combining results of studies, if done, including measures of consistency (e.g., I^2) for each meta-analysis.	4–5

Table 2 Common characteristics of selected human studies of cardiac shock wave therapy

Author (year)	Study population	Stress test, used to detect myocardial ischemia	Patients, Total control (n)	Age (years)	Sex, male, n (%)	Follow up, months
Non-controlled studies						
Caspari G. H. et al. (1999) [19]	Stable angina	SPECT	9/-	65 ± 7	nd	6[d]
Gutersohn A. et al. (2003) [51]	Stable angina	SPECT, ET	25/-	66 ± 7.3	nd	6[d]
Gutersohn A. et al. (2005) [52]	Stable angina	SPECT	14/-	66	nd	12[e]
Gutersohn A. et al. (2006) [53]	Stable angina	SPECT	23/-	66	nd	60[d]
Fukumoto Y. et al. (2006) [54]	Stable angina	ET, SPECT	9/-	67.8	5 (55.5%)	12[d]
Lyadov K. et al. (2006) [55]	Stable angina	DSE, CPET	13/-	59.6 ± 6.9	11 (85%)	1[e]
Naber C. et al. (2007) [56]	Stable angina	SPECT	25/-	63.8 ± 8.2	nd	3[d]
KhattabA.A. et al. (2007) [57]	Stable angina	SPECT	10/-	nd	nd	1[d]
Naber C. et al. (2008) [58]	Stable angina	SPECT	24/-	63.8 ± 8.2	18 (75%)	3[d]
Takayama T. et al. (2008) [28]	Stable angina	SPECT	17/-	67.5	17 (100%)	6[d]
Wang Y. et al. (2010) [59]	Stable angina	DSE, SPECT	9/-	63.7 ± 5.7	9 (100%)	1[d]
Faber L. et al. (2010) [60]	Stable angina	PET, CPET	16/-	66 ± 10	nd	1[d]
Vainer J. et al. (2010) [61]	Stable angina	ET, SPECT	22/-	69 ± 7	18 (81.8%)	4[d]
Vasyuk Y. A. et al. (2010) [25]	Ischemic HF	DSE, SPECT	24/-	63.3 ± 6.1	20 (83.3%)	6[d]
Alunni G. et al. (2011) [62]	Stable angina	SPECT	16/-	71 ± 5.6	12 (80%)	12
Vainer J. et al. (2012) [63]	Stable angina	SPECT	50/-	68 ± 9	40 (80%)	4[d]
Alunni G. et al. (2013) [64]	Stable angina	SPECT	25/-	nd	nd	6[d]
Gabrusenko S.A. et al. (2013) [29]	Stable angina	SPECT	17/-	67.4 ± 8.6	14 (82.4%)	1[e]
Zuoziene G. et al. (2013) [65]	Stable angina	DSE, SPECT	40/-	67.7 ± 7	30 (75%)	3[d]
Prinz C. et al. (2013) [66]	Stable angina	ET, PET	43/-	67 ± 10	nd	1[d]
Cassar A. et al. (2014) [27]	Stable angina	ET, SPECT	15/-	65.0 ± 12.1	13 (86.7)	4[d]
Faber L. et al. (2014) [67]	Stable angina	PET	47/-	67 ± 10	nd	1,5[d]
Prasad M. et al. (2015) [68]	Stable angina	SPECT, ET	111/-	62.9 ± 10.9	98 (83.7)	3–6[e]
Kaller M. et al. (2015) [49]	Stable angina	PET, ET	21/-	65 ± 10	13 (61.9%)	1.5–2[d]
Cai HY et al. (2015) [30]	Stable angina	ET	26/-	63 ± 10	23 (88.5%)	4[d]
Liu BY et al. (2015) [69]	Stable angina	SPECT	11/-	nd	nd	12[d]
Vainer J. et al. (2016) [70]	Stable angina	ET, SPECT	33/-	69.7 ± 8	27 (82%)	4[d]
Non-randomized, controlled studies						
Kikuchi Y. et al. (2010)[c] [31]	Stable angina	CPET	8/8	70 ± 3	5 (62.5%)	3[d]
Kazmi W.H. et al. (2012) [71]	Stable angina	SPECT	86/43	57.7 ± 10.5	73 (84.5%)	6[d]
Alunni G. et al. (2014) [72]	Stable angina	SPECT	72/29	70 ± 5.3	60 (83.3%)	6[d]
Nirala S. et al. (2016) [73]	Stable angina	ET, DSE	52/11	63.4 ± 10.8	43 (82.7%)	72[d]
Randomized, controlled studies						
Peng Y.Z. et al. (2012) [26]	Ischemic HF	SPECT	50/nd	nd	nd	1[d]
Wang Y. et al. (2012)[a] [24]	Stable angina	DSE, SPECT	55/14	64.1 ± 9.8	47 (85%)	12[e]
Zhao L. et al. (2015)[b] [74]	Stable angina	SPECT, ET	87/27	66.8 ± 8.4	68 (78%)	12[e]
Randomized, placebo controlled studies						
Schmid J.P. et al. (2006) [75]	Stable angina	SPECT	15/8	68 ± 8	14 (60%)	3[d]
Yang P. et al. (2012)[a] [76]	Stable angina	SPECT	45/20	67 ± 8.3	36 (80%)	3[e]
Leibowitz D. et al. (2012)[a] [77]	Stable angina	ET, SPECT	28/10	63.3 ± 9.2	24 (85.7%)	3[d]
Schmid J.P. et al. (2013) [78]	Stable angina	CPET	21/10	68.2 ± 8.3	19 (90.5%)	3[d]
Yang P. et al. (2013)[a] [79]	Stable angina	SPECT	25/11	65.1 ± 8.5	18 (72%)	6[d]

Continuous variables were expressed as mean value ± standard deviation (SD), whereas categorical variables were expressed as percentages

ET ECG Exercise test, *CPET* cardiopulmonary exercise test, *DSE* dobutamine stress echocardiography, *PET* positron emission tomography, *SPECT* single photon emission computed tomography; nd = no data; [a]double blind; [b]single blind; [c]double blind, placebo controlled, crossover design; [d]time after the end of treatment (treatment ends at 9th treatment week); [e]time from the treatment initiation

of allocation and random sequence generation, blinding of participants and personnel, incomplete outcome data and selective reporting. For risk of bias assessments the low/unclear/high scale was used.

The effect sizes used in each study are presented as standardized mean difference (SMD) with 95% confidence interval (CI) to allow for combination of different measurements of exercise capacity. In line with Cohen's classification [22], effect sizes were divided into trivial (Cohen's d ≤0.2), small (<0.5), moderate (<0.8), and large (>0.8).

Heterogeneity was assessed by using the chi-square test for heterogeneity and the I^2 statistic to determine the proportion of variation attributable to heterogeneity among studies. Values of I^2 considered as low (<25%), moderate (25–50%) and high (>50%) heterogeneity. Meta-analysis results are presented as forest plots. Random effects model according to Der Simonian-Laird was used to verify the significant evidence of heterogeneity between the results of studies. Publication bias was estimated by drawing funnel plot. The analysis was performed using RevMan 5.3 software (Copenhagen, The Nordic Cochrane Centre) [23].

Results

Study characteristics and patient population

From 590 identified publications after exclusion of irrelevant, experimental, animal and non-English studies 39 studies were selected for review following the PRISMA statement [20] (Fig. 1, Table 1); their common characteristics are summarized in Table 2.

In total, 1189 patients were included with 1006 patients treated with CSWT (483 patients underwent CSWT in controlled studies), 183 patients entered control groups. The mean age of patients was 66 ± 6.7 years, 80.8% were men. Study sample size was from 8 to 111 patients; duration of follow up lasted from 1 to 72 months.

No procedure related adverse events and good treatment tolerance were reported.

Studies did not include patients with acute coronary syndromes at least 3 months before enrolment, recent revascularization and thrombus in the left ventricle.

In most studies the treatment protocol consisted of nine sessions conducted over a 9-week period with three treatment series performed on the 1st, 5th and 9th week. Shock waves were applied to targeted area of myocardial ischemia detected by imaging stress tests. Wang showed that a modified regimen of nine treatment sessions within 1 month had similar therapeutic effect, as compared to the standard treatment protocol [24]; only a standard treatment group from this study was included in meta-analysis in order to reduce possible heterogeneity.

Risk of bias and quality assessment of controlled studies is shown in Table 3.

Cardiac shock wave therapy effect on clinical variables

All selected studies demonstrated positive effect of CSWT on clinical variables (results of controlled studies are shown in Table 4). In CSWT patients CCS angina scale (31 studies) and NYHA class (13 studies) have reduced by 1 (1, 1) and 1 (0, 1), respectively, compared with the baseline values. The frequency of weekly nitroglycerine use declined from 40 to 75% (in 16 related studies).

Meta-analysis of cardiac shock wave therapy effect on exercise capacity

Two studies investigating ischemic heart failure population were excluded from meta-analysis [25, 26].

From remaining 37 studies only 22 studies provided data suitable to be included in meta-analysis to evaluate the impact of CSWT on the parameters of exercise

Table 3 Quality and risk of bias assessment for randomized studies

	Wang Y. 2012 [24]	Zhao L. 2015 [74]	Yang P. 2012 [76]	Leibowitz D. 2012 [77]	Schmid J.P. 2013 [78]	Yang P. 2013 [79]
Random sequence generation	high risk	low risk	high risk	high risk	high risk	high risk
Allocation concealment	high risk	high risk	high risk	high risk	high risk	high risk
Blinding of participants	high risk	low risk	high risk	low risk	low risk	high risk
Blinding of personnel who provide CSWT treatment	high risk	high risk	high risk	high risk	high risk	high risk
Blinding of outcome assessment	unclear risk	high risk	high risk	high risk	high risk	high risk
Incomplete outcome data	high risk	high risk	low risk	high risk	high risk	low risk
Selective reporting	low risk	low risk	low risk	low risk	low risk	low risk
Blinding of CWST procedure	high risk	low risk	high risk	low risk	low risk	high risk
Endpoints were based on sample size calculation	high risk	high risk	high risk	high risk	high risk	high risk
Complete testing in both groups	low risk	low risk	low risk	low risk	low risk	low risk

CSWT cardiac shock wave therapy

Table 4 Effect of cardiac shock wave therapy in human controlled studies: clinical and quality of life parameters

		Period	CCS angina class	Nitroglycerine consumption	NYHA class	Seattle angina questionnaire
P. Yang 2013 [79]	Test group (N=14)	Baseline	2.0 (1.0, 3.0)	2.0 (0.0, 3.0)	2.0 (1.0, 2.0)	73.5 (60.5, 81.0)
		Post treatment	1.0 (1.0, 2.0)*	1.0 (0.0, 2.0)	1.0 (1.0, 1.0)*	82.0 (74.5, 88.0)*
	Placebo group (N=11)	Baseline	2.0 (1.0, 3.0)	2.0 (1.0, 3.0)	1.0 (1.0, 2.0)	73.0 (63.0, 80.0)
		Post treatment	2.0 (1.0, 2.0)	2.0 (0.0, 2.0)	2.0 (1.0, 2.0)	78.0 (69.0, 85.0)
Y. Wang 2012 [24]	I group (standard treatment) (N=20)	Baseline	2 (1, 2)	1 (0, 2)	1.5 (1, 3)	64.9±11.72
		Post treatment	1 (1, 1)*	0 (0, 1)	1 (1, 1)	75.0±10.45*
	II group (modified treatment) (N=21)	Baseline	3 (2, 3)	2 (0, 3)	2 (1, 2.5)	67.9±13.0
		Post treatment	2 (1, 2)	0 (0, 1)	1 (1, 1)	76.14±12.28
	Control group (N=14)	Baseline	2 (2, 3)	1 (0, 4)	2 (1, 3)	63.21±11.89
		Post treatment	2 (1, 2.3)	0 (0, 2)	1 (1, 2.3)	60.14±12.82
P. Yang 2012 [76]	Test group (N=25)	Baseline	2.72±0.46	2.35±0.86	2.16±0.69	65.96±11.78
		Post treatment	1.46±0.58*	1.0±0.73*	1.48±0.65*	76.4±11.78*
	Placebo group (N=20)	Baseline				
		Post treatment	No significant changes	No significant changes	No significant changes	No significant changes
S. Nirala 2016 [73]	Test group (N=41)	Baseline	2.21±0.85	1.34±1.35	1.85±0.96	66.34±12.34
		Post treatment	1.14±0.57	0.21±0.82*	1.04±0.49**	79.92±25.14**
	Control group (N=11)	Baseline	1.81±0.75	1.36±1.62	1.36±0.67	84±7.61
		Post treatment	2.18±0.75	2±1.18	2.09±0.94	72.72±12.33
Y. Kikuchi 2010 [31]	Test group (N=8)	Baseline	3.0	4.0	-	-
		Post treatment	2.25*	1.0*	-	-
	Placebo group (N=8)	Baseline	2.75	4.0	-	-
		Post treatment	2.75	3.0*	-	-
W.H. Kazmi 2012 [71]	Test group (N=43)	Baseline	2.63±0.7	-	2.48±0.6	-
		Post treatment	1.95±0.8**	-	1.95±0.5**	-
	Control group (N=43)	Baseline	2.63±0.7	-	2.48±0.6	-
		Post treatment	2.63±0.7	-	2.46±0.6	-
G. Alunni 2014 [72]	Test group (N=43)	Baseline	2.67±0.75	26(60.5%)	2.51±0.74	-
		Post treatment	1.33±0.57**	9 (20%)*	1.23±0.42**	-
	Control group (N=29)	Baseline	2.52±0.78	18 (41%)*	2.32±0.79	-
		Post treatment	1.92±0.69	13 (44.8%)*	1.73±0.59	-

CCS Canadian Cardiovascular Society Angina Class, nitroglycerine consumption is expressed as number of tablets per day, *NYHA* New York Heart Association class, * = $p<0.05$ compared to baseline, ** = $p<0.001$ compared to baseline

tolerance (mean and standard deviation or standard error of mean values, both baseline and post procedure), (Fig. 2, Table 5).

Across 22 contributing studies (596 participants) the exercise capacity was significantly improved after CSWT, as compared with the baseline values (SMD = −0.74; 95% CI, −0.97 to −0.5; $p < 0.001$, $I^2 = 70\%$, Fig. 2); mean follow up period made 8 months (range 1–72 months).

In order to explain heterogeneity, we performed sensitivity analysis by removing from analysis one of the studies at a time. Overall effect changed to −0.61, 95% CI (−0.78 to −0.44), $p < 0.001$ when excluding study of Zhao L. et al.

(2015) and to −0.77, 95% CI (−1.01 to −0.52), $p < 0.001$ when excluding study of Prinz C. et al (2013).

Funnel plot analysis was performed in order to evaluate publication bias (Fig. 3). The funnel plot graph was asymmetrical and three outliers were identified representing studies of Caspari, Gutersohn and Zhao group. Without these studies heterogeneity decreased to $I^2 = 0\%$, $p = 0.57$ with SMD = −0.54; 95% CI, −0.66 to −0.42; $p < 0.001$.

Interestingly, in uncontrolled studies treatment effect was smaller than in controlled studies (SMD -0.59 (−0.81, −0.36) vs -0.93 (−1.44, −0.42)).

Study or Subgroup	before ESMR Mean	SD	Total	after ESMR Mean	SD	Total	Weight	Std. Mean Difference IV, Random, 95% CI	Year	Std. Mean Difference IV, Random, 95% CI
1.1.1 Main group										
Lyadov K. et al. 2006	11.9	2.2	13	14.1	2.8	13	3.9%	-0.85 [-1.65, -0.04]	2006	
Fukumoto Y. et al. 2006	3.9	1.89	6	5	1.69	6	2.6%	-0.57 [-1.73, 0.60]	2006	
Schmid J.P. et al. 2006	98	27	7	115	15	7	2.8%	-0.73 [-1.82, 0.37]	2006	
Naber C. et al. 2008	66.6	33.3	24	95.8	24.5	24	4.9%	-0.98 [-1.58, -0.38]	2008	
Faber L. et al. 2010	80	45	16	90	39	16	4.4%	-0.23 [-0.93, 0.46]	2010	
Vainer J. et al. 2010	7.8	4	22	8.5	3	22	5.0%	-0.19 [-0.79, 0.40]	2010	
Kikuchi Y. et al. 2010	44.7	16.2	8	50.5	16.2	8	3.2%	-0.34 [-1.33, 0.65]	2010	
Vainer J. et al. 2012	8.2	3.2	50	9.6	3.8	50	6.0%	-0.40 [-0.79, 0.00]	2012	
Kazmi W.H. et al. 2012	12.2	7.8	43	20.1	15.7	43	5.8%	-0.63 [-1.07, -0.20]	2012	
Yang P. et al. 2012	339.44	83.37	25	427.92	63.32	25	4.9%	-1.18 [-1.78, -0.57]	2012	
Wang Y. et al.(Standard CSWT) 2012	344.25	106.44	20	434.25	99.7	20	4.7%	-0.86 [-1.51, -0.20]	2012	
Schmid J.P. et al.. 2013	91.2	29.1	11	94.1	35.2	11	3.8%	-0.09 [-0.92, 0.75]	2013	
Prinz C. et al. 2013	78	53	43	90	46	43	5.9%	-0.24 [-0.66, 0.18]	2013	
Cassar A. et al. 2014	319.8	157.2	15	422.1	183.3	15	4.3%	-0.58 [-1.32, 0.15]	2014	
Cai H.I. et al. 2015	360.69	116.79	26	434.15	86.29	26	5.1%	-0.70 [-1.27, -0.14]	2015	
Kaller M. et al. 2015	93	44	16	101	41	16	4.4%	-0.18 [-0.88, 0.51]	2015	
Prasad M. et al., 2015	252.1	51.6	111	313.5	164.3	111	6.6%	-0.50 [-0.77, -0.24]	2015	
Vainer J 2016	7.4	2.8	33	8.8	3.6	33	5.5%	-0.43 [-0.92, 0.06]	2016	
Nirala S. 2016	336.65	120.46	52	445.8	172.41	52	6.0%	-0.73 [-1.13, -0.33]	2016	
Subtotal (95% CI)			541			541	90.0%	-0.54 [-0.66, -0.42]		
Heterogeneity: Tau² = 0.00; Chi² = 16.36, df = 18 (P = 0.57); I² = 0%										
Test for overall effect: Z = 8.64 (P < 0.00001)										
1.1.2 Outliers										
Caspari G. H. et al.1999	58	18	9	111	18	9	2.1%	-2.80 [-4.19, -1.42]	1999	
Gutersohn A. et al.. 2005	70	15.3	14	100	16.8	14	3.5%	-1.81 [-2.71, -0.91]	2005	
Zhao L. et al. (Standard CSWT) 2015	343.91	85.03	32	558.41	67.67	32	4.4%	-2.76 [-3.45, -2.06]	2015	
Subtotal (95% CI)			55			55	10.0%	-2.44 [-3.09, -1.79]		
Heterogeneity: Tau² = 0.11; Chi² = 2.92, df = 2 (P = 0.23); I² = 32%										
Test for overall effect: Z = 7.34 (P < 0.00001)										
Total (95% CI)			596			596	100.0%	-0.74 [-0.97, -0.50]		
Heterogeneity: Tau² = 0.20; Chi² = 70.56, df = 21 (P < 0.00001); I² = 70%										
Test for overall effect: Z = 6.15 (P < 0.00001)										
Test for subgroup differences: Chi² = 31.63, df = 1 (P < 0.00001), I² = 96.8%										

-4 -2 0 2 4
Favours [experimental] Favours [control]

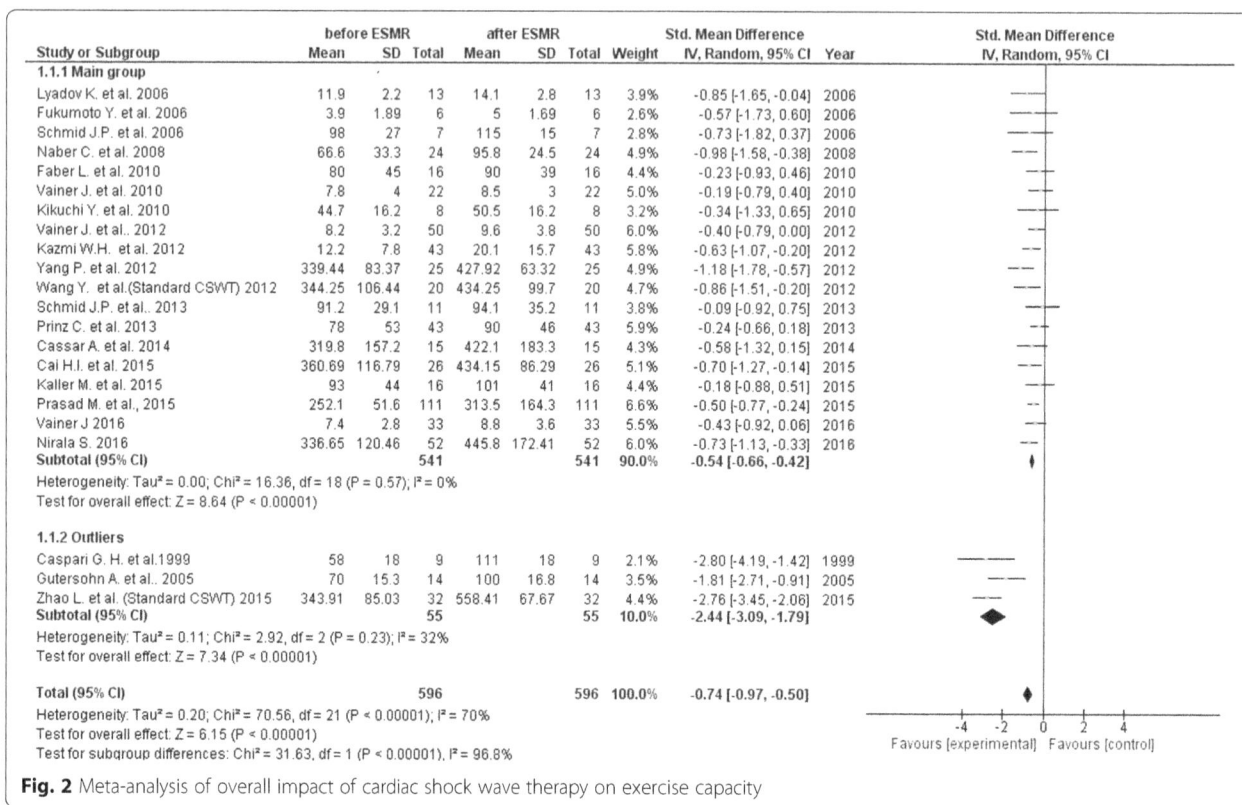

Fig. 2 Meta-analysis of overall impact of cardiac shock wave therapy on exercise capacity

Cardiac shock wave therapy effect on left ventricular function

Figures 4 and 5 demonstrate changes of rest left ventricular (LV) function by echocardiography and magnetic resonance imaging (MRI), respectively. Changes of LV end diastolic diameter are shown in Fig. 6. Seven studies demonstrated significant LV function improvement due to CSWT, while in eight studies no statistically significant changes were found.

Cardiac shock wave therapy effect on myocardial perfusion

During SPECT significant improvement of myocardial perfusion was demonstrated in 27 of 32 studies, during PET in two of four studies. Beneficial changes of myocardial perfusion were associated with increase of LVEF in seven of 13 studies with modest effect of 3.58% (2.0, 4.57). Cassar et al. [27] compared segments that were treated with CSW and those that were not, and found that after 4 months of follow–up the progression of ischemic burden of untreated segments was significantly greater.

Cardiac shock wave therapy effect on angiogenesis markers

Angiogenesis markers were assessed in four studies. Increased VEGF concentration was revealed after CSWT [28–30]. Kikuchi et al. found that the number of circulating progenitor cells (CD $34^+/KDR^+$ and CD $34^+/KDR^+/c-kit^+$) in peripheral blood remained unchanged [31]. Cai et al. observed significant increase in the number of circulating progenitor cells ($CD45^{low}/CD34^+/VEGFR2$) in peripheral blood [30].

Generation of shock waves and cardiac shock wave treatment

Shock waves (SW) belong to acoustic waves that can be transmitted through a liquid medium and focused with a precision of several millimetres to any intended treatment area inside the body.

In CAD patients, SW can be delivered to the border of the ischemic area to potentially induce neovascularization from the healthy area to the ischemic zone. Shock waves can be generated by discharge of a high-voltage spark under water or electromagnetic impulse. CSWT is performed using a SW generator system coupled with a cardiac ultrasound imaging system that is traditionally used to target the treatment to area with previously documented ischemia (Fig. 7). SW are delivered via a special applicator through the anatomical acoustic window to the treatment area under electrocardiographic R-wave gating. For optimal therapy, the treatment area is divided into target zones corresponding to the size of the focal zone of the SW applicator (Fig. 7).

Table 5 Effect of cardiac shock wave therapy on the parameters of exercise capacity

Study (year)	Study type	Number of patients who underwent CSWT	Value before CSWT	Value after CSWT	Measurement unit
Caspari G.H. et al. (1999) [19]	Single arm	9	58±18	111±18	Wt
Gutersohn A. et al. (2005) [52]	Single arm	14	70±15.3	100±16.8	Wt
Lyadov K. et al. (2006) [55]	Single arm	13	11.9±2.2	14.1±2.8	VO_2 ml/kg/min
Fukumoto Y. et al. (2006) [54]	Single arm	9	3.9±1.9	5±1.7	Met
Schmid J.P. et al. (2006) [75]	Randomized, Placebo controlled	7	98±27	115±15	Wt
Naber C. et al. (2008) [58][a]	Single arm	24	66.6±33.3	95.8±24.5	Wt
Faber L. et al. (2010) [60]	Single arm	16	80±45	90±39	Wt
Vainer J. et al. (2010) [61]	Single arm	22	7.8±4	8.5±3	Minutes
Kikuchi Y. Et al. (2010) [31]	Placebo controlled	8	44.7±16.2	50.5±16.2	Wt
Vainer J. et al. (2012) [63]	Single arm	50	8.2±3.2	9.6±3.8	Minutes
Kazmi W.H. et al. (2012) [71]	Controlled	43	12.2±7.8	20.1±15.7	Minutes
Yang P. et al. (2012) [79]	Randomized, Placebo controlled	25	339.44±83.3	427.9±63.3	Meters
Wang Y. et al. (2012) [24][b]	Randomized, controlled	31	344.3±106.4	434.3±99.7	Meters
Schmid J.P. et al. (2013) [78]	Randomized, Placebo controlled	11	91.2±29.1	94.1±35.2	Wt
Prinz C. et al. (2013) [66]	Single arm	43	78±53	90±46	Wt
Cassar A. et al. (2014) [27]	Single arm	15	319.8±157.2	422.1±183.3	Seconds
Zhao L. et al. (2015) [74][b]	Randomized, controlled	32	343.9±85.0	489.4±72.2	Seconds
Prasad M. et al. (2015) [68]	Single arm	111	252.1±51.6[c]	313.5±164.3	Seconds
			457.0±146.8[d]	606.0±126.4	
Kaller M. et al. (2015) [49]	Single arm	16	93±44	101±41	Wt
Cai HY. et al. (2015) [30]	Single arm	26	360.7±116.8	434.2±86.3	Meters
Nirala S. et al. (2016) [73]	Controlled	41	336.7±120.5	445.8±172.4	Meters
Vainer J. et al. (2016) [70]	Single arm	33	7.4±2.8	8.8±3.6	Minutes

All valuables presented as mean ± SD, [a]valuable presented as mean ± SE, SE calculated into SD using standard formulas; [b]group with standard CSWT protocol, [c]Bruce protocol, [d]modified Bruce protocol

Discussion

Clinical research in intriguing CSWT field continues since 1999, and several new trials are being published every year. The aim of this study was to summarize the results and also to evaluate the quality of currently accumulated evidence on the efficacy of CSWT on CAD treatment. This systematic review expands previously published analysis [32] by including 23 recent studies, and confirms the beneficial effects of CSWT in a larger pooled sample size of patients with stable CAD. The strength of this paper is a systematic character of review, an inclusion in meta-analysis studies with single clinical indication and a uniform treatment protocol, and assessment of bias risk in randomised trials.

In contrast to our study, recently published meta-analysis of Wang and co-authors covered only a limited period of publications, from 2010 to 2014, and included not only English but also Chinese articles [33]. As a result, our work presents the largest contemporary review of human CSWT trials incorporating all the research period.

Like in the previous analyses the majority of detected trials are relatively small, single centre, single arm, some of them insufficiently report methodology and results. In order to avoid substantial heterogeneity and publication bias reported by Wang, we excluded from meta-analysis studies, which targeted at different population of ischemic heart failure, and also non-English articles as potentially producing more beneficial results. Our study focused on the stable CAD patients and confirmed consistent positive anti-anginal effect of CSWT.

In medical field high-energy extracorporeal shock wave therapy (ESWT) was introduced more than 30 years ago as a treatment option for urinary tract stones [34]. ESWT has changed the treatment of urinary calculi, and even today it remains the primary treatment in most non-complicated cases [35]. ESWT has also been applied in biliary tract [36], pancreatic [37] and salivary stones treatment [38]. Low energy ESWT has regenerative features and has been developed as a treatment standard for a variety of orthopedic and soft tissue diseases [39], including wound healing in diabetic patients [40].

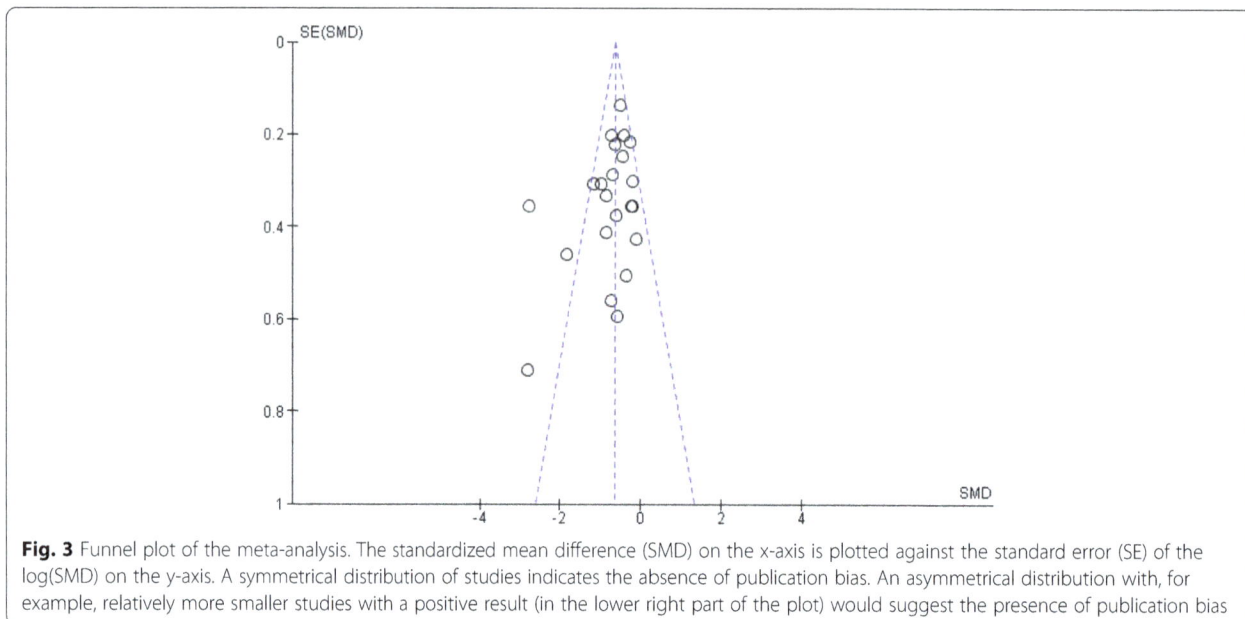

Fig. 3 Funnel plot of the meta-analysis. The standardized mean difference (SMD) on the x-axis is plotted against the standard error (SE) of the log(SMD) on the y-axis. A symmetrical distribution of studies indicates the absence of publication bias. An asymmetrical distribution with, for example, relatively more smaller studies with a positive result (in the lower right part of the plot) would suggest the presence of publication bias

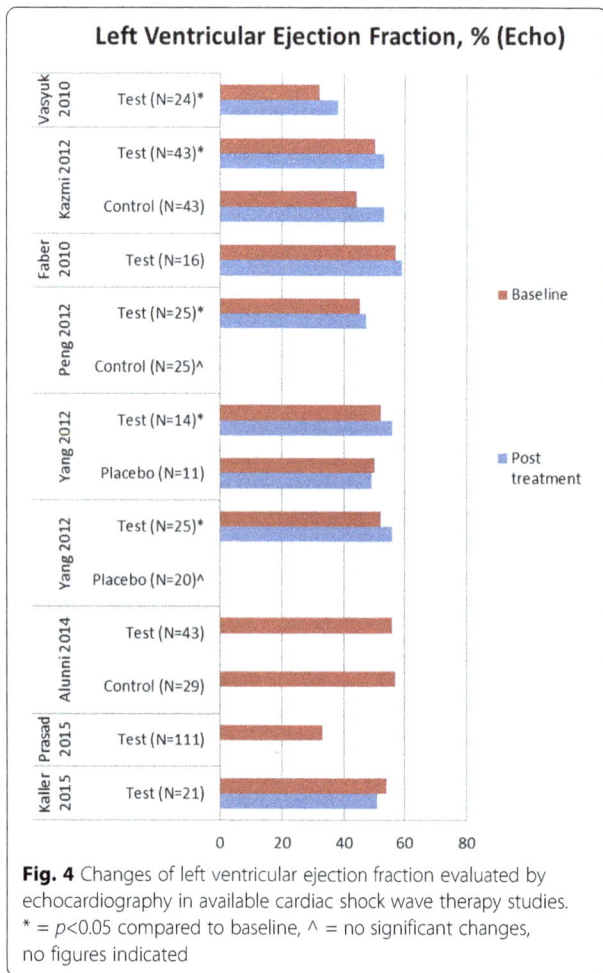

Fig. 4 Changes of left ventricular ejection fraction evaluated by echocardiography in available cardiac shock wave therapy studies. * = p<0.05 compared to baseline, ^ = no significant changes, no figures indicated

Furthermore, shockwaves have been used for treatment chronic pelvic pain syndrome [41] and erectile dysfunction. The observed immediate increase in blood flow due to local vasodilatation and the formation of new capillaries in the treated tissue [16, 17] has led to one of its more promising application in cardiovascular medicine as a possible treatment for patients with stable angina.

The mechanism of CSWT action is multifactorial. SW induces tissue cavitation, leading to a variety of biochemical effects, including shear stress on cell membranes [42], an increase in nitric oxide synthesis [43–46], an upregulation of vascular endothelial growth factor (VEGF), [14], acceleration of bone marrow cell differentiation into endothelial cells [47], an increase of the amount of circulating endothelial progenitor cells [15]. Thus, CSWT may enhance angiogenesis, reduce inflammatory response, oxidative stress, cellular apoptosis and fibrosis [14, 47, 48].

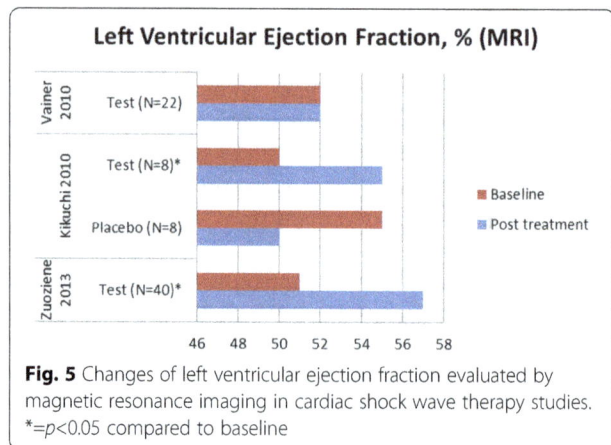

Fig. 5 Changes of left ventricular ejection fraction evaluated by magnetic resonance imaging in cardiac shock wave therapy studies. *=p<0.05 compared to baseline

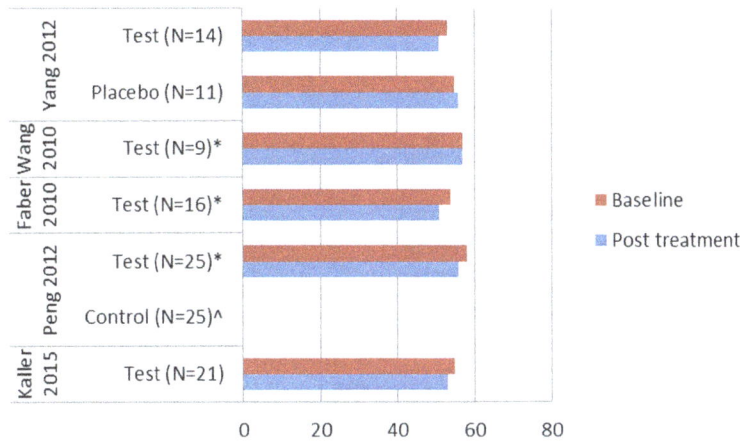

Fig. 6 Changes of left ventricular end diastolic diameter in cardiac shock wave therapy studies. *=$p<0.05$ compared to baseline, ^ = no significant changes, no figures indicated

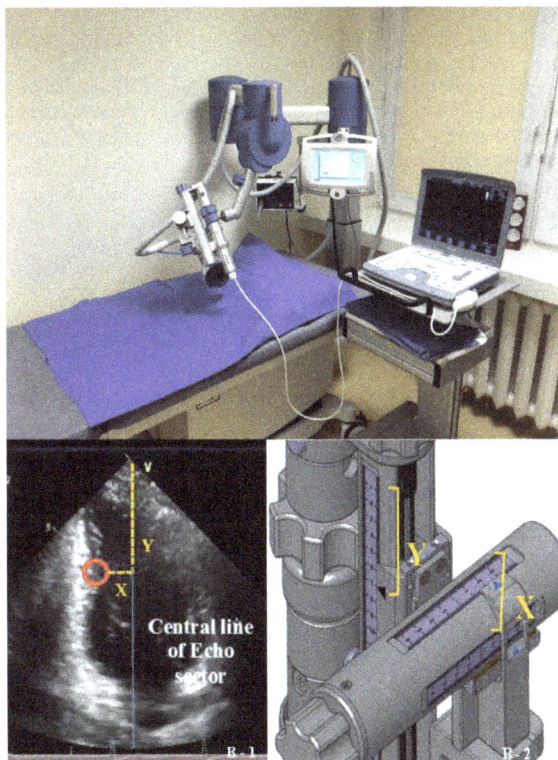

Fig. 7 The methodology of cardiac shock wave therapy. **a** Shock wave generator system (Medispec, Germantown, MD, USA) and cardiac imaging system (Vivid i, GE Healthcare, Horten, Norway). **b** Shock wave focal zone alignment: Position of the sub-segment on the 2-dimensional image determined by X and Y coordinates (1). The shockwave applicator position is identically adjusted along X- and Y-axes corresponding to the X and Y coordinates of the ultrasound image (2)

It is presumed that these mechanisms demonstrated in experimental settings could be translated into clinical effects of improvement of symptoms and myocardial perfusion in CAD patients.

Our review and meta-analysis show that in the majority of published CSWT studies, nitroglycerine consumption and angina frequency decreases, CCS, SAQ scores and NYHA class improves, myocardial perfusion and exercise capacity increases significantly. Most benefits could be observed as early as in the first month, suggesting the contribution of an early local vasodilating effect of SW. Those beneficial effects persisted during the 1-year of follow up, probably related to angiogenesis and other tissue reactions [49, 50].

Total exercise capacity is one of the most important variables used to assess efficacy of any anti-anginal treatment. We evaluated data from randomized clinical studies along with several non-controlled studies of good quality, though certain extent of heterogeneity is not avoided. Our meta-analysis of 596 participants suggests at least a moderate improving effect of CSWT on exercise tolerance.

However, most of the studies included in the review and meta-analysis are single-centre and uncontrolled, making the likelihood of bias towards larger intervention effect substantial. Different methodological quality, inadequate design or unbalanced analysis compels cautious interpretation of the real CSWT effect. Moreover, Wang assessment of methodology confirms our findings that quality of published controlled trials methodology was low [33]. The majority of the randomised studies were evaluated as having high risk if bias in terms of attribution, sample size calculation, blinding of participants and outcome assessment.

Despite very well tolerance, virtually absence of side effects, considerable symptomatic effect and non-invasive nature of CSWT it has not been widely put into practice. This may be associated with the need of special average cost equipment, particular skills of ultrasound scanning and CSWT application, and with the significant time consumption for the whole therapy course as well. Therefore, CSWT can be considered not as a substitutive but as adjunct therapy in case of limited efficacy of optimal medical treatment.

It seems that the tentative phase of this novel treatment lasted enough, and still there is a lack of high quality evidence. This warrants to perform adequately powered double blind, randomized, placebo controlled study in patients with CAD. Currently appropriately designed multicentre study is ongoing with the aim to confirm the additional improvement of exercise tolerance due to CSWT (NCT02339454).

Conclusions

Systematic review of CSWT studies in stable CAD demonstrated a clinically significant improvement of clinical variables including angina class and quality of life, as well as positive changes in LV function and perfusion. Meta-analysis showed moderate improvement in exercise capacity. Overall, CSWT is a potentially effective new non-invasive option for patients with CAD, but evidence is limited to small low/moderate quality single-centre studies. Multicentre adequately powered randomised double blind studies are warranted.

Abbreviations

CAD: Coronary artery disease; CCS: Canadian Cardiology Society; CI: Confidence interval; CSWT: Cardiac shock wave therapy; LV: Left ventricular; LVEF: Left ventricular ejection fraction; MRI: Magnetic resonance imaging; NYHA: New York Heart Association; OMT: Optimal medical treatment; PET: Positron emission tomography; RFA: Refractory angina; SAQ: Seattle Angina Questionnaire; SMD: Standardized mean difference; SPECT: Single photon emission computed tomography; SW: Shock waves; VEGF: Vascular endothelial growth factor

Acknowledgements

Not applicable.

Funding

No funding.

Author's contributions

GB participated in conception and design creation, collection and interpretation of data, drafting the manuscript. ES participated in conception and design creation, collection and interpretation of data, drafting the manuscript and revising it critically for important intellectual content and final approval of the manuscript submission. JC participated in conception and design creation, collection and interpretation of data, drafting the manuscript and revising it critically for important intellectual content. GZ participated in analysis and interpretation of data, drafting the manuscript. IB participated in analysis and interpretation of data, drafting the manuscript. BP participated in analysis and interpretation of data, drafting the manuscript. PS participated in analysis and interpretation of data, drafting the manuscript. AL participated in conception and design creation, analysis and interpretation of data, drafting the manuscript and revising it critically for important intellectual content and final approval of the manuscript submission. AL participated in analysis and interpretation of data, drafting the manuscript and revising it critically for important intellectual content and final approval of the manuscript submission. All authors read and approved the final manuscript.

Competing interests

GB has received investigator fees from Sanofi and Janssen Research; has received travel fee from Servier; has received research support from Medispec (applicators for study NCT02339454). ES has received consulting fee and research support from Medispec (applicators for study NCT02339454); has received speaker fee from Servier, GE Healthcare; has received investigator fees from Servier and Bayer. JC is a member of advisory board for Novartis; has received investigator fees from Amgen and Servier; has received research support from Medispec (applicators for study NCT02339454). GZ has received travel fee from Servier; has received research support from Medispec for Cardiac Shock wave study. IB has received investigator fee from Bioventrix. BP is a member of steering committee for Novartis and Janssen Research; has received speaker fees from Remedica, Astra Zeneca, Pfizer, Bayer and Beohringer-Ingelheim. PS has no competing interest. AL is a member of steering committee for Servier and Sanofi; has received research support from Medispec for Cardiac Shock wave study. AL has no competing interest.

Author details

[1]Clinic of Cardiac and Vascular Diseases, Faculty of Medicine, Vilnius University, Vilnius, Lithuania. [2]Centre of Cardiology and Angiology, Vilnius University Hospital Santariskiu Klinikos, Vilnius, Lithuania. [3]Moscow State University of Medicine and Dentistry, Moscow, Russia. [4]Yale- New Haven Health Bridgeport Hospital, Connecticut, United States of America. [5]Centre of Innovative Medicine, Vilnius, Lithuania. [6]Division of Cardiovascular Diseases, Mayo Clinic, Rochester, Minnesota, United States of America. [7]Room No A311, Santariskiu str. 2, 08661 Vilnius, Lithuania.

References

1. Williams B, Menon M, Satran D, Hayward D, Hodges JS, Burke MN, et al. Patients with coronary artery disease not amenable to traditional revascularization: prevalence and 3-year mortality. Catheter Cardiovasc Interv. 2010;75:886–91.
2. McGillion M, Arthur H, Cook A, Carroll SL, Victor JC, L'allier PL, et al. Management of patients with refractory angina: Canadian Cardiovascular Society/Canadian Pain Society Joint Guidelines. Can J Cardiol. 2012;28:S20–41.
3. Henry TD. A new option for the "no-option" patient with refractory angina? Catheter Cardiovasc Interv. 2009;74:395–7.
4. Henry TD, Satran D, Hodges JS, Johnson RK, Poulose AK, Campbell AR, et al. Long-term survival in patients with refractory angina. Eur Heart J. 2013;34:2683–8.
5. Briones E, Lacalle JR, Marin I. Transmyocardial laser revascularization versus medical therapy for refractory angina. Cohrane Database Syst Rev. 2009;1, CD003712.
6. Oesterele SN, Sanborn TA, Ali N, Resar J, Ramee SR, Heuser R, et al. Percutaneus transmyocardial laser revascularization for severe angina: the PACIFIC randomized trial. Potential class improvement from intramyocardial channels. Lancet. 2000;356:1705–10.
7. Salem M, Rotevatn S, Nordrehaug JE. Long-term results following percutaneous myocardial laser therapy. Coron Artery Dis. 2006;17:385–90.
8. Taylor RS, De Vries J, Bucher E, Dejongste MJ. Spinal cord stimulation in the treatment of refrctory angina: systematic review and metaanalysis of randomised controlled trials. BMC Cardiovasc Disord. 2009;9:13.
9. Van Ramshorst J, Bax JJ, SI B, Dibbets-Schneider P, Roes SD, Stokkel MP, et al. Intramyocardial bone marrow cell injection for chronic myocardial ischemia: a randomised controlled trial. JAMA. 2009;301:1997–2004.
10. Assmus B, Schachinger V, Teupe C, Britten M, Lehmann R, Döbert N, et al. Transplantation of Progenitor Cells and Regeneration Enhancement in Acute Myocardial Infarction (TOPCARE-AMI). Circulation. 2002;106:3009–17.

11. Wollert KC, Meyer GP, Lotz J, Ringes-Lichtenberg S, Lippolt P, Breidenbach C, et al. Intracoronary autologous bone-marrow cell transfer after myocardial infarction: the BOOST randomised controlled clinical trial. Lancet. 2004;364:141–8.

12. Loh PH, Cleland JG, Louis AA, Kennard ED, Cook JF, Caplin JL, et al. Enhanced external counterpulsation in the treatment of chronic refractory angina: A long-term follow-up outcome from the international enhanced external counterpulsation patient registry. ClinCardiol. 2008;31:159–64.

13. Kumar A, Aronow WS, Vadnerkar A, Sindhu P, Mittal S, Kasliwal RR, et al. Effect of enhanced external counterpulsation on clinical symptoms, quality of life, 6-min walking distance, and echocardiographic measurements of left ventricular systolic and diastolic function after 35 days of treatment and at 1-year follow up in 47 patients with chronic refractory angina pectoris. Am J Ther. 2009;16:116–8.

14. Nishida T, Shimokawa H, Oi K, Tatewaki H, Uwatoku T, Abe K, et al. Extracorporeal cardiac shock wave therapy markedly ameliorates ischemia-induced myocardial dysfunction in pigs in vivo. Circulation. 2004;110:3055–61.

15. Fu M, Sun CK, Lin YC, Wang CJ, Wu CJ, Ko SF, et al. Extracorporeal shock wave therapy reverses ischemia-related left ventricular dysfunction and remodeling: molecular-cellular and functional assessment. PLoS One. 2011;6, e24342.

16. Young SR, Dyson M. The effect of therapeutic ultrasound on angiogenesis. Ultrasound Med Biol. 1990;16:261–9.

17. Wang CJ, Huang HY, Pai CH. Shock wave-enhanced neovascularization at the tendon-bone junction: an experiment in dogs. J Foot Ankle Surg. 2002;41:16–22.

18. Song J, Qi M, Kaul S, Price RJ. Stimulation of arteriogenesis in skeletal muscle by microbuble destruction with ultrasound. Circulation. 2002;106:1550–5.

19. Caspari GH, Erbel R. Revascularization with extracorporeal shock wave therapy: first clinical results. Circulation. 1999;100 Suppl 18:84–9.

20. Moher D, Liberati A, Tetzlaff J, Altman DG, The PRISMA Group. Preferred reporting items for systematic reviews and meta- analyses: the PRISMA statement. PLoS Med. 2009;6(7), e1000097. doi:10.1371/journal.pmed. 1000097.

21. Higgins JPT, Altman DG, Gøtzsche PC, Jüni P, Moher D, Oxman A, on behalf of Cochrane Bias Methods Group; Cochrane Statistical Methods Group, et al. The Cochrane Collaboration's tool for assessing risk of bias in randomized trials. BMJ. 2011;343:d5928.

22. Cohen J. Statistical power analysis for the behavioral sciences. 2nd ed. New Jersey: Lawrence Erlbaum; 1988. p. 567.

23. 2014 Review Manager (RevMan) [Computer program]. Version 5.3. Copenhagen: The Nordic Cochrane Centre, The Cochrane Collaboration. http://community. cochrane.org/tools/review-production-tools/revman-5/about.

24. Wang Y, Guo T, Ma T, Cai H, Tao S, Peng Y, et al. A modified regimen of extracorporeal cardiac shock wave therapy for treatment of coronary artery disease. Cardiovasc Ultrasound. 2012;10:35.

25. Vasyuk Y, Hadzegova A, Shkolnik E, Kopeleva M, Krikunova O, Iouchtchouk E, et al. Initial clinical experience with extracorporeal shock wave therapy in treatment of ischemic heart failure. Congest Heart Fail. 2010;16:226–30.

26. Peng YZ, Guo T, Yang P, Yang HW, Zhou P, Wang Y, et al. Effects of extracorporeal cardiac shock wave therapy in patients with ischemic heart failure. Zhonghua Xin Xue Guan Bing Za Zhi. 2012;40:141–6.

27. Cassar A, Prasad M, Rodriguez-Porcel M, Reeder GS, Karia D, DeMaria AN, et al. Safety and efficacy of extracorporeal shock wave myocardial revascularization therapy for refractory angina pectoris. Mayo Clin Proc. 2014;89:346–54.

28. Takayama T, Saito S, Hirayama A, Honye J, Chiku M, Yoda T, et al. Investigation into effectiveness of Shock Wave treatment for Angina Pectoris patients post-bypass surgery. Eur Heart J. 2008;29:200.

29. Gabrusenko S, Malakhov V, Shitov V, Sankova A, Sergienko V, Masenko V, et al. An experience of the use of a curative metod of cardiac shock wave therapy in patients with ischemic heart disease. Kardiologiya. 2013;53:20–6.

30. Cai HY, Li L, Guo T, Wang Y, Ma TK, Xiao JM, et al. Cardiac shockwave therapy improves myocardial function in patients with refractory coronary artery disease by promoting VEGF and IL-8 secretion to mediate the proliferation of endothelial progenitor cells. Exp Ther Med. 2015;10:2410–6.

31. Kikuchi Y, Ito K, Ito Y, Shiroto T, Tsuburaya R, Aizawa K, et al. Double-blind and placebo-controlled study of the effectiveness and safety of extracorporeal cardiac shock wave therapy for severe angina pectoris. Circ J. 2010;74:589 -91.

32. Ruiz-Garcia J, Lerman A. Cardiac shock-wave therapy in the treatment of refractive angina pectoris. Interv Cardiol. 2011;3(2):191-201.

33. Wang J, Zhou C, Liu L, Pan X, Guo T. Clinical effect of cardiac shock wave therapy on patients with ischemic heart disease: a systematic review and meta-analysis. Eur J Clin Invest. 2015;45(12):1270–85.

34. Chaussy C, Brendel W, Schmiedt E. Extracorporeally induced destruction of kidney stones by shock waves. Lancet. 1980;2:1265–8.

35. Turk C, Knoll T, Petrik A, Sarica K, Skolarikos A, Straub M, Seitz C. European Association of Urology, Guidelines on Urolithiasis. 2015. p. 1–71.

36. Tandan M, Reddy DN, Santosh D, Reddy V, Koppuju V, Lakhtakia S, et al. Extracorporeal shock wave lithotripsy of large difficult common bile duct stones: efficacy and analysis of factors that favour stone fragmentation. J Gastroenterol Hepatol. 2009;24:1370–4.

37. Parsi MA, Stevens T, Lopez R, Vargo JJ. Extracorporeal shock wave lithotripsy for prevention of recurrent pancreatitis caused by obstructive pancreatic stones. Pancreas. 2010;39:153–5.

38. Capaccio P, Torreta S, Pignataro L. Extracorporeal lithotripsy techniques for salivary stones. Otorungol Clin North Am. 2009;42:1139–59.

39. Zelle BA, Gollwitzer H, Zlowodzki M, Buhren V. Extracorporeal shock wave therapy:current evidence. J Orthop Trauma. 2010;24 Suppl 1:S66–70.

40. Wang CJ, Cheng JH, Kuo YR, Schaden W, Mittermayr R. Extracorporeal shockwave therapy in diabetic foot ulcers. Int J Surg. 2015. doi:10.1016/j.ijsu. 2015.06.024.

41. Vahdatpour B, Alizadeh F, Moayednia A, Emadi M, Khorami MH, Haghdani S. Efficacy of extracorporeal shock wave therapy for the treatment of chronic pelvic pain syndrome: a randomized, controlled trial. ISRN Urology. 2013: 972601. doi: 10.1155/2013/972601..

42. Maisonhaute E, Prado C, White PC, Compton RG. Surface acoustic cavitation understood via nanosecond electrochemistry. Part III: shear stress in ultrasonic cleaning. Ultrason Sonochem. 2002;9:297–303.

43. Ito Y, Ito K, Shiroto T, Tsuburaya YGJ, Takeda M, et al. Cardiac shock wave therapy ameliorates left ventricular remodeling after myocardial ischemia-reperfusion injury in pigs in vivo. Coron Artery Dis. 2010;21:304–11.

44. Gotte G, Amelio E, Russo S, Marlinghaus E, Musci G, Suzuki H. Short-time non-enzmatic nitric oxide synthesis from L-arginine and hydrogen peroxide induced by shock waves treatment. FEBS Lett. 2002;520:153–5.

45. Mariotto S, Cavalieri E, Amelio E, Ciampa AR, de Prati AC, Marlinghaus E, et al. Extracorporeal shock waves: from lithotripsy to anti-inflamatory action by NO production. Nitric Oxide. 2005;12:89–96.

46. Mariotto S, de Prati AC, Cavalieri E, Amelio E, Marlinghaus E, Suzuki H. Extracorporeal shock wave therapy in inflammatory diseases: molecular mechanism that triggers anti-inflammatory action. Curr Med Chem. 2009;16:2366–72.

47. Yip JK, Chang LT, Sun CK, Youssef AA, Sheu JJ, Wang CJ. Shock wave therapy applied to rat bone marrow-derived mononuclear cells enhances formation of cells stained positive for CD31 and vascular endothelial growth factor. Circ J. 2008;72:150–6.

48. Ciampa AR, de Prati AC, Amelio E, Cavalieri E, Persichini T, Colasanti M, et al. Nitric oxide mediates anti-inflammatory action of extracorporeal shock waves. FEBS Lett. 2005;579:6839–45.

49. Kaller M, Faber L, Bogunovic N, Horstkotte D, Burchert W, Lindner O. Cardiac shock wave therapy and myocardial perfusion in severe coronary artery disease. Clin Res Cardiol. 2015;104(10):843–9.

50. Zuoziene G, Laucevicius A, Leibowitz D. Extracorporeal shockwave myocardial revascularization improves clinical symptoms and left ventricular function in patients with refractory angina. Coron Artery Dis. 2012;23:62–7.

51. Gutersohn A, Caspari G, Erbel R. Cardiac shock wave therapy: new option for endstage cardiovascular disease. Atherosclerosis Suppl. 2003;4(2):3P-0626.

52. Gutersohn A, Caspari G, Erbel R. Autoangiogenesis induced by Cardiac Shock Wave Therapy (CSWT) increases perfusion and exersice tolerance in endstage CAD patients with refractory angina. Presented at the 69th Annual Scientific Meeting of the Japanese Circulation Society 2005.

53. Gutersohn A, Caspari G, Erbel R. Short and long term clinical improvement in patients with refractory angina using Cardiac Shock Wave Therapy (CSWT). Presented at the ACC 2006.

54. Fukumoto Y, Ito A, Uwatoku T, Matoba T, Kishi T, Takeshita A, et al. Extracorporeal cardiac shock wave therapy ameliorates myocardial ischemia in patients with severe coronary artery disease. Coron Artery Dis. 2006;17(1):63–70.

55. Lyadov K, Uvarov A. Cardiac shock-wave therapy: First Experience. Presented at the 6th Mediterranean congress of PRM. 2006;181–2.

56. Naber C, Ebralidze T, Lammers S, Hakim G, Erbel R. Non invasive cardiac angiogenesis shock wave therapy increases perfusion and exercise tolerance in endstage CAD patients. Eur J Heart Fail. 2007;7:71.

57. Khattab A, Brodersen B, Schuermann-Kuchenbrandt D, Beurich H, Tölg R, Geist V, et al. Extracorporeal cardiac shock wave therapy: First experience in the everyday practice for treatment of chronic refractory angina pectoris. Int J Cardiol. 2007;121(1):84–5.

58. Naber C, Lammers S, Lind T, Müller N, Hakim G, Erbel R. Safety and efficacy of extracorporeal low energy shockwave application for the treatment of refractory angina pectoris and myocardial ischemia in patients with end-stage coronary artery disease. Medispec. 2008;1–16.

59. Wang Y, Guo T, Cai HY, Ma TK, Tao SM, Sun S, et al. Cardiac shock wave therapy reduces angina and improves myocardial function in patients with refractory coronary artery disease. Clin Cardiol. 2010;33:693–9.

60. Faber L, Lindner O, Prinz C, Fricke E, Hering D, Burchert W, et al. Echo-guided extracorporeal shock wave therapy for refractory angina improves regional myocardial blood flow as assessed by PET imaging. J Am Coll Cardiol. 2010;55(10A):A120.

61. Vainer J, Habets J, Lousberg A, Brans B, Schalla S, Waltenberger J. Cardiac shockwave therapy in patients with end-stage coronary artery disease and chronic refractory angina pectoris – mid term results. Eur Heart J. 2010;31(Abstract Supplement):198.

62. Alunni G, D'amico M, Meynet I, Andriani M, Giraudi E, Giorgi M, et al. A new treatment for patients with refractory angina: extracorporeal shockwave myocardial revascularization. Eur Heart J. 2011;32(Abstract Supplement):575.

63. Vainer J, Habets J, De Pont C, Lousberg A, Schalla S, Brans B, et al. Extracorporeal shockwave myocardial revascularization therapy (ESMR): an alternative for patients with end-stage coronary artery disease and chronic refractory angina pectoris? Eur Heart J. 2012;33(Abstract Supplement):782.

64. Alunni G, Meynet I, D'Amico M, Garrone P, Checco L, Marra S. Extracorporeal shockwave myocardial revascularization: a promising therapy for refractory angina. Cardiology. 2013;126 Suppl 2:390.

65. Zuoziene G. Evaluation of myocardium revascularization y cardiac shock wave therapy applying multimodal image analysis. Summary of doctoral dissertation. Vilnius University, 2013

66. Prinz C, Faber L, Lindner O, Bogunovic N, Hering D, Burchert D, et al. Echo-guided extracorporeal shock wave therapy for refractory angina improves regional myocardial blood flow as assessed by PET imaging. Eur Heart J. 2013;34 suppl 1:4007.

67. Faber L, Prinz C, Lindner O, Bogunovic N, Hering D, Burchert D, et al. Echo-guided extracorporeal shock wave therapy for refractory angina improves regional left ventricular function along with myocardial blood flow. Eur Heart J. 2014;35(Abstract Supplement):658.

68. Prasad M, Wan Ahmad WA, Sukmawan R, Magsombol EB, Cassar A, Vinshtok J, et al. Extracorporeal shockwave myocardial therapy is efficacious in improving symptoms in patients with refractory angina pectoris – a multicenter study. Coron Artery Dis. 2015;26:194–200.

69. Liu BY, Li WC, Zhang RS, Chen CX, Yao ZM, He Q. Application of extracorporeal cardiac shock wave therapy in treating coronary heart disease in the elderly. J Am Geriatr Soc. 2015;63:S408.

70. Vainer J, Habets JHM, Schalla S, Lousberg AHP, dePont CDJM, Voo SA, et al. Cardiac shockwave therapy in patients with chronic refractory angina pectoris. Neth Heart J. 2016;24:343–9.

71. Kazmi WH, Rasheed SZ, Ahmed S, Saadat M, Altaf S, Samad A. Noninvasive therapy for the management of patients with advanced coronary artery disease. Coron Artery Dis. 2012;23:549–54.

72. Alunni G, Marra S, Meynet I, D'amico M, Elisa P, Fanelli A, et al. The beneficial effect of extracorporeal shockwave myocardial revascularization in patients with refractory angina. Cardiovasc Revasc Med. 2015;16:6–11.

73. Nirala S, Wang Y, Peng YZ, Yang P, Guo T. Cardiac shock wave therapy shows better outcomes in the coronary artery disease patients in a long term. Eur Rev Med Pharmacol Sci. 2016;20:330–8.

74. Zhao L, Yang P, Tang Y, Li R, Peng Y, Wang Y, et al. Effect of cardiac shock wave therapy on the microvolt T wave alternans of patients with coronary artery disease. Int J Clin Exp Med. 2015;8:16463–71.

75. Schmid JP, Capoferri M, Schepis T, Siegrist P, Schroeder V, Kaufmann P, et al. Extracorporeal shock wave for therapy of refractory angina pectoris: the shock trial. Presented at the American College of Cardiology 55th Annual Scientific Session 2006.

76. Yang P, Peng Y, Guo T, Wang Y, Cai H, Zhou P. A clinical study of the extracorporeal cardiac shock wave therapy for coronary artery disease. Heart. 2012;98 Suppl 2:E163–4.

77. Leibowitz D, Weiss AT, Rott D, Durst R, Lotan C. The efficacy of cardiac shock wave therapy in the treatment of refractory angina: a pilot prospective, randomized, double-blind trial. Int J Cardiol. 2013;167:3033–4.

78. Schmid JP, Capoferri, Wahl A, Eshtehardi P, Hess OM. Cardiac shock wave therapy for chronic refractory angina pectoris. a prospective placebo-controlled randomized trial. Cardiovasc Ther. 2013;31:e1–6.

79. Yang P, Guo T, Wang W, Peng YZ, Wang Y, Zhou P, et al. Randomized and double-blind controlled clinical trial of extracorporeal cardiac shock wave therapy for coronary heart disease. Heart Vessels. 2013;28:284–91.

16

Modified mallampati classification in determining the success of unsedated transesophageal echocardiography procedure in patients with heart disease: simple but efficient

Jureerat Khongkaew[1*], Dujdao Sahasthas[2], Tharrittawadha Potat[1] and Phatchara Thammawirat[1]

Abstract

Background: The transesophageal echocardiograhpy (TEE) has been studied worldwide. However, identifying additional factors on top of operator's experience and patient's cooperation which could influence the success of the procedure in unsedated patients with heart disease is not well documented.

Methods: Under the cross-sectional descriptive design, 85 target patients were fulfilling the criteria: being Thai national at the age of at least 20-year-old, being performed TEE by the study participant's cardiologists, being able to communicate verbally. Seven outcomes were recorded, including gag reflex, insertion attempt, insertion time, vital signs (heart rate, oxygen saturation and mean arterial blood pressure), visible blood on TEE probe tip, and oropharyngeal pain at 1 h and 24-h.

Results: There were 85 eligible patients during June 2013 to June 2014. The major participants were male (46, 54 %) and the mean age was 51.2 ± 12.5 years. The MMC class III was mostly found (33, 38.80 %). TEE probe insertion time and gag reflex were indicated statistical significance ($P < 0.05$). Linear regression revealed that MMC class III (b 3.718; SD $\pm$ 1.077; $P = 0.001$) and class IV (b 5.15; SD $\pm$ 1.286; $P = 0.000$) were statistically associated with TEE probe insertion time, whereas MMC class II was no statistically significant (b 2.348; SD $\pm$ 1.405; $P = 0.099$) according to constant value in MMC class I (5.318 s). Similarly, logistic regression indicated that the patients with high grade MMC were more likely to have gagging than the low grade MMC patients (MMC 2 OR 0.567, 95 % CI 0.09–3.42, $P = 0.536$; MMC 3 OR 5.231, 95 % CI 1.55–17.67, $P = 0.008$; MMC 4 OR 3.4, 95 % CI 0.84–13.76, $P = 0.086$).

Conclusions: Modified Mallampati Classification is one of determining factors in the success of unsedated TEE procedure in patients with heart disease, especially for assessment of gagging and successful TEE probe insertion time.

Keywords: Modified Mallampati Classification, Unsedated transesophageal echocardiography, Heart disease patient

Background

In the non-invasive cardiac diagnostic settings worldwide, a transesophageal echocardiography (TEE) can be performed with or without conscious sedation. According to the guidelines for performing a TEE, the procedure is well tolerated by an unsedated patient who is adequately given oral anaesthesia [1]. Comparing with a sedated TEE, the unsedated patients show a lower incidence of cardiopulmonary complications and also receive more in benefit in terms of recovery time and medical care cost [1, 2]. However, performing a TEE without sedation requires a well cooperative patient since the procedure can easily injure organs, including lips, teeth, oropharynx, larynx, esophagus and stomach [3, 4]. In addition, the patients who show gagging during the procedure tend to have more oropharygeal injury than the absent gagging group [5, 6].

---

* Correspondence: jureerat2545@hotmail.com
[1]Queen Sirikit Heart Center of the Northeast, Faculty of Medicine, Khon Kaen University, Khon Kaen, Thailand
Full list of author information is available at the end of the article

As gagging is a significant obstacle to succeed in performing an unsedated TEE, oropharynx assessment should be considered as an important process. However, previous studies mention that only operator's experience and patient's cooperation are the two influencing factors [1, 4]. In the field of gastrointestology, Huang, et al. compare the tolerance in esophagogastroduodenoscopy (EGD) among the patients based on Modified Mallampati Classification (MMC) [6]. The result clearly shows that the patients with MMC class III and class IV mostly present gagging during the procedure which leads the patient to be intolerant and be given sedation. Also, in the field of anaesthesiology, the MMC has been accepted as one of the factors affecting a successful endotracheal tube intubation [7–9]. Focusing on the field of cardiology, there is a lack of data supporting the correlation between MMC and the TEE outcomes. Even though TEE probe insertion is technically easier than endotracheal tube intubation, some complications can occur since the long probe has to be passed oropharynx before being inserted into the esophagus. From this point of view, our present study aims to identify additional factors on top of operator experience and patient co-operation which can influence the success of a TEE procedure in unsedated patients with heart disease.

Methods
Population
This study was approved by the Human Research Ethics Committee of Khon Kaen University, Thailand. The patients who were considered for the study's inclusion would meet specific criteria, including being a Thai national at the age of 20-year-old or more, being performed the TEE by the participant's cardiologist, being able to communicate verbally in Thai language, and willing to have the unsedated TEE as well as willing to be the study's participant. The excluded patients were those younger than 20-year-old, unwilling to have the unsedated TEE and to participate in the study, incomplete informed consent form, unable to communicate verbally in Thai language, having a history of dysphagia or bleeding disorder, undergoing oropharyngeal surgery, unable to be assessed MMC, and being given sedation before or during the procedure.

Data collection
The data was collected using the specific form, consisted of three significant parts: demographic data, factors involving TEE procedure, and the seven TEE outcomes (insertion attempt, successful insertion time, gag reflex during insertion, vital signs' change, oropharyngeal pain at 1-h and 24-h, and visible blood on probe tip). Initially, the informed consent form must be completed. Throughout the procedure, neither the cardiologists

together with the two collecting data nurses nor the patient themselves knew the patient's MMC class, except the two well-trained MMC assessment nurse who graded patients' MMC class using the MMC chart as shown in Fig. 1.

According to our hospital TEE preparation, the patient would be orally anaesthetized receiving lidocaine (Astra Zeneca) both 10 % spray and 2 % jelly. With a total safe dosage of less than 400 mg [10], 150 mg of lidocaine jelly was orally given to the patient twice; the second dose was administered five minutes following the first. The patient would be then evaluated the gag reflex and would be given 2 more puffs (20 mg) of lidocaine spray if gagging was presented. When the oropharyngeal preparation was completed, the patient was placed in left lateral decubitus position.

Before TEE probe insertion, a bite guard was already put in place. While the patient was lying in the specific position under the safety setting, the operator gently entered a lubricated TEE probe (model GE 6Tc) into the patient oral cavity. Once the probe being passed through the patient' mouth until being placed into the esophagus, presented gagging, vital signs, successful TEE probe insertion time and attempt were noted in agreement of the two collecting data nurses.

After the procedure had been completed, the transducer was slowly pulled out of the patient mouth and was placed on a white towel in order to evaluate blood on the transducer tip. The patient vital signs were continuously monitored for 30 min. Oropharyngeal pain at 1 h and 24-h were assessed by means of a phone call asking the patient to state a 0–10 oropharyngeal pain score, adapted from visual analog scale (VAS) as shown in Fig. 2.

Definition of terms

1. Patient's cooperation refers to a willingness to have unsedated TEE procedure which is evaluated by observation of the patient's compliance with topical anaesthesic agent given and facial expression. The criteria are below.
   1.1 Excellent cooperation is rated for the patient who shows smiling face and truly willingness to be anaesthetized for the unsedated TEE procedure.
   1.2 Good cooperation is described as the patient presents with neutral face and actions.
   1.3 Poor cooperation refers to the patient showing unhappy face and being difficult to give topical anaesthesic agent.
2. Insertion attempt means the number of attempt to insert the TEE probe into the patient's esophagus successfully.

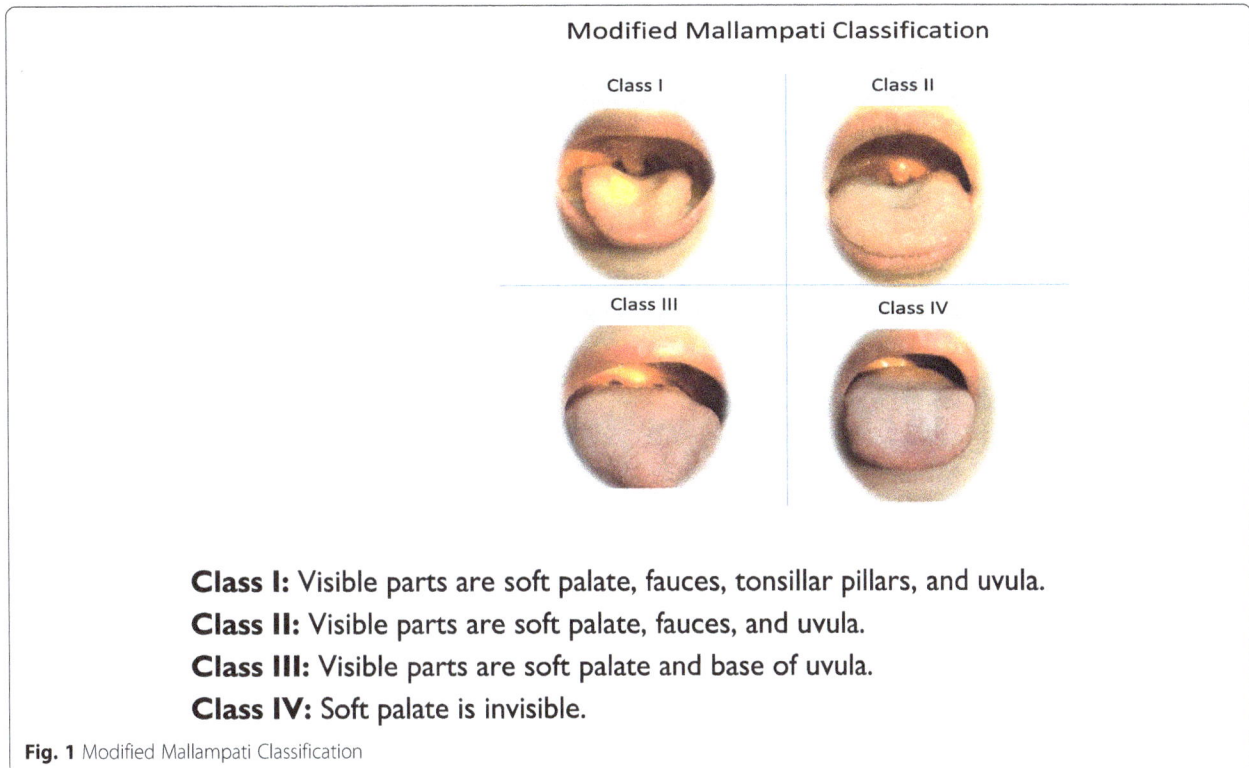

Modified Mallampati Classification

Class I   Class II

Class III   Class IV

Class I: Visible parts are soft palate, fauces, tonsillar pillars, and uvula.

Class II: Visible parts are soft palate, fauces, and uvula.

Class III: Visible parts are soft palate and base of uvula.

Class IV: Soft palate is invisible.

Fig. 1 Modified Mallampati Classification

3. Successful probe insertion time refers to the specific time when the TEE probe can be in place.
4. Gag reflex during insertion refers to a gagging which is stimulated by the touching of the TEE probe on the patient's oropharynx before being placed into the esophagus.
5. Vital signs' change is noted if there is a decrease of oxygen saturation less than 90 % or a 20 % change of either heart rate (HR) or mean arterial pressure (MAP).

Statistical analysis

The raw data was analyzed using SPSS for windows version 17.0. The continuous data were presented as mean ± standard deviation (SD) while all categorical data were shown as absolute number and percentage (%). The difference and correlation between the MMC and seven related variables (insertion attempt, successful probe insertion time, gag reflex, vital signs' change, visible blood on probe tip, and oropharyngeal pain score at 1-h and at 24- h) were analyzed using one-way ANOVA and simple linear regression analysis for continuous data, whereas chi square and logistic regression analysis were used for analyzing categorical variables. P value < 0.05 was considered as statistic significant.

Results

Patient's demographic characteristics

Throughout a year (June 2013-June 2014), a total of 147 heart disease patients underwent the TEE procedure at Queen Sirikit Heart Center of the Northeast, Faculty of Medicine, Khon Kaen University. There were 86 patients who met the study inclusion criteria. Only one case was excluded due to left jaw pain which affected mouth opening. Out of 85 eligible patients, most of them were

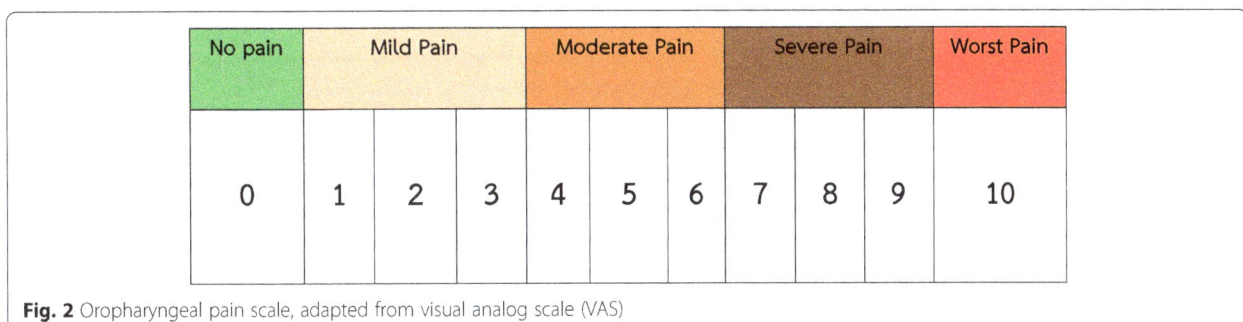

No pain	Mild Pain			Moderate Pain			Severe Pain			Worst Pain
0	1	2	3	4	5	6	7	8	9	10

Fig. 2 Oropharyngeal pain scale, adapted from visual analog scale (VAS)

male (46, 54 %). The mean age and BMI were 51.2 ± 12.48 and 23.95 ± 4.72, respectively. Sixty-one patients (71.8 %) had no experience with the TEE, but showed good cooperation (59, 64.40 %). Also, nearly half of them took anticoagulant medications (42, 49.40 %). MMC class III was the most presented class (33, 38.80 %) and was mostly found in women (20, 60.6 %). All parameters are shown in Table 1.

Comparison of TEE outcomes among the patients based on MMC

Out of the seven outcomes, only the gag reflex and the successful TEE probe insertion time indicated statistical significance ($P = 0.005$). Among the four groups, the patient with MMC class III (20, 60.6 %) and MMC IV (8, 50.0 %) were the first two group which mostly presented gagging while the less presented gagging were the patients with MMC class I (5, 22.7 %) and class II (2, 14.3 %). Similar to gag reflex, the patients with MMC class III and class IV (9.04 ± 3.72, 10.48 ± 6.53) had longer successful insertion time than the patients with MMC class I and class II (5.32 ± 1.67, 7.67 ± 2.50). Contrary to the insertion attempt, although MMC class IV showed the highest number of attempt (1.38 ± 1.09), the differences number of attempt among MMC classes showed no statistical significance ($P = 0.133$).

Focusing on the vital signs' change, there was no statistically significant difference between MMC and each of the three vital signs, including mean arterial pressure (MAP), heart rate (HR), and oxygen saturation (O2sat). However, the percentage of HR change was increased in each higher MMC classes as follows: MMC class I was 36.36 %, MMC class II was 42.90 %, MMC class III was 45.45 % and MMC class IV was 56.25 %. Also, the MAP in the patients with MMC class III (6, 18.18 %) and MMC class IV (5, 31.25 %) showed higher percentages than the patients with MMC class I (2, 9.10) and MMC class II (1, 7.14 %) while there was an unremarkable change of the O2sat (≤90 %) throughout the procedure.

The last three outcomes, recorded after pulling the TEE probe out of the patient's mouth were oropharyngeal pain (OP) at 1-h, oropharyngeal pain (OP) at 24-h, and visible blood on probe tip. According to the OP score 0–10, the mean score of both OP at 1 h (1.31 ± 1.23) and 24-h (0.78 ± 1.15) showed mild pain score and no statistically significant difference ($P = 0.086$, $P = 0.950$). Likewise, 21 (24.71 %) patients were found to have blood on probe tip as well as no statistically significant difference ($P = 0.983$). The data are presented in Table 2.

Correlation between the outcomes and the MMC

Having been identified as statistically significant variables, gag reflex and successful TEE probe insertion time were further analyzed using regression analysis.

Table 1 Patient's demographic characteristics

Demographic Characteristics	Total (*n* = 85)	MMC 1 (*n* = 22)	MMC 2 (*n* = 14)	MMC 3 (*n* = 33)	MMC 4 (*n* = 16)
MMC class No. (%)	85 (100)	22 (25.9)	14 (16.5)	33 (38.8)	16 (18.8)
Age (Mean ± SD)	51.20 ± 12.48	48.82 ± 14.53	50.86 ± 10.54	49.12 ± 12.05	59.06 ± 9.33
BMI (Mean ± SD)	23.95 ± 4.72	23.20 ± 3.50	23.20 ± 3.60	24.35 ± 5.40	24.90 ± 5.70
Gender- No. (%)					
Male	46 (54.1)	14 (63.6)	9 (64.3)	13 (39.4)	10 (62.5)
Female	39 (45.9)	8 (36.4)	5 (35.7)	20 (60.6)	6 (37.5)
Education - No. (%)					
Elementary	47 (55.3)	11 (50.0)	8 (57.1)	17 (51.5)	11 (68.8)
High School	18 (21.2)	8 (36.4)	2 (14.3)	7 (21.2)	1 (6.3)
Higher Education	20 (23.5)	3 (13.6)	4 (28.6)	9 (27.3)	4 (25.0)
Previous TEE - No. (%)					
Yes	24 (28.2)	5 (22.7)	4 (28.6)	9 (27.3)	6 (37.5)
No	61 (71.8)	17 (77.3)	10 (71.4)	24 (72.7)	10 (62.5)
Cooperation - No. (%)					
Poor	5 (5.9)	2 (9.1)	1 (7.1)	2 (6.1)	0 (0.0)
Good	59 (69.4)	14 (63.6)	11 (78.6)	26 (78.8)	8 (50.0)
Excellent	21 (24.7)	6 (27.3)	2 (14.3)	5 (15.2)	8 (50.0)
Anticoagulation - No. (%)					
Yes	42 (49.4)	14 (63.6)	4 (28.6)	12 (36.4)	12 (75.0)
No	43 (50.6)	8 (36.4)	10 (71.4)	21 (63.6)	4 (25.0)

Table 2 Comparison of TEE outcomes among Modified Mallampati Classification

Outcomes	Total (n = 85)	MMC 1 (n = 22)	MMC 2 (n = 14)	MMC 3 (n = 33)	MMC 4 (n = 16)	P-value
Gag Reflex - No. (%)	35 (41.18)	5 (22.7)	2 (14.3)	20 (60.6)	8 (50.0)	0.005
Attempt (Mean ± SD)	1.12 ± 0.52	1.14 ± 00.35	1.00 ± 0.00	1.03 ± 0.03	1.38 ± 1.09	0.133
Time (Mean ± SD)	8.13 ± 4.28	5.32 ± 1.67	7.67 ± 2.50	9.04 ± 3.72	10.48 ± 6.53	0.003
Vital Signs' Change						
MAP - No. (%)	14 (16.47)	2 (9.10)	1 (7.14)	6 (18.18)	5 (31.25)	0.224
O2sat - No. (%)	0 (0.0)	0 (0.0)	0 (0.0)	0 (0.0)	0 (0.0)	-
HR - No. (%)	38 (44.71)	8 (36.36)	6 (42.90)	15 (45.45)	9 (56.25)	0.680
Throat Pain Score						
1-h (Mean ± SD)	1.31 ± 1.23	1.09 ± 0.97	1.29 ± 1.54	1.55 ± 1.28	1.13 ± 1.20	0.086
24-h (Mean ± SD)	0.78 ± 1.15	0.64 ± 1.23	0.57 ± 1.02	1.06 ± 1.17	0.56 ± 1.09	0.950
Bleeding - No. (%)	21 (24.71)	5 (22.73)	4 (28.57)	8 (24.24)	4 (25.00)	0.983
Operator A	38 (44.70)	11 (28.95)	5 (13.16)	15 (39.48)	7 (18.43)	
Insertion attempt	1.05 ± 0.23	1.09 ± 0.30	1.00 ± 0.00	1.07 ± 0.26	1.07 ± 0.26	0.810
Insertion time	6.85 ± 2.37	4.82 ± 1.25	7.80 ± 2.59	7.95 ± 2.03	7.00 ± 2.58	0.003
Gag Reflex	16 (42.11)	3 (27.28)	0 (0.0)	10 (66.67)	3 (42.86)	0.039
Bleeding	5 (13.16)	1 (9.09)	1 (20.00)	1 (6.67)	2 (28.58)	0.499
Operator B	47 (55.30)	11 (23.40)	7 (14.90)	20 (42.56)	9 (19.14)	
Insertion Attempt	1.15 ± 0.68	1.18 ± 0.41	1.00 ± 0.00	1.00 ± 0.00	1.67 ± 1.41	0.085
Insertion Time	9.21 ± 5.18	5.82 ± 1.94	7.57 ± 2.64	9.94 ± 4.56	13.18 ± 7.50	00.007
Gag Reflex	22 (48.90)	2 (18.19)	1 (12.50)	13 (72.23)	6 (66.67)	0.004
Bleeding	16 (34.79)	4 (36.37)	3 (37.50)	7 (38.89)	2 (22.23)	0.850

Based on logistic regression, comparing gag reflex between MMC class I and the others, while the patients with MMC class II were indicated non statistical significance (OR 0.567; 95 % CI 0.094–3.423; $P = 0.536$), the high grade MMC such as class III was found to be statistically significant associated with gag reflex during the TEE probe insertion (OR 5.231; 95 % CI 1.548–17.670; $P = 0.008$). Moreover, although the association was no statistically significant, the patients with MMC class IV also had a tendency to have gagging (OR 3.4; 95 % CI 0.840–13.761; $P = 0.086$). The data is shown in Table 3.

Simple linear regression was performed in order to identify the association between successful TEE probe insertion time and the MMC as shown in Table 4. By using the successful time of MMC class I as the constant (5.318 s), the results indicated that the high grade MMC class III (b 3.718; SD ± 1.077; $P = 0.001$) and IV (b 5.15; SD ± 1.286; $P = 0.000$) were statistically significant correlated with the successful TEE probe insertion time, whereas the patients with MMC class II were no statistically significant (b 2.348; SD ± 1.405; $P = 0.099$). The data is shown in Table 4.

Discussion

Based on the study results, the high grade MMC (class III and class IV) was statistically significant associated with the gag reflex and the insertion time. These findings are additional clinical information for performing a TEE since previous studies mention only operator's experience and patient's cooperation as the key success factors [1, 4]. However, one of the most important problems in performing a TEE is insertion of the probe, especially in the unsedated patients.

During the TEE probe insertion, even though topical anaesthetic agent has been applied throughout the oropharynx, gagging still remains in some cases. This physical reaction is induced by the touch of the transducer on any six sensitive oropharyngeal parts, including soft palate, uvula, fauces, posterior pharyngeal wall, back of the tongue and epiglottis [5, 6]. The effect of gagging can cause a failure of the probe insertion or aspiration during the procedure [5]. As reported by Huang, et al., the patients who have gagging are tended to have lower tolerance for esophagogastroduodenoscopy (EGD) than the patients in the opposite group. They also find out that the patients with high grade MMC (classes III and IV) are found to have more gagging than the low grade MMC patients (classes I and II) [6]. In agreement with our results, the patients who presented with MMC class III and class IV had a 5.2–fold and 3.4-fold more gagging than MMC class I patients. This finding was similar to the insertion time which also associated with MMC.

Table 3 Correlation between MMC and gag reflex

MMC	Wald	df	P-value	Exp (B)	95 % CI Lower	95 % CI Upper
MMC 1	11.640	3	0.009	1		
MMC 2	0.383	1	0.536	0.567	0.094	3.423
MMC 3	7.097	1	0.008	5.231	1.548	17.670
MMC 4	2.934	1	0.086	3.400	0.840	13.761
Constant	5.786	1	0.016	0.294		

In reference to our results, the mean time of the fastest probe insertion was 5.32 ± 1.67 s which was found in the group of MMC I while the other three groups of the higher classes showed longer times as in MMC class II was 2.35 ± 2.5 s ($P = 0.099$), MMC class III was 3.72 ± 3.72 s ($P = 0.001$) and MMC class IV was 5.16 ± 6.53 s ($P = 0.000$).

Therefore, according to regression equation, $Y = ax + b$ [11, 12], the successfully inserted time of the patients with MMC class II, class III and class IV are as follows: 7.67 ± 2.5 s, 9.04 ± 3.72 s, and 10.48 ± 6.53 s. Comparing to the another study, there is a lack of data on the TEE probe insertion time, but an approximation is within 1 min [13].

To the best of our knowledge, even though all participants were successfully performed the TEE without sedation, MMC should be considered as one of determining factors affecting the unsedated TEE's outcome since it is related to gagging and probe insertion time. These correlations may be explained using MMC criteria classified by oropharyngeal cavity [14–19]. By the view of fully opened mouth and protruded tongue without any sounds, MMC class III and class IV allow the examiner to see only soft palate and maybe uvular because the size and position of the tongue which are larger and farther than MMC class I and class II [15]. This specific anatomy is an obstacle to performing the TEE because of the compression of the probe which spontaneously creates a direct pressure on the posterior of the tongue leading to a spasm of the pharynx, a natural mechanism of choking prevention [20–23]. Moreover, the narrow oropharyngeal cavity also affects the procedure in terms of difficulty passing the TEE probe into esophagus. For these two reasons, the patients with the narrow oral cavity (MMC class III and class IV) are tended to experience

longer successful insertion time than those who have wider oral cavity (MMC class I and class II).

The other interesting finding was the patients with MMC class III and class IV had a tendency to have oropharyngeal pain at 1 h after the procedure ($P = 0.086$). This result could be explained based on the successful insertion time and gagging which were related to MMC. As mentioned above, the patients with high grade MMC had narrow oral cavity which might be abraded easily on oropharyngeal mucous membrane by the TEE probe during insertion, especially when having gagging. That is, the patients who present more gagging during the TEE procedure are likely to experience more oropharyngeal pain at 1 h after the procedure than others [13, 24, 25]. This finding supports the TEE is not only a safe procedure but also a non-admitted procedure. According to the TEE guideline, an outpatient can be discharged if there is non-serious complication after the procedure [26].

The reduction of gagging during performing endoscopic procedure has been studied worldwide in order to increase patients' tolerance and comfort [17, 18],such as using a micro TEE probe and intra cardiac echocardiography probe (ICE) instead of using a conventional probe [27, 28]. Moreover, Tsuboi et al., claim that performing an unsedated EGD by passing the EGD probe through nasal cavity shows better outcomes than passing through oral cavity [15]. Apart from the equipment and the passage, Ulusoy and Kucukarslan state that the sitting position can help the patient to be successfully inserted the TEE probe [6]. Similar to Samsoon and Young, in the field of anesthesiology, neck flexion and head extension are the two important factors facilitating the operator to successfully intubate endotracheal tube.

However, in a busy non-invasive cardiac testing setting or a non-anesthesiology setting, the TEE may be performed without sedation as well as using the conventional probe and technique. In such a limited resource setting, MMC can be used for a quick assessment of gagging which will be helpful in terms of administrating topical anaesthesia. Moreover, the patients with MMC class III and class IV may need to be placed in a particular position of head and neck instead of placing them on the conventional left lateral decubitus position which focuses only on aspiration prevention [28]. In summary, optimizing the unsedated TEE outcomes, the patients with high grade MMC should be given effective oropharyngeal anaesthesia and be placed in a proper position.

Limitations of the study

The three main points being considered as the study limitations are sample size, other factors affecting gagging, and the subjects' age. First, our data were unavoidably analyzed from a small number of patients from single heart center and the totally unequal subject

Table 4 Association between successful TEE probe insertion time and MMC

MMC	B	SD	Mean + SD	Mean-SD	P-value
Constant	5.318	0.835	6.02	4.35	0.000
MMC 2	2.348	1.405	3.76	0.90	00.099
MMC 3	3.718	1.077	4.80	2.65	0.001
MMC 4	5.517	1.286	6.45	3.88	0.000

numbers in each group. Further study may need to investigate in a larger sample size. Next, the other factors affecting gaging apart from the MMC were not included in the study protocol. These factors may also affect gagging during TEE probe insertion in the patients with MMC classes I and II. Last, our results might not be generally used as a reference for the heart disease patients of all ages because most participants were middle aged and cooperative.

Conclusion

Our study demonstrates that MMC is positively associated with the successful TEE probe insertion time. Moreover, the high grade MMC patients (MMC class III and class IV) are found to be correlated with gagging during the TEE probe insertion and found to have a tendency toward oropharyngeal pain at 1 h after the TEE. From these reasons, MMC should be considered as one of determining factors in the success of unsedated TEE procedure in the patients with heart disease. Therefore, in order to optimize unsedated TEE outcomes, the patients should be assessed MMC which will benefit in terms of administrating topical anaesthesia.

Abbreviations

EGD: Esophagogastroduodenoscopy; HR: Heart rate; ICE: Intra cardiac echocardiography probe; MAP: Mean arterial pressure; MMC: Modified mallampati classification; SD: Standard deviation; TEE: Transesophageal echocardiography; TN-EGD: Transnasal esophagogastroduodenoscopy; TO-EGD: Ransoral esophagogastroduodenoscopy

Acknowledgments

Not applicable.

Funding

Queen Sirikit Heart Center of the Northeast Faculty of Medicine Khon Kaen University.

Authors' contributions

Miss JK carried out the study, participated in the design of the study and performed the statistical analysis, participated in the sequence alignment and drafted the manuscript. Dr. DS was the study consultant. Mrs. TP participated in the sequence alignment. Mrs. PT conceived of the study, and participated in its design and coordination. All authors read and approved the final manuscript.

Competing interests

The authors declare that we have no competing interests.

Author details

[1]Queen Sirikit Heart Center of the Northeast, Faculty of Medicine, Khon Kaen University, Khon Kaen, Thailand. [2]Division of Cardiology, Department of Medicine, Khon Kaen University, Khon Kaen, Thailand.

References

1. Khalid O, Srivastava R, Mulhall A, Paladugu A, Stoddard M, Lippmann S. Conscious sedation: for a TEE, is it always required? Echocardiography. 2010; 27(1):74–6.
2. Daniel WG, Erbel R, Kasper W, Visser CA, Engberding R, Sutherland GR, et al. Safety of transesophageal echocardiography: A multicenter survey of 10,419 examinations. Circ. 1991;83:817–21.
3. Mathur KS, Singh P. Transesophageal echocardiography related complications. Indian J Anaesth. 2009;53:567–74.
4. Kallmeyer JI, Collard CD, Fox JA, Body SC, Sherman SI. The safety of intraoperative transesophageal echocardiography: A case series of 7200 cardiac surgical patients. Anesth Analg. 2001;92:1126–30.
5. Hilberath JN, Oakes DA, Shernan SK, Bulwer BE, D'Ambra MN, Eltzschig HK. Safety of transesophagealechocardiography: Comprehensive review. J Am Soc Echocardiogr. 2010;23:1115–27.
6. Ulusoy ER, Kucukarslan N. Novel intubation technique for transesophageal echocardiography examination. Eur J Echocardiogr. 2009;10:227–8.
7. Huang HH, Lee MS, Shih YL, Chu HC, Huang TY, Hsieh TY. Modified mallampati classification as a clinical predictor of peroral esophagogastroduodenoscopy tolerance. BMC Gastroenterol. 2011;11:1–7.
8. Berkow CL. Strategies for airway management. Best Pract Res Clin Anaesthesiol. 2004;18:531–48.
9. Adamus M, Fritscherovaa S, Hrabalekb L, Gabrhelika T, Zapletalovac J, Janoutd V. Mallampati test as a predictor of laryngoscopic view. Biomed Pap Med Fac Univ Palacky Olomouc Czech Repub. 2010;154: 339–44.
10. Marchiondo K. Tranesophageal and interventions: Nursing implications. Crit Care Nurse. 2007;27:25–35.
11. Flynn AJ, Choi JM, Wooster DL. Oxford American Handbook of Clinical Medicine. USA: Oxford University Press; 2013. p. 719.
12. Crawley MJ. Statistics: an introduction using R. New York: Wiley; 2005. p. 117.
13. Chee ST, Quek SSS, Ding PZ, Chua SM. Clinical utility, safety, acceptability and complications of transoesophageal echocardiography (TEE) in 901 patients. Singapore Med J. 1995;36:479–83.
14. Mike JW. Symptomatic care pending diagnosis: Pain. In: Bope ET, Kellerman R, Rakel RE, editors. Conn's Current Therapy 2011. Philadelphia: Saunders/Elsevier; 2010. p. 5.
15. Tsuboi M, Arai M, Maruoka D, Matsumura T, Nakagawa T, Katsuno T, et al. Utility and stability of transnasal endoscopy for examination of the pharynx - A prospective study and comparison with transoral endoscopy. Int J Med Sci. 2013;10(9):1085–91.
16. Samsoon GLT, Young JRB. Difficult tracheal intubation: a retrospective study. Anaesth. 1987;42:487–90.
17. Lee A, Fan L, Gin T, Karmakar M, Ngan Kee WD. A systematic review (Meta-Analysis) of the accuracy of the Mallampati tests to predict the difficult airway. Anesth Analg. 2006;102:1867–78.
18. Restelli L, Moretti MP, Todaro C, Banfi L. The Mallampati's scale: a study of reliability in clinical practice. Minerva Anestesiol. 1993;59(5):261–5.
19. Gupta S, Sharma R, Jain D. Airway Assessment: Predictors of difficult airway. Indian J Anaesth. 2005;49(4):257–62.
20. Chhabra B, Kiran S, Malhotra N, Bharadwaj M, Thakur A. Risk stratification in anaesthesia practice. Indian J Anaesth. 2002;46(5):347–52.
21. Malik P, Rathee M. Gagging and its management: A review volume. Int J Sci Res. 2014;3(1):357–8.
22. Goyal G. Gag Reflex: Causes and management. Int J Dent Med Res. 2014; 1(3):163–6.
23. Naeem A, Taseer B, Arti S, Shilpi C, Vijay K, Monu Y. Gag Reflex: A Situational challenge. Int J Sci Res Pub. 2014;4(10):1–2.
24. Cote G, Denault A. Transesophageal echocardiography-related complications. Can J Anaesth. 2008;55(9):622–47.
25. Sutton DC, Kluger R. Intraoperative transoesophageal echocardiography: impact on adult cardiac surgery. Anaesth Intensive Care. 1998;26:287–93.
26. Hahn RT, Abraham T, Adams MS, Bruce CJ, Glas KE, Lang RM, et al. Guidelines for performing a comprehensive transesophageal echocardiographic examination: recommendations from the American Society of Echocardiography and the Society of Cardiovascular Anesthesiologists. J Am Soc Echocardiogr. 2013;26:921–6.
27. Mitchell-Heggs L, Lellouche N, Deal L, Hamdaoui B, Castanie JB, Dubois-Rande JL, et al. Transseptal puncture using minimally invasive echocardiography during atrial fibrillation ablation. Europace. 2010;12: 1435 8.

17

3D vena contracta area after MitraClip© procedure: precise quantification of residual mitral regurgitation and identification of prognostic information

Alexander Dietl[1,2]* ⓘ, Christine Prieschenk[1], Franziska Eckert[1], Christoph Birner[1], Andreas Luchner[1,3], Lars S. Maier[1] and Stefan Buchner[1,4]

Abstract

Background: Percutaneous mitral valve repair (PMVR) is increasingly performed in patients with severe mitral regurgitation (MR). Post-procedural MR grading is challenging and an unsettled issue. We hypothesised that the direct planimetry of vena contracta area (VCA) by 3D–transoesophageal echocardiography allows quantifying post-procedural MR and implies further prognostic relevance missed by the usual ordinal scale (grade I-IV).

Methods: Based on a single-centre PMVR registry containing 102 patients, the association of VCA reduction and patients' functional capacity measured as six-minute walk distance (6 MW) was evaluated. 3D–colour-Doppler datasets were available before, during and 4 weeks after PMVR.

Results: Twenty nine patients (age 77.0 ± 5.8 years) with advanced heart failure (75.9% NYHA III/IV) and severe degenerative (34%) or functional (66%) MR were eligible. VCA was reduced in all patients by PMVR (0.99 ± 0.46 cm^2 vs. 0.22 ± 0.15 cm^2, $p < 0.0001$). It remained stable after median time of 33 days ($p = 0.999$). 6 MW improved after the procedure (257.5 ± 82.5 m vs. 295.7 ± 96.3 m, $p < 0.01$). Patients with a decrease in VCA less than the median VCA reduction showed a more distinct improvement in 6 MW than patients with better technical result ($p < 0.05$). This paradoxical finding was driven by inferior results in very large functional MR.

Conclusions: VCA improves the evaluation of small residual MR. Its post-procedural values remain stable during a short-term follow-up and imply prognostic information for the patients' physical improvement. VCA might contribute to a more substantiated estimation of treatment success in the heterogeneous functional MR group.

Keywords: Percutaneous mitral valve repair, MitraClip, 3D echocardiography, Vena contracta area, Six-minute walk test, NT-proBNP, Prognosis, Functional mitral regurgitation

Background

Percutaneous mitral valve repair (PMVR) by the MitraClip©-system (Abbott Vascular) has evolved as successful alternative to surgery for the treatment of severe mitral regurgitation (MR) in patients at high surgical risk [1]. Due to edge-to-edge technique at least two neo-orifices are created by the procedure. Therefore, established parameters of grading MR recommended by current guidelines like width of vena contracta and effective regurgitant orifice area [2–4] are not appropriate for the complex post-procedural mitral valve anatomy. The few existing recommendations for MR grading after PMVR get by with a multimodal approach integrating parameters as visual assessment of regurgitant jet [5], which are semi-quantitative and subjectively influenced. However, vena contracta area (VCA) cannot only be approximated by the PISA method, but also be directly measured by cardiac magnetic resonance imaging [6, 7] or three-dimensional transoesophageal echocardiography

* Correspondence: Alexander.dietl@ukr.de
[1]Department of Internal Medicine II, University Hospital Regensburg, Franz-Josef-Strauss Allee 11, D-93053 Regensburg, Germany
[2]Comprehensive Heart Failure Center Würzburg, University Hospital and University of Würzburg, Würzburg, Germany
Full list of author information is available at the end of the article

(3D–TEE) [8]. As 3D–TEE was known to be reliable in multiple VCA [9], its use for the MR assessment after PMVR appeared reasonable. Recently, the feasibility of direct VCA measurement in multiple neo-orifices was demonstrated with a significant decrease of VCA by PMVR [10, 11]. Post-procedural VCA is supposed to be more precise than an ordinal scaled MR grading - as if the imaging resolution in grade I and II MR is increased. However, this incremental parameter will serve little purpose, unless it implies any prognostic information. To date, data on the prognostic relevance of VCA reduction for the patients' functional outcome after PMVR is lacking. Therefore, we analysed the data of a single-centre registry containing 102 patients, who underwent PMVR, in order to examine the association of VCA-reduction and patients' functional capacity measured as six-minute walking distance.

Methods
Study population
The PMVR registry of the University Hospital Regensburg, Germany, comprises 102 patients, who underwent the procedure between 04/2012 and 12/2015 and were screened for eligibility. Inclusion criteria for this study were a standardised six-minute walk test before and after PMVR as well as stored 3D–TEE colour Doppler datasets before and during PMVR. For this investigation, we excluded 73 patients (unavailable six-minute walk test, 48 subjects; unavailable 3D–TEE colour Doppler dataset, 17 subjects; insufficient quality of stored echocardiography for VCA determination, 8 subjects), yielding 29 cases for this analysis.

Clinical parameters
Further information concerning the patients' health status was derived from medical records. EuroScoreII and logEuroScore were calculated [12]. A six-minute walk test (6MW) was recorded before PMVR and 4 weeks after the procedure. The test was performed according to the current statement of the American Thoracic Society [13] indoors, along a flat, straight, enclosed, seldom travelled corridor with a hard surface by a trained nurse. The percutaneous-repair procedure was performed under general anaesthesia with the MitraClip System (Abbott Vascular, Lake Bluff, USA) as previously described [1, 14].

Echocardiography
Two-dimensional transthoracic echocardiography (iE-33 ultrasound system with S5–1 transducer; Philips Medical Systems, Amsterdam, The Netherlands) was performed in all patients before and 4 weeks after PMVR. Left ventricular volumes and left ventricular ejection fraction were calculated by Simpson's rule according to recent guidelines [15]. MR was quantified in an integrative view according to the

Endovascular Valve Edge-to-Edge REpair STudy (EVEREST) criteria [16]. Information on valve morphology, colour flow doppler, presence or absence of systolic pulmonary vein flow, regurgitant volume and regurgitant fraction was gathered according to recent guidelines [2–4] and combined to grade MR on a scale from mild to severe (I to IV) [16] to assure comparability to previously published registries [1, 17–21]. MR immediately after PMVR was graded from I to IV according to the recommendations of the German Cardiac Society (DGK, Additional file 1).

All patients underwent TEE for screening ("before PMVR") purpose and during the catheter intervention providing a dataset immediately after Clip release ("immediately after PMVR"). In a subgroup, a follow-up TEE was performed 4 weeks after PMVR ("Follow up"). All images were acquired using an iE-33 ultrasound system equipped with a 3D–matrix array transducer (X7-2 t). Screening and follow-up examinations were done in conscious sedation using benzodiazepines. General anaesthesia was established for PMVR. The aetiology of mitral regurgitation was described as degenerative (DMR) or functional (FMR).

3D–colour Doppler datasets of the mitral valve were obtained from mid-oesophageal views. Seven electrocardiographically triggered sequential 3D–scans were composed for a 3D–colour full volume dataset. A post-hoc analysis was performed using commercially available software packages (Xcelera R3.2 L1, version 3.2.1.820–2011; Qlab, version 10.5, Philips Medical Systems, Amsterdam, Netherlands) according to current guidelines [2]. Tissue priority and tissue threshold were set to factory settings. All recorded 3D–colour full volume datasets were checked for lines of disagreement between neighbouring 3D subvolumes ("stitching artefacts") within the VCA borders or "dropouts" within the dataset. Care was taken to identify blooming effects, rendering the Doppler signal larger than the laminar jet core itself [2]. If artefacts were present, the patients were excluded from further analyses (8 subjects). The median 3D frame rate came to 18 Hz, as recommended [22], with a narrow interquartile range (15 to 18 Hz; minimum 8 Hz in 1 subject). VCA was defined as the cross-sectional area of the narrowest portion of the proximal regurgitant jet through the closed mitral valve in early-to mid-systole [8, 23]. The datasets were manually cropped to provide a direct en-face view perpendicular to the jet direction. The Nyquist limit was stepwise reduced to a median of 41.1 cm/s (30.8;41.1) to visualise the colour flow regurgitant jet with maximum clarity as previously described [24, 25]. To identify the level of the narrowest portion of the regurgitant jet, the datasets were tomographically sliced. A manual planimetry of the colour Doppler signal was performed (Fig. 1). Care was taken to measure only the central laminar jet core [26] of highest, similar, transverse velocity and to

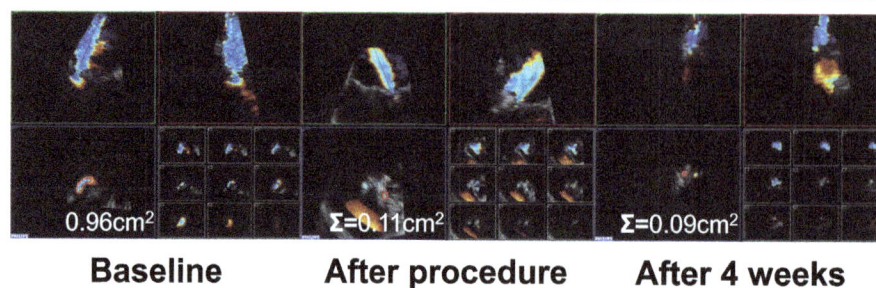

Fig. 1 Vena contracta area determination by 3D–TEE is exemplarily shown for a DMR patient. Shown are MPR views at three time points. Each MPR view is based on one recorded data set and composed of a fourfold table. Top left (green box): midoesophageal long axis view. Top right (red): orthogonal plane to green box. Bottom left (blue): 3D–en face view to VCA (traced by red line). Bottom right: multislice representation of 9 evenly distributed slices parallel to 3D–en face view, used to find actual VCA plane. VCA was defined as the central laminar jet core (within red lines) as defined by current ASE guidelines [2]. Immediately after PMVR the residual regurgitant jet was split into at least two. VCA of each jet was determined separately and summed up. After PMVR, measurement of one jet is exemplarily shown. VCA: vena contracta area. DMR: degenerative mitral regurgitation. MR: mitral regurgitation. Σ: two residual jets were summed up. ASE: American Society of Echocardiography

exclude low-velocity eddies as recommended by previous publications and the current guidelines [2, 27]. As after PMVR there used to be multiple jets, VCA of each jet was determined separately and summed up as for complex mitral regurgitation [9].

Statistical analysis

Categorical data are expressed as percentages. Their differences were tested for significance by Pearson's chi-squared test. The distributions of continuous variables were assessed for normality by Shapiro-Wilk test. If normally distributed, they are expressed as mean ± standard deviation. Significance of differences was tested by Student's t-test for dependent or independent variables, respectively. Two-way analysis of variance (two-way ANOVA) was computed to analyse the influence of categorical independent variables on left ventricular volumes and ejection fraction, respectively. When normal distribution was rejected, median and interquartile range (P25; P75) are given and variables are shown as Turkey box plots. Mann-Whitney U test, Wilcoxon signed-rank test and Friedman's test with consecutive Dunn's multiple comparison test were performed, as appropriate. Effect size was approximated as Cohen's d or Hedges's g [28] using dedicated software [29]. To assess the reduction in VCA, the ratio (VCAr) was calculated as quotient (VCAr = VCA PMVR/VCA at baseline). The absolute area of VCA reduction (VCAdiff) was defined as difference (VCAdiff = VCA baseline–VCA PMVR). VCAdiff gives the VCA reduction in absolute numbers [cm^2]. Six-minute walk change (6MWc) was calculated as difference (6MWc = distance after–before PMVR) [30]. Kendall rank correlation coefficient (τ) was calculated to measure the degree of correlation of non-parametric data.

All statistical analyses were performed using SPSS statistics version 22 (IBM, Armonk, New York, USA) and GraphPad Prism Version 6.00 (GraphPad software, La Jolla, California, USA). Statistical significance was assigned at a two-sided p-value of less than 0.05.

Power calculation analysis

For post-hoc power analysis G-Power [31] (version 3.1.9.2) was employed. A post-hoc power calculation was performed for the two main readouts (decrease in VCA and six-minute walking distance). It revealed sufficient power ($\beta < 0.0001/0.01$) for decrease in VCA/6 MW (Additional file 2).

Results

Patients' characteristics

Baseline characteristics of the registry of the University Hospital Regensburg, Germany, are depicted in Table 1. Twenty nine patients were included for further analyses (Table 2). Patients were characterised by higher age (77.0 ± 5.8 years), advanced heart failure (75.9% in NYHA class III or IV), severely limited physical capacity in terms of short 6 MW (257.5 ± 82.5 m), high-burden of comorbidities and elevated estimated surgical risk. As depicted by Table 3, Vena contracta width (7.6 ± 1.8 mm) and effective regurgitant orifice area according to PISA method (0.45 ± 0.25 cm^2) were measured elevated by the initial TEE. The aetiology of severe MR was considered DMR in one third ($n = 10$) and FMR in two thirds ($n = 19$) of patients. Four of 10 DMR cases were due to flail leaflet. In 7 patients, a follow-up 3D–TEE was available 41 (35;48) days after PMVR.

Effect of PMVR on MR, 6 MW and NT-proBNP levels

The effects of PMVR are depicted in Table 4. MR was decreased from median grade 4 to 1 in the total study sample. The effect was also significant analysing

Table 1 Regensburg registry and other published trials and registries including patients treated by the MitraClip system

	Regensburg	GRASP [17]	TRAMI [19]	MitraSWISS [18]	Pilot Registry [21][a]	ACCESS-EU [20]	EVEREST-II [1]
Year of publication		2016	2016	2014	2014	2013	2011
Participants	102	180	749	74	628	567	184
Female [%]	42.2	38.3	38.6	27	36.9	36.2	38
Age [years]	77.0 ± 5.8	71.6 ± 9.8	76 (10)[b]	72 ± 12	74.2 ± 9.7	73.7 ± 9.6	67.3 ± 12.8
MR grade III/IV [%]	100	–	93.8	100	86.1[c]	97.7	96
DMR [%]	28.4	18.3	27.8	38	22.8	20.6	74
FMR [%]	71.6	81.7	71.3	62	72.0	69.3	27
NYHA III/IV [%]	75.5	81.1	89	–	85.5	84.9	52
EuroScore II	5.1 ± 5.9	7.6 ± 6.4	–	–	–	–	–
LogEuroScore [%]	26.6 ± 18.0	–	20 (19)f	21 ± 17	20.4 ± 16.7	23.0 ± 18.3	–
Regurgitant orifice area [cm²]	0.40 ± 0.18	–	–	–	0.43 ± 0.16	–	0.56 ± 0.38

Shown are mean and standard deviation or proportions (if not indicated otherwise)
[a]Transcatheter Valve Treatment Sentinel Pilot Registry, [b]median (IQR), [c]severe (graded as mild, moderate, severe). *MR* mitral regurgitation, *DMR* degenerative mitral regurgitation, *FMR* functional mitral regurgitation, *NYHA* New York Heart Association functional classification

Table 2 Baseline characteristics of the study sample

Age [years]	77.0 ± 5.8
Female	41.4 (12/29)
Heart rate [bpm]	74 ± 9
Systolic blood pressure [mmHg]	119 ± 19
Diastolic blood pressure [mmHg]	67 ± 14
Body mass index [kg/m²]	25.8 ± 4.2
NT-proBNP [pg/ml] median(P25;75)	3618 (1619; 5782)
Serum creatinine [mg/dl] median(P25;75)	1.1 (1.0; 1.6)
logEuroScore [%] median(P25;75)	18.5 (12.7; 32.2)
NYHA functional class	
I	0 (0/29)
II	24.1 (7/29)
III	62.1 (18/29)
IV	13.8 (4/29)
Comorbidities	
DCM	10.3 (3/29)
Coronary artery disease	62.1 (18/29)
Diabetes mellitus II	34.5 (10/29)
Medical/Device treatment	
High-ceiling diuretics	100 (29/29)
ACE inhibitors	48.3 (14/29)
MRA	62.1 (18/29)
Beta-blocker	89.7 (26/29)
CRT	6.9 (2/29)

Shown are percentage of subjects (number of subjects / total number of subjects in parentheses) or mean ± standard deviation, if not indicated otherwise
NYHA New York Heart Association, *DCM* dilated cardiomyopathy, *ACE* angiotensin- converting enzyme, *MRA* mineralocorticoid receptor antagonist, *CRT* cardiac resynchronization therapy

DMR (decrease from grade 4 (3.5;4.0) to 1 (1;1.5); $p < 0.01$) and FMR separately (decrease from grade 4 (3;4) to 1 (0.5;1.5); $p < 0.001$). Largest residual MR was graded 2.5 ($n = 1$).

6MW was significantly improved by PMVR. The effect was particularly pronounced in patients suffering from DMR (240.4 ± 80.3 m vs. 296.1 ± 63.0 m, Cohen's d 0.97, $p = 0.013$, $n = 10$). In FMR, effect size was smaller and slightly missed significance (266.5 ± 84.4 m, Cohen's d = 0.47, $p = 0.053$, $n = 19$). In consequence, PMVR achieved as early as 4 weeks after the procedure a significant improvement of 6 MW with a more distinct effect for DMR.

NT-proBNP blood levels, left-ventricular volumes and ejection fraction did not show a significant change (Table 4).

Reduction of VCA by PMVR and consistency between intra-procedural measurement and follow-up examination

VCA determination was independent of age, sex, left ventricular ejection fraction, NYHA class and EuroScore.

Table 3 Mitral regurgitation in the study sample

MR aetiology	Degenerative	34.5 (10/29)
	Functional	65.5 (19/29)
MR grading	III	17.2 (5/29)
	IV	82.8 (24/29)
Vena contracta width [mm]	Degenerative	7.30 ± 1.34
	Functional	7.79 ± 2.04
ERO [cm²] median (P25;P75)	Degenerative	0.45 (0.33; 0.61)
	Functional	0.36 (0.27;0.60)
Number of implanted clips	1	51.7 (15/29)
	2	48.3 (14/29)

Percentage of subjects (number of subjects / total number of subjects in parentheses). *MR* mitral regurgitation, *ERO* effective regurgitant orifice calculated by the Proximal- isovelocity surface area (PISA) method

Table 4 Effect of PMVR on mitral regurgitation, 6-min walk and LV remodelling

	Before PMVR	After PMVR	p-value
MR grade median (P25;P75)	4 (3.5;4.0)	1 (0.5;1.5)	< 0.001
6 min walk [m]	257.5 ± 82.5	295.7 ± 96.3	< 0.01
VCA (3D) [cm^2] median (P25;P75)	0.89 (0.65;1.33)	0.17 (0.09;0.37)	< 0.0001
NT-proBNP [pg/ml] median(P25;75)	3618 (1619;5782)	3247 (2273;4693)	0.954
LV end-diastolic volume [ml/m^2]	85.0 ± 26.5	79.4 ± 23.2	0.17
LV end-systolic volume [ml/m^2]	49.8 ± 22.2	44.7 ± 17.4	0.11
LV ejection fraction [%]	42.5 ± 12.5	43.6 ± 10.1	0.51

PMVR decreased mitral regurgitation and improved six-minute walking distance in a follow-up examination 4 weeks after the intervention. NT-proBNP and left-ventricular volumes and ejection fraction remained unchanged. Shown are mean ± standard deviation, if not indicated otherwise
PMVR percutaneous mitral valve repair, *LV* left ventricular, *MR* mitral regurgitation, *VCA (3D)* vena contracta area determined by direct planimetry in a 3D–coulor Doppler full volume

Baseline VCA was significantly reduced from 0.89cm^2 to 0.17cm^2 after PMVR (Table 4). Median VCAr was 0.19 (0.09;0.42). In the subgroup of patients with follow-up 3D–TEE, VCA did not vary between the measurements immediately after PMVR and during follow-up ($p = 0.999$, Fig. 2). Their characteristics did not differ from the group missing a follow-up 3D–TEE examination with respect to sex, age or clinical manifestation of MR (Additional file 3).

Correlation of intra-procedural VCA measures and grading of residual MR

Common ordinal scaled MR grading (1 to 4) and VCA were compared for evaluating residual MR. There was significant but weak correlation ($\tau = 0.361$; $p = 0.01$). As seen in Fig. 3, the VCAs of all ordinal scaled MR grades after PMVR spread widely.

VCA reduction as predictor of clinical outcome

The link of MR reduction (VCAr) and an improvement of the patients' physical capacity (6MWc) is depicted by Fig. 4. Using the median VCAr of 0.19 as cut-off value, patients with a more pronounced procedural VCA reduction, mirrored by a VCAr below the median, had a significantly smaller 6 MWc. Contrary to expectations, data imply a more modest success for functional improvement in patients, whose technical success in VCA reduction was essentially more distinct.

To scrutinize possible underlying causes, two groups divided by the median VCAr were compared. Explorative data analysis did not yield significantly differing results between groups except for the absolute area of VCA change (VCAdiff) (Additional file 4). VCAr and VCAdiff were correlated with a negative Kendall rank correlation coefficient ($\tau = -0.51$, $p = 0.0001$). Thus, as VCAr decreases, VCAdiff increases, which seems quite conclusive.

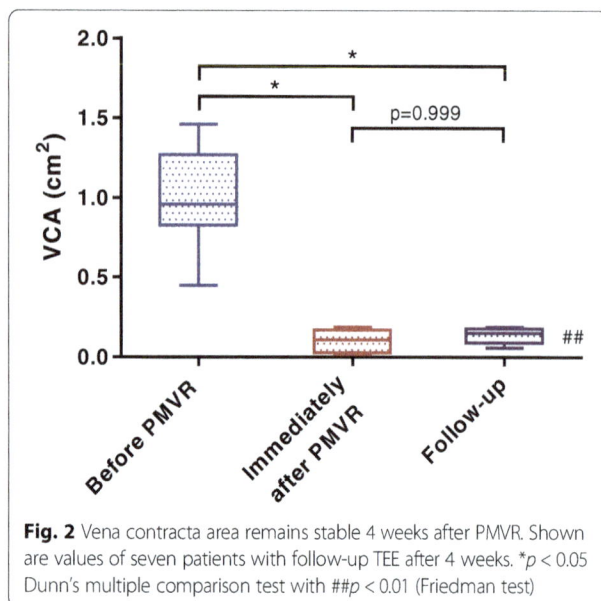

Fig. 2 Vena contracta area remains stable 4 weeks after PMVR. Shown are values of seven patients with follow-up TEE after 4 weeks. *$p < 0.05$ Dunn's multiple comparison test with ##$p < 0.01$ (Friedman test)

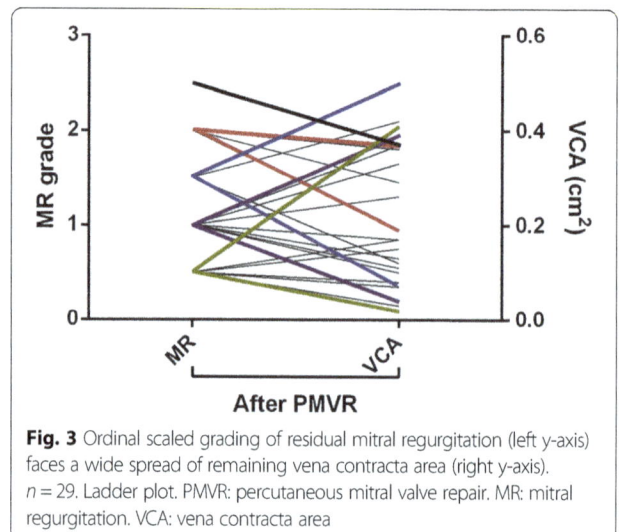

Fig. 3 Ordinal scaled grading of residual mitral regurgitation (left y-axis) faces a wide spread of remaining vena contracta area (right y-axis). $n = 29$. Ladder plot. PMVR: percutaneous mitral valve repair. MR: mitral regurgitation. VCA: vena contracta area

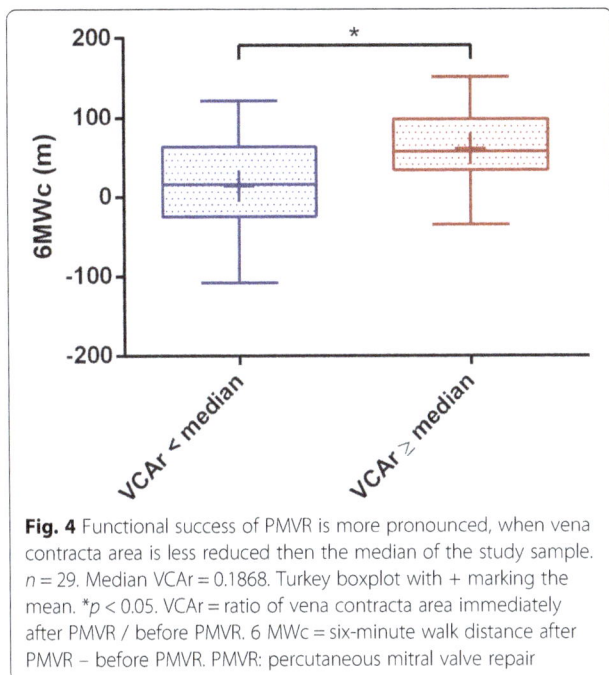

Fig. 4 Functional success of PMVR is more pronounced, when vena contracta area is less reduced then the median of the study sample. $n = 29$. Median VCAr = 0.1868. Turkey boxplot with + marking the mean. *$p < 0.05$. VCAr = ratio of vena contracta area immediately after PMVR / before PMVR. 6 MWc = six-minute walk distance after PMVR – before PMVR. PMVR: percutaneous mitral valve repair

Based on these observations, we speculated, whether effects of very large VCA could drive our results. The 75% quantile of VCAdiff was used as cut-off to differ between low and high VCAdiff (75% quantile = 1.05 cm^2). Patients, who were suffering from FMR and exhibited a VCAdiff below the 75% quantile, had a post-procedural increase in six-minute walking distance ($+43.57 \pm 49.53$ m, $n = 14$). By contrast, patients with larger VCAdiff came to a decreased six-minute walk distance after PMVR (-12.20 ± 76.59 m, $n = 5$). The difference showed a strong effect (Hedges's $g = -0.977$) slightly missing significance ($p = 0.078$).

There was no difference between small and large VCAdiff regarding changes in post-procedural left ventricular volumes or function compared to baseline (p for end-diastolic volume/end-systolic volume/ejection fraction = 0.97/0.68/0.45, 2-way ANOVA).

Thus, in large, potentially long-standing FMR, our data was indicative for a less beneficial effect than in smaller FMR with regard to the patients' functional outcome.

Discussion

In this study assessing prognostic implications of VCA reduction, we observed the following key findings:

1) Patients' six-minute walking distance was improved already 4 weeks after PMVR with a more pronounced effect for DMR.

2) VCA is significantly reduced by PMVR and its dimensions remain stable during a short-term follow-up.

3) VCA measurement immediately after PMVR improves the evaluation of small remaining MR by implying prognostic relevance for the patients' physical capacity measured as 6MWc.

Study sample and treatment success in the context of published literature

The baseline characteristics of the Regensburg PMVR Registry reported for the first time by our study were quite comparable to currently published results of several registries [1, 17–21] (Table 1) mirroring the real-life practice. The use in FMR was consistently reported higher than in the initial EVEREST-II trial [1]. Remarkably, in our data the effect of PMVR on patients' functional capacity (6 MW) was more pronounced in DMR. NT-proBNP as marker of left ventricular wall stress and predictor of cardiovascular outcome [32] was elevated before and after PMVR without significant change in line with a current publication reporting no benefit of PMVR with regard to NT-proBNP levels in 144 patients [33]. Nevertheless, the field is still not settled due to contrary results in smaller samples [34]. Heterogeneous comorbidities might explain nonresponse of NT-proBNP after PMVR [35].

VCA as independent measurement for quantifying residual MR after PMVR

In patients with high grade MR and elevated surgical risk, PMVR is increasingly used leading to significant improvements in clinical outcome [1, 14, 19]. The edge-to-edge technique of PMVR alters the complex anatomy of the mitral valve in DMR [36] and FMR [10] and creates at least two neo-orifices. The remaining MR is split into often very eccentric regurgitant jets (Fig. 1) and common parameters of echocardiographic MR assessment as width of vena contracta and effective regurgitant orifice area are not applicable. The sparse existing guidelines (e.g. of the German Cardiac Society [5], Additional file 1) recommend a multimodal approach integrating parameters determined by echocardiography (visual grading of regurgitant jet), right-heart catheterization (v-wave) and left ventriculography (regurgitant volume) with echocardiography as mainstay. Though in real-life most often used during PMVR, the qualitative as well as quantitative assessment of the regurgitant jets using colour-Doppler is imprecise and tents to an overestimation of remaining MR in the situation of multiple jets [37]. Even before the launch of PMVR, VCA was known for several strengths in the assessment of high-grade MR [8]: In an in vitro model of MR, VCA provided the strongest correlation with known orifice area ($r = 0.92$, $p < 0.001$) compared to other echocardiographic measurements, which could be translated to a prospective study comprising 61 patients with at least mild MR of different aetiology: feasibility and reproducibility was established yielding satisfying interobserver agreement ($r = 0.96$; 0.05 ± 0.02 cm^2) [38]. In the same year, a further prospective study including 57 patients with relevant MR of different aetiologies [39] reported feasible measurements in all patients within 2.6 ± 0.7 min of measuring time and ruled out significant interobserver variability ($r = 0.97$, 0.04 ± 0.09 cm^2). VCA is reliable in multiple jet areas, too [9].

Considering VCA measurement after PMVR, Altiok et al. set the stage by using VCA determined by 3-D-TEE to analyse the procedural effects of PMVR in FMR [11] with acceptable feasibility and reproducibility. In 2017, these data were confirmed [10] by a retrospective study comprising 97 heart failure patients with severe MR undergoing MitraClip therapy reporting adequate interobserver variability ($r = 0.95$, $p < 0.001$). Comparing VCA to the common ordinal scale of MR grading, our data show that within each MR grade VCA still spreads. It highlights the potential of VCA measurement to increase the resolution of residual MR grading.

The intraprocedural TEE has to face the inherent problem of anaesthesia, which changes cardiac pre- and afterload influencing mitral valve function [40]. Interestingly, VCA did not change in our dataset between the intraprocedural TEE in general anaesthesia and a follow-up examination, which has been done in conscious sedation using benzodiazepines 4 weeks later. These results might indicate a quite comparability of both examinations regarding particularly VCA measurement.

VCA as predictor of post-procedural outcome

The need for a reliable measurement of residual MR is underscored by its prognostic importance: data from the MitraSWISS registry revealed residual MR severity after PMVR as significant predictor of reduced survival after 2 years [18]. They suggested that MR should be reduced as far as possible. It has to be stressed that these analyses relied on ordinal scaled grading of residual MR by combined methods. In 2017, Alessandrini et al. measured VCA in FMR patients after PMVR. Dichotomised VCA (≥ 0.25cm^2, upper vs. lower and middle tertile of their sample) was associated with mortality during a median follow-up of 13.4 months (HR = 3.8, CI 1.9–7.8) [10]. Our data confirm prognostic implication of remaining MR. However, since MR severity is very dynamic, we hypothesised beyond previous published analyses, that there might be differences in outcome depending on pre-procedural MR anatomy. Therefore, we wanted to assess the association of decreasing VCA (ratio post/pre-procedural) and the patients' outcome, which was measured as gain in 6 MW. Strikingly, we observed a more pronounced increase in 6 MW 4 weeks after PMVR in patients, whose VCA was less reduced by PMVR. This paradoxical result was predominantly driven by the negative outcome of patients suffering from FMR with a large absolute difference between their VCA before and immediately after PMVR (> 75% quantile, > 1.05cm^2). These patients lacking functional improvement after PMVR had considerably large functional regurgitant jets measured as VCA 2.5-fold higher than the cut-off value defining the edge between moderate and high-grade disease [8, 39, 41]. It is tempting to speculate whether PMVR strictly decreasing VCA might be less beneficial in very-large, presumably chronic and long-standing FMR than at an earlier point of intervention as additionally suggested by recent data [42]. For FMR comprises a variety of entities as a result of cardiac remodelling [43–46]. Thus, our study might suggest with VCA an interesting, objective, measurable pre-procedural criterion for PMVR planning. Nonetheless, this issue awaits further, strongly required prospective evaluation as patient selection in FMR for PMVR is a central and current problem and valid parameters for this purpose are strongly needed.

Strengths and limitations

Strengths of our study include precise measurement of MR by the direct planimetry of VCA using 3D–TEE, which has already been shown to be accurate [8] and feasible in multiple jets [9] even after PMVR [10, 11]. However, data on DMR has been lacking to date. Furthermore, nor VCA neither another method has been used until now to assess prognostic implication of residual MR concerning functional treatment success. Thus, a novel approach was chosen and provided new insights. Furthermore, the recorded follow-up 3D–TEE examinations permitted an analysis of stability during short-term follow-up.

However, some limitations warrant consideration: reduction in regurgitant volume immediately after PMVR could similarly be discussed as another potential marker of later clinical outcome. Regurgitant volume is estimated as difference of stroke volumes measured at the LVOT and mitral valve level [47] or alternatively, by magnetic resonance imaging. Both methods are applicable even after MitraClip [48]. Unfortunately, we do not have this data to compare it with VCA reduction. This issue awaits future studies.

The retrospective design with a moderate-sized number of participants limits analytic options. Nevertheless, it is the first study in the field addressing this current and highly relevant issue by testing a clear and unambiguous hypothesis and using a precise measuring method as well as a quantifiable, relevant outcome variable. Thus, it allowed a thorough statistical analysis even in a medium-sized sample with appropriate statistical power.

Still, due to the small sample size, little effects can be missed and non-significant results do not rule out a potentially overseen small effect. Nonetheless, our study may report on significant effects yielded by PMVR. However, albeit significance was computed, some justified concerns about generalizability might remain because of the small sample size and should by answered by further research. To offer valid information at the moment, we provide also estimates of effect sizes beside *p*-values, which could facilitate a-priori power calculation for future prospective studies.

The study emphasised the importance of precise echocardiographic imaging in PMVR, although all large registries ignore new measurements of residual MR as VCA (Table 1). It is our hope that our results will help to design future prospective studies, which further elucidate the prognostic meaningfulness of residual MR particularly in outsized FMR.

Conclusions

The current study confirms direct planimetry of VCA by 3D–TEE as a feasible method to quantify DMR as well as FMR in the situation of multiple neo-orifices after PMVR. PMVR reduces VCA and improves significantly 6 MWc as early as 4 weeks after the procedure with a more pronounced effect in DMR. The values of VCA determined immediately after Clip release remain stable during a short-term follow-up of 4 weeks and they imply prognostic relevance for the patients' physical capacity measured as 6 MWc. There is some evidence that in FMR as heterogeneous disease VCA might contribute to a more substantiated estimation of treatment success.

Acknowledgements
Not applicable.

Funding
AD is supported by a research grant of the German Cardiac Society (DGK – Deutsche Gesellschaft für Kardiologie, Herz- und Kreislaufforschung).

Authors' contributions
AD designed this study, performed partially the transthoracic and transoesophageal echocardiograms, did the post-hoc assessment of 3D datasets, analysed and interpreted data and wrote the first draft of the manuscript. CP analysed and interpreted data. FE did the post-hoc assessment of left ventricular volumes and function, analysed and interpreted data. CB analysed and interpreted data. AL performed most PMVR interventions, validated proper data storage, initiated the analysis, analysed and interpreted data and reviewed and edited the manuscript. LSM analysed and interpreted data and reviewed the manuscript. SB performed partially the transthoracic and transoesophageal echocardiograms and partially the PMVR interventions, supervised and validated the entire study, analysed and interpreted data and was a major contributor to critical review and editing of the manuscript. All authors read and approved the final manuscript.

Competing interests
LSM has received speaker honorarium from Abbott Vascular. AD, CP, CB, AL, SB: None.

Author details
[1]Department of Internal Medicine II, University Hospital Regensburg, Franz-Josef-Strauss Allee 11, D-93053 Regensburg, Germany. [2]Comprehensive Heart Failure Center Würzburg, University Hospital and University of Würzburg, Würzburg, Germany. [3]Department of Internal Medicine I, Klinikum St. Marien, Amberg, Germany. [4]Department of Internal Medicine II, Sana Kliniken Cham, Cham, Germany.

References
1. Feldman T, Foster E, Glower DD, Glower DG, Kar S, Rinaldi MJ, et al. Percutaneous repair or surgery for mitral regurgitation. N Engl J Med. 2011; 364:1395–406.
2. Zoghbi WA, Adams D, Bonow RO, Enriquez-Sarano M, Foster E, Grayburn PA, et al. Recommendations for noninvasive evaluation of native Valvular regurgitation: a report from the American Society of Echocardiography developed in collaboration with the Society for Cardiovascular Magnetic Resonance. J Am Soc Echocardiogr. 2017;30:303–71.
3. Nishimura RA, Otto CM, Bonow RO, Carabello BA, Erwin JP, Fleisher LA, et al. 2017 AHA/ACC focused update of the 2014 AHA/ACC guideline for the Management of Patients with Valvular Heart Disease: a report of the American College of Cardiology/American Heart Association task force on clinical practice guidelines. J Am Coll Cardiol. 2017;135:e1159–95.
4. Baumgartner H, Falk V, Bax JJ, De Bonis M, Hamm C, Holm PJ, et al. 2017 ESC/EACTS guidelines for the Management of Valvular Heart Disease: the task force for the management of Valvular heart disease of the European Society of Cardiology (ESC) and the European Association for Cardio-Thoracic Surgery (EACTS). Eur Heart J. 2017;38:2739–91.
5. Boekstegers P, Hausleiter J, Baldus S, von Bardeleben R, Beucher H, Butter C, et al. Interventionelle Behandlung der Mitralklappeninsuffizienz mit dem MitraClip®-Verfahren. Kardiologe. 2013;7:91–104.
6. Buchner S, Poschenrieder F, Hamer OW, Jungbauer C, Resch M, Birner C, et al. Direct visualization of Regurgitant orifice by CMR reveals differential asymmetry according to etiology of mitral regurgitation. JACC Cardiovasc Imaging. 2011;4:1088–96.
7. Buchner S, Debl K, Poschenrieder F, Feuerbach S, Riegger GAJ, Luchner A, et al. Cardiovascular magnetic resonance for direct assessment of anatomic regurgitant orifice in mitral regurgitation. Circ Cardiovasc Imaging. 2008;1:148–55.
8. Buck T, Plicht B. Real-time three-dimensional Echocardiographic assessment of severity of mitral regurgitation using proximal Isovelocity surface area and vena Contracta area method. Lessons we learned and clinical implications. Curr Cardiovasc Imaging Rep. 2015;8:38.
9. Hyodo E, Iwata S, Tugcu A, Arai K, Shimada K, Muro T, et al. Direct measurement of multiple vena Contracta areas for assessing the severity of mitral regurgitation using 3D TEE. JACC Cardiovasc Imaging. 2012;5:669–76.
10. Alessandrini H, Kreidel F, Schlüter M, Frerker C, Schmidt T, Thielsen T, et al. Prognostic implication of post-MitraClip vena contracta area in heart failure patients with functional mitral regurgitation. EuroIntervention. 2017;12:1946–53.
11. Altiok E, Hamada S, Brehmer K, Kuhr K, Reith S, Becker M, et al. Analysis of procedural effects of Percutaneous edge-to-edge mitral valve repair by 2D and 3D echocardiography. Circ Cardiovasc Imaging. 2012;5:748–55.
12. Nashef SAM, Roques F, Sharples LD, Nilsson J, Smith C, Goldstone AR, et al. EuroSCORE II. Eur J Cardiothorac Surg. 2012;41:734–45.
13. ATS Committee on Proficiency Standards for Clinical Pulmonary Function Laboratories. ATS statement: guidelines for the six-minute walk test. Am J Respir Crit Care Med. 2002;166:111–7.
14. Buchner S, Dreher A, Resch M, Schach C, Birner C, Luchner A. Simplified method for insertion of steerable guide into the left atrium using a pigtail guide wire during the MitraClip(®) procedure: a technical tip. J Interv Cardiol. 2015;28:472–8.
15. Lang RM, Badano LP, Mor-Avi V, Afilalo J, Armstrong A, Ernande L, et al. Recommendations for cardiac chamber quantification by echocardiography in adults: an update from the American Society of Echocardiography and the European Association of Cardiovascular Imaging. Eur. Hear. J. – Cardiovasc. Imaging. 2015;16:233–71.
16. Foster E, Wasserman HS, Gray W, Homma S, Di Tullio MR, Rodriguez L, et al. Quantitative assessment of severity of mitral regurgitation by serial

echocardiography in a multicenter clinical trial of Percutaneous mitral valve repair. Am J Cardiol. 2007;100:1577–83.

17. Scandura S, Capranzano P, Caggegi A, Grasso C, Ronsivalle G, Mangiafico S, et al. Percutaneous mitral valve repair with the MitraClip system in the elderly: one-year outcomes from the GRASP registry. Int J Cardiol. 2016;224:440–6.

18. Toggweiler S, Zuber M, Sürder D, Biaggi P, Gstrein C, Moccetti T, et al. Two-year outcomes after percutaneous mitral valve repair with the MitraClip system: durability of the procedure and predictors of outcome. Open Hear. 2014;1:e000056.

19. Puls M, Lubos E, Boekstegers P, von Bardeleben RS, Ouarrak T, Butter C, et al. One-year outcomes and predictors of mortality after MitraClip therapy in contemporary clinical practice: results from the German transcatheter mitral valve interventions registry. Eur Heart J. 2016;37:703–12.

20. Maisano F, Franzen O, Baldus S, Schäfer U, Hausleiter J, Butter C, et al. Percutaneous mitral valve interventions in the real world: early and 1-year results from the ACCESS-EU, a prospective, multicenter, nonrandomized post-approval study of the MitraClip therapy in Europe. J Am Coll Cardiol. 2013;62:1052–61.

21. Nickenig G, Estevez-Loureiro R, Franzen O, Tamburino C, Vanderheyden M, Lüscher TF, et al. Percutaneous mitral valve edge-to-edge repair: in-hospital results and 1-year follow-up of 628 patients of the 2011-2012 pilot European sentinel registry. J Am Coll Cardiol. 2014;64:875–84.

22. Lang RM, Badano LP, Tsang W, Adams DH, Agricola E, Buck T, et al. EAE/ASE recommendations for image acquisition and display using three-dimensional echocardiography. J Am Soc Echocardiogr. 2012;25:3–46.

23. Khanna D, Vengala S, Miller AP, Nanda NC, Lloyd SG, Ahmed S, et al. Quantification of mitral regurgitation by live three-dimensional transthoracic Echocardiographic measurements of vena Contracta area. Echocardiography. 2004;21:737–43.

24. Heß H, Eibel S, Mukherjee C, Kaisers UX, Ender J. Quantification of mitral valve regurgitation with color flow Doppler using baseline shift. Int J Cardiovasc Imaging. 2013;29:267–74.

25. Buck T. Valvular heart disease – insufficiencies. Three-dimensional Echocardiogr. Berlin: Springer Berlin Heidelberg; 2011. p. 109–54.

26. Diebold B, Delouche A, Delouche P, Guglielmi JP, Dumee P, Herment A. In vitro flow mapping of regurgitant jets. Systematic description of free jet with laser Doppler velocimetry. Circulation. 1996;94:158–69.

27. Plicht B, Kahlert P, Goldwasser R, Janosi RA, Hunold P, Erbel R, et al. Direct quantification of mitral Regurgitant flow volume by real-time three-dimensional echocardiography using Dealiasing of color Doppler flow at the vena Contracta. J Am Soc Echocardiogr. 2008;21:1337–46.

28. Ellis PD. The essential guide to effect sizes - statistical power, meta-analysis, and the interpretation of research results. 1st ed. New York: Cambridge University Press; 2010.

29. Lenhard W, Lenhard A. Calculation of effect sizes. 2016. https://www.psychometrica.de/effect_size.html. Accessed: 12 Dec 2016.

30. Galiè N, Barberà JA, Frost AE, Ghofrani H-A, Hoeper MM, McLaughlin VV, et al. Initial use of Ambrisentan plus Tadalafil in pulmonary arterial hypertension. N Engl J Med. 2015;373:834–44.

31. Faul F, Erdfelder E, Lang A-G, Buchner A. G*power 3: a flexible statistical power analysis program for the social, behavioral, and biomedical sciences. Behav Res Methods. 2007;39:175–91.

32. Dietl A, Stark K, Zimmermann ME, Meisinger C, Schunkert H, Birner C, et al. NT-proBNP predicts cardiovascular death in the general population independent of left ventricular mass and function: insights from a large population-based study with long-term follow-up. PLoS One. 2016;11: e0164060.

33. Yoon J-N, Frangieh AH, Attinger-Toller A, Gruner C, Tanner FC, Taramasso M, et al. Changes in serum biomarker profiles after percutaneous mitral valve repair with the MitraClip system. Cardiol J. 2016;23:384–92.

34. Franzen O, Baldus S, Rudolph V, Meyer S, Knap M, Koschyk D, et al. Acute outcomes of MitraClip therapy for mitral regurgitation in high-surgical-risk patients: emphasis on adverse valve morphology and severe left ventricular dysfunction. Eur Heart J. 2010;31:1373–81.

35. Kaneko H, Neuss M, Weissenborn J, Butter C. Role of right ventricular dysfunction and diabetes mellitus in N-terminal pro-B-type Natriuretic peptide response of patients with severe mitral regurgitation and heart failure after MitraClip. Int Heart J. 2017;58:225–31.

36. Sturla F, Redaelli A, Puppini G, Onorati F, Faggian G, Votta E. Functional and biomechanical effects of the edge-to-edge repair in the setting of mitral regurgitation: consolidated knowledge and novel tools to gain insight into its Percutaneous implementation. Cardiovasc Eng Technol. 2015;6:117–40.

37. Lin BA, Forouhar AS, Pahlevan NM, Anastassiou CA, Grayburn PA, Thomas JD, et al. Color Doppler jet area overestimates Regurgitant volume when multiple jets are present. J Am Soc Echocardiogr. 2010;23:993–1000.

38. Little SH, Pirat B, Kumar R, Igo SR, McCulloch M, Hartley CJ, et al. Three-dimensional color Doppler echocardiography for direct measurement of vena contracta area in mitral regurgitation: in vitro validation and clinical experience. JACC Cardiovasc Imaging. 2008;1:695–704.

39. Kahlert P, Plicht B, Schenk IM, Janosi R-A, Erbel R, Buck T. Direct assessment of size and shape of noncircular vena Contracta area in functional versus organic mitral regurgitation using real-time three-dimensional echocardiography. J Am Soc Echocardiogr. 2008;21:912–21.

40. Patzelt J, Zhang Y, Seizer P, Magunia H, Henning A, Riemlova V, et al. Effects of mechanical ventilation on heart geometry and mitral valve leaflet Coaptation during Percutaneous edge-to-edge mitral valve repair. JACC Cardiovasc Interv. 2016;9:151–9.

41. Zeng X, Levine RA, Hua L, Morris EL, Kang Y, Flaherty M, et al. Diagnostic value of vena contracta area in the quantification of mitral regurgitation severity by color Doppler 3D echocardiography. Circ Cardiovasc Imaging. 2011;4:506–13.

42. Pighi M, Estevez-Loureiro R, Maisano F, Ussia GP, Dall'Ara G, Franzen O, et al. Immediate and 12-month outcomes of ischemic versus nonischemic functional mitral regurgitation in patients treated with MitraClip (from the 2011 to 2012 pilot sentinel registry of Percutaneous edge-to-edge mitral valve repair of the European Society of Cardiology). Am J Cardiol. 2017;119:630–7.

43. Dietl A, Winkel I, Deutzmann R, Schröder J, Hupf J, Riegger G, et al. Interatrial differences of basal molecular set-up and changes in tachycardia-induced heart failure-a proteomic profiling study. Eur J Heart Fail. 2014;16: 835–45.

44. Birner C, Dietl A, Deutzmann R, Schröder J, Schmid P, Jungbauer C, et al. Proteomic profiling implies mitochondrial dysfunction in tachycardia-induced heart failure. J Card Fail. 2012;18:660–73.

45. Dietl A, Maack C. Targeting mitochondrial calcium handling and reactive oxygen species in heart failure. Curr Heart Fail Rep. 2017;14:338–49.

46. Heusch G, Libby P, Gersh B, Yellon D, Böhm M, Lopaschuk G, et al. Cardiovascular remodelling in coronary artery disease and heart failure. Lancet. 2014;383:1933–43.

47. Enriquez-Sarano M, Bailey KR, Seward JB, Tajik AJ, Krohn MJ, Mays JM. Quantitative Doppler assessment of valvular regurgitation. Circulation [internet]. American Heart Association, Inc. 1993;87:841–8.

48. Hamilton-Craig C, Strugnell W, Gaikwad N, Ischenko M, Speranza V, Chan J, et al. Quantitation of mitral regurgitation after percutaneous MitraClip repair: comparison of Doppler echocardiography and cardiac magnetic resonance imaging. Ann Cardiothorac Surg. 2015;4:341–51.

18

Tricuspid annular plane systolic excursion and central venous pressure in mechanically ventilated critically ill patients

Hongmin Zhang[1], Xiaoting Wang[1], Xiukai Chen[2], Qing Zhang[1] and Dawei Liu[1]*

Abstract

Background: The tricuspid annular plane systolic excursion (TAPSE) is commonly recommended for estimating the right ventricular systolic function. The central venous pressure (CVP), which is determined by venous return and right heart function, was found to be associated with right ventricular outflow fractional shortening. This study thus aimed to investigate the relationship between the TAPSE and CVP in mechanically ventilated critically ill patients.

Methods: This is a prospective observational study. From October 1 to December 31, 2017, patients admitted to the intensive care unit with CVP monitoring and controlled mechanical ventilation were screened for enrolment. Echocardiographic parameters, including the TAPSE, mitral annular plane systolic excursion (MAPSE), left ventricular ejection fraction (LVEF), and internal diameter of inferior vena cava (dIVC), and haemodynamic parameters, including the CVP, were collected.

Results: Seventy-four patients were included. Thirty-one were included in the low LVEF (< 55%) group, and 43 were included in the high LVEF (≥55%) group. In the high LVEF group, the TAPSE and CVP were not correlated ($r = -0.234$, $P = 0.151$). In the low LVEF group, partial correlation analysis indicated that the TAPSE and CVP were correlated ($r = -0.516$, $P = 0.006$), and multivariable linear regression analysis indicated that the TAPSE was independently associated with the CVP (standard coefficient: -0.601, $p < 0.001$). Additionally, in the low LVEF group, a ROC analysis showed that the area under the curve of the TAPSE for the detection of CVP greater than 8 mmHg was 0.860 (95% confidence interval: 0.730–0.991; $P = 0.001$). The optimum cut-off value was 1.52 cm, which resulted in a sensitivity of 75.0%, a specificity of 86.7%, a positive predictive value of 84.6% and a negative predictive value of 77.8%.

Conclusions: The TAPSE is inversely correlated with the CVP in mechanically ventilated critically ill patients who have a LVEF less than 55%.

Keywords: Echocardiography, Tricuspid annulus plane systolic excursion, Central venous pressure, Critically ill

Background

Echocardiography is a noninvasive diagnostic tool and can provide important information regarding certain haemodynamic parameters [1]. Among the measures of the right ventricle (RV) systolic function, the tricuspid annular plane systolic excursion (TAPSE) is easily applied and has low inter-observer variability [2, 3]. The American Society of Echocardiography recommend using the TAPSE routinely as a simple method to estimate the RV systolic function [4]. The TAPSE has also been shown to have prognostic value both in patients with pulmonary hypertension and heart failure and in noncardiac critically ill patients [5–7].

The Central venous pressure (CVP) is widely recognized as a useful parameter for managing critically ill patients. The CVP is determined by venous return and RV function and plays an important role in the monitoring and management of right ventricular failure patients [8–11]. Even though the CVP can only provide information about fluid responsiveness in extreme values, it is still useful when it is followed over time [12, 13]. Furthermore, the CVP can be used as a safety limit to avoid

* Correspondence: pumchicuky@163.com
[1]Department of Critical Care Medicine, Peking Union Medical College Hospital, Chinese Academy of Medical Sciences, 1# Shuai Fu Yuan, Dong Cheng District, Beijing 100730, China
Full list of author information is available at the end of the article

extra thoracic organ oedema because the risks for peripheral oedema, renal impairment and liver impairment are related to the absolute CVP value [14, 15]. Additionally, the CVP is of great value in the prognosis of critically ill patients [16, 17].

A previous study found that right ventricular outflow fractional shortening, which is used to assess right ventricular systolic function, can be used to predict the central venous pressure [18]. In a large cohort of healthy subjects, Ferrara F et al. noted that the TAPSE was correlated with echo-Doppler indices reflecting preload [19]. However, the relationship between the CVP and TAPSE has rarely been reported in the critically ill. The present study aimed to investigate the relationship between the TAPSE and CVP in mechanically ventilated critically ill patients.

Methods

Study population

Consecutive patients admitted to Peking Union Medical College Hospital Intensive Care Unit (ICU) from October 1 to December 31, 2017, were screened for enrolment within the first 24 h of being admitted.

Patients were included if they had central venous pressure monitoring and mechanically ventilation without spontaneous breath effort.

The exclusion criteria were post-cardiac surgery, acute Cor Pulmonale or severe pulmonary arterial hypertension (PAH), severe valvular disease, dilated or hypertrophic cardiomyopathy, constrictive pericarditis, Takotsubo syndrome, acute myocardial infarction, a non-sinus rhythm, intra-abdominal hypertension and an inadequate echocardiographic image for measurement.

This study was conducted according to the Declaration of Helsinki and was approved by the ethics committee of our institution. Written informed consent was obtained from the next of kin of each patient because all of the patients were in a state of unconscious.

Echocardiography

Echocardiograms were performed using an echocardiograph (CX50, PHILIPS, USA) with a 2.5-MHz phased-array probe within the first 24 h of ICU admission. ECG was recorded continuously during the echo examination. Three cardiac cycles were analysed and averaged. The patients were in the semi left lateral position during the examination. Echocardiographic M-mode and Doppler measurements were taken in a standard manner. The images were recorded for offline analysis. Two intensivists with experience in echocardiography performed the examination.

The left ventricular ejection fraction (LVEF) was obtained using a modified biplane Simpson's method from the apical two- and four-chamber views. Indexes of longitudinal systolic function measurements were taken from the apical four-chamber view. The mitral annular plane systolic excursion (MAPSE) was obtained by putting the cursor along the mitral ring and measuring the difference between the highest and lowest points of the M-mode sinusoid wave. The tricuspid annular plane systolic excursion (TAPSE) was obtained by putting the M-mode cursor along the lateral part of the tricuspid valve ring (Fig. 1). The ratio of end diastolic area of the

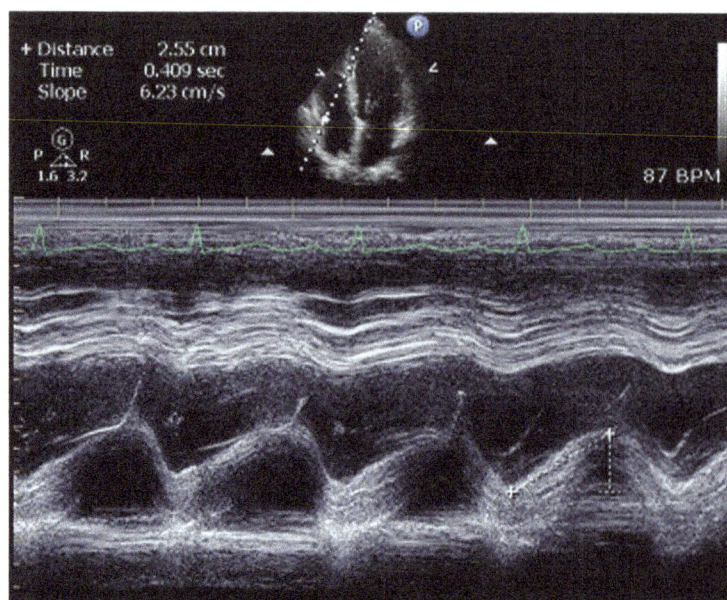

Fig. 1 The measurement of TAPSE

right ventricle and left ventricle (R/LVEDA) was measured at an apical 4-chamber view during end-diastole. The left ventricular outflow tract (LVOT) velocity-time integral (VTI) was obtained from pulsed Doppler by putting the sample volume at the LVOT approximately 0.5 cm below the aortic valve [20]. The IVC was examined subcostally in the longitudinal view, and its diameter was measured at the end of expiration just upstream of the origin of the suprahepatic vein.

Other parameters collected

The demographics, Acute Physiology and Chronic Health Evaluation (APACHE) II score, Sequential Organ Failure Assessment (SOFA) score, reason for admission and comorbidities were collected for each patient. A central line was placed in the internal jugular vein for all patients to allow for the CVP measurement. We recorded the heart rate (HR), mean arterial pressure (MAP), CVP, vasoactive agents and ventilator settings at the onset of the echo examination.

Statistical analysis

The statistical analysis was performed using the SPSS 13.0 statistical software package (SPSS Inc., Chicago, Illinois, USA). Continuous data were expressed as the mean ± SD or as the median and the interquartile range. Categorical variables were presented as the number and the percentages. Normal distribution of the continuous values was assessed by the Kolmogorov-Smirnov test.

Group comparisons were performed by Students' t test, Mann-Whitney U test or Chi-squared test or Fisher's exact test where appropriate. A partial correlation test was used to assess univariate relations. Multivariable linear regression analysis, including all echocardiographic parameters from the univariate analysis, was constructed to assess the independent associations of these variables with the CVP. Receiver-operating characteristic (ROC) curves were analysed, and the areas under each respective curve were calculated and compared. All p-values were two tailed and were considered significant when p < 0.05. Intraobserver and interobserver variability on TAPSE, dIVC, LVEF were assessed in 20 randomly selected patients and were tested using both paired t tests and intraclass correlation coefficients (ICCs). An ICC '0.8 was considered excellent agreement.

Results
General characteristics of all patients

A total of 146 patients were screened for enrolment in the study and 74 were included; of them, 31 patients were placed in the low LVEF (< 55%) group and the remaining 43 were placed in the high LVEF (≥55%) group (Fig. 2). The general characteristics of the patients are illustrated in Table 1. The reasons for admission to ICU included sepsis, high risk surgery and others (stoke, renal failure, and severe electrolyte disturbances). No difference was found between the two groups in terms of age, sex, reason for admission and comorbidities. The

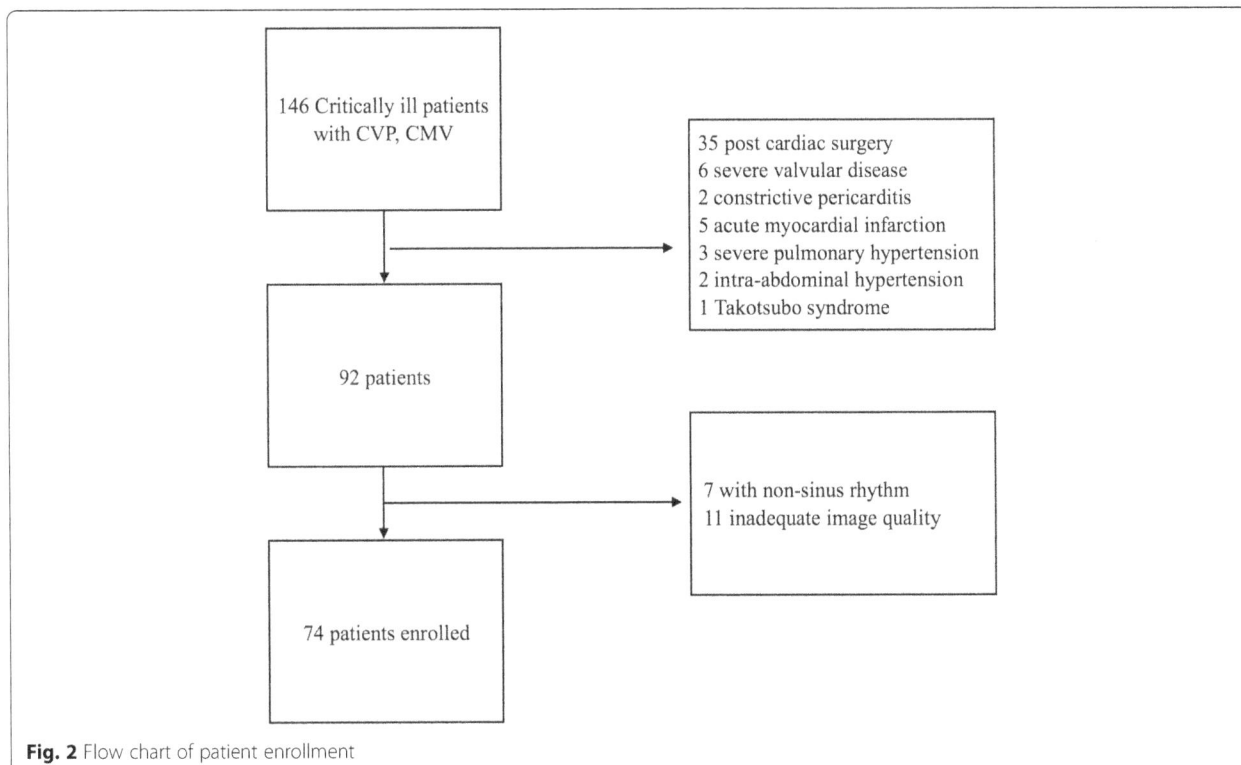

Fig. 2 Flow chart of patient enrollment

Table 1 General Characteristics

Categories	LVEF<55%(n = 31)	LVEF≥55%(n = 43)	p
Age (yr)	67.4 ± 16.5	61.1 ± 15.5	0.096
Sex (male, %)	23 (71.9%)	26 (60.5%)	0.303
APACHEII	20.6 ± 8.1	16.9 ± 6.2	0.032
SOFA	9.5 ± 2.6	7.4 ± 3.0	0.005
Reason for admission (n, %)			
Sepsis	18 (56.3%)	22(51.2%)	0.674
High-risk Surgery	10 (31.3%)	19(44.2%)	0.250
Others	4 (12.5%)	2 (4.7%)	0.220
Comorbidities (n, %)			
HTN	13 (40.6%)	14 (32.6%)	0.466
CAD	4 (12.5%)	4 (9.3%)	0.650
DM	6 (18.7%)	7 (16.3%)	0.762
Stroke	2 (6.3%)	1 (2.3%)	0.405
NE (n, %)	23 (71.9%)	20 (46.5%)	0.027
NE dose (µg/kg/min)	0.35 (0.19, 0.60)	0.18 (0.06, 0.30)	0.008
ARDS (n, %)	7 (22.6%)	5 (11.6%)	0.201
PEEP (mmHg)	6.1 ± 1.9	5.7 ± 1.4	0.310
Pplat (mmHg)	16.1 ± 4.7	15.9 ± 2.9	0.798

*Others: stroke, renal failure, severe electrolyte disturbances
APACHE acute physiology and chronic health evaluation, SOFA sequential organ failure assessment, HTN hypertension, CAD coronary arterial disease, DM diabetes mellitus, NE norepinephrine, ARDS acute respiratory distress syndrome, PEEP positive end expiratory pressure, Pplat plateau pressure

Table 2 Hemodynamics and echocardiographic parameters

Categories	LVEF<55%(n = 31)	LVEF≥55%(n = 43)	p
HR (bpm)	95 ± 19	90 ± 21	0.351
MAP (mmHg)	87 ± 15	91 ± 16	0.240
CVP (mmHg)	9 (8, 10)	8 (5, 10)	0.056
R/LVEDA (n, %)			
>1	0	0	–
0.6–1	20 (64.5%)	23(53.5%)	0.351
<0.6	11 (35.5%)	20 (46.5%)	0.351
TAPSE (cm)	1.61 ± 0.49	2.15 ± 0.37	<0.001
MAPSE (cm)	1.17 ± 0.42	1.55 ± 0.37	<0.001
dIVC (cm)	1.8 ± 0.3	1.6 ± 0.4	0.017
VTI (cm)	16.3 ± 4.5	20.9 ± 5.7	<0.001
LVEF (%)	45 ± 9	69 ± 6	<0.001

HR heart rate, MAP mean arterial pressure, CVP central venous pressure, R/LVEDA ratio of end diastolic area between right and left ventricle, TAPSE tricuspid annular plane systolic excursion, MAPSE mitral annular plane systolic excursion, dIVC internal diameter of inferior vena cava, VTI velocity-time integral, LVEF left ventricular ejection fraction

different. No difference was found in the HR and MAP between the groups (Table 2).

Correlation between the CVP and echocardiographic parameters in the high LVEF group

In the univariate analysis, the CVP was positively correlated with the dIVC ($r = 0.414$, 95% confidence interval [CI]: 0.061–0.680, $p = 0.009$). No significant correlation was found between the CVP and other parameters, including the TAPSE, MAPSE, VTI and LVEF. In a multivariable analysis, the dIVC was the only independent variable associated with the CVP (standard coefficient 0.522, $p < 0.001$) (Table 3).

Correlation between the CVP and echocardiographic parameters in the low LVEF group

In the univariate analysis, the CVP was positively correlated with the dIVC ($r = 0.390$, 95%CI: 0.012 to 0.689, $p = 0.044$) and negatively correlated with the TAPSE ($r = -0.516$, 95%CI: -0.132 to -0.799, $P = 0.006$) (Fig. 3).

low LVEF group had higherAPACHE II and SOFA scores, 20.6 vs 16.9, $p = 0.032$ and 9.5 vs 7.4, $p = 0.005$, respectively. The low LVEF group had more patients being administered norepinephrine (NE) and had a larger dose, 71.9% vs 46.5%, $p = 0.027$ and 0.35 µg/kg/min vs 0.18 µg/kg/min, $p = 0.008$, respectively. No differences were found in the proportion of ARDS patients, positive end expiration pressure (PEEP) and plateau pressure (Pplat) between the two groups.

Haemodynamic and echocardiographic parameters

The mean LVEFs in the low LVEF group and high LVEF group were 45 and 69%, respectively. The low LVEF group had a higher CVP than the high LVEF group did, but this difference was not statistically significant (9 mmHg vs 8 mmHg, $p = 0.056$). Compared with the high LVEF group, the low LVEF group had a significantly lower VTI, 16.3 cm vs 20.9 cm, $p < 0.001$. The low LVEF group also had a significantly lower TASPE and MAPSE, 1.61 cm vs 2.15 cm, p < 0.001 and 1.17 cm vs 1.55 cm, p < 0.001, respectively. The low LVEF group had a greater dIVC, 1.8 cm vs 1.6 cm, $p = 0.017$. None of the patients in the two groups were found to have a R/LVEDA>1, and the proportion of patients with a R/LVEDA 0.6–1 and R/LVEDA < 0.6 between the groups was not significantly

Table 3 Significant independent relation of CVP with echocardiographic variables in high LVEF group

Variables	Univariate analysis			Multivariate analysis	
		95%CI	P	Std coefficient (β)	P
TAPSE	−0.234	−0.516 to 0.161	0.151	−0.215	0.107
dIVC	0.414	0.061 to 0.680	0.009	0.522	<0.001
MAPSE	−0.014	−0.292 to 0.287	0.932	−0.134	0.347
VTI	0.283	0.017 to 0.516	0.081	0.230	0.118
LVEF	0.133	−0.200 to 0.475	0.420	0.107	0.430

TAPSE tricuspid annular plane systolic excursion, MAPSE mitral annular plane systolic excursion, dIVC internal diameter of inferior vena cava, VTI velocity-time integral, LVEF left ventricular ejection fraction, Std standard

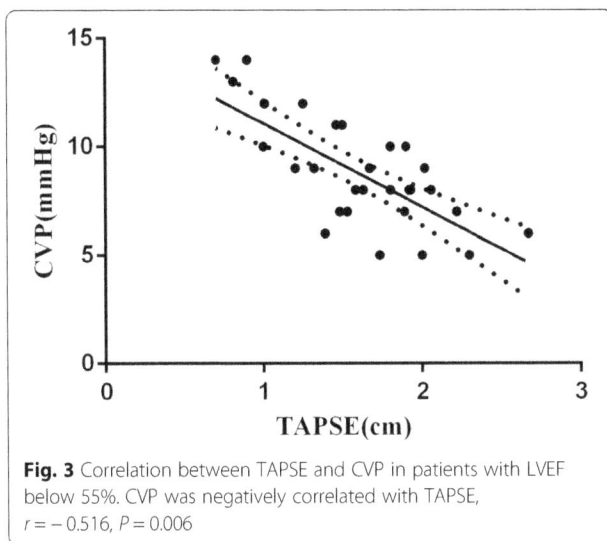

Fig. 3 Correlation between TAPSE and CVP in patients with LVEF below 55%. CVP was negatively correlated with TAPSE, $r = -0.516$, $P = 0.006$

No significant correlation was observed between the CVP and other parameters, including the MAPSE, VTI and LVEF. In a multivariable analysis, the TAPSE and dIVC were independent variables associated with the CVP (standard coefficient -0.601, $p < 0.001$ and standard coefficient 0.300, $p = 0.030$, respectively) (Table 4).

To evaluate the sensitivity and specificity of the two parameters for detecting a CVP greater than 8 mmHg, ROC curves were calculated (Fig. 4). The ROC analysis showed that the TAPSE was a good marker, with an area under the curve (AUC) of 0.860 (95% CI: 0.730–0.991, $P = 0.001$). The AUC of the dIVC was 0.723 (95%CI: 0.533–0.913, $p = 0.034$). The two AUCs were not statistically different ($Z = -1.162$, $p = 0.245$).

For the TAPSE, the optimum cut-off value was 1.52 cm, which resulted in a sensitivity of 75.0%, a specificity of 86.7%, a positive predictive value (PPV) of 84.6% and a negative predictive value (NPV) of 77.8%. For the dIVC, the optimum cut-off value was 1.8 cm, which resulted in a sensitivity of 68.8%, a specificity of 73.3%, a PPV of 64.2% and an NPV of 76.5%.

Table 4 Significant independent relation of CVP with echocardiographic variables in low LVEF group

Variables	Univariate analysis			Multivariate analysis	
	r	95%CI	P	Std coefficient (β)	P
TAPSE	−0.516	−0.132 to −0.799	0.006	−0.601	<0.001
dIVC	0.390	0.012 to 0.689	0.044	0.300	0.030
MAPSE	0.021	−0.447 to 0.546	0.918	0.004	0.978
VTI	−0.239	−0.489 to 0.018	0.231	−0.170	0.763
LVEF	−0.067	−0.455 to 0.274	0.741	−0.029	0.886

TAPSE tricuspid annular plane systolic excursion, *MAPSE* mitral annular plane systolic excursion *dIVC* internal diameter of inferior vena cava, *VTI* velocity-time integral, *LVEF* left ventricular ejection fraction, *Std* standard

Measurement variability

The intraobserver variabilities on TAPSE, dIVC and LVEF were minimal. The interobserver variability analysis revealed that ICCS regarding TAPSE, dIVC and LVEF were respectively: 0.937 (95%CI:0.824–0.978), 0.987 (95%CI:0.948–0.997) and 0.925 (95%CI:0.792–0.974).

Discussion

TAPSE is a clinically feasible parameter of the RV and has been proven to be a valuable prognostic marker in various cardiac diseases [5, 21, 22]. Interestingly, in this study, we observed striking differences on the relationship between the CVP and TASPE in patients with a LVEF below 55% and in those with a LVEF of 55% and greater. We observed that the TAPSE was inversely correlated with the CVP in critically ill patients who had a LVEF below 55%. When adjusting for other possible confounding factors, the TAPSE remained an independent predictor of the CVP, and it was proven to be a good marker for discriminating whether the CVP was greater than 8 mmHg.

Volume is among the first steps of shock therapy [23]. Although dynamic parameters of volume responsiveness are recommended, they have their own innate weaknesses. Pulse pressure variation or stroke volume variation can only be used reliably in a subset of patients, i.e., those who are mechanically ventilated, sedated and without arrhythmias [24]. The passive leg raising test has fewer limitations but is not as simple to perform as it may seem at first glance; it also requires a close monitoring of stroke volume [25]. As a parameter, the CVP is far from perfect but is of great value in fluid therapy of the critically ill [26]. Our results suggest that TAPSE has the potential to predict the CVP in low LVEF patients and provides a noninvasive way to assess the right atrial pressure. The reliability of IVC respiratory variation to assess volume responsiveness has long been debated. No decisive conclusions on the accuracy of IVC respiratory variation can be drawn [27–29]. In consistency with prior studies, we found that dIVC is directly correlated with the CVP [30, 31]. However, dIVC has its own limitations. In a group of cardiac surgical patients, Lorsomradee S, et al. noted that the correlation between the dIVC and CVP was poor when the CVP was greater than 11 mmHg [32]. Other researchers also noted that the IVC dimension and collapsibility have limited utility in identifying the magnitude of CVP elevation [33, 34]. Thus, the TAPSE could be an alternative parameter in assessing right atrial pressure for low LVEF patients.

RV function, which is often compromised when facing an elevated afterload, could lead to elevation of the CVP. A linear inverse relationship was observed between the TAPSE and pulmonary vascular resistance in a group of

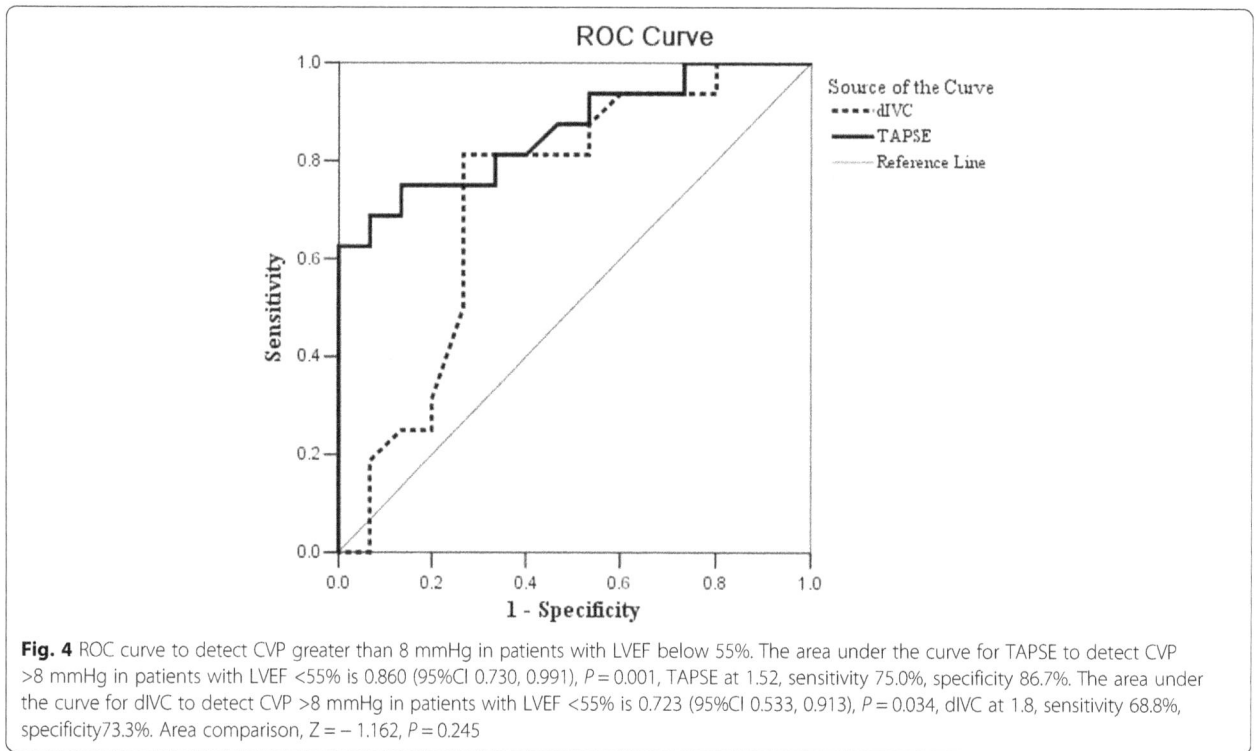

Fig. 4 ROC curve to detect CVP greater than 8 mmHg in patients with LVEF below 55%. The area under the curve for TAPSE to detect CVP >8 mmHg in patients with LVEF <55% is 0.860 (95%CI 0.730, 0.991), $P = 0.001$, TAPSE at 1.52, sensitivity 75.0%, specificity 86.7%. The area under the curve for dIVC to detect CVP >8 mmHg in patients with LVEF <55% is 0.723 (95%CI 0.533, 0.913), $P = 0.034$, dIVC at 1.8, sensitivity 68.8%, specificity73.3%. Area comparison, $Z = -1.162$, $P = 0.245$

PAH patients who had a mean systolic pulmonary pressure of 75 mmHg [5]. However, no such relationship was found among healthy subjects [19]. In this study, patients with severe PAH were excluded. No difference was found between the groups regarding the proportion of ARDS patients and the levels of PEEP and Pplat. We did include the measurement of the R/LVEDA and no difference was found between high and low LVEF patients. These results suggest that the two groups had the same risk for RV afterload elevation. Left ventricle (LV) dysfunction could also precipitate pulmonary arterial pressure through an elevated left atrial pressure [35]. However, in a group of heart failure patients, no relation was discovered between the TAPSE and maximal tricuspid regurgitation pressure gradient [22]. Therefore, the correlation of the TAPSE and CVP cannot be explained by RV afterload elevation in these low LVEF patients.

To date, the accepted definition of septic myocardiopathy is based on a depressed LVEF, but several studies reported that the RV function was also compromised [36, 37]. However, a significant part of the RV systolic function depends on the LV systolic function, and its incidence is difficult to identify [38]. The right ventricle is bounded by its free wall with transverse fibre orientation in the septum; this is essential for ventricular twisting, which is the vital mechanism for RV ejection [39]. An experimental study demonstrated that 30% of the contraction force of the RV comes from the LV [40]. A previous study reported that the TAPSE is reduced with LV

dysfunction in heart failure patients, particularly with reduced septal longitudinal motion [41]. We speculated that the TAPSE was determined, to a greater degree, by the right ventricular function in patients with a low LVEF. Therefore, it is likely that TAPSE can reflect the RV function and volume load more precisely when treating patients with low LVEF. Although the mechanism needs further study to confirm it, the result of this study indicated that monitoring of the TAPSE in these patients holds greater value.

There are several limitations to this study. First, TAPSE is a load- and angle-dependent parameter that is reflective of both the right and left ventricle function. Furthermore, this is a single-centre study, and the sample size is insufficient to provide a definite conclusion. Nevertheless, it represents a useful pilot study for further prospective investigations with larger numbers of patients. Second, pulmonary arterial pressure was not measured directly through techniques like Swan-Ganz catheter, and only a few patients were found with measurable tricuspid regurgitation on echocardiography. This may limit the direct interpretation of RV afterload. Third, the subjects in this study were heterogeneous, and the cause of LV dysfunction was not addressed. Previous studies demonstrated that LV dysfunction was very common in ICU patients and that a variety of conditions could result in LV dysfunction, including severe sepsis, prolonged hypoxia, severe metabolic and multiorgan insults, and even tachyarrhythmias [42, 43]. Chockalingam A et al.

noted that, to present a unified management approach, acute left ventricular dysfunction could be classified into global LV dysfunction, acute coronary syndrome, stress cardiomyopathy and myocardial injury with minor troponin elevations [42]. The present study excluded patients with severe valvular disease, severe pulmonary hypertension, acute myocardial infarction and Takotsubo syndrome. Therefore, only patients with normal LV function or patients with global LV dysfunction were enrolled. Moreover, the patients in this study reflected the makeup of the population referred for critical care in clinical practice.

Conclusion

TAPSE is inversely correlated with CVP in mechanically ventilated critically ill patients who have a LVEF less than 55%.

Abbreviations

CVP: Central venous pressure; TAPSE: Tricuspid annular plane systolic excursion; MAPSE: Mitral annular plane systolic excursion; dIVC: Internal diameter of inferior vena cava; LVEF: Left ventricular ejection fraction; RV: Right ventricle; ICU: Intensive care unit; PAH: Pulmonary arterial hypertension; R/LVEDA: Ratio of end diastolic area of the right ventricle and left ventricle; LVOT: Left ventricular outflow tract; VTI: Velocity-time integral; APACHE Ⅱ score: Acute Physiology and Chronic Health Evaluation Ⅱ score; SOFA: Sequential Organ Failure Assessment; HR: Heart rate; MAP: Mean arterial pressure; NE: Norepinephrine; PEEP: Positive end expiration pressure; Pplat: Plateau pressure; LV: Left ventricle

Acknowledgements

This study was performed at Critical Care Department of Peking Union Medical College Hospital.
We would like to thank Dr. Wei He, from Beijing Tongren Hospital, for his good advice on the study design. We would also like to thank Prof. Fuhai Shen, from Department of Epidemiology North China University of Science and Technology, for his kind suggestions on the statistical issue.

Funding

Nil.

Authors' contributions

HZ conceived and designed the study, analyzed and interpreted data, performed the statistical analysis, and drafted the manuscript. XW analyzed data and revised the manuscript. XC analyzed data and revised the manuscript. QZ obtained data and revised manuscript. DL designed the study, interpreted data and revised the manuscript. All authors read and approved the final manuscript.

Competing interests

The authors declare that they have no competing interests.

Author details

Department of Critical Care Medicine, Peking Union Medical College Hospital, Chinese Academy of Medical Sciences, 1# Shuai Fu Yuan, Dong Cheng District, Beijing 100730, China. ²Pittsburgh Heart, Lung, Blood and Vascular Medicine Institute, University of Pittsburgh, Pittsburg, PA 15261, USA.

References

1. Beigel R, Cercek B, Arsanjani R, Siegel RJ. Echocardiography in the use of noninvasive hemodynamic monitoring. J Crit Care. 2014;29:184. e181–8
2. Kopecna D, Briongos S, Castillo H, Moreno C, Recio M, Navas P, et al. Interobserver reliability of echocardiography for prognostication of normotensive patients with pulmonary embolism. Cardiovasc Ultrasound. 2014;12:29.
3. Aloia E, Cameli M, D'Ascenzi F, Sciaccaluga C, Mondillo S. TAPSE: an old but useful tool in different diseases. Int J Cardiol. 2016;225:177–83.
4. Rudski LG, Lai WW, Afilalo J, Hua LQ, Handschumacher MD, Chandrasekaran K, et al. Guidelines for the echocardiographic assessment of the right heart in adults: a report from the American Society of Echocardiography endorsed by the European Association of Echocardiography, a registered branch of the European Society of Cardiology, and the Canadian Society of Echocardiography. J Am Soc Echocardiog. 2010;23:685–713.
5. Forfia PR, Fisher MR, Mathai SC, Housten-Harris T, Hemnes AR, Borlaug BA, et al. Tricuspid annular displacement predicts survival in pulmonary hypertension. Am J Respir Crit Care Med. 2006;174:1034–41.
6. Damy T, Kallvikbacka-Bennett A, Goode K, Khaleva O, Lewinter C, Hobkirk J, et al. Prevalence of, associations with, and prognostic value of tricuspid annular plane systolic excursion (TAPSE) among out-patients referred for the evaluation of heart failure. J Card Fail. 2012;18:216–25.
7. Demirkol S, Ozturk C, Unlu M, Arslan Z, Celik T. Tricuspid annular plane systolic excursion and its association with mortality in critically ill patients: right ventricular function in critically ill patients. Echocardiography. 2015;32:1330.
8. Guyton AC. Determination of cardiac output by equating venous return curves with cardiac response curves. Physiol Rev. 1955;35:123–9.
9. Cecconi M, Aya HD, Geisen M, Ebm C, Fletcher N, Grounds RM, et al. Changes in the mean systemic filling pressure during a fluid challenge in postsurgical intensive care patients. Intensive Care Med. 2013;39:1299–305.
10. Green EM, Givertz MM. Management of acute right ventricular failure in the intensive care unit. Curr Heart Fail Rep. 2012;9:228–35.
11. Haddad F, Hunt SA, Rosenthal DN, Murphy DJ. Right ventricular function in cardiovascular disease, part I: anatomy, physiology, aging, and functional assessment of the right ventricle. Circulation. 2008;117:1436–48.
12. Magder S. Understanding central venous pressure: not a preload index? Curr Opin Crit Care. 2015;21:369–75.
13. Eskesen TG, Wetterslev M, Perner A. Systematic review including re-analyses of 1148 individual data sets of central venous pressure as a predictor of fluid responsiveness. Intensive Care Med. 2016;42:324–32.
14. Legrand M, Dupuis C, Simon C, Gayat E, Mateo J, Lukaszewicz AC, et al. Association between systemic hemodynamics and septic acute kidney injury in critically ill patients: a retrospective observational study. Crit Care. 2013;17:R278.
15. Chen KP, Cavender S, Lee J, Feng M, Mark RG, Celi LA, et al. Peripheral edema, central venous pressure, and risk of AKI in critical illness. Clin J Am Soc Nephrol. 2016;11:602–8.
16. Wang XT, Yao B, Liu DW, Zhang HM. Central venous pressure dropped early is associated with organ function and prognosis in septic shock patients: a retrospective observational study. Shock. 2015;44:426–30.
17. Long Y, Su L, Zhang Q, Zhou X, Wang H, Cui N, et al. Elevated mean airway pressure and central venous pressure in the first day of mechanical ventilation indicated poor outcome. Crit Care Med. 2017;45:e485–92.
18. Unluer EE, Yavasi O, Akoglu H, Kara HP, Bayata S, Yurekli I, et al. Bedside assessment of central venous pressure by sonographic measurement of right ventricular outflow-tract fractional shortening. Eur J Emerg Med. 2013;20:18–22.
19. Ferrara F, Rudski LG, Vriz O, Gargani L, Afilalo J, D'Andrea A, et al. Physiologic correlates of tricuspid annular plane systolic excursion in 1168 healthy subjects. Int J Cardiol. 2016;223:736–43.
20. MA Q, CM O, Stoddard M, Waggoner A, WA Z, Nomenclature DQTFot, et al. Recommendations for quantification of Doppler echocardiography: a report from the Doppler quantification task force of the nomenclature and standards Committee of the American Society of echocardiography. J Am Soc Echocardiog. 2002;15:167–84.
21. Gajanana D, Seetha Rammohan H, Alli O, Romero-Corral A, Purushottam B, Ponamgi S, et al. Tricuspid annular plane systolic excursion and its association with mortality in critically ill patients. Echocardiography. 2015;32:1222–7.
22. Kjaergaard J, Akkan D, Iversen KK, Kober L, Torp-Pedersen C, Hassager C. Right ventricular dysfunction as an independent predictor of short- and long-term mortality in patients with heart failure. Eur J Heart Fail. 2007;9:610–6.

23. Vincent JL, De Backer D. Circulatory shock. N Engl J Med. 2013;369:1726–34.

24. Yang X, Du B. Does pulse pressure variation predict fluid responsiveness in critically ill patients? syst rev meta-analysis Crit Care. 2014;18:650.

25. He HW, Liu DW. Passive Leg Raising in Intensive Care Medicine. Chin Med J (Engl). 2016;129:1755–8.

26. De Backer D, Vincent JL. Should we measure the central venous pressure to guide fluid management? Ten answers to 10 questions. Crit Care. 2018;22:43.

27. Orso D, Paoli I, Piani T, Cilenti FL, Cristiani L, Guglielmo N. Accuracy of Ultrasonographic Measurements of Inferior Vena Cava to Determine Fluid Responsiveness: A Systematic Review and Meta-Analysis. J Intensive Care Med. 2018;55:1–10.

28. Long E, Oakley E, Duke T, Babl FE. Does respiratory variation in inferior vena cava diameter predict fluid responsiveness: a systematic review and meta-analysis. Shock. 2017;47:550–9.

29. Zhang Z, Xu X, Ye S, Xu L. Ultrasonographic measurement of the respiratory variation in the inferior vena cava diameter is predictive of fluid responsiveness in critically ill patients: systematic review and meta-analysis. Ultrasound Med Biol. 2014;40:845–53.

30. Ommen SR, Nishimura RA, Hurrell DG, Klarich KW. Assessment of right atrial pressure with 2-dimensional and Doppler echocardiography: a simultaneous catheterization and echocardiographic study. Mayo Clin Proc. 2000;75:24–9.

31. Schefold JC, Storm C, Bercker S, Pschowski R, Oppert M, Kruger A, et al. Inferior vena cava diameter correlates with invasive hemodynamic measures in mechanically ventilated intensive care unit patients with sepsis. J Emerg Med. 2010;38:632–7.

32. Lorsomradee S, Lorsomradee S, Cromheecke S, ten Broecke PW, De Hert SG. Inferior vena cava diameter and central venous pressure correlation during cardiac surgery. J Cardiothorac Vasc Anesth. 2007;21:492–6.

33. Beigel R, Cercek B, Luo H, Siegel RJ. Noninvasive evaluation of right atrial pressure. J Am Soc Echocardiogr. 2013;26:1033–42.

34. Moreno FLL, Hagan AD, JRH M, Pryor TA, Strickland RD, Castle CH. Evaluation of size and dynamics of the inferior vena cava as an index of right-sided cardiac function. Am J Cardiol. 1984;53:579–85.

35. Hansmann G. Pulmonary hypertension in infants, children, and young adults. J Am Coll Cardiol. 2017;69:2551.

36. Pulido JN, Afessa B, Masaki M, Yuasa T, Gillespie S, Herasevich V, et al. Clinical spectrum, frequency, and significance of myocardial dysfunction in severe sepsis and septic shock. Mayo Clin Proc. 2012;87:620–8.

37. Harmankaya A, Akilli H, Gul M, Akilli NB, Ergin M, Aribas A, et al. Assessment of right ventricular functions in patients with sepsis, severe sepsis and septic shock and its prognostic importance: a tissue Doppler study. J Crit Care. 2013;28:e7–11.

38. Vieillard-Baron A, Cecconi M. Understanding cardiac failure in sepsis. Intensive Care Med. 2014;40:1560–3.

39. Saleh S, Liakopoulos OJ, Buckberg GD. The septal motor of biventricular function. Eur J Cardiothorac Surg. 2006;29(Suppl 1):S126–38.

40. Santamore WP, Dell'Italia LJ. Ventricular interdependence: significant left ventricular contributions to right ventricular systolic function. Prog Cardiovasc Dis. 1998;40:289–308.

41. Kjaergaard J, Iversen KK, Akkan D, Moller JE, Kober LV, Torp-Pedersen C, et al. Predictors of right ventricular function as measured by tricuspid annular plane systolic excursion in heart failure. Cardiovasc Ultrasound. 2009;7:51.

42. Chockalingam A, Mehra A, Dorairajan S, Dellsperger KC. Acute left ventricular dysfunction in the critically ill. Chest. 2010;138:198–207.

43. Marcelino PA, Marum SM, Fernandes AP, Germano N, Lopes MG. Routine transthoracic echocardiography in a general intensive care unit: an 18 month survey in 704 patients. Eur J Intern Med. 2009;20:e37–42.

19

Post-operative left atrial volume index is a predictor of the occurrence of permanent atrial fibrillation after mitral valve surgery in patients who undergo mitral valve surgery

Min-Kyung Kang[1], Boyoung Joung[2], Chi Young Shim[2], In Jeong Cho[2], Woo-In Yang[3], Jeonggeun Moon[4], Yangsoo Jang[2], Namsik Chung[2], Byung-Chul Chang[2] and Jong-Won Ha[2]*

Abstract

Background: Atrial fibrillation (AF) can occur even after the correction of mitral valve (MV) pathology in patients who have pre-operative sinus rhythm and undergo MV surgery. However, the factors associated with the occurrence of AF after MV surgery are still unclear. The aim of this retrospective study was to investigate the factors determining the occurrence of permanent AF after MV surgery in patients with preoperative sinus rhythm who underwent MV surgery.

Methods: Four hundred and forty-two patients (mean age 46 ± 12, 190 men) who underwent MV surgery and sinus rhythm were investigated retrospectively. Transthoracic echocardiography was performed before and after MV surgery at the time of dismissal.

Results: Permanent post-operative AF occurred in 81 (18%) patients even after successful MV surgery and preoperative sinus rhythm. It was more common in rheumatic etiology, a presence of mitral stenosis, lower pre- and post-operative left ventricular ejection fraction, higher post-operative mean diastolic pressure gradient across mitral prosthesis, larger post-operative left atrial volume index (LAVI) and lesser degrees of reduction in LAVI after surgery. In multiple regression analysis, post-operative LAVI was found to be an independent predictor for occurrence of AF. Post-operative LAVI > 39 ml/m2 was the cut-off value for best prediction of new onset permanent AF (sensitivity: 79%, AUC: 0.762, SE: 0.051, $p < 0.001$).

Conclusion: New-onset permanent post-operative AF is not uncommon, even after successful MV surgery despite pre-operative sinus rhythm. Larger post-operative LAVI was an independent predictor for the occurrence of AF.

Keywords: Atrial fibrillation, Mitral valve, Left atrium

Background

Increased left atrial (LA) size is associated with the occurrence of atrial fibrillation (AF) [1]. Therefore, AF is frequently observed in patients with chronic mitral valve (MV) disease, which invariably induces LA remodeling [2–4]. On the other hand, reduction of LA size (reverse LA remodeling) can also occur after correction of MV pathology [3, 5]. It has been shown that the degree of reverse LA remodeling varies, particularly according to pre-operative cardiac rhythm. Moreover, pre-operative sinus rhythm is associated with larger degrees of reverse LA remodeling [3]. In addition, this structural reversal can also induce reversal of electrophysiologic abnormalities that are predisposed to the occurrence of AF. Therefore, reversal of these changes by treatment, i.e., MV surgery, could potentially have important implications for the prevention of AF [5, 6]. Nevertheless AF can occur even after correction of MV pathology in patients who have undergone MV surgery [7–17]. However, the incidence and

* Correspondence: jwha@yuhs.ac
[2]Division of Cardiology and Cardiovascular Surgery, Severance Cardiovascular Hospital, Yonsei University College of Medicine, 134 Shinchon-dong, Seodaemun-gu, Seoul 120-752, Republic of Korea
Full list of author information is available at the end of the article

predictors of new onset permanent AF after MV surgery have not been clearly defined. Therefore, the aim of this study is to investigate the prevalence and predictors of the occurrence of new onset permanent AF in patients with MV diseases who have undergone MV surgery and sinus rhythm pre-operatively.

Methods

Study design and participants

A total of 1841 patients underwent MV surgery from June 1982 to February 2009. Among them, patients with pre-existing AF, concomitant MAZE procedure during surgery ($n = 1189$), patients with permanent pacemaker implantation ($n = 20$), and patients unknown pre-operative rhythm ($n = 190$) were excluded. The remaining 442 patients (mean age 46 ± 12, 191 men) comprised the study population (Fig. 1). We reviewed the medical records to define the etiology of MV pathology and reason for valve surgery in addition to pre- and post-operative transthoracic echocardiography (TTE) and electrocardiogram (ECG). ECG was taken pre- and post-operatively and at follow up once a year thereafter. New onset permanent AF was defined as the occurrence of AF post-operatively detected by post-operative ECG during the hospital stay and that persisted thereafter.

Echocardiography

TTE was performed by standard techniques with a 2.5-MHz transducer. Two-dimensional echocardiographic images were obtained in the standard parasternal long-axis and apical 2 and 4 chamber views. Left ventricular (LV) ejection fraction (EF) was assessed by the modified Quinones method. Mediolateral (ML) and superior/inferior (SI) dimensions of LA were measured from the apical 4 chamber view, and anteroposterior (AP) dimensions were measured from the parasternal long axis view

at the end-systole. Maximal LA volume was calculated using the prolate ellipsoid model3 and indexed to the body surface area (LA volume index; LAVI). Measurement of LA volume was available in 200 of 442 patients at pre- and post-operative periods. In those patients, the LA volume change and the percentage of LA volume change were calculated [18]. Assessment of valvuar heart diseases were based on the guidelines [19].

Statistical analysis

Continuous variables are presented as means $\pm$ standard deviation (SD) and compared using Student's unpaired t test or Mann-Whitney's U test. Categorical variables are presented as numbers or percentages, and used the Chi-square test. To determine the variables associated with the occurrence of AF, logistic regression analysis was performed separately using clinical variables and echo-cardiographic findings. The predictive ability of the LAVI was determined by the area under the receiver-operating characteristic curves (ROC). Kaplan-Meier estimator was used for AF free survival curves. P value < 0.05 was considered statistically significant.

Results

The enrolled patients were classified into the two groups according to the occurrence of permanent AF or maintained sinus rhythm after MV surgery (normal sinus rhythm [NSR] group vs. AF group). Post-operative new onset permanent AF occurred in 81 (18%) patients. Baseline characteristics of the study subjects are shown in Table 1. The mean age at the time of surgery was similar in both groups. The majority of patients (81%) had rheumatic etiology and others (19%) had non-rheumatic etiology, such as infective endocarditis, MV prolapse, or chordae rupture. The proportion of rheumatic valve disease was significantly higher in patients

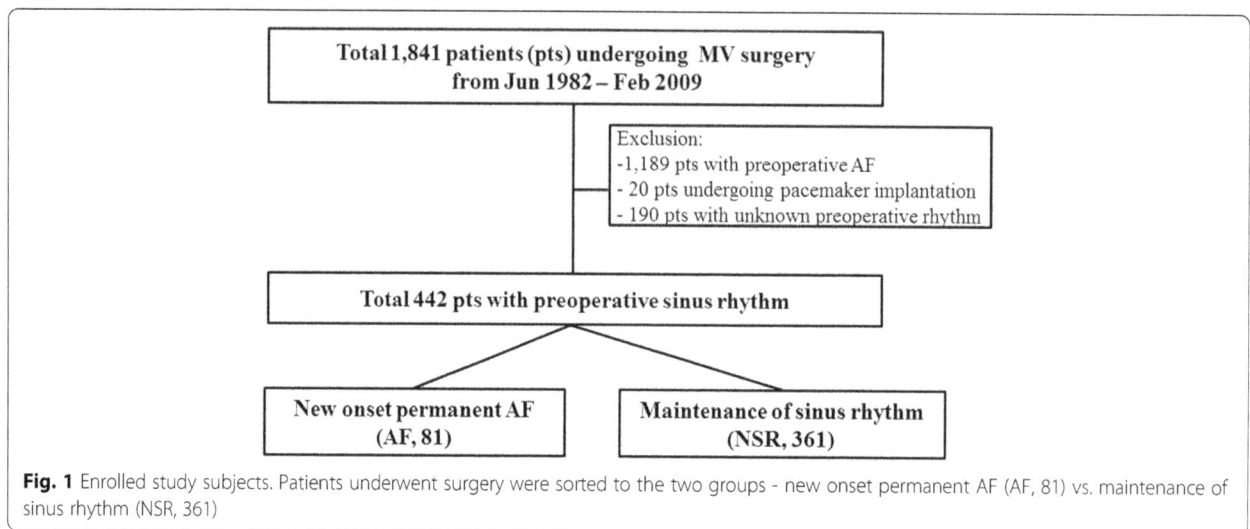

Fig. 1 Enrolled study subjects. Patients underwent surgery were sorted to the two groups - new onset permanent AF (AF, 81) vs. maintenance of sinus rhythm (NSR, 361)

Table 1 Baseline characteristics of the patients

Variables	NSR (n = 361)	AF (n = 81)	p
Age at surgery (years)	41 ± 13	41 ± 11	0.782
Male gender	151 (42%)	39 (49%)	0.264
Body surface area (m²)	1.65 ± 0.16	1.64 ± 0.16	0.967
Etiology			0.018
Rheumatic etiology	284 (79%)	73 (90%)	
Non-rheumatic valvular disease	77 (21%)	8 (10%)	
Diagnosis			0.065
Pure mitral regurgitation	205 (57%)	37 (46%)	
Presence of mitral stenosis	156 (43%)	44 (54%)	
Combined with other valve	180 (58%)	44 (70%)	0.091
Type of surgery			0.478
Mitral valve replacement	348 (96.4%)	79 (97.5%)	
Bioprosthesis	7 (2.0%)	2 (2.5%)	
Mechanical	341 (98.0%)	77 (97.5%)	
Mitral valve repair	13 (3.6%)	2 (2.5%)	
Annular size	28.4 ± 2.1	29.0 ± 2.6	0.070
Preoperative heart rate (bpm)	76 ± 19	75 ± 15	0.762
Preoperative blood pressure (mmHg)			
Systolic blood pressure	121 ± 17	123 ± 16	0.825
Diastolic blood pressure	75 ± 13	74 ± 10	0.623
Postoperative HR	73 ± 18	72 ± 14	0.854
Postoperative blood pressure			
Systolic blood pressure	119 ± 15	120 ± 15	0.718
Diastolic blood pressure	73 ± 11	74 ± 11	0.777

Table 2 Echocardiographic parameters before and after surgery

	NSR (n = 361)	AF (n = 81)	p
Before surgery			
LV end diastolic dimension (mm)	56.6 ± 10.8	55.0 ± 10.9	0.375
LV end systolic dimension (mm)	38.4 ± 9.2	38.7 ± 9.9	0.863
LV ejection fraction (%)	62.7 ± 10.0	58.9 ± 14.1	0.026
LA antero-posterior dimension (AP) (mm)	50.7 ± 8.7	53.1 ± 6.9	0.080
LA medio-lateral dimension (ML) (mm)	56.2 ± 10.6	58.6 ± 9.9	0.339
LA supero-inferior dimension (SI) (mm)	62.4 ± 9.7	60.4 ± 9.1	0.372
LA volume index (ml/m²)ᵃ	58.4 ± 24.9	62.9 ± 22.8	0.399
TR grade	0.4 ± 0.8	1.2 ± 1.1	0.005
Estimated PAP	39.2 ± 17.5	44.5 ± 18.4	0.252
After surgery			
LV end diastolic dimension (mm)	48.9 ± 5.3	50.1 ± 8.9	0.126
LV end systolic dimension (mm)	33.8 ± 5.8	35.9 ± 10.8	0.015
LV ejection fraction (%)	60.9 ± 9.5	57.2 ± 13.8	0.006
LA AP dimension (mm)	42.9 ± 6.0	50.7 ± 8.1	< .001
LA ML dimension (mm)	50.3 ± 6.8	56.3 ± 7.5	< .001
LA SI dimension (mm)	57.3 ± 27.5	61.8 ± 8.2	0.172
LA AP change (mm)	7.7 ± 8.4	4.1 ± 7.9	0.011
LA ML change (mm)	6.7 ± 10.4	3.4 ± 10.1	0.197
LA SI change (mm)	7.4 ± 9.0	1.3 ± 8.3	0.005
LA volume index (ml/m²)	37.9 ± 12.6	52.1 ± 15.6	< .001
LA volume change (ml/m²)	20.5 ± 21.3	10.8 ± 23.4	0.041
LA volume change %	28.1 ± 27.9	9.5 ± 36.8	< .001
MDPG of the MV (mmHg)	3.5 ± 1.4	3.9 ± 1.5	0.023
Residual mitral regurgitation			0.337
No	352 (97.5%)	77 (95.1%)	
Trivial	8 (2.2%)	3 (3.7%)	
More than grade I	1 (0.3%)	1 (1.2%)	
TR grade	0.3 ± 0.6	1.0 ± 1.0	< 0.001
Estimated PAP	26.4 ± 6.6	29.8 ± 7.1	0.001
TAP or TVR	33 (7.5%)	6 (1.4%)	0.828

ᵃLA volume index was available only in 200 patients (176 of NSR, 24 of AF); NSR normal sinus rhythm, AF atrial fibrillation, LV left ventricular, LA left atrial, MDPG mean diastolic pressure gradient, TR tricuspid regurgitation, PAP pulmonary artery pressure, TAP tricuspid valve repair with an annuloplasty ring, TVR tricuspid valve replacement

with new onset permanent AF ($p = 0.018$). The median interval from the surgery to the occurrence of AF was 9.2 years ($110.6 ± 78.9$ months), and the mean follow-up duration was not significantly different in both groups ($9.8 ± 5.9$ years in the NSR vs. $9.4 ± 6.5$ years in the AF, $p = 0.566$). The TTE parameters before and after surgery are listed in Table 2. Pre- and post-operative LV EF were significantly lower in the AF group ($63 ± 10\%$ in the NSR vs. $59 ± 14\%$ in the AF, $p = 0.026$ & $61 ± 10\%$ in the NSR vs. $57 ± 14\%$ in the AF, $p = 0.006$), although the LV EF of both groups were in normal range. Pre-operative LA AP dimension ($51 ± 9$ mm in the NSR vs. $53 ± 7$ mm in the AF, $p = 0.080$) and LAVI ($58 ± 25$ ml/m² in the NSR vs. $63 ± 23$ ml/m² in the AF, $p = 0.399$) were not significantly different in both groups. However, the degree of reduction of LAVI ($21 ± 21$ ml/m² in the NSR vs. $11 ± 23$ ml/m² in the AF, $p = 0.041$) and percentage reduction of LAVI ($28 ± 28\%$ in the NSR vs. $10 ± 37\%$ in the AF, $p < .001$) were significantly smaller in the AF group (Fig. 2). Therefore, post-operative LA size was significantly larger in the AF group, shown as AP dimension ($43 ± 6$ mm in the NSR vs. $51 ± 8$ mm in the AF, $p < .001$) and LAVI ($38 ± 13$ ml/m² in the NSR vs. $52 ± 16$ ml/m² in

the AF, $p < .001$). When the degree of reduction of LA dimension was compared according to the direction (AP, ML or SI), the change in SI direction was most prominent (Table 2). Regarding the hemodynamic variables, the post-operative mean diastolic pressure gradient (MDPG) of the MV was significantly higher in patients with permanent AF group ($3.5 ± 1.4$ mmHg in the NSR vs. $3.9 ± 1.5$ mmHg in the AF, $p = 0.023$). The grade of pre and post-operative tricuspid regurgitation (TR) were slightly higher in the AF

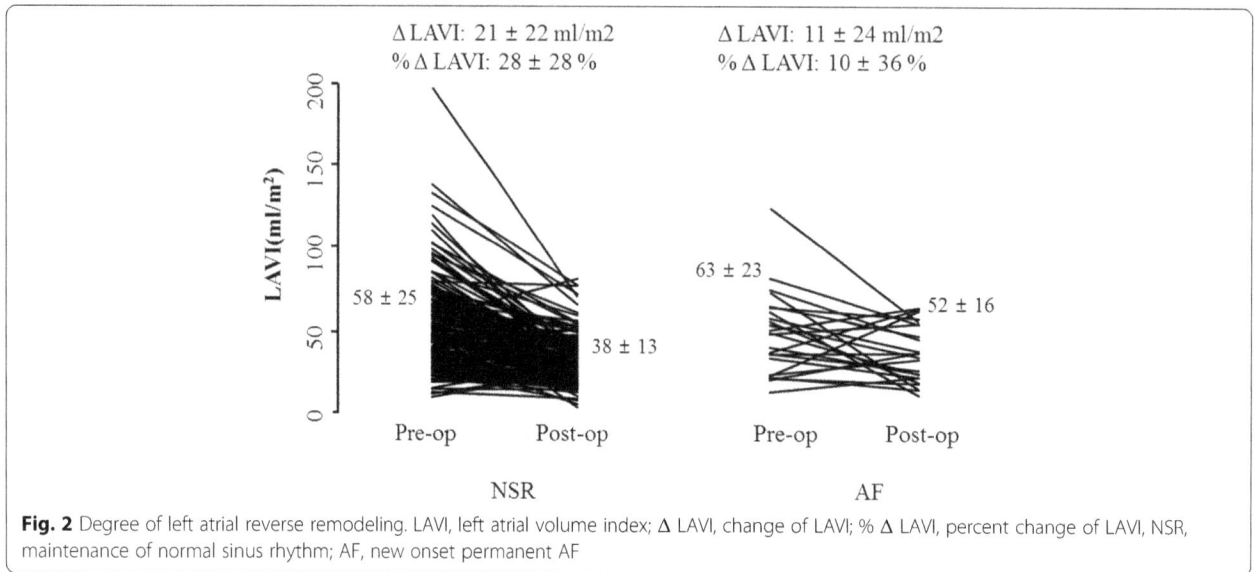

Fig. 2 Degree of left atrial reverse remodeling. LAVI, left atrial volume index; Δ LAVI, change of LAVI; % Δ LAVI, percent change of LAVI, NSR, maintenance of normal sinus rhythm; AF, new onset permanent AF

group. Post-operative estimated pulmonary artery pressure (PAP) was also slightly higher in the AF group. In univariate analysis, rheumatic etiology (odds ratio [OR] = 2.474, 95% confidence interval [CI] = 1.143–5.355, $p = 0.021$), lower pre (OR = 0.971, 95% CI = 0.945–0.997, $p = 0.028$) and post-operative LV EF (OR = 0.970, 95% CI = 0.949–0.992, $p = 0.007$), higher post-operative MDPG across mitral prosthesis (OR = 1.212, 95% CI = 1.024–1.434, $p = 0.025$), lesser degree of reduction in LA size after surgery (OR = 0.790, 95% CI = 0.960–0.980, $p < 0.001$), and large post-operative LA size (OR = 1.064, 95% CI = 1.045–1.083, $p < 0.001$) were risk factors for the occurrence of AF. Presence of MS rather than pure MR (OR = 1.767, 95% CI = 0.981–3.182, $p = 0.058$) was associated with the occurrence of AF with borderline significance (Table 3). Interestingly, none

of the parameters reflecting pre-operative LA size was associated with post-operative AF. Pre and post-operative TR (OR = 1.864, 95% CI = 1.328–2.617, $p < 0.001$ & OR = 2.641, 95% CI = 1.922–3.630, $p < 0.001$) and postoperative higher PAP (OR = 1.067, 95% CI = 1.025–1.110, $p = 0.001$) were associated with the occurrence of AF. In multivariate analysis, post-operative LAVI was an independent predictor for the occurrence of AF (Table 4). The predictive ability of the LAVI was determined by the area under the curve of the receiver operating curve and post-operative LAVI > 39 ml/m² (cut-off value) was associated with new onset permanent AF (sensitivity: 79%, AUC: 0.762, SE: 0.051, $p < 0.001$). The AF-free survival curves of patients with post-op LAVI < 39 ml/m2 or ≥39 ml/m2 are shown in Fig. 3 ($p = 0.06$).

Table 3 Factors determining the occurrence of atrial fibrillation after surgery (univariate analysis)

Variables	Odds ratio	95% confidence interval	p
Rheumatic VHD	2.474	1.143–5.355	0.021
Presence of MS	1.767	0.981–3.182	0.058
Preoperative LV EF	0.971	0.949–0.992	0.028
Postoperative LV EF	0.970	0.949–0.992	0.007
Δ LAVI	0.960	0.940–0.990	0.007
% Δ LAVI	0.790	0.960–0.980	< .001
Postoperative LAVI	1.064	1.045–1.083	< .001
Postoperative MDPG	1.212	1.024–1.434	0.025
Preoperative TR	1.864	1.328–2.617	< 0.001
Postoperative TR	2.641	1.922–3.630	< 0.001
Postoperative PAP	1.067	1.025–1.110	0.001

VHD valvular heart disease, MS mitral stenosis, LV Left ventricular, EF ejection fraction, Δ change, LAVI left atrial volume index, MDPG mean diastolic pressure gradient, TR tricuspid valve regurgitation, PAP pulmonary artery pressrue

Table 4 Factors determining the occurrence of atrial fibrillation after surgery (multivariate analysis)

Variables	Odds ratio	95% confidence interval	p
Rheumatic VHD	4.683	0.716–30.460	0.107
Presence of MS	3.534	0.884–14.125	0.074
Preoperative LV EF	0.997	0.953–1.043	0.815
Postoperative LV EF	1.004	0.957–1.054	0.863
% Δ LAVI	0.993	0.976–1.010	0.409
Postoperative LAVI	1.098	1.047–1.153	< .001
Postoperative MDPG of MV	0.902	0.557–1.459	0.673
Preoperative TR	0.686	0.181–2.596	0.579
Postoperative TR	2.274	0.896–5.773	0.084
Postoperative PAP	0.930	0.788–1.097	0.389

VHD valvular heart disease, MS mitral stenosis, LV Left ventricular, EF ejection fraction, Δ change, LAVI left atrial volume index, MDPG mean diastolic pressure gradient, MV mitral valve, TR tricuspid valve regurgitation, PAP pulmonary artery pressrue

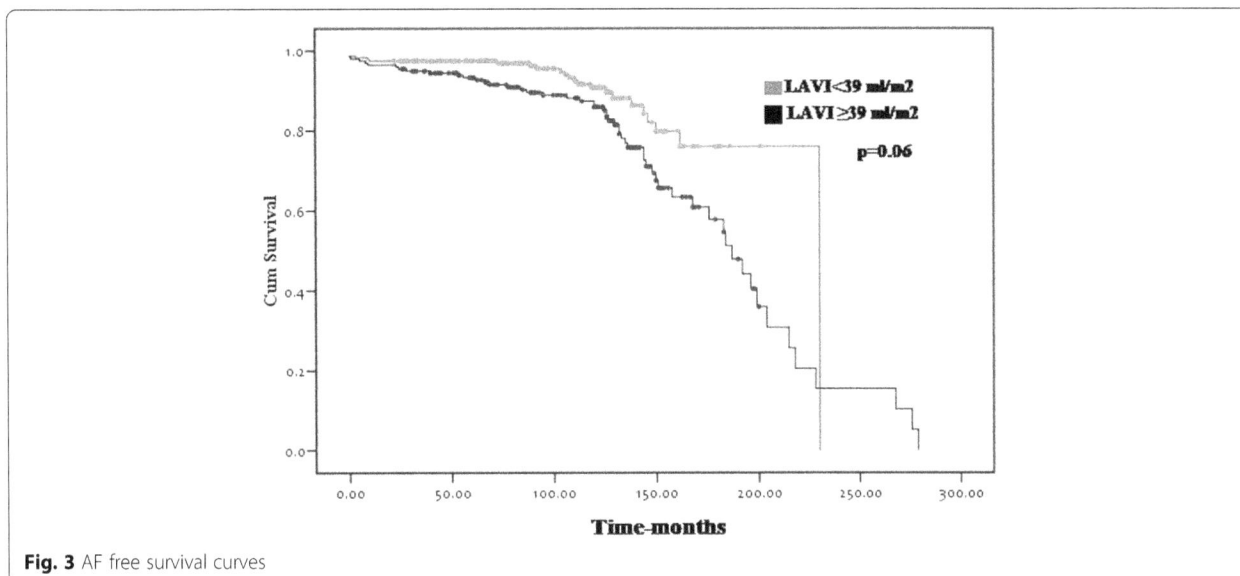

Fig. 3 AF free survival curves

Discussion

In the present study, the prevalence and predictors of new onset permanent AF after MV surgery were investigated. The results showed that new onset permanent AF is not uncommon, occurring in about 20% of patients even after successful MV surgery and pre-operative sinus rhythm. Although several parameters, such as rheumatic etiology of MV, presence of mitral stenosis (MS), lower LV EF, higher post-operative mean diastolic pressure gradient across mitral prosthesis, and lesser degree of reverse LA remodeling after surgery, were shown to be associated with the occurrence of post-operative AF, post-operative LAVI was found to be an independent predictor for the occurrence of AF in multivariate analysis. Interestingly, none of the parameters reflecting pre-operative LA size was associated with post-operative AF. These findings underscore the importance of post-operative echocardiographic assessment before dismissal of the evaluation of LV function and LA size even in patients who have undergone successful MV surgery and pre-operative sinus rhythm.

Factors associated with new onset permanent AF
Reverse LA remodeling and post-operative AF
The degree of LA reverse remodeling was different in the two groups and showed that the reduction of LAVI and decrease in percentage of LAVI were smaller in the post-op AF group. Accordingly, post-operative LA size was significantly larger in the post-op AF group. In a previous study, post-operative LAVI ≥60 ml/m² was shown to be associated with adverse clinical outcomes in patients with organic mitral regurgitation (MR) [19]. In our study, 9 (47%) of 19 patients who had post-operative LAVI ≥60 ml/m² developed new onset permanent AF, whereas 15 (8%) of 181 patients who had post-operative

LAVI < 60 ml/m2 had new onset AF ($p < 0.001$). These findings are consistent with previous research [20]. However, in our study, post-operative LAVI ≥39 ml/m² was selected as a cut-off value for new onset AF. It had a sensitivity of 79% as well as the largest AUC (0.762). The smaller cut-off value of LAVI in our study was probably due to the inclusion of the patients with MS in our study. Regarding the direction of LA reverse remodeling, the change in SI dimension was the most prominent when compared with that of the AP and ML dimensions. Therefore, assessing the change in LA size only in the AP dimension may not accurately reflect the change in LA size. Thus, the degree of LA reverse remodeling could be underestimated.

Impact of LV systolic function on post-operative AF
In our study, lower pre- and post-operative LV EF was also associated with new onset AF. Despite similar pre-operative LAVI, lesser degrees of reduction in LAVI and decreases in percentage of LAVI occurred in patients with LV EF < 60%. LV systolic dysfunction usually accompanies LV diastolic dysfunction and elevated LV filling pressures. Despite similar LA size, the presence of LV systolic dysfunction and concomitant LV diastolic dysfunction with elevated LV filling pressure might interfere with LA reverse remodeling.

Pre-operative etiology of MV pathology
New onset permanent AF occurred more frequently in patients with rheumatic etiology and presence of MS rather than pure MR. Because LA kinetic energy is different in MS and MR, a long-standing pressure overload of the LA in MS might be associated with higher LA kinetic energy than volume overload in MR. Therefore, increased LA work in MS may result in further LA

fatigue and failure over time, which may disturb LA reverse remodeling [2, 21].

Role of post-operative echocardiography before dismissal

Although successful intervention was performed on diseased MV, AF can occur in patients with post-operative LAVI ≥ 39 ml/m^2 according to the results from our study. Therefore, it is imperative to not only focus on the successful results of valve surgery but also perform post-operative echocardiography to evaluate post-operative LAVI to predict the occurrence of AF.

Echocardiography has a different role in the evaluation of valvular heart disease (VHD) at different stages before and after surgery. Pre-operative TTE should provide an accurate diagnosis to determine the possible cause of valvular diseases [22, 23]. In addition, quantitative echocardiographic evaluation of LV size and function is a key factor in clinical decision making in adults with VHD [24–27]. Other key echocardiographic data includes LV diastolic function, LA enlargement, and the presence of intra-cardiac thrombus, pulmonary artery pressures, and so on [28]. Despite the important information obtained from pre-operative echocardiography, none of the pre-operative echocardiographic parameters provides predictive information regarding post-operative permanent AF in this study. Intra-operatively, transesophageal echocardiography (TEE) provides a roadmap for the surgeons regarding the location and severity of MV pathologic lesions, enhancing the ability to detect unexpected associated lesions. In addition, intra-operative TEE is used to confirm results of surgical procedures on the MV, which can result in improved surgical outcomes [28, 29]. Therefore, the American College of Cardiology and the American Heart Association have established guidelines for the management of patients with VHD, which state that the use of intra-operative TEE in MV repair is a class I indication [30].

Although the importance of pre-operative and intra-operative echocardiographic evaluations of MV disease has been well recognized, the role of post-operative pre-discharge TTE has been overlooked in patients undergoing MV surgery. Unlike pre-operative echocardiographic parameters, post-operative LAVI measured before dismissal was able to predict the occurrence of post-operative permanent AF in patients undergoing MV surgery. Based on these results, the importance of post-operative echocardiographic assessment is emphasized not only for assessing the results of MV surgery but also for evaluating cardiac chamber size and function, particularly LA volume.

Limitations

The current study has several limitations. First, it was a retrospective study, so the data collection was done by reviewing medical charts and recorded echocardiographic data. Therefore, the measurement of LAVI was available in only 200 of 442 patients, and only echocardiographic report was available in the remainder. And, the majority of the study patients had undergone MVR rather than MV repair. Anticoagulation is one of the most important treatments for AF. However, all patients should have life-long anticoagulation therapy for the implanted valve, except for MV reconstructions and bioprosthetic valve implantation. Therefore, our results cannot apply to patients who have undergone MV repair.

Conclusions

Newly developed postoperative permanent AF is not uncommon, occurring in 18% of patients who have undergone successful MV surgery despite pre-operative sinus rhythm. Rheumatic etiology, the presence of MS, lower LV EF, lesser degree of LA reverse remodeling, and larger post-operative LAVI were associated with new onset permanent AF. Post-operative LAVI > 39 ml/m2 was an independent predictor for the occurrence of AF.

Abbreviations

AF: atrial fibrillation; AP: anteroposterior; CI: confidence interval; ECG: electrocardiogram; EF: ejection fraction; LA: left atrial; LAVI: left atrial volume index; LV: left ventricular; MDPG: mean diastolic pressure gradient; ML: mediolateral; MR: mitral regurgitation; MS: mitral stenosis; MV: mitral valve; NSR: normal sinus rhythm; OR: odds ratio; ROC: receiver-operating-characteristic; SD: standard deviation; SI: superior/inferior; TEE: transesophageal echocardiography; TTE: transthoracic echocardiography; VHD: valvular heart disease

Acknowledgements

There is nothing to declare with this study.

Funding

This research received no specific grant from any funding agency.

Author's contributions

MKK and JWH designed this study as the first author and corresponding author. BYJ confirmed ECG. CYS, IJC, WIY, and JM made the SPSS data together. YJ, NC, and BCC were involved in data acquisition and analysis in this study. All authors read and approved the final manuscript.

Competing interests

There are no conflicts of interest in this study.

Author details

[1]Division of Cardiology, Kangnam Sacred Heart Hospital, Hallym University Medical Center, Seoul, South Korea. [2]Division of Cardiology and Cardiovascular Surgery, Severance Cardiovascular Hospital, Yonsei University College of Medicine, 134 Shinchon-dong, Seodaemun-gu, Seoul 120-752, Republic of Korea. [3]Division of Cardiology, CHA Bundang Medical Center, CHA University, Seongnam, South Korea. [4]Division of Cardiology and Cardiovascular Surgery, Department of Internal Medicine, Gachon University of Medicine and Science, Incheon, South Korea.

References

1. Henry WL, Morganroth J, Pearlman AS, Clark CE, Redwood DR, Itscoitz SB, et al. Relation between echocardiographically determined left atrial size and atrial fibrillation. Circulation. 1976;53:273–9.
2. Cho DK, Ha JW, Chang BC, Lee SH, Yoon SJ, Shim CY, et al. Factors determining early left atrial reverse remodeling after mitral valve surgery. Am J Cardiol. 2008;101:374–7.
3. Tsang TS, Abhayaratna WP, Barnes ME, Miyasaka Y, Gersh BJ, Bailey KR, et al. Prediction of cardiovascular outcomes with left atrial size: is volume superior to area or diameter? J Am Coll Cardiol. 2006;47:1018–23.
4. Abhayaratna WP, Seward JB, Appleton CP, Douglas PS, Oh JK, Tajik AJ, et al. Left atrial size: physiologic determinants and clinical applications. J Am Coll Cardiol. 2006;47:2357–63.
5. John B, Stiles MK, Kuklik P, Brooks AG, Chandy ST, Kalman JM, et al. Reverse remodeling of the atria after treatment of chronic stretch in humans: implications for the atrial fibrillation substrate. J Am Coll Cardiol. 2010;55:1217–26.
6. Guffi M, Visconti Brick A, Seixas T, Portilho C, Klier Peres A, Vieira JJ Jr, et al. Intraoperative treatment of chronic atrial fibrillation with ultrasound. J Cardiovasc Surg. 2005;46:69–75.
7. Maisel WH, Rawn JD, Stevenson WG. Atrial fibrillation after cardiac surgery. Ann Intern Med. 2001;18(135):1061–73.
8. Mathew JP, Fontes ML, Tudor IC, Ramsay J, Duke P, Mazer CD, et al. Investigators of the Ischemia Research and Education Foundation; multicenter study of perioperative ischemia research group. A multicenter risk index for atrial fibrillation after cardiac surgery JAMA. 2004;291:1720–9.
9. Angelini P, Feldman MI, Lufschanowski R, Leachman RD. Cardiac arrhythmias during and after heart surgery: diagnosis and management. Prog Cardiovasc Dis. 1974;16:469–95.
10. Tchervenkov CI, Wynands JE, Symes JF, Malcolm ID, Dobell AR, JEI M. Persistent atrial activity during cardioplegic arrest: a possible factor in the etiology of post-operative supraventricular tachyarrhythmias. Ann Thorac Surg. 1983;36:437–43.
11. Chen X, Newman M, Rosenfeldt FL. Internal cardiac cooling improves atrial preservation: electrophysiological and biochemical assessment. Ann Thorac Surg. 1988;46:406–11.
12. Smith PK, Buhrman WC, Levett JM, Ferguson TB Jr, Holman WL, Cox JL. Supraventricular conduction abnormalities following cardiac operations: a complication of inadequate atrial preservation. J Thorac Cardiovasc Surg. 1983;85:105–15.
13. White HD, Antman EM, Glynn MA, Collins JJ, Cohn LH, Shemin RJ, et al. Efficacy and safety of timolol for prevention of supraventricular tachyarrhythmias after coronary artery bypass surgery. Circulation. 1984;70:479–84.
14. Kalman JM, Munawar M, Howes LG, Louis WJ, Buxton BF, Gutteridge G, et al. Atrial fibrillation after coronary artery bypass grafting is associated with sympathetic activation. Ann Thorac Surg. 1995;60:1709–15.
15. Klemperer JD, Klein IL, Ojamaa K, Helm RE, Gomez M, Isom OW, et al. Triiodothyronine therapy lowers the incidence of atrial fibrillation after cardiac operations. Ann Thorac Surg. 1996;61:1323–9.
16. Dunning J, Treasure T, Versteegh M, Nashef SA, Audit EACTS, Committee G. Guidelines on the prevention and management of de novo atrial fibrillation after cardiac and thoracic surgery. Eur J Cardiothorac Surg. 2006;30:852–72.
17. Kinoshita T, Asai T, Nishimura O, Hiramatsu N, Suzuki T, Kambara A, et al. Statin for prevention of atrial fibrillation after off-pump coronary artery bypass grafting in Japanese patients. Circ J. 2010;74:1866–72.
18. Lang RM, Bierig M, Devereux RB, Flachskampf FA, Foster E, Pellikka PA, et al. Chamber quantification writing group; American Society of Echocardiography's guidelines and standards committee; European Association of Echocardiography. Recommendations for chamber quantification: a report from the American Society of Echocardiography's guidelines and standards committee and the chamber quantification writing group, developed in conjunction with the European Association of Echocardiography, a branch of the European Society of Cardiology. J Am Soc Echocardiogr. 2005;18:1440 63.
19. American College of Cardiology/American Heart Association Task Force on Practice Guidelines; Society of Cardiovascular Anesthesiologists; Society for Cardiovascular Angiography and Interventions; Society of Thoracic Surgeons, Bonow RO, Carabello BA, Kanu C, de Leon AC Jr, Faxon DP, et al. ACC/AHA 2006 guidelines for the management of patients with valvular heart disease: a report of the American College of Cardiology/American Heart Association task force on practice guidelines (writing committee to revise the 1998 guidelines for the Management of Patients with Valvular Heart Disease): developed in collaboration with the Society of Cardiovascular Anesthesiologists: endorsed by the Society for Cardiovascular Angiography and Interventions and the Society of Thoracic Surgeons. Circulation. 2006;115:e84–231.
20. Le Tourneau T, Messika-Zeitoun D, Russo A, Detaint D, Topilsky Y, Mahoney DW, et al. Impact of left atrial volume on clinical outcome in organic mitral regurgitation. J Am Coll Cardiol. 2010;56:570–8.
21. Boudoulas H, Boudoulas D, Sparks EA, Pearson AC, Nagaraja HN, Wooley CF. Left atrial performance indices in chronic mitral valve disease. J Heart Valve Dis. 1995;4Suppl(2):S242–7.
22. Vahanian A, Baumgartner H, Bax J, Butchart E, Dion R, Filippatos G, et al. Task force on the Management of Valvular Hearth Disease of the European Society of Cardiology; ESC Committee for practice guidelines. Guidelines on the management of valvular heart disease: the task force on the management of Valvular heart disease of the European Society of Cardiology. Eur Heart J. 2007;28:230–68.
23. American College of Cardiology; American Heart Association Task Force on Practice Guidelines (Writing Committee to revise the 1998 guidelines for the management of patients with valvular heart disease); Society of Cardiovascular Anesthesiologists, Bonow RO, Carabello BA, Chatterjee K, et al. ACC/AHA 2006 guidelines for the management of patients with valvular heart disease: a report of the American College of Cardiology/American Heart Association task force on practice guidelines (writing committee to revise the 1998 guidelines for the management of patients with valvular heart disease) developed in collaboration with the Society of Cardiovascular Anesthesiologists endorsed by the Society for Cardiovascular Angiography and Interventions and the Society of Thoracic Surgeons. J Am Coll Cardiol. 2006;48:e1–148.
24. Rosenhek R, Rader F, Klaar U, Gabriel H, Krejc M, Kalbeck D, et al. Outcome of watchful waiting in asymptomatic severe mitral regurgitation. Circulation. 2006;113:2238–44.
25. Enriquez-Sarano M, Avierinos JF, Messika-Zeitoun D, Detaint D, Capps M, Nkomo V, et al. Quantitative determinants of the outcome of asymptomatic mitral regurgitation. N Engl J Med. 2005;352:875–83.
26. Grigioni F, Tribouilloy C, Avierinos JF, Barbieri A, Ferlito M, Trojette F, et al. MIDA investigators. Outcomes in mitral regurgitation due to flail leaflets a multicenter European study. JACC Cardiovasc Imaging. 2008;1:133–41.
27. Enriquez-Sarano M, Sundt TM 3rd. Early surgery is recommended for mitral regurgitation. Circulation. 2010;121:804–11.
28. Otto CM, Bonow RO, et al. Valvular heart disease. Third edition. 431–436.
29. Miller D, Farah MG, Liner A, Fox K, Schlucher M, Hoit BD. The relation between quantitative right ventricular ejection fraction and indices of tricuspid annular motion and myocardial performance. J Am Soc Echocardiogr. 2004;17:443–7.
30. Bonow RO, KC CBAC, de Leon AC Jr, Faxon DP, Freed MD, et al. ACC/AHA 2006 guideline for the management of patients with valvular heart disease: a report of the American college of cardiology/American heart association task force on practice guidelines (writing committee to revise the 1998 guidelines for the management of patients with Valvular heart disease): developed in collaboration with the Society of Cardiovascular Anestheiologists: endorsed by the Society for Cardiovascular Angiography and Intervention and the Society of Thoracic Surgeons. Circulation. 2006; 114:e84–231.

20

Echocardiographic characteristics of primary malignant pericardial mesothelioma and outcomes analysis: a retrospective study

Lingyun Kong[1], Ziwang Li[2], Jingrui Wang[3] and Xiuzhang Lv[1*]

Abstract

Background: Little is known about the echocardiographic characteristics of primary malignant pericardial mesothelioma (PPM) due to its rarity. The aim of this study was to explore the sex-specific echocardiographic patterns of PPM and risk factors for in-hospital mortality.

Methods: A retrospective information retrieval was conducted for cases of PPM reported from China during 1981 and 2015. The diagnosis was made by histopathological examinations and only cases with echocardiographic descriptions were included. Data on the clinical and echocardiographic findings were collected. Difference in clinical, sex-specific echocardiographic characteristics and findings across different time periods were assessed. Logistic regression analysis was performed to explore echocardiographic risk factors for in-hospital mortality.

Results: A total of 64 patients with PPM were included, with a mean age of 39.2 ± 15.6 years and minor male dominance (40, 62.5%). The most common echocardiographic presentations were pericardial effusion (55, 85.9%), pericardial masses (36.4%) and thickening (17.3%), respectively. The positive rate of pericardiocentesis was only 20.9%. Six patients (15.4%) died among 39 cases reporting in-hospital outcome. Logistics analysis identified no clinical or echocardiographic parameters associated with in-hospital mortality (all $P > 0.05$).

Conclusions: The echocardiographic signs of PPM are basically nonspecific with massive pericardial effusion as the most common sign, although no echocardiographic gender differences or association with in-hospital mortality could be identified.

Keywords: Pericardial mesothelioma, Echocardiography, Diagnosis, Prognosis

Background

Primary malignant pericardial mesothelioma (PPM) is an extremely rare malignancy originating from the pericardium, with an incidence < 0.0022% [1, 2]. Little is known about the echocardiographic characteristics of PPM due to its rarity. This study was aimed to investigate the echocardiographic patterns of PPM, explore potential gender difference, the changes with time periods and echocardiographic risk factors for in-hospital mortality based on literature

review of histologically proven PPM cases reported in China mainland.

Methods

Data sources and study population

The Chinese medical literature database including Wan Fang database, VIP database and China National Knowledge Infrastructure (CNKI) database as well as PubMed database were searched for cases of histopathologically diagnosed PPM reported from China mainland between January 1981 and December 2015. We used "pericardial mesothelioma", "heart and mesothelioma" and "mesothelioma" as the keywords. References from the identified case reports were also reviewed. The diagnosis was based on

* Correspondence: lvxzcyh@163.com
[1]Echocardiography Department of Heart Center, Beijing Chao-Yang Hospital, Capital Medical University, 8 Gongren Tiyuchang Nanlu, Chaoyang District, Beijing 100020, China
Full list of author information is available at the end of the article

detection of malignant mesothelial cells upon histopathological examinations including exploratory thoracotomy, biopsy and autopsy. Cases with extractable individual clinical and echocardiographic data were included. The cases may be reported in the form of case report, series or conference papers. Exclusion criteria included metastatic pericardial tumors, primary pericardial tumor of other pathological origin, repeat reports and cases diagnosed with pericardial effusion cytological tests. Particular attention was paid to cases from the same author or institution to rule out repeat cases, but patient information was extracted from all relevant publications to supplement data.

Clinical and echocardiographic parameters

We collected clinical data including age, gender, blood pressure and heart rate. Echocardiographic data were obtained from the publications and the images, where available, provided in the literature. The signs collected included: presence, amount and color of pericardial effusion, presence, location and echodensity of pericardial mass, presence of pericardial wall thickening. The size of pericardial effusion was recorded mainly according to the reports, and the largest amount was extracted for analysis in patients having more than one echocardiogram. In the cases not describing the amount straightforward, we defined it as large ≥ 2 of the following signs were present: swimming heart, the amount > 500 mL at one pericardiocentesis/ > 1000 mL at two, or flask-like cardiomegaly on chest radiograph. The color of effusion was confirmed by both pericardiocentesis and surgery or autopsy. The frequency of pericardial mass and pericardial thickening was recorded from both echocardiography and other examinations: imaging tests like cardiac computed tomography (CT), magnetic resonance (CMR) and Positron Emission Tomography–Computed Tomography (PET-CT), and invasive exploratory thoracotomy and autopsy. The myocardial infiltration and hemodynamic complications including cardiac tamponade and constrictive pericarditis were also recorded.

The anatomical classification of PPM, including diffuse and localized type, was established according to the scale of pericardial wall involvement and presence of pericardial mass. Patients with diffuse pericardial wall thickening as evidenced by surgery, autopsy, CT, CMR or PET-CT were grouped into the diffuse type whether the mass was present or not. Patients without pericardial mass, whether there was pericardial effusion or not, were also considered as the diffuse type. Cases reported as having one or more masses in the pericardial cavity and no evidence of diffuse pericardial wall thickening were grouped into the localized type. The pathological classification was based on histopathological examinations, including epithelioid, sarcomatous and mixed (biphasic) type. Cases with pathological descriptions of nestle-like, gland-like or papillary arrangement of

malignant mesothelial cells were considered as the epithelioid type.

The outcome information was retrieved when available. The primary endpoint was defined as in-hospital mortality. Two reviewers were responsible for collecting the data using the same data abstraction form. For judgment in doubt, discussion and consensus were obtained for analysis.

Statistical analyses

Continuous data are expressed as mean ± SD, and categorical data as frequency (percentage, %). Patients were grouped according to sex to explore sex-specific difference. Considering that the study covered a relatively long range of time (35 years), during which echocardiography has undergone marked technical progress, the patients were split into two groups according to publication years: from 1981 to 2000 and from 2001 to 2015. Continuous data were compared using Student's t test and categorical data were compared using χ^2 or Fisher's exact test. For patients with both echocardiography and other examinations, the ability of detecting pericardial thickening and mass were compared using exact McNemar test. Agreement between the echocardiography and other examinations in detecting the two signs was assessed using simple kappa (κ). Binary logistic regression analysis was used to identify risk factors for in-hospital mortality. The results were reported as Odds ratio (OR) and 95% confidence interval (CI). Analyses were performed with IBM SPSS 23.0. $P < 0.05$ was considered statistically significant.

Results

Retrieval information and patients demographics

A total of 119 articles containing 242 PPM patients were retrieved. After exclusion of 77 articles (178 patients) not meeting the inclusion criteria: individual data unavailable 11 articles (30 patients); metastatic pericardial mesothelioma or unclear primary lesion 4 articles (5 patients); repeat reports 11 articles (22 patients); unavailable echocardiographic data 26 articles (64 patients); cytological diagnosis 19 articles (34 patients) and unspecified age or gender 6 articles (23 patients), finally 49 articles (64 patients) were enrolled (Fig. 1), among whom, 51 (79.7%, containing one case diagnosed also by biopsy) patients were diagnosed with exploratory thoracotomy, 10 (15.6%) with biopsy and 4 (6.2%) with autopsy. The clinical features and inter-gender difference of the study population is presented in Table 1. The study revealed a male/female ratio of 1.7:1 in PPM, with an increasing trend for female prevalence, which was 18.2% during 1981 and 2000, and rising to 47.6% during 2001 and 2015. The mean age was 39.5 ± 15.5 years, covering a wide range from 2 to 77 years. Notably, the age group from 19~ 65 years was mostly affected (55, 85.9%), with

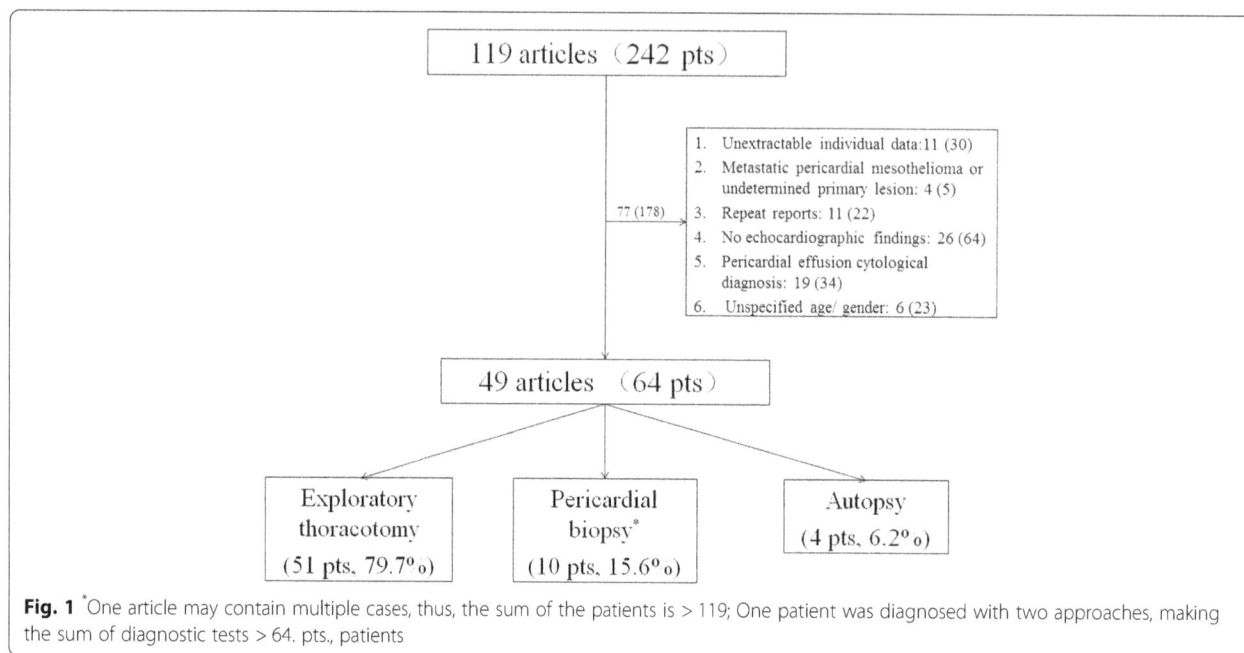

Fig. 1 *One article may contain multiple cases, thus, the sum of the patients is > 119; One patient was diagnosed with two approaches, making the sum of diagnostic tests > 64. pts., patients

7 (10.9%) patients in the 2~18 years group and 2 (3.1%) in the >65 years group. There was no significant sex difference in clinical characteristics except for a lower systolic blood pressure in female patients ($P = 0.03$). In 58 patients whose morphological phenotype could be determined, the diffuse type was more common than the localized type (69.0% vs.31.0%, $P < 0.05$). 28 cases provided pathologic diagnosis or detailed description, of which the epithelioid type was most frequently found (15, 53.6%), followed by the mixed (9, 32.1%) and sarcomatous type

Table 1 Clinical characteristics of patients with PPM

Parameters	All (n = 64)	Group based on sex			Group based on publishing year		
		Male (n = 40)	Female (n = 24)	P	1981 to 2000 (n = 22)	2001 to 2015 (n = 42)	P
Female	24 (37.5%)	NA	NA	NA	4 (18.2%)	20 (47.6%)	0.03*
Age (yrs.)	39.5 ± 15.5	38.2 ± 16.4	41.5 ± 13.8	0.41	40.6 ± 16.4	38.9 ± 15.1	0.83
Anatomical type	n = 58	n = 37	n = 21	0.40	n = 21	n = 37	0.38
Diffuse	40 (69.0%)	24 (64.9%)	16 (76.2%)		13 (61.9%)	27 (73.0%)	
Localized	18 (31.0%)	13(35.1%)	5 (23.8%)		8 (38.1%)	10 (27.0%)	
Histopathological type	n = 28	n = 20	n = 8	0.40	n = 7	n = 21	0.97
Epithelioid	15 (53.6%)	8 (40.0%)	7 (87.8%)		4 (57.1%)	11 (52.4%)	
Sarcomatous	4 (14.3%)	4 (20.0%)	0 (0.0%)		1 (14.3%)	3 (7.1%)	
Mixed	9 (32.1%)	8 (40.0%)	1 (12.5%)		2 (28.6%)	7 (16.7%)	
Complications	n = 51	n = 31	n = 20		n = 18	n = 33	
Tamponade	19 (37.3%)	11 (35.5%)	8 (40.0%)	0.77	9 (50.0%)	10 (30.3%)	0.23
Constriction	14 (27.5%)	9 (29.0%)	5 (25.0%)	0.75	6 (33.3%)	8 (24.2%)	0.71
Pleural effusion	n = 38	n = 23	n = 15		n = 11	n = 27	0.76
Left	9 (23.7%)	7 (30.4%)	2 (13.3%)		3 (27.3%)	6 (22.2%)	
Right	3 (7.9%)	0	3 (20.0%)		0 (0%)	3 (11.1%)	
Bilateral	21 (55.3%)	13 (56.5%)	8 (53.3%)		6 (54.5%)	15 (55.6%)	
None	5 (13.2%)	3 (13.0%)	2 (13.3%)		2 (18.2%)	3 (11.1%)	

HR heart rate, *SBP* systolic blood pressure, *DBP* diastolic blood pressure, *NA* not applicable
*indicates $P < 0.05$ between male and female patients

(4, 14.3%). Pleural effusion was found in 33 (86.8%) of 38 patients, affecting mostly bilateral pleural cavity. One case reported initial onset as systematic erythroderma.

Echocardiographic characteristics

The echocardiographic sings of the study population are presented in Table 2. No difference was found between male and female patients or across time periods (all $P > 0.05$). Of all, pericardial effusion was the most frequent finding (55, 85.9%), most (43/55, 67.2%) of which was massive. Notably, PPM with no pericardial effusion was reported in > 10% of the population. Forty-three cases reported pericardiocentesis, of whom 9 (20.9%) detected malignant mesothelial cells from pericardial effusion cytological examinations. In 44 cases describing the color of pericardial effusion, 42 (95.4%) was bloody (including one case alternating with bloody and faint yellow, and another one mixed with purulent component), and the other 2 (4.5%) purely faint yellow. Twenty-six cases reported subsequent response to pericardiocentesis: 19 (73.1%) showed rapid re-accumulation in short term after pericardiocentesis, 4 (15.4%) showed temporary decrease in effusion amount but rapid progression of pericardial wall thickening and constrictive pericarditis, and the other 3 (11.5%) reported decreased amount. On the other hand, 22 cases were initially misdiagnosed as tuberculous pericarditis and received antituberculosis therapy. All these patients received pericardiocentesis and 17 cases reported the response of antituberculosis therapy: 11 (64.7%) showed rapid re-accumulation after several weeks of therapy, one of whom developed constrictive pericarditis and 6

(35.3%) showed decreased effusion and development of constrictive pericarditis.

Pericardial wall thickening was reported in 12 (18.8%) and pericardial cavity mass was found in 21 (32.8%) of all 64 patients, far less than the rate of pericardial effusion (85.9%). Particularly, we focused on the cases having echocardiogram and ≥ 1 another examination to assess the efficacy of echocardiography in identifying pericardial wall thickening and pericardial cavity masses in PPM (Table 2). In 52 cases that pericardial thickening could be determined by both echo and other examinations, the frequency of pericardial wall thickening was 63.5% (33/52) on non-echo exams, contrasting with an echocardiographic positive rate of only 17.3% (9/52, $P = 0.000$).

In 55 cases that pericardial mass could be identified by non-echo examinations (3 cases more than the counting of pericardial thickening were confirmed by histopathological description), 32 (58.2%) recorded pericardial masses, while echocardiography was positive in only 20 (36.4%) of the 55 patients ($P = 0.000$). Notably, 5 cases were detected on repeat echocardiography after pericardiocentesis when the amount of effusion decreased. In 43 cases reporting the location of masses: 5 (11.6%) had masses at > 3 or multiple sites, 12 (27.9%) located around the left ventricle, 8 (18.6%) around the right ventricle, 3 (6.9%) around the left atrium and 4 (9.3%) around (including one extending into) the right atrium, and the remaining 11 (25.6%) around the cardiac base, surrounding or compressing the major vessels, of which two reported thrombosis in the superior vena cava. Furthermore, 17 cases reported the echodensity of masses: 10 (58.8%) were solid, 4 (23.5%) were of mixed echodensity, and 3 (17.6%) were echolucent.

Table 2 Echocardiographic findings of PPM

Parameters	All patients (n = 64)	Group based on sex		P	Group based on publishing year		P
		Male (n = 40)	Female (n = 24)		1981 to 2000 (n = 22)	2001 to 2015 (n = 42)	
Pericardial effusion (n = 64)		n = 40	n = 24	0.86	n = 22	n = 42	0.48
Mild	6 (9.4%)	3 (7.5%)	3 (12.5%)		0 (0%)	6 (14.3%)	
Moderate	6 (9.4%)	6 (15.0%)	0 (0%)		1 (4.5%)	5 (11.9%)	
Massive	43 (67.2%)	26 (65.0%)	17 (70.8%)		17 (77.3%)	26 (61.9%)	
None	9 (14.1%)	5 (12.5%)	4 (16.7%)		4 (18.2%)	5 (11.9%)	
Echo-Pericardial thickening (n = 64)	12 (18.8%)	7 (17.5%)	5 (20.8%)	0.83	4 (18.2%)	8 (19.0%)	0.61
Echo- Pericardial mass (n = 64)	21 (32.8%)	13 (32.5%)	8 (33.3%)	0.94	4 (18.2%)	17 (40.5%)	0.09
Comparable Pericardial wall thickening (n = 52)[a]		n = 32	n = 20		n = 20	n = 32	
Frequency on echo	9 (17.3%)	5 (15.6%)	4 (20.0%)	0.94	3 (15.0%)	6 (18.8%)	0.73
Frequency on other exams	33 (63.5%)	21 (65.6%)	12 (60.0%)	0.72	12 (60%)	21 (65.6%)	0.77
Comparable pericardial mass (n = 55)[a]		n = 35	n = 20		n = 20	n = 35	
Frequency on echo	20 (36.4%)	13(37.1%)	7 (35.0%)	0.87	4 (20.0%)	16 (38.1%)	0.06
Frequency on other exams	32 (58.2%)	19 (54.3%)	13 (65.0%)	0.57	10 (50.0%)	22 (62.8%)	0.40

[a]Referring to the patients with both echocardiography and at least one another examination including cardiac CT, CMR, PET-CT, exploratory thoracotomy and autopsy

The coexistence of pericardial effusion, thickening and mass was also assessed. Based on the echocardiographic data, among 55 cases of pericardial effusion, only 2 (3.6%) cases had both pericardial thickening and mass.

Agreement analysis showed poor agreement of echocardiography and non-echo examinations in identifying pericardial wall thickening (Kappa = 0.21, P = 0.02) and pericardial mass (Kappa = 0.58, P = 0.000). Sex stratified analysis also revealed a lower detectable rate of echocardiography in identifying pericardial thickening and pericardial mass (Table 2).

Ventricular wall hypokinesis was observed in 3 (4.7%) of all patients on echocardiography. While in 44 patients providing detailed description on thoracotomy (n = 42) or autopsy (n = 2), 20 (45.4%) found adhesion of malignant mesothelial tissue to ventricular wall, among whom only one (5.0%) reported wall motion hypokinesis by echocardiography.

Furthermore, we analyzed the 58 patients whose anatomic classifications could be determined. No statistically significant difference in clinical measures or occurrence of pericardial effusion was found between the diffuse and localized groups (Table 3). The detection rate of pericardial thickening in patients with diffuse type was significantly higher than that of the localized type (Table 3). The occurrence of pericardial mass was higher in patients with localized type than the diffuse type PPM on both echocardiography and non-echo examinations (P < 0.05).

Survival analysis

Thirty-nine cases reported in-hospital mortality, of whom 6 (15.4%) died. Logistics analysis of parameters associated with in-hospital mortality is presented in Table 4. Potential clinical confounders (age, gender, cardiac tamponade, constrictive pericarditis and treatment with surgery) and echocardiographic parameters were included into analysis, but no predictive parameter was found (all P > 0.05). The analysis did not include histopathological type (n = 28) as all the 16 cases reporting histopathological type and outcome survived the index hospitalization.

Discussion

In the present study, the echocardiographic characteristics of patients with histologically diagnosed PPM in China mainland in the past 35 years were systematically reviewed. According to our observations, pericardial effusion was the most common echocardiographic finding of PPM, followed by masses in the pericardial sac and pericardial thickening. The coexistence of these findings, however, is uncommon. No sex difference of prognostic echocardiographic parameters was identified.

PPM is an extremely rare but highly aggressive primary pericardial malignant tumor [1, 3–6]. Most relevant literature thus far has been case reports, resulting in poor knowledge about its echocardiographic findings. We enrolled only cases having histopathological diagnoses, as the definitive diagnosis of PPM relies on histopathological examinations [7]. This study also showed that the positive rate of pericardial effusion is low (20.9%), similar to previous report (24%) [8].

The analyzed patients showed a male/female ratio of 1.7:1, similar to a recent study by Mensi et al., who reported a male/female ratio of 1.79 in 4442 patients with

Table 3 Echocardiographic features of PPM patients with two anatomic classifications

Parameter	Diffuse type (n = 40)	Localized type (n = 18)	P value
Age (years)	39.3 ± 16.4	38.6 ± 14.0	0.88
Gender (male, %)	24 (60%)	13 (72.2%)	0.39
Pericardial effusion Size (n = 58)			
Mild	2 (5.0%)	3 (16.7%)	
Moderate	6 (15.0%)	0 (0%)	
Massive	26 (65.0%)	11 (61.1%)	
None	6 (15.0%)	4 (22.2%)	0.58
Pericardial wall thickening (n = 48)[a]	n = 33	n = 15	
Frequency on echo	9 (27.3%)	0 (0%)	0.04
Frequency on other exams	31 (93.9%)	2 (13.3%)	0.00
Pericardial cavity mass (n = 51)[a]	n = 34	n = 17	
Frequency on echo	8 (23.5%)	9 (52.9%)	0.04
Frequency on other exams	11 (32.4%)	17 (100%)	0.00
In-hospital mortality (n = 36)	n = 24	n = 12	
	5 (20.8%)	1 (8.3%)	0.64

[a]including cases with at least one another cardiac examinations

Table 4 Binary Logistics analysis for predictors of in-hospital mortality

Variables	OR (95% CI)	P value
Age	1.00 (0.96–1.08)	0.52
Gender	1.33 (0.21–8.58)	0.76
Anatomical type	0.34 (0.04–3.35)	0.36
Echocardiographic signs		
Pericardial effusion	2.27 (0.46–11.3)	0.31
Pericardial thickening	1.22 (0.11–13.97)	0.87
Pericardial mass	2.75 (0.33–22.92)	0.35
Signs confirmed by other examinations[a]		
Pericardial wall thickening	1.67 (0.15–18.2)	0.67
Pericardial cavity mass	0.67 (0.08–4.08)	0.70
Cardiac tamponade	0.71 (0.11–4.51)	0.71
Constrictive pericarditis	1.11 (0.17–7.2)	0.91
Surgery	0.57 (0.08–4.08)	0.58

[a]including CT, CMR, PET-CT and invasive procedures (thoracotomy and autopsy)

malignant mesothelioma [3]. We also found that the middle-aged group was mostly affected (85.9%) with a mean age of 39.5 years. PPM of diffuse (69.0%) and epithelioid type (53.6%) was more commonly seen. Our study confirmed that the hemodynamic complications of cardiac tamponade and constrictive pericarditis in PPM were quite common (37.3% and 27.5% respectively), which have been reported frequently [9–11]. It has been suggested that the presence of cardiac tamponade increases the likelihood of malignancy [11]. This may be associated with the diffuse mesothelial cell proliferations and myocardial infiltration which may decrease the relaxation and compliance of left ventricle.

Pericardial effusion

This study showed that the most common echocardiographic sign of PPM, regardless of gender or morphological type, is pericardial effusion (85.9%), which is often massive (67.2%), bloody (95.4%) and associated with hemodynamic instability. When determining the etiology of pericardial effusion, it is crucial to exclude other more commonly seen causes, such as metastatic malignant effusion or inflammatory pericardial diseases [12, 13], considering the rarity of PPM. Timely pericardiocentesis helps to stabilize hemodynamics, and yet we found that rapid reaccumulation of massive effusion after days or weeks of pericardiocentesis is quite common (73.1%). This phenomenon may suggest the malignancy of etiology, helpful for differentiating with tuberculosis [14]. Interestingly, there is also a number of patients (15.4%) who showed temporarily decreased effusion but rapid progression into pericardial thickening and development of constrictive pericarditis. This may be caused by the mechanical injury with pericardiocentesis, which might stimulate malignant mesothelial cells proliferation. However, whether this response to pericardiocentesis is specific to PPM could not be determined from this retrospective study.

It should be noted that PPM with no or minimal pericardial effusion, and significant pericardial thickening, constriction or even occlusion of pericardial cavity was not uncommon (> 10%). Lee et al [10] reported a similar case in a 59-year-old woman of epitheliod PPM, who had marked pericardial thickening but no fluid on echocardiography. This may be associated with the multi-differentiating potential of mesothelial cells, different percentiles of the fibrous component takes or tumor invasiveness of the vessels.

Pericardial mass

According to our data, the pericardial mass may develop in any place around the visceral or parietal pericardium. Notably, masses around the cardiac base (25.6%) tend to be large and aggressive for adjacent structures. In the analyzed patients, two cases developed superior vena caval thrombosis [14]. Nguyen et al [5] observed that patients with mesothelioma are susceptible to thromboembolic events (27.7%), probably correlated with excessive release of procoagulant factors. Also, we found that the echocardiographic detectable rate of pericardial mass is less than that of other examinations performed in the same patients (36.4% vs.58.2%, $P = 0.000$). In consideration of the indicative value of detecting pericardial mass in narrowing down differential diagnoses, this finding supports the routine screening for pericardial mass when assessing pericardial fluid.

Pericardial thickening

Our data showed that the majority (93.9%) of diffuse type PPM patients have diffused pericardial thickening, more than that of the localized type (13.3%). This may result from the difference in mesothelial cell growth and proliferation velocity between the two phenotypes. The frequency of echo identified pericardial thickening is no more than 20%, far less than the rate (63.5%) confirmed by other examinations, supporting the superiority of cardiac CT and CMR in determining the thickening or tissue characteristics of pericardial walls [15]. Jiang et al. [16] reported a patient with sarcomatoid PPM whose echocardiogram indicated only pericardial mass and effusion, while both cardiac CT and PET scan confirmed a thickened pericardium. The suboptimal pericardial wall visualization of echocardiogram, difficulty to discern between pericardial thickening and epicardial fat or masses of other nature is responsible for its low detection rate, particularly under emergency bedside condition when more attention was given to the effusion or ventricular function assessment.

Myocardial involvement

It is noteworthy that myocardial infiltration confirmed by open heart surgery is as high as 45.4% in the present study, in contrast with only 5.0% of wall motion hypokinesis on echocardiography. This finding not only indicates the aggressive nature of PPM but implies the insensitivity of conventional echocardiographic parameters to detect myocardial lesions in PPM. The use of speckle tracking imaging to assess cardiac strain has been confirmed to be sensitive of detecting subclinical myocardial impairment by a large body of evidence, and might be helpful to detect early subtle myocardial lesions in PPM [17]. Severe case with myocardial necrosis was reported in one 77-year-old male, manifesting as severe dyspnea, ST segment elevation, increased cardiac troponin level and hypokinetic ventricular wall motion in the patient cohort, similar to a 75-year-old woman with suspected ST-elevation myocardial infarction reported by Barroso et al. [18].

It is difficult to define the "typical" of "classical" signs of PPM from this study. The coexistence of massive pericardial effusion, pericardial mass, thickening and signs of cardiac tamponade seems to be indicative of malignant etiology but is uncommon and nonspecific [19]. PPM should be considered after excluding the much more frequent metastatic or benign pericardial tumors. The present study found an in-hospital mortality of 15.4% of PPM, but no prognostic clinical or echocardiographic parameters could be determined, possibly limited by the relatively small population and end-point events.

Study limitations

Due to the extreme rarity of PPM incidence, we can only perform a retrospective analysis and included a limited number of patients. Thus, the association between asbestos exposure and PPM, which has been controversial [8, 20], cannot be determined. Besides, Selection bias that is inherent to retrospective study and the fact that complete information was not available in each and all patient, represent a major limitation of the study. However, for diseases of rare incidence, retrospective review of cases from multiple institutions or across a wide time range is valuable for accumulating knowledge about the index disease [21]. Consequently, we enrolled only histopathologically diagnosed cases and cases with individual clinical and echocardiographic information as these may have relatively complete data. However, only inclusion of patients with echocardiographic data might limit the extrapolation of our results. Further prospective nation-wide registry study of PPM is required. It is also noteworthy that the echocardiographic findings of PPM described in our study are all nonspecific. The definitive diagnosis of PPM remains to be histopathological tests.

Conclusion

Our study revealed the echocardiographic features of PPM and showed that massive pericardial effusion is the most common echocardiographic sign, although the signs are generally nonspecific and had no gender-specific difference or association with in-hospital mortality. The detecting ability of echocardiogram for pericardial wall lesions and the yield of pericardiocentesis are not perfect, indicating the necessity for timely histopathological examinations to confirm diagnosis in suspected cases.

Abbreviations

CMR: magnetic resonance; CT: computed tomography; PET: Positron Emission Tomography; PPM: Primary malignant pericardial mesothelioma

Acknowledgements
We thank the authors who originally published the cases so that we can get a glimplse of this rare cardiac neoplasm.

Authors' contributions
LK (first author) study concept and design, acquisition of data, analysis and interpretation of data, drafting/revising the manuscript, control and guarantee that all aspects of the work was investigated and resolved. LK approved the final manuscript. ZL acquisition of data, analysis and interpretation of data, drafting/revising the manuscript, control and guarantee that all aspects of the work was investigated and resolved. ZL approved the final manuscript. JW acquisition of data, analysis and interpretation of data, drafting/revising the manuscript, control and guarantee that all aspects of the work was investigated and resolved. JW approved the final manuscript. XL (corresponding author) study concept and design, interpretation of data, revising the manuscript, control and guarantee that all aspects of the work was investigated and resolved, critical revision of the manuscript for important intellectual content, study supervision. XL approved the final manuscript.

Competing interests
The authors declare that they have no competing interests.

Author details
[1]Echocardiography Department of Heart Center, Beijing Chao-Yang Hospital, Capital Medical University, 8 Gongren Tiyuchang Nanlu, Chaoyang District, Beijing 100020, China. [2]Department of Cardiology, Jiang Xi Yichun Hospital of Traditional Chinese Medicine, Jiang Xi, China. [3]Department of Cardiology, Beijing Daxing District people's Hospital, Beijing, China.

References
1. Ramachandran R, Radhan P, Santosham R, Rajendiran S. A rare case of primary malignant pericardial mesothelioma. J Clin Imaging Sci. 2014;4:47.
2. Feng X, Zhao L, Han G, Khalil M, Green F, Ogilvie T, et al. A case report of an extremely rare and aggressive tumor: primary malignant pericardial mesothelioma. Rare Tumors. 2012;2:e21.
3. Mensi C, De Matteis S, Dallari B, Riboldi L, Bertazzi PA, Consonni D. Incidence of mesothelioma in Lombardy, Italy: exposure to asbestos, time patterns and future projections. Occup Environ Med. 2016;9:607–13.
4. Mensi C, Romano A, Berti A, Dore R, Riboldi L. A second case of pericardial mesothelioma mimicking systemic lupus erythematosus in the literature in over 30 years: a case report. J Med Case Rep. 2017;1:85.
5. Nguyen D, Lee S-J, Libby E, Verschraegen C. Rate of thromboembolic events in mesothelioma. Ann Thorac Surg. 2008;3:1032–8.
6. Adler Y, Charron P, Imazio M, Badano L, Barón-Esquivias G, Bogaert J, et al. 2015 ESC guidelines for the diagnosis and management of pericardial diseases: the task force for the diagnosis and management of pericardial diseases of the European Society of Cardiology (ESC)endorsed by: the European Association for Cardio-Thoracic Surgery (EACTS). Eur Heart J. 2015;42:2921–64.
7. Takeshima Y, Inai K, Amatya VJ, Gemba K, Aoe K, Fujimoto N, et al. Accuracy of pathological diagnosis of mesothelioma cases in Japan: clinicopathological analysis of 382 cases. Lung Cancer. 2009 Nov;2:191–7.
8. Nilsson A, Rasmuson T. Primary pericardial mesothelioma: report of a patient and literature review. Case Rep Oncol. 2009 Jul;2:125–32.
9. Belli E, Landolfo K. Primary pericardial mesothelioma: a rare cause of constrictive pericarditis. Asian Cardiovasc Thorac Ann. 2015;5:599–600.
10. Lee MJ, Kim DH, Kwan J, Park KS, Shin SH, Woo SI, et al. A case of malignant pericardial mesothelioma with constrictive pericarditis physiology misdiagnosed as pericardial metastatic Cancer. Korean Circ J. 2011;6:338–41.
11. de Ceuninck M, Demedts I, Trenson S. Malignant cardiac tamponade. Acta Cardiol. 2013;5:505–7.
12. Lam KY, Dickens P, Chan AC. Tumors of the heart. A 20-year experience with a review of 12,485 consecutive autopsies. Arch Pathol Lab Med. 1993;10:1027–31.
13. Yusuf SW, Bathina JD, Qureshi S, Kaynak HE, Banchs J, Trent JC, et al. Cardiac tumors in a tertiary care cancer hospital: clinical features, echocardiographic findings, treatment and outcomes. Heart Int. 2012;1:e4.
14. Gong W, Ye X, Shi K, Zhao Q. Primary malignant pericardial mesothelioma—a rare cause of superior vena cava thrombosis and constrictive pericarditis. J Thorac Dis. 2014;12:E272–5.
15. Miller CA, Schmitt M. Epicardial Lipomatous hypertrophy mimicking pericardial effusion: characterization with cardiovascular magnetic resonance. Circ Cardiovasc Imaging. 2011;1:77–8.

21

Evaluation of a commercial multi-dimensional echocardiography technique for ventricular volumetry in small animals

Jana Grune[1,2,7], Annelie Blumrich[1,2], Sarah Brix[1,2], Sarah Jeuthe[2,5,6], Cathleen Drescher[2,3], Tilman Grune[2,3,4], Anna Foryst-Ludwig[1,2], Daniel Messroghli[2,5,6], Wolfgang M. Kuebler[2,7], Christiane Ott[2,3] and Ulrich Kintscher[1,2*]

Abstract

Background: The assessment of ventricular volumes using conventional echocardiography methods is limited with regards to the need of geometrical assumptions. In the present study, we aimed to evaluate a novel commercial system for three-dimensional echocardiography (3DE) in preclinical models by direct comparison with conventional 1D- and 2D-echocardiography (1DE; 2DE) and the gold-standard technique magnetic resonance imaging (MRI). Further, we provide a standard operating protocol for image acquisition and analysis with 3DE.

Methods: 3DE was carried out using a 30 MHz center frequency transducer coupled to a Vevo®3100 Imaging System. We evaluated under different experimental conditions: 1) in vitro phantom measurements served as controlled setting in which boundaries were clearly delineated; 2) a validation cohort composed of healthy C57BL/6 J mice and New Zealand Obese (NZO) mice was used in order to validate 3DE against cardiac MRI; 3) a standard mouse model of pressure overload induced-heart failure was investigated to estimate the value of 3DE.

Results: First, in vitro volumetry revealed good agreement between 3DE assessed volumes and the MRI-assessed volumes. Second, cardiac volume determination with 3DE showed smaller mean differences compared to cardiac MRI than conventional 1DE and 2DE. Third, 3DE was suitable to detect reduced ejection fractions in heart failure mice. Fourth, inter- and intra-observer variability of 3DE showed good to excellent agreement regarding absolute volumes in healthy mice, whereas agreement rates for the relative metrics ejection fraction and stroke volume demonstrated good to moderate observer variabilities.

Conclusions: 3DE provides a novel method for accurate volumetry in small animals without the need for spatial assumptions, demonstrating a technique for an improved analysis of ventricular function. Further validation work and highly standardized image analyses are required to increase reproducibility of this approach.

Keywords: 3D echocardiography, Heart failure, Volumetry, Preclinical imaging, Small animals

Background

Echocardiography provides a reliable, cost-effective and widely available technique for evaluation of cardiac function in both human and small animal imaging. However, the assessment of cardiac wall- and chamber dimensions by conventional echocardiography methods is limited with regards to the need of geometrical assumptions for formula-based computation of three-dimensional volumes [1, 2]. Therefore, cardiac magnetic resonance imaging (MRI) is considered as gold standard measurement for left ventricular (LV) volumetry even in rodents, since it allows the assessment of the entire heart in multiple planes [3, 4]. Nevertheless, high expenses and consecutively restricted availability of MRI together with a time-consuming image acquisition process limit its widespread application [3–6]. Recently, matrix array transducers for clinical three-dimensional echocardiography (3DE) have been developed that allow "real-time" volumetry with a superior precision compared to two-dimensional echocardiography

* Correspondence: ulrich.kintscher@charite.de

[1]Institute of Pharmacology, Center for Cardiovascular Research, Charité
-Universitaetsmedizin Berlin, Hessische Str. 3-4, 10115 Berlin, Germany
[2]German Center for Cardiovascular Research (DZHK), partner site Berlin,
10117 Berlin, Germany
Full list of author information is available at the end of the article

(2DE) [7]. Albeit limitations are comparable between clinical and small animal echocardiography, a comprehensive evaluation of a novel, commercially available 3DE in small animals is currently lacking.

Due to their high temporal resolution, linear M-Mode measurements (one-dimensional echocardiography; 1DE) have been widely applied in small animal imaging, especially to determine LV wall thicknesses and −mass [8, 9]. However, with respect to clinical guidelines, 1DE-derived volumetry is obsolete since it is highly vulnerable against misestimations, especially in case of asymmetric LV shape [2, 10]. Increased temporal and spatial resolutions of ultrasound transducers allow assessment of appropriate 2D B-Mode images of the LV and consecutive volumetry by method of disks [11, 12]. Several studies reported on tomographic reconstruction of such 2DE images as potential technique for 3DE in small animals [13, 14]. Albeit this experimental approach has been successfully validated against MRI [14, 15], its widespread application was limited with regards to procedural standardization, ECG-gated synchronization, a rather low spatial resolution and the lack of corresponding post-procession software.

Recently, these pioneering studies paved the way for a commercially available rodent 3DE system that allows automated respiratory-gated acquisition of high-resolution 2D B-Mode images at different levels of the heart and at every point of the cardiac cycle (Fig. 1a-c) [16, 17]. 3DE data sets are built by tomographic multi-slice reconstruction of acquired 2D images up to a step size of 50 µm, and can be analyzed with a dedicated software package allowing visualization and calculation of LV volumes along the cardiac cycle (Fig. 1d-f).

In this study, we aimed to evaluate this automated commercial 3DE system against MRI and standard 2DE under different experimental conditions: 1) in vitro phantom measurements served as controlled setting in which boundaries were clearly delineated; 2) a validation cohort composed of healthy C57BL/6 J mice and New Zealand Obese (NZO) mice was used in order to validate 3DE against cardiac MRI as gold standard measurement; 3) a mouse model of pressure overload-induced heart failure was investigated to estimate the incremental value of 3DE for a standard application in the field of applied research.

Materials and methods

In vitro Volumetry

Round-shaped, oval latex balloons between 0.6 and 1.0 cm in size ($n = 6$; 176–300 µL; Fig. 2a) mimicking mice hearts, served as phantoms for ultrasound- and MRI measurements, as described before [18]. Balloons were filled with tap water before being embedded in a 1% agarose gel matrix.

Phantoms were scanned in a 3 Tesla small animal magnetic resonance system (MR Solutions, Guildford, United Kingdom) with a quadrature birdcage cardiac volume coil as previously reported by us [19]. A T2-weighed fast spin echo sequence with following parameters was applied: repetition time, 4800 ms; echo time, 68 ms; flip angle, 90°; field of view, 40.00\40.00\0.30 mm; pixel spacing 0.16\0.16; number of signal averages, 3; slice thickness 0.3 mm. Volumes were calculated by multi-slice tracing using Osirix software (version 7.0.3; Pixmeo SARL, Geneva, Switzerland).

For 2DE, B-Mode images of the maximum dimension of the round-shaped phantoms were acquired and volumes were calculated using the monoplane method of disks.

3DE image acquisition was started at the maximum dimension of the phantom at a slice thickness of 0.3 mm (equivalent to MRI).

Validation cohort

All animal procedures were performed in accordance with the guidelines of the German Law on the Protection of Animals and were approved by the local authorities (Landesamt für Gesundheit und Soziales, Berlin, Germany). Animals used in this study served as controls in ongoing projects and were kept under identical housing conditions (12 h light/dark cycle, standard diet ad libitum, 21 °C room temperature).

A cohort of 5 male C57BL/6 J and 5 male NZO mice ($n = 10$ total) was analyzed regarding cardiac volumes and ejection fraction (EF). All mice underwent echocardiography (1DE, 2DE and 3DE) and cardiac magnetic resonance (CMR) examination at the age of 22 weeks as described below. All data sets were acquired prospectively and analyzed for this study in a retrospective manner.

Heart failure cohort

Male C57BL/6 J mice (8–9 weeks) were anesthetized by intra-peritoneal injection of ketamine/xylazine (100 mg/kg/d, 20 mg/kg/d) (Sigma-Aldrich, Steinheim, Germany) before partial sternotomy was performed. Transverse aortic constriction (TAC) was induced by placing a silk suture around the aorta between right and left carotid arteries and a 26 gauge needle as previously reported by us ($n = 9$) [20]. Same procedure was performed on SHAM-operated animals ($n = 7$) except for the aortic banding. Echocardiography (1DE, 2DE and 3DE) was performed 10 weeks after TAC or SHAM-surgery.

CMR measurements in vivo

Similar to in vitro measurements, C57BL/6 J and NZO mice were scanned using a 3 Tesla small animal MRI system (MR Solutions, Guildford, United Kingdom) with a quadrature birdcage cardiac volume coil [19]. After induction of inhalative anesthesia with isoflurane-oxygen

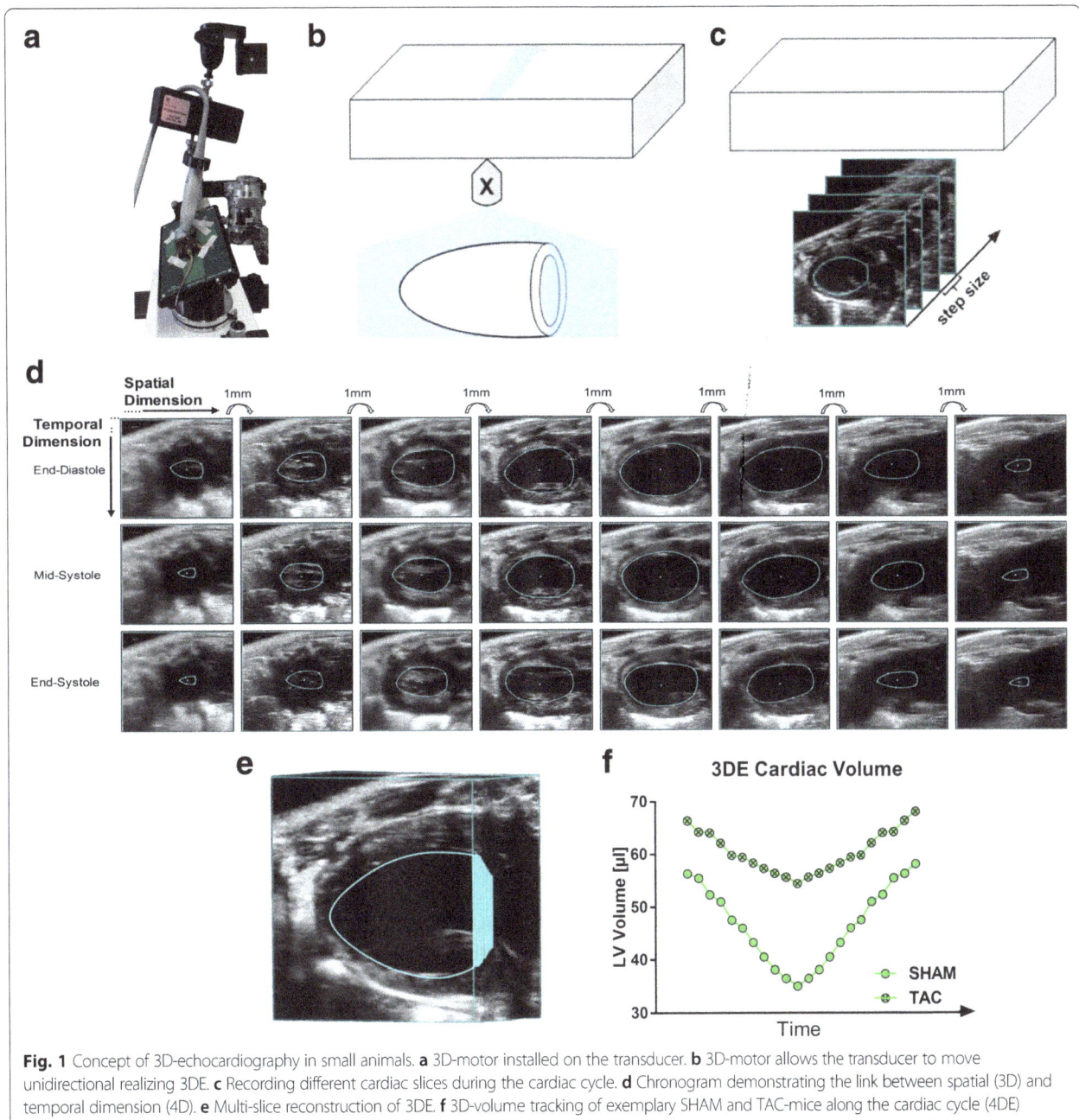

Fig. 1 Concept of 3D-echocardiography in small animals. **a** 3D-motor installed on the transducer. **b** 3D-motor allows the transducer to move unidirectional realizing 3DE. **c** Recording different cardiac slices during the cardiac cycle. **d** Chronogram demonstrating the link between spatial (3D) and temporal dimension (4D). **e** Multi-slice reconstruction of 3DE. **f** 3D-volume tracking of exemplary SHAM and TAC-mice along the cardiac cycle (4DE)

(4–5%) animals were positioned in a coil head first position and ECG electrodes were placed on the mice' feet. Anesthesia was maintained throughout the examination via inhalation of 1–2% isoflurane-oxygen to achieve heart rates around 400 beats per minutes. Mice were positioned in a heat-controlled animal bed (Equipment Veterinaire Minerve, Esternay, France) to maintain body temperature at 37 °C. Images were acquired using respiratory and ECG-gated gradient-echo cine sequences resulting in a LV cine short-axis stack with five to eight short-axis planes completely covering the LV (phases, 16; repetition time, 10 ms; echo time, 3 ms; flip angle,

20°; field of view, 40.00\40.00\1.00 mm; pixel spacing 0.16\0.16 mm; number of signal averages, 3; slices, 8; slice thickness 1.0 mm). Cardiac volumes and ejection fraction (EF) were assessed using CMR42 software package (version 3.4.1; Circle Cardiovascular Imaging Inc., Calgary, Alberta, Canada).

1D and 2D echocardiography

Echocardiography was performed using a MX400 ultra-high frequency linear array transducer (18–38 MHz, center transmit: 30 MHz, axial resolution: 50 μm) together with a Vevo® 3100 high-resolution Imaging System (both

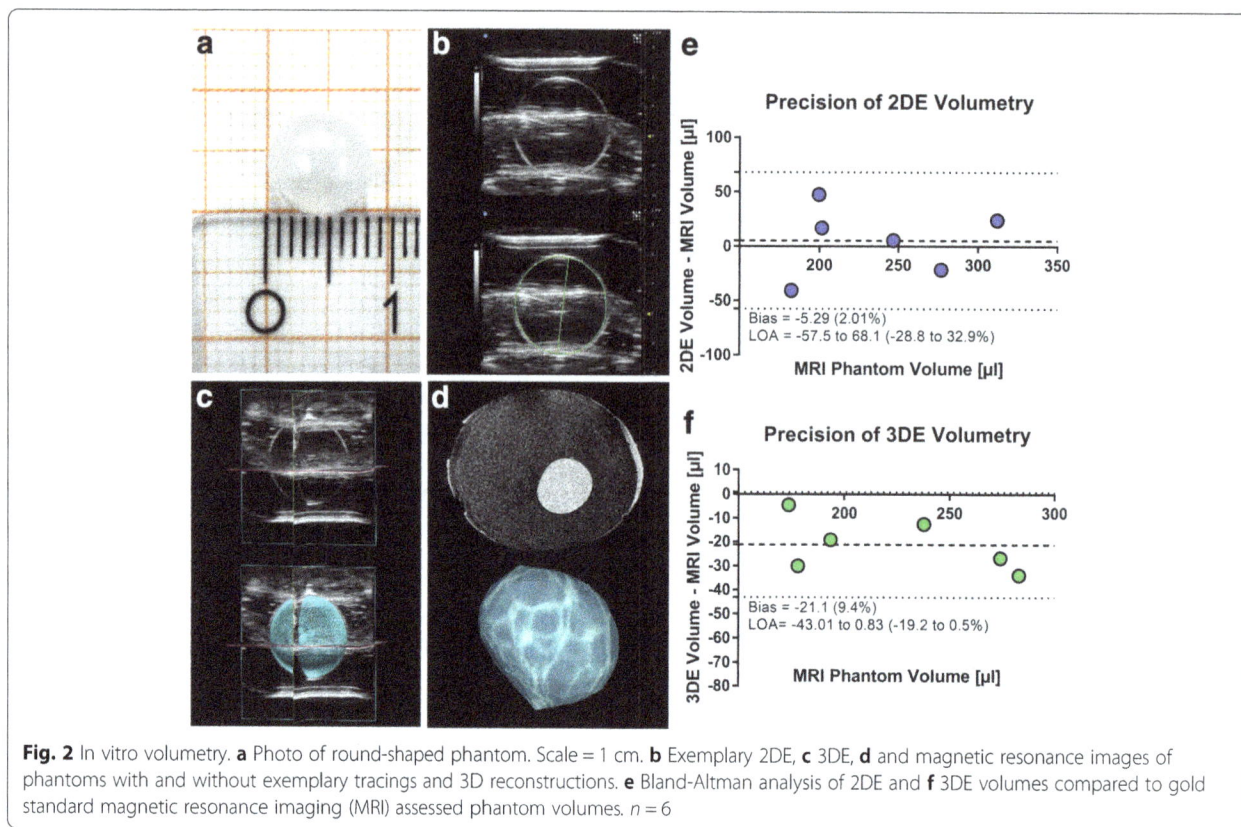

Fig. 2 In vitro volumetry. **a** Photo of round-shaped phantom. Scale = 1 cm. **b** Exemplary 2DE, **c** 3DE, **d** and magnetic resonance images of phantoms with and without exemplary tracings and 3D reconstructions. **e** Bland-Altman analysis of 2DE and **f** 3DE volumes compared to gold standard magnetic resonance imaging (MRI) assessed phantom volumes. $n = 6$

FUJIFILM VisualSonics, Toronto, Ontario, Canada). Mice were sedated with 3% isoflurane (Baxter International, Deerfield, Illinois, USA) and fixed in dorsal position on a heated pad at 37 °C (FUJIFILM VisualSonics, Toronto, Ontario, Canada), for body temperature maintenance of mice. After depilation, pre-warmed ultrasound gel (Parker Laboratories Fairfield, New Jersey, USA) was applied on the chest. Isoflurane concentration was reduced to a minimum (1–2%) to achieve constant and comparable heart rates during examination (Additional file 1: Table S1).

For 1DE, M-Mode images of the maximum dimension of the LV in parasternal long axis view were acquired as recently described by us [21]. Care was taken to visualize the LV in its maximum dimension from apex to base while recording B-mode images in parasternal long axis view for 2DE analyses. Additionally, velocity profiles of the heart failure cohort of the ascending and descending aorta were carried out using pulsed-wave Doppler mode. All acquired images were digitally stored in raw format (DICOM) for further offline-analyses.

Image analyses were performed by a single observer using the dedicated software package VevoLAB Version 3.0 (FUJIFILM VisualSonics, Toronto, Ontario, Canada). For inter-observer analysis data was analyzed by a second independent observer. Both observers had comparable long-time experience in performing and analyzing small animal echocardiography, including 1DE, 2DE and

speckle-tracking echocardiography, but no experience with 3DE.

Cardiac parameters of the heart failure cohort like diastolic wall thicknesses, LV inner diameter (LVID), and fractional shortening (FS) were evaluated in acquired 1DE M-Mode images. LV mass (LVM) was calculated according to the manufacturer's instructions. Gradient P assessing the degree of aortic stenosis was calculated from velocity parameters 10 weeks post-TAC as described previously [22, 23]. Corresponding 1DE-assessed cardiac volumes and EF were calculated according to the Teichholz formula for both cohorts as followed [24]:

$$EDV = \left(\frac{7.0}{2.4 + LVID; d} \right) x \, LVID; d^3$$

$$ESV = \left(\frac{7.0}{2.4 + LVID; s} \right) x \, LVID; s3$$

2DE analysis of both cohorts was determined by using the *LVtrace*-tool of VevoLAB for planimetry in B-Mode images derived from parasternal long axis view. Endocardial borders were traced during end-diastole and end-systole from LV outflow tract to apex. Calculations of 2DE-assessed cardiac volumes and EF were based on monoplane Simpson's method of discs. All analyses were performed according to the guidelines for cardiac chamber quantification provided by the American Society of Echocardiography [2].

3D echocardiography

A detailed standard operating procedure for 3DE can be found in the Online Supplement (Additional file 1). For generation of 3DE datasets, the ultrasound probe was clamped into a specialized 3D-motor (FUJIFILM VisualSonics, Toronto, Ontario, Canada), allowing automated and stepwise movement of the probe. The linear movement of the transducer facilitates image acquisition at multiple levels of the heart with step sizes on a micrometer scale. The parasternal long axis view in maximum dimension from apex to base served as starting point for consecutive image recordings. The system generates 4D data in terms of automatically respiration-gated cine loops to avoid respiratory motion artifacts. Images were recorded with the following settings: scan distance: 0.8–1.2 cm (depending on heart size covering the whole LV); step size: 100 μm, acquisition type: quick; process quality: sharp; frame rate: 200 fps. This resulted in 79–119 scan steps/heart slices and an acquisition time of 3–6 min per animal. All acquired images were digitally stored in raw format (DICOM) for further offline-analyses.

3D-volumes and EF were investigated by multi-slice reconstruction starting the analysis with a picture at maximum expansion of the LV. The distance between analyzed images amounts to 1 mm (Fig. 1D). Manual tracing of the images was performed, leading to 5–8 analyzed images (depending on heart size) at one time point of the cardiac cycle (spatial dimension, 3D). In total, three different time periods of the cardiac cycle (end-diastolic, mid-systolic and end-systolic) (temporal dimension, 4D), automatically chosen by VevoLAB software tool, were analyzed (Fig. 1D). LV volumes and corresponding EF were calculated, using a disc summation without assumptions. Exemplary tracings and 3D reconstructions of the cardiac volume can be found in the Additional files 2, 3 and 4.

For calculation of inter- and intra-observer variabilities, identical echocardiographic images (SHAM: $n = 7$, TAC: $n = 9$) were analyzed with 1DE, 2DE and 3DE by the same observer twice or by another investigator, respectively.

Statistical analysis

All analyses were performed using GraphPad Prism 7. A p-value of < 0.05 was assumed as statistically significant. Results are shown as mean ± standard error of mean (SEM). Normal distribution of variables was verified in advance of further statistical analysis, using the Kolmogorov Smirnov Normality Test. Statistical analyses were performed using unpaired two-tailed Student's t-test, one-way-ANOVA for multiple comparisons followed by Uncorrected Fisher's LSD posttest or two-way-ANOVA for multiple comparisons followed by Tukey's multiple comparisons test, as appropriate. Method comparisons and inter- and intra-observer variabilities were analyzed using Bland-Altman plots. Results of Bland-Altman analysis were expressed as bias and agreement intervals. The rate of agreement was defined by the percent difference to gold standard MRI values (method comparison) or the first observer (inter-observer variability) as follows: $\leq \pm 5\%$ excellent, $\leq \pm 10\%$ good, $\leq \pm 20\%$ moderate, $\leq \pm 30\%$ poor.

Results
Validation of 3DE in vitro

In a first step, we evaluated the accuracy of 3DE in vitro, by assessing the volumes of round-shaped phantoms in comparison to conventional 2DE and MRI as gold standard measurement (Fig. 2). To this end, latex balloons (Fig. 2a) were scanned and analyzed with conventional 2DE (Fig. 2b), novel 3DE tomographic multi-slice reconstructions (Fig. 2c) and MRI (Fig. 2d). 1DE was not applied since the underlying Teichholz formula is based on an ellipsoid geometric shape not being fulfilled by the used round-shaped phantoms [25]. Bland-Altman analysis of 2DE and 3DE in comparison to gold standard MRI measurements revealed that 3DE tended to underestimate phantom volumes, whereas 2DE misestimated in both directions (Fig. 2e, f). This effect might be due to MRI artifacts caused by the agarose gel matrix. Further, 3DE showed good agreement when compared to gold standard MRI measurements, whereas conventional 2DE showed excellent values for mean differences, but large agreement intervals, misestimating strongly in both directions (Fig. 2e, f).

Validation of 3DE in vivo

In a second step, we validated 3DE against conventional 2DE and cardiac magnetic resonance (CMR) imaging under in vivo conditions in a validation cohort consisting of C57/BL6 and NZO mice, aiming for a broad range of cardiac performance (Table 1). NZO mice are known to develop severe obesity and therefore show increased blood pressure levels, heart and body weights [26, 27]. The cardiac phenotype of NZO mice is reflected by significantly enhanced end-diastolic (EDV) and end-systolic volumes (ESV), stroke volumes (SV) and decreased EFs, when compared to CMR-assessed parameters of healthy control mice (Table 1). In addition to CMR measurements, we applied 1DE, 2DE and novel 3DE to the validation cohort and compared the results to CMR-derived volumetric data (Fig. 3). Figure 3 shows exemplary pictures of the compared imaging modalities A) M-Mode (1DE), B) B-Mode (2DE), C) tomographic multi slice reconstruction (3DE) and D) CMR (Fig. 3a-d).

Table 1 CMR-characteristics of validation cohort

	C57BL/6 J	NZO
n-number (%)	5 (50)	5 (50)
CMR Data		
ESV, µl	13.22 ± 1.9	52.42 ± 16.5*
EDV, µl	34.61 ± 3.1	90.22 ± 18.6*
EF, %	62.5 ± 2.6	47.76 ± 7.5*
SV, µl	21.39 ± 1.4	37.81 ± 2.1***

Mean ± SEM. Student's t-test. *$p < .05$; ***$p < .001$ vs. C57BL/6 J cohort. ESV = end-systolic volume; EDV = end-diastolic volume; EF = ejection fraction; SV = stroke volume

3DE-assessed ESVs and EDVs showed significant smaller mean differences to CMR-assessed volumes, when compared to 1DE and 2DE-assessed volumes (ESV - 1DE: 16.5 ± 2.9 µl, 2DE: 14.3 ± 2.6 µl, 3DE: 4.3 ± 3.9 µl; EDV – 1DE: 36.7 ± 4.5 µl, 2DE: 24.9 ± 5.2 µl, 3DE: 8.8 ± 6.3 µl) (Fig. 3e, f). Of note, all echocardiographic modalities tended to overestimate the true LV volumes. Based on the values of EDV and ESV the relative measures SV and EF

were calculated. SVs assessed by 3DE showed the smallest mean difference to the CMR-assessed SVs (Fig. 3g). Significant differences among the echocardiographic modalities were found between 1DE and 3DE, but not between 2DE and 3DE (Fig. 3g). The clinical relevant measure EF was underestimated by all echocardiographic techniques (Fig. 3h). However, no significant differences were observed between the echocardiographic modalities (Fig. 3h).

Application of 3DE in experimental heart failure

To test whether novel commercially available 3DE is suitable to detect expected alterations of cardiac performance, we applied 3DE in a standard mouse model of pressure overload-induced heart failure realized by TAC-surgery. Successful TAC-surgery was proven by increased pressure gradients (*Gradient P*) measured across the aortic banding (Table 2). TAC induced a marked cardiac hypertrophy in terms of LV wall thickening and increased internal diameters pointing towards a dilatation of the LV (1DE, M-mode) (Table 2). All echocardiography modalities

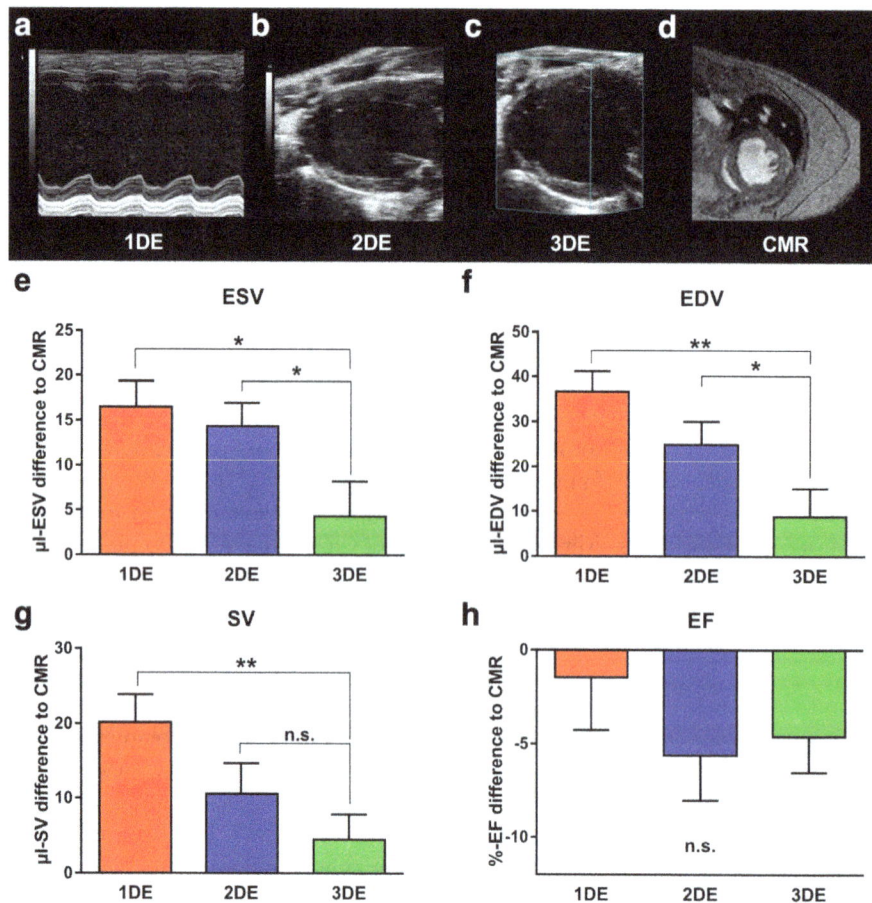

Fig. 3 In vivo volumetry. **a** Exemplary 1DE, **b** 2DE, **C** 3DE and **d** cardiac magnetic resonance (CMR) images of left ventricles of NZO mice. Mean differences of echocardiographic-assessed **e** ESV, **f** EDV, **G** SV and **h** EF to values assessed with gold standard CMR (CMR) imaging. $n = 10$. *$p < .05$, **$p < .01$ vs. 3DE

Table 2 Phenotypic characterization of heart failure cohort

	SHAM (n = 7)	TAC (n = 9)
Stenosis		
Aortic peak velocity desc, mm/s	− 945.7 ± 74.4	− 3107 ± 142.4****
Aortic peak velocity asc, mm/s	1200 ± 72.0	1268 ± 139
Gradient P	−2.17 ± 1.1	32.22 ± 3.2****
1DE		
Heart rate, bpm	489.2 ± 24.7	512.5 ± 16.5
LVAW, d, mm	0.61 ± 0.04	0.84 ± 0.03***
LVPW, d, mm	0.63 ± 0.02	0.73 ± 0.02**
LVID, d, mm	3.99 ± 0.1	4.34 ± 0.12*
LVM, mg	66.91 ± 3.2	105.2 ± 5.9***
FS, %	27.68 ± 2.1	17.98 ± 2.5*

Mean ± SEM. Student's t-test. *p < .05. **p <.01. ***p <.001. ****p <.0001. SHAM: n = 7, TAC: n = 9. Asc = ascendens; desc = descendens; LVAW, d = left ventricular anterior wall (diastole); LVPW, d = left ventricular posterior wall (diastole); LVID, d = left ventricular inner diameter (diastole); FS = fractional shortening

reliably detected the presence of a significantly reduced EF among TAC-operated animals (Table 3). Additionally, the extent of EF reduction was similar among the methods used (Table 3). Interestingly, however, only 3DE detected a significant increase in EDV after TAC, whereas 1DE and 2DE failed to reach statistical significance (Table 3). All methods detected a significant increase of ESV after TAC without significant differences among the techniques (Table 3). Within SHAM- and TAC-groups, we observed no significant differences of ESV or EF values determined by the different echocardiographic techniques (Fig. 4). In direct comparison of values derived from the different echocardiographic methods, 3DE showed significantly lower EDVs and SVs in healthy mice and TAC mice (independent from disease status) when compared to 1DE and 2DE (Fig. 4).

Reproducibility of measures

All echocardiographic modalities were tested for inter- and intra-observer variability (Table 4). In general, healthy SHAM-mice showed good to excellent inter- and intra-observer variabilities regarding the absolute

measures ESV and EDV, whereas TAC-mice demonstrated moderate to good agreement, independent of the echocardiographic technique (Table 4). Further, we observed poorer agreement rates for the relative metrics EF and SV than for total volumes, independent of SHAM or TAC intervention (Table 4). When we compared novel 3D with the conventional echocardiographic techniques 1DE and 2DE, agreement rates for inter-observer variabilities were comparable between imaging modalities, whereas 3DE intra-observer variability appeared to be slightly inferior. Representative planimetric tracings (Fig. 5a) and corresponding reconstructed 3D-volumes (Fig. 5b) of two different observers exemplify the challenge of unambiguous identification of endocardial borders in 3DE. In detail, corresponding Bland-Altman analysis of SHAM and TAC-mice demonstrated good and excellent agreement between observers when analyzing ESV and EDV of healthy SHAM-mice, respectively (Fig. 5c). However, the agreement between observers for the relative metrics of SV and EF was only moderate in healthy mice. When analyzing data of heart failure mice, the inter-observer variability for 3DE metrics was moderate, indicating a difficulty to analyze heart failure mice (Fig. 5d).

Discussion

In the present study, we evaluated a recently launched commercially available 3DE system for small animals in various experimental settings. We were able to show that (1) 3DE-derived volumetry under in vitro conditions is in good agreement with MRI as gold standard measurement; (2) cardiac volume determination with 3DE demonstrates smaller mean differences to CMR-assessed volumes, when compared with conventional echocardiographic techniques; (3) 3DE was suitable to detect reduced EFs in a standard mouse model of pressure overload; (4) Inter- and intra-observer variability of 3DE showed good to excellent agreement regarding absolute volumes in healthy mice, whereas agreement rates for the relative metrics EF and SV demonstrated good to moderate observer variabilities.

Our results in the cardiac phantoms demonstrated that under controlled conditions with clearly delineated boundaries and comparable step sizes between 3DE and MRI,

Table 3 Method comparison of imaging modalities in the heart failure cohort

Method	1DE		2DE		3DE	
	SHAM	TAC	SHAM	TAC	SHAM	TAC
ESV, μl	33.15 ± 4.3	55.72 ± 7.6*	34.63 ± 4.4	58.4 ± 8.6*	26.95 ± 2.6	41.57 ± 3.7**
EDV, μl	70.01 ± 4.2	85.53 ± 5.5	65.24 ± 5.2	83.54 ± 6.8	48.84 ± 2.1	58.31 ± 3.2*
EF, %	53.85 ± 3.4	36.89 ± 4.8*	47.96 ± 3.0	32.4 ± 4.1*	45.29 ± 3.8	28.9 ± 4.1*
SV, μl	36.87 ± 1.0	29.8 ± 3.5	30.62 ± 1.6	25.2 ± 2.5	21.89 ± 1.6	16.7 ± 2.6

Mean ± SEM. Student's t-test. *p <.05. **p <.01. SHAM: n = 7, TAC: n = 9. EDV = end-diastolic volume; ESV = end-systolic volume; EF = ejection fraction; SV = stroke volume

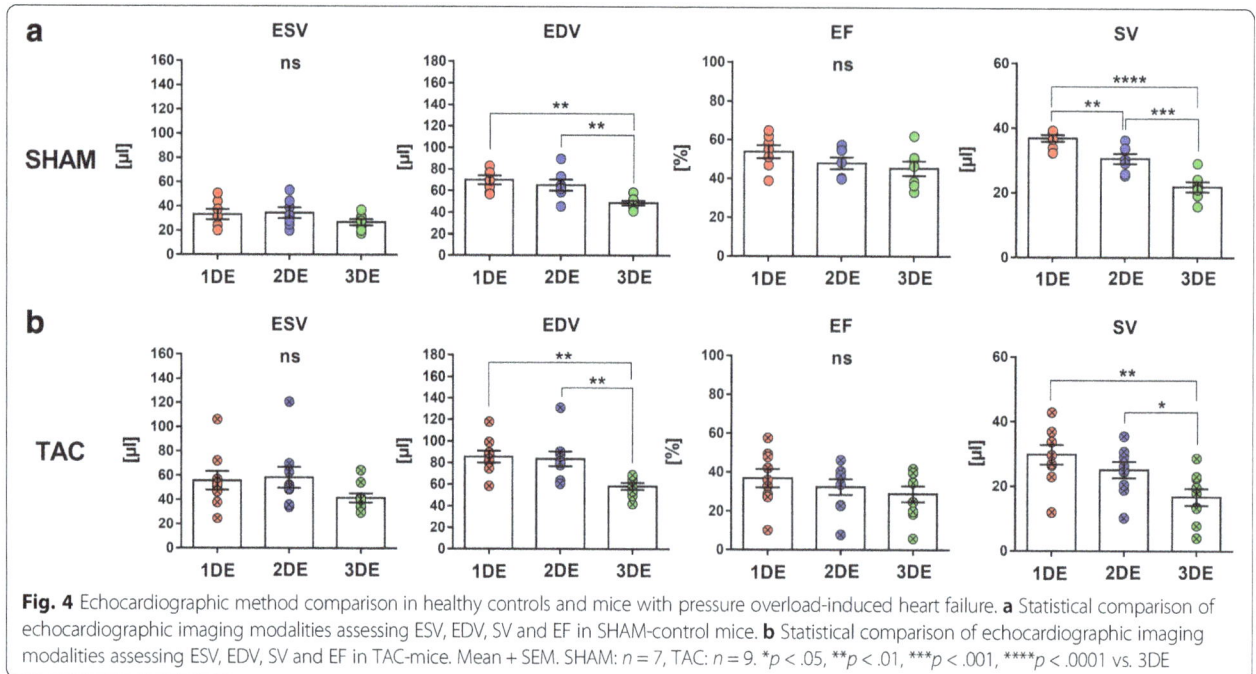

Fig. 4 Echocardiographic method comparison in healthy controls and mice with pressure overload-induced heart failure. **a** Statistical comparison of echocardiographic imaging modalities assessing ESV, EDV, SV and EF in SHAM-control mice. **b** Statistical comparison of echocardiographic imaging modalities assessing ESV, EDV, SV and EF in TAC-mice. Mean + SEM. SHAM: $n = 7$, TAC: $n = 9$. *$p < .05$, **$p < .01$, ***$p < .001$, ****$p < .0001$ vs. 3DE

3DE consistently underestimated phantom volumes, whereas 2DE misestimated in both directions. One explanation for this result might be that tiny air bubbles, emerging at the outer phantom rim within the agarose gel matrix, may cause small MRI artifacts, which consequently generates a halo-like effect during MRI border identification. This would consequently lead to an overestimation of MRI-assessed phantom volumes. A direct method comparison between MRI and echocardiographic-assessed volumes would therefore result in allegedly volume underestimation of echocardiography. However, we only observed consistently underestimation of phantom volumes with 3DE, but not conventional 2DE. We believe that the missing echocardiographic underestimation of 2DE (in comparison to MRI), might be due to the angle-dependency of 2DE, masking the underestimation effect of echocardiography, depending on the positioning of phantoms within the agarose gel matrix and the angle of the transducer. Albeit we cannot prove this hypothetical limitation of 2DE, one of the major advantages of 3DE is to outdistance the angle-dependency of conventional echocardiography and therefore misestimating only in one direction.

Our results demonstrate that 3DE is suitable to determine cardiac volumes in vivo. These findings are in line with pioneering studies, evaluating non-commercially available 3DE-techniques [14, 15]. In 1999, Scherrer-Crosbie and colleagues demonstrated for the first time that multidimensional imaging allows precise LV volumetry and ventricular function, comparable to flow-probe measurements in a mouse model of myocardial infarction [14]. *Dawson* et al. applied ECG- and respiration-gated 3DE in small

animals and were the first, who demonstrated excellent agreement by comparison with the current gold standard volumetric technology (MRI) [15]. However, the widespread application of these non-commercially 3DE approaches was limited with regards to standardization, post-processing software and spatial resolutions. Based on these pioneering studies, the present commercially available 3DE system for small animals was launched [16]. Very recently, Damen and colleagues analyzed the novel commercially available 3DE-system in a genetic model of LV hypertrophy and healthy controls in comparison to 1DE and CMR [16]. The authors found no significant differences between 3DE and CMR measured mean values of cardiac volumetry and corresponding relative metrics, whereas 1DE on average overestimated cardiac volumes [16]. In contrast, our results demonstrated a moderate overestimation of 3DE-assessed cardiac volumes when compared to CMR values. This effect might be explained by the differences in step size used for 3DE (step size: 0.1 mm) and CMR (step size: 1.0 mm) analysis in our study. A reduction of CMR-slice thickness will increase spatiotemporal resolution of the acquired images, but will consequently lead to prolonged acquisition time, which further can cause problems with anesthesia. It is known from the clinics that a coarsely chosen resolution of CMR-image lines can lead to partial volume effects, in case the last part of the apex (short axis orientation) is located between two slices and therefore not included during endocardial border tracing [28, 29]. This effect has already been reported for other imaging techniques like positron emission tomography (PET) in preclinical animal models [30, 31]. In terms of our findings, the 10-fold difference in

Table 4 Inter- and intra-observer variabilities

			Inter-observer variability		Intra-observer variability	
			Mean diff. ± SD	LOA	Mean diff. ± SD	LOA
1DE	ESV	SHAM	3.8 ± 6.0	−9.4 to 17.0	2.3 ± 6.0	− 10.8 to 15.5
		TAC	2.8 ± 11.2	−20.9 to 26.6	− 0.8 ± 11.0	− 24.0 to 22.5
	EDV	SHAM	6.2 ± 6.2	− 7.3 to 19.7	2.1 ± 5.8	− 10.6 to 14.8
		TAC	7.2 ± 8.6	− 11.0 to 25.5	− 0.3 ± 7.9	− 17.0 to 16.5
	EF	SHAM	−1.4 ± 4.5	− 11.2 to 8.4	−2.1 ± 4.3	− 11.4 to 7.2
		TAC	2.2 ± 6.5	− 11.5 to 15.9	1.3 ± 5.8	− 11.0 to 13.5
	SV	SHAM	−1.1 ± 5.9	−1.1 to 5.9	−0.03 ± 1.5	− 3.2 to 3.2
		TAC	4.4 ± 3.9	− 3.8 to 12.6	1.8 ± 4.4	− 7.5 to 11.2
2DE	ESV	SHAM	−1.9 ± 5.7	− 14.3 to 10.4	0.3 ± 6.2	− 13.2 to 13.9
		TAC	− 5.4 ± 11.7	− 30.1 to 19.4	− 0.5 ± 12.4	− 26.9 to 25.8
	EDV	SHAM	−4.6 ± 6.2	−18.1 to 9.0	−2.2 ± 7.3	− 18.2 to 13.7
		TAC	− 7.0 ± 9.2	− 26.4 to 12.4	− 0.9 ± 10.0	− 22.0 to 20.3
	EF	SHAM	−1.1 ± 4.6	− 11.1 to 9.0	−2.1 ± 4.3	−11.4 to 7.2
		TAC	−0.6 ± 5.9	− 11.9 to 13.1	1.3 ± 5.8	− 11.0 to 13.5
	SV	SHAM	−3.9 ± 2.6	− 9.5 to 1.7	−2.6 ± 2.3	−7.6 to 2.5
		TAC	− 1.8 ± 3.8	− 9.9 to 6.3	− 0.3 ± 3.7	− 8.1 to 7.5
3DE	ESV	SHAM	−1.72 ± 3.5	−9.4 to 5.9	−2.6 ± 2.9	− 9.0 to 3.7
		TAC	6.18 ± 4.3	− 3.0 to 15.4	4.0 ± 3.9	− 4.3 to 12.2
	EDV	SHAM	1.06 ± 3.6	− 6.8 to 8.9	− 0.3 ± 3.4	−7.7 to 7.2
		TAC	4.87 ± 4.5	− 4.7 to 14.4	1.0 ± 4.4	− 8.2 to 10.3
	EF	SHAM	5.44 ± 5.3	−6.2 to 17.1	5.7 ± 4.3	− 3.7 to 15.1
		TAC	− 4.23 ± 5.4	− 15.7 to 7.2	− 5.6 ± 5.4	− 17.1 to 5.9
	SV	SHAM	2.78 ± 2.6	−2.8 to 8.4	2.4 ± 2.2	− 2.4 to 7.1
		TAC	−1.31 ± 3.7	− 9.2 to 6.5	− 2.9 ± 3.7	− 10.8 to 5.0

SHAM: n = 7, TAC: n = 9. SD = standard deviation; LOA = limits of agreement; ESV = end-systolic volume (µl); EDV = end-diastolic volume (µl); EF = ejection fraction (%); SV = stroke volume (µl)

resolution between 3DE and CMR may lead to an ostensible overestimation of 3DE-assessed volumes, but might also be reasoned by a CMR-based partial volume effect. Our findings are in contrast to the data of Damen and colleagues, who detected no significant differences for mean values of cardiac volumes [16], although they also used different slice thicknesses during image acquisition (3DE: 0.076 mm vs CMR: 1.00 mm).

When comparing gold standard CMR to echocardiographic imaging modalities, it turned out that the variability of measurements was lower for absolute cardiac volumes, than for relative metrics. One of the difficulties facing LV functional assessment is that EF varies with changes in blood pressure, heart rate and body temperature [32]. Since major differences regarding physiological and technical conditions between preclinical CMR and echocardiography still exist (e.g. positioning of mice (prone vs. supine position), spatiotemporal resolution (1.0 mm vs. 0.1 mm step sizes)), it seems unlikely to assess identical values for LV volumes with these methods. While our study was designed to keep these parameters constant between different imaging methods by the use of similar anesthesia strategies, especially the difference in positioning of mice between preclinical CMR and echocardiography most probably has a

significant impact on hemodynamics that cannot be avoided. Thus, it is mandatory to examine all animals under the same conditions within one modality to increase reproducibility and minimize variations between measurements [32]. However, feasibility of this set up is often restrained by financial and time by financial and temporal requirements. Today, CMR data are widely accepted as the gold standard method for the assessment of cardiac volumes in humans and small animals. Both 3DE and CMR do not rely on geometrical assumptions for formula-based computation of 3D volumes and should therefore be preferred over 1D and 2D methods to avoid inaccuracy when assessing cardiac volumes and function.

A precursor of the present 3DE system has already been validated against Micro-CT and 1DE in a murine model of muscular dystrophy [33]. The authors found that although each aforementioned imaging modality measured decreased cardiac function as disease progresses in genetically modified mice, 3DE had higher agreement with gold standard measurements acquired by gated micro-CT and smaller variability [33]. These data are in line with our findings from the heart failure cohort, showing that all echocardiographic modalities are suitable to detect a decrease of ventricular function, but smallest standard deviation was recognized for

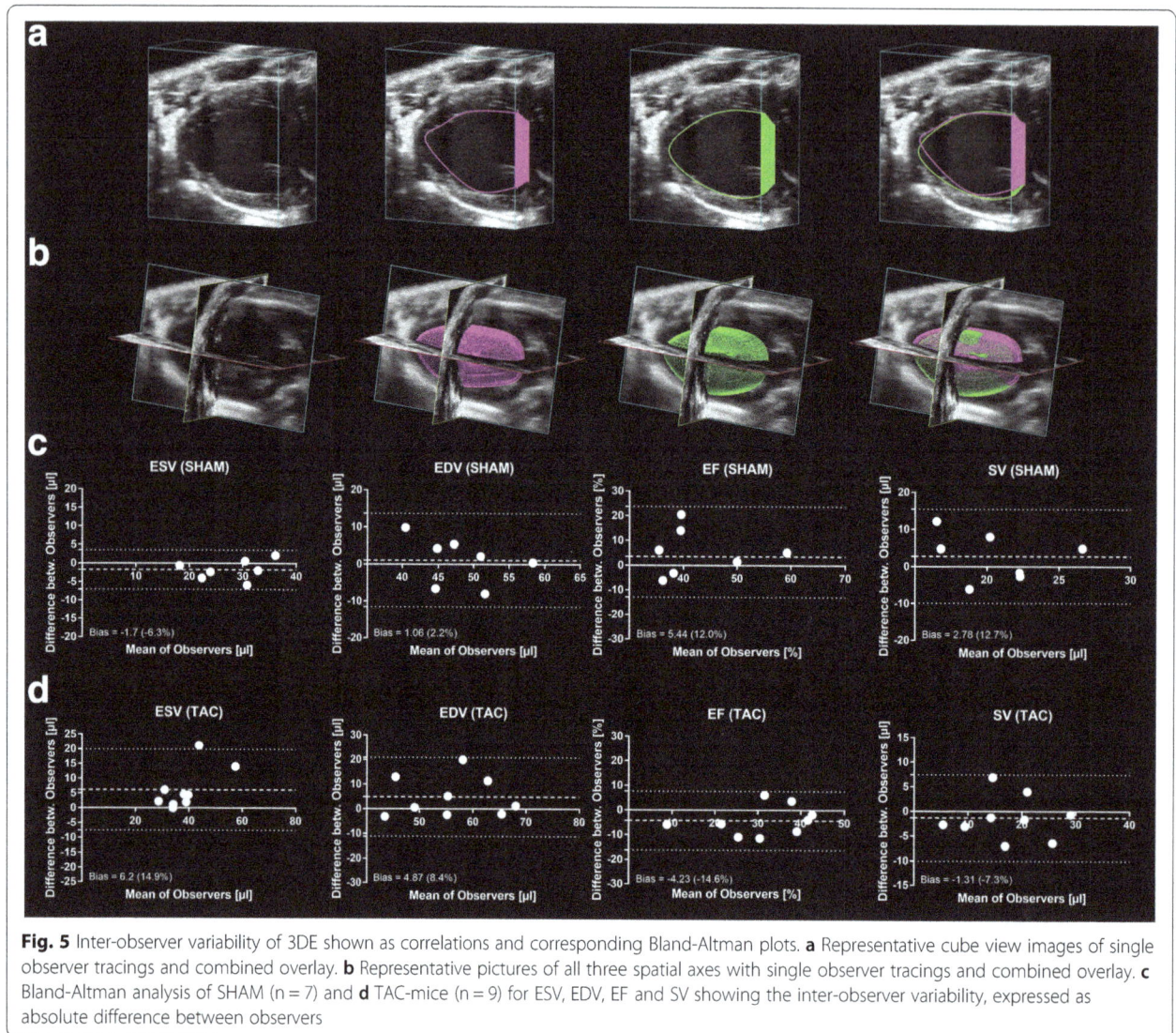

Fig. 5 Inter-observer variability of 3DE shown as correlations and corresponding Bland-Altman plots. **a** Representative cube view images of single observer tracings and combined overlay. **b** Representative pictures of all three spatial axes with single observer tracings and combined overlay. **c** Bland-Altman analysis of SHAM (n = 7) and **d** TAC-mice (n = 9) for ESV, EDV, EF and SV showing the inter-observer variability, expressed as absolute difference between observers

3DE-derived volumetry. In contrast to 1DE and 2DE, 3DE was able to detect expected alterations of EDVs in mice suffering from pressure overload-induced heart failure after TAC-surgery [29]. Cardiac remodeling plays a crucial role during development of heart failure and therefore influences LV volumes [30]. Further, LV volumes were demonstrated as superior predictors of cardiac outcome in heart failure patients, when compared to LVEF [31]. The incremental value of 3DE for the diagnosis of patients has been shown decades ago and became apparent in high accuracy and good feasibility [32]. Especially the diagnoses of cardiac valve diseases and ventricular asynchrony on the basis of LV volume quantification has been demonstrated as great advantage of novel 3DE over conventional echocardiographic approaches in the clinics [7, 33, 34]. Indeed, 3DE used in the clinics is technically based on matrix array transducers, which are currently not available for small animals,

hampering the direct translation of results from "bedside to bench". However, robust assessment of impaired ventricular function, based on altered cardiac volumetry, demonstrates the useful potential of 3DE and the certain advantage over conventional echocardiographic approaches in small animal models.

Further, Bondoc et al. detected only minor standard deviation for 3DE measurements and good reproducibility, while 1DE exhibited considerably greater variability [33]. We found good to moderate inter- and intra-observer variabilities for 3DE, which were comparable or slightly inferior when compared to conventional echocardiography using a different imaging system. This finding might be explained by relevant limitations recognized during image acquisition and analysis of 3DE: The automated image processing algorithm implemented by the VevoLab software does not allow for manual corrections of the chosen time periods for the cardiac cycle or the visualization of endocardial borders for 3DE image acquisition and analysis. In contrast, the analysis of 1DE and 2DE images is based on manual selection of cardiac cycle time periods and also of clearly delineated endocardial borders. In general, automated image processing algorithms are preferred in order to strengthen reproducibility of obtained data sets. However, it appears as a major limitation that the operator cannot verify if the software has chosen the time points for cardiac volume assessment correctly, which also hampers the comparability between conventional echocardiographic imaging modalities and novel 3DE. In addition, the identification of myocardial boundaries in the consecutive tracing seems to be a general and major limitation of the novel 3DE approach. Starting from the maximum dimension of the LV long axis, the problem aggravates when reaching outer regions in which no myocardial borders are visible in most cases. Nevertheless, tracing at these outer slices is required for reconstruction of realistic LV volumes. We included in our study only images with acceptable image quality, enabling us to perform reliable 3DE analysis. A large meta-analysis of 3DE in clinical trials revealed that the inclusion of all 3D datasets, regardless of image quality, increased the variability of 3DE-derived data (as defined by elevated 95% confidence intervals) when compared to studies with pre-selected high image quality [7]. Future studies exclusively focusing on 3DE data sets with high image quality will reveal the impact of image quality on 3DE data in small animal models.

Besides, it should be stressed that valid, precise and robust assessment of cardiac volumetry using a novel software package requires experienced observers, which remains challenging due to the novelty of the imaging technique in small animals. Additionally, a highly standardized protocol for the tracing procedure is required in order to assure comparability between different observers.

In summary, our data indicates that 3DE may provide additional value for basic research, especially in preclinical models in which precise LV volumetry is of interest. However, an extensive evaluation of this currently available commercial 3DE approach is still lacking and only little is known about the ideal field of application. For instance, asymmetric ventricular shape (e.g. after myocardial infarction) represents a major limitation of calculation-based 1DE and 2DE and might be a field of application for 3DE in future [2, 17]. Therefore, 3DE is expected to have add-on value especially when being applied to experimental models in which a non-symmetric LV geometry is expected. Further investigations are required in order to identify suitable indications for usage of 3DE in basic research.

Limitations

First, all echocardiographic examinations were performed under inhaled anesthesia which might have had an impact on heart rate and function and hampers comparison to CMR-assessed values. Further, echocardiographic examination, including novel 3DE, is always limited due to sternum, rib and lung artifacts, which can blur endocardial borders. Second, the choice of end-diastolic, mid-systolic and end-systolic time periods during the cardiac cycle is automatically done by the VevoLab software. Therefore, the user is dependent on the correct selection with no option for the user to validate the choice of cardiac cycle time periods. This may become relevant when investigating cardiac pathologies with arrhythmias. Third, the sample size of the present study was relatively low and only two animal cohorts were used to evaluate novel 3DE. Thus, future validation using larger sample sizes and different animal models is still required. Fourth, tracing of MRI/CMR data was performed manually, whereas ultrasound images were analyzed with semiautomatic software tools. Fifth, we found moderate inter- and intra-observer variabilities for 3DE in diseased mice, which were comparable or slightly inferior when compared to conventional echocardiography. Sixth, we only acquired images from mice during a single ultrasound session. Future studies will reveal reproducibility of novel 3DE when screening the same animal in multiple ultrasound sessions. Lastly, it should be taken into account that we used a suboptimal setting of body temperature controlling during image acquisition and did not monitor body temperature of mice directly. Therefore, we cannot prove whether body temperature variations had potential confounding effects on the assessment of cardiac volumetry in our study.

Conclusion

In conclusion, we report here the evaluation of a newly available technique for 3DE in experimental conditions. 3DE-derived volumetry under in vitro conditions was in good agreement with MRI measurements, consistently underestimating phantom volumes. In vivo, 3DE showed smaller mean differences in LV volumes compared to CMR than conventional echocardiography. Further, 3DE was found to be suitable for the detection of altered LV volumes and assessment of impaired cardiac function. The application of 3DE was characterized by rapid acquisition time (compared to CMR), low costs and high spatiotemporal resolutions. However, difficulties with endocardial border tracing and a moderate reproducibility appear as relevant limitations. To achieve the full potential of 3DE for the assessment of LV volumes, further standardization processes for image acquisition and analysis are needed to obtain a valid and robust method, providing a reliable tool for diagnosis of systolic dysfunction.

Abbreviations
1DE: One-dimensional echocardiography; 2DE: Two-dimensional echocardiography; 3DECMR: Three-dimensional echocardiography cardiac magnetic resonance; EDV: End-diastolic volume; EF: Ejection fraction; ESV: End-systolic volume; FS: Fractional shortening; LOA: Limits of agreement; LV: Left ventricular; LVID: Left ventricular inner diameter; LVM: Left ventricular mass; MRI: Magnetic resonance imaging; NZO: New Zealand Obese; SEM: Standard error of mean; SV: Stroke volume; TAC: Transverse aortic constriction

Acknowledgements
We thank Niklas Beyhoff for excellent support in literature research and enlightening discussions. Dr. Magdalena Steiner, Dr. Katrin Suppelt and Dr. Dieter Fuchs (FUJIFILM VisualSonics) for helpful support during image acquisition. Beata Höft, Christiane Sprang and Manuela Sommerfeld for their excellent technical assistance.

Funding
JG, TG and CO were supported by DynAge, FU Berlin. CD and TG were supported by NZOcardio (100290384) and the Gesundheitscampus Brandenburg. SB was supported by the Deutsche Stiftung für Herzforschung. AFL was supported by the DFG (KFO 218/2), the Deutsche Stiftung für Herzforschung, and the DZHK (BER 5.4 PR). UK was supported by the DFG (KFO 218/2), the Else Kröner-Fresenius Stiftung (2014_A100), and the DZHK (BER 5.4 PR).

Authors' contributions
The authors contributed to this work as follows: JG: animal treatment, echocardiographic data acquisition and –analysis, statistics, preparation of manuscript. AB: preparation/review of manuscript, statistics. SB: animal treatment, echocardiographic data acquisition. SJ: CMR/MRI measurements, preparation/review of manuscript. CD: animal treatment. TG: preparation/review of manuscript, funding. AFL: preparation/review of manuscript. DM: preparation/review of manuscript. WMK: preparation/review of manuscript. CO: conception and design of study, funding of study. UK: conception and design of study, funding of study. All authors read and approved the final manuscript.

Ethics approval
All animal procedures were performed in accordance with the guidelines of the German Law on the Protection of Animals and were approved by the local authorities (Landesamt für Gesundheit und Soziales, Berlin, Germany).

Competing interests
The authors declare that they have no competing interests.

Author details
[1]Institute of Pharmacology, Center for Cardiovascular Research, Charité -Universitaetsmedizin Berlin, Hessische Str. 3-4, 10115 Berlin, Germany. [2]German Center for Cardiovascular Research (DZHK), partner site Berlin, 10117 Berlin, Germany. [3]Department of Molecular Toxicology, German Institute of Human Nutrition Potsdam-Rehbruecke (DIfE), 14558 Nuthetal, Germany. [4]German Center for Diabetes Research (DZD), 85764 Muenchen-Neuherberg, Germany. [5]Internal Medicine/Cardiology, Deutsches Herzzentrum Berlin, Augustenburger Platz 1, 13353 Berlin, Germany. [6]Department of Cardiology, Charité University Medicine Berlin, Augustenburger Platz 1, 13353 Berlin, Germany. [7]Institute of Physiology, Charité University Medicine Berlin, Charitéplatz 1, 10117 Berlin, Germany.

References
1. Dekker DL, Piziali RL, Dong E. A system for ultrasonically imaging the human heart in three dimensions. Comput Biomed Res. 1974;7:544–53.
2. Lang RM, Badano LP, Mor-Avi V, Afilalo J, Armstrong A, Ernande L, et al. Recommendations for cardiac chamber quantification by echocardiography in adults: an update from the American Society of Echocardiography and the European Association of Cardiovascular Imaging. J Am Soc Echocardiogr 2015;28:1–39.e14.
3. Amundsen BH, Ericsson M, Seland JG, Pavlin T, Ellingsen Ø, Brekken C. A comparison of retrospectively self-gated magnetic resonance imaging and high-frequency echocardiography for characterization of left ventricular function in mice. Lab Anim. 2011;45:31–7.
4. Stuckey DJ, Carr CA, Tyler DJ, Clarke K. Cine-MRI versus two-dimensional echocardiography to measure in vivo left ventricular function in rat heart. NMR Biomed. 2008;21:765–72.
5. Azam S, Desjardins CL, Schluchter M, Liner A, Stelzer JE, Yu X, et al. Comparison of velocity vector imaging echocardiography with magnetic resonance imaging in mouse models of cardiomyopathy. Circ Cardiovasc Imaging. 2012;5:776–81.
6. Urboniene D, Haber I, Fang Y-H, Thenappan T, Archer SL. Validation of high-resolution echocardiography and magnetic resonance imaging vs. high-fidelity catheterization in experimental pulmonary hypertension. Am J Physiol Lung Cell Mol Physiol. 2010;299:L401–12.
7. Dorosz JL, Lezotte DC, Weitzenkamp DA, Allen LA, Salcedo EE. Performance of 3-dimensional echocardiography in measuring left ventricular volumes and ejection fraction. J Am Coll Cardiol. 2012;59:1799–808.
8. Ram R, Mickelsen DM, Theodoropoulos C, Blaxall BC. New approaches in small animal echocardiography: imaging the sounds of silence. AJP: Heart and Circulatory Physiology. 2011;301:H1765–80.
9. Respress JL, Wehrens XHT. Transthoracic Echocardiography in Mice. J Vis Exp [Internet]. 2010 [cited 2017 Dec 22]; Available from: https://www.ncbi.nlm.nih.gov/pmc/articles/PMC3144600/
10. Ponikowski P, Voors AA, Anker SD, Bueno H, Cleland JGF, Coats AJS, et al. ESC guidelines for the diagnosis and treatment of acute and chronic heart failure: the task force for the diagnosis and treatment of acute and chronic heart failure of the European Society of Cardiology (ESC)developed with the special contribution of the heart failure association (HFA) of the ESC. Eur Heart J. 2016:2016.
11. Lindsey ML, Kassiri Z, Virag JAI, de Castro Brás LE, Scherrer-Crosbie M. Guidelines for measuring cardiac physiology in mice. Am J Phys Heart Circ Phys. 2018;314:H733–52.
12. Stypmann J, Engelen MA, Troatz C, Rothenburger M, Eckardt L, Tiemann K. Echocardiographic assessment of global left ventricular function in mice. Lab Anim. 2009;43:127–37.
13. Kanno S, Lerner DL, Schuessler RB, Betsuyaku T, Yamada KA, Saffitz JE, et al. Echocardiographic evaluation of ventricular remodeling in a mouse model of myocardial infarction. J Am Soc Echocardiogr. 2002;15:601–9.
14. Scherrer-Crosbie M, Steudel W, Hunziker PR, Liel-Cohen N, Ullrich R, Zapol WM, et al. Three-dimensional echocardiographic assessment of left Ventricular Wall motion abnormalities in mouse myocardial infarction. J Am Soc Echocardiogr. 1999;12:834–40.
15. Dawson D, Lygate CA, Saunders J, Schneider JE, Ye X, Hulbert K, et al. Quantitative 3-dimensional echocardiography for accurate and rapid cardiac phenotype characterization in mice. Circulation. 2004;110:1632–7.
16. Damen FW, Berman AG, Soepriatna AH, Ellis JM, Buttars SD, Aasa KL, et al. High-frequency 4-dimensional ultrasound (4DUS): a reliable method for assessing murine cardiac function. Tomography. 2017;3:180–7.
17. Soepriatna AH, Damen FW, Vlachos PP, Goergen CJ. Cardiac and respiratory-gated volumetric murine ultrasound. Int J Cardiovasc Imaging. 2017;
18. Aurich M, André F, Keller M, Greiner S, Hess A, Buss SJ, et al. Assessment of left ventricular volumes with echocardiography and cardiac magnetic resonance imaging: real-life evaluation of standard versus new semiautomatic methods. J Am Soc Echocardiogr. 2014;27:1017–24.
19. Lapinskas T, Grune J, Zamani SM, Jeuthe S, Messroghli D, Gebker R, et al. Cardiovascular magnetic resonance feature tracking in small animals – a preliminary study on reproducibility and sample size calculation. BMC Med Imaging [Internet]. 2017 [cited 2017 Sep 21];17. Available from: http://bmcmedimaging.biomedcentral.com/articles/10.1186/s12880-017-0223-7
20. Grune J, Benz V, Brix S, Salatzki J, Blumrich A, Höft B, et al. Steroidal and nonsteroidal mineralocorticoid receptor antagonists cause differential cardiac gene expression in pressure overload-induced cardiac hypertrophy. J Cardiovasc Pharmacol. 2016;67:402–11.

Evaluation of a commercial multi-dimensional echocardiography technique for ventricular volumetry in small...

205

21. Beyhoff N, Brix S, Betz IR, Klopfleisch R, Foryst-Ludwig A, Krannich A, et al. Application of speckle-tracking echocardiography in an experimental model of isolated subendocardial damage. J Am Soc Echocardiogr. 2017;30:1239–1250.e2.

22. Garcia-Menendez L, Karamanlidis G, Kolwicz S, Tian R. Substrain specific response to cardiac pressure overload in C57BL/6 mice. Am J Physiol Heart Circ Physiol. 2013;305:H397–402.

23. Zhao M, Fajardo G, Urashima T, Spin JM, Poorfarahani S, Rajagopalan V, et al. Cardiac pressure overload hypertrophy is differentially regulated by -adrenergic receptor subtypes. AJP: Heart and Circulatory Physiology. 2011; 301:H1461–70.

24. Mihalef V, Ionasec RI, Sharma P, Georgescu B, Voigt I, Suehling M, et al. Patient-specific modelling of whole heart anatomy, dynamics and haemodynamics from four-dimensional cardiac CT images. Interface Focus. 2011;1:286–96.

25. Chengode S. Left ventricular global systolic function assessment by echocardiography. Ann Card Anaesth. 2016;19:S26–34.

26. Ortlepp JR, Kluge R, Giesen K, Plum L, Radke P, Hanrath P, et al. A metabolic syndrome of hypertension, hyperinsulinaemia and hypercholesterolaemia in the New Zealand obese mouse. Eur J Clin Investig. 2000;30:195–202.

27. Radavelli-Bagatini S, Blair AR, Proietto J, Spritzer PM, Andrikopoulos S. The New Zealand obese mouse model of obesity insulin resistance and poor breeding performance: evaluation of ovarian structure and function. J Endocrinol. 2011;209:307–15.

28. González Ballester MA, Zisserman AP, Brady M. Estimation of the partial volume effect in MRI. Med Image Anal. 2002;6:389–405.

29. Chen JJ, Smith MR, Frayne R. The impact of partial-volume effects in dynamic susceptibility contrast magnetic resonance perfusion imaging. J Magn Reson Imaging. 2005;22:390–9.

30. Soret M, Bacharach SL, Buvat I. Partial-volume effect in PET tumor imaging. J Nucl Med. 2007;48:932–45.

31. Mannheim JG, Judenhofer MS, Schmid A, Tillmanns J, Stiller D, Sossi V, et al. Quantification accuracy and partial volume effect in dependence of the attenuation correction of a state-of-the-art small animal PET scanner. Phys Med Biol. 2012;57:3981–93.

32. Wood PW, Choy JB, Nanda NC, Becher H. Left ventricular ejection fraction and volumes: it depends on the imaging method. Echocardiography. 2014; 31:87–100.

33. Bondoc AB, Detombe S, Dunmore-Buyze J, Gutpell KM, Liu L, Kaszuba A, et al. Application of 3-D echocardiography and gated micro-computed tomography to assess cardiomyopathy in a mouse model of Duchenne muscular dystrophy. Ultrasound Med Biol. 2014;40:2857–67.

34. Lang RM, Badano LP, Tsang W, Adams DH, Agricola E, Buck T, et al. EAE/ASE recommendations for image acquisition and display using three-dimensional echocardiography. Eur Heart J Cardiovasc Imaging. 2012;13:1–46.

22

Cardiac fluid dynamics meets deformation imaging

Matteo Dal Ferro[1], Davide Stolfo[1], Valerio De Paris[1], Pierluigi Lesizza[1], Renata Korcova[1], Dario Collia[2], Giovanni Tonti[3], Gianfranco Sinagra[1] and Gianni Pedrizzetti[2]* (iD)

Abstract

Cardiac function is about creating and sustaining blood in motion. This is achieved through a proper sequence of myocardial deformation whose final goal is that of creating flow. Deformation imaging provided valuable contributions to understanding cardiac mechanics; more recently, several studies evidenced the existence of an intimate relationship between cardiac function and intra-ventricular fluid dynamics. This paper summarizes the recent advances in cardiac flow evaluations, highlighting its relationship with heart wall mechanics assessed through the newest techniques of deformation imaging and finally providing an opinion of the most promising clinical perspectives of this emerging field. It will be shown how fluid dynamics can integrate volumetric and deformation assessments to provide a further level of knowledge of cardiac mechanics.

Keywords: Cardiac fluid dynamics, Speckle tracking, Deformation imaging, Hemodynamic forces, Intraventricular pressure gradient

Background

The evaluation of blood flow velocity inside the heart has a pivotal role in all echocardiographic studies. For example, the pattern of pulsed wave Doppler (PW) of mitral inflow, when combined with other measurements, allows a good estimate of the diastolic function of left ventricle (LV), moreover Doppler derived pressure gradient (PG) across the valves and Color Doppler representation of flow are currently used to estimate valvular stenosis o regurgitation. Evolving technologies allow now a deeper access to the three-dimensional pattern of blood motion inside the heart and recent literature unveil novel, startling, physiological aspects of cardiac fluid dynamics.

This paper aims to give a thoughtful summary of the latest advances in cardiac flow evaluations. The overall literature in this field is multidisciplinary and a thorough review of the many aspects involved is out of the scope of this manuscript. Here, literature and recent imaging methods are used for driving the reader toward prospective clinical applications of cardiac fluid dynamics, highlighting the relationship with wall mechanics

assessed through the newest techniques of deformation imaging. The eventual objective of this paper is that of providing an opinion of the most promising clinical perspectives of this emerging field.

To this aim, the manuscript is organized in an unconventional way. It starts with a review of the main lines of research in cardiac fluid dynamics, deformation imaging and their interrelation. However, fluid dynamics and myocardial deformation are found in literature as separate topics only. Therefore, the paper proceeds presenting preliminary results of two original applications, as instructive examples where both flow and strain are analyzed at the same time. Afterwards, a unitary discussion reporting authors' viewpoint is provided.

Lines of research in literature

In a pioneering letter to Nature [1] the asymmetric sinuous flow paths around a vortex in the human left ventricle (LV) were accurately described using magnetic resonance sequences. It was suggested therein that the observed asymmetric vortical arrangement of flow was the functional counterpart of the looped heart structure that enhances the atrium-ventricular mechanical synergy supporting the transfer of momentum from the entry mitral jet to the systolic ejection. The combination of

* Correspondence: giannip@dia.units.it
[2]Department of Engineering and Architecture, University of Trieste, P.le Europa 1, 34127 Trieste, Italy
Full list of author information is available at the end of the article

physics and physiology allowed revealing the dynamical balance between LV asymmetrical shape, vortex formation and longitudinal filling-emptying mechanism [2]. Following these initial observations, more recently, several studies evidenced the existence of an intimate relationship between cardiac function and the behavior of intraventricular fluid dynamics. Based on these findings most researchers initially paid particular attention to the risk of thrombus formation due to the increased time of blood persistence in the LV associated with wall motion abnormalities from any causes [3–5]. More recently, attention was directed toward the efficiency of blood-tissue dynamical interaction [3, 6] as a way to detect pathological conditions well before overt clinical manifestation, in a phase during which appropriate therapeutic interventions can prevent the progression of the disease or even reverse its outcome [7, 8]. The latter topic will be careful discussed here for its potential clinical relevance that requires thoughtful and knowledgeable developments.

Initial clinical applications of cardiac fluid dynamics

Blood is an incompressible medium that interacts with the surrounding tissue by the exchanges of forces and momentum in consequence of the displacement of tissue regions. In different terms, tissue deformation creates intraventricular pressure gradients (IVPGs) that drive blood motion and, the other way round, flow-mediated IVPGs create forces on the tissue that affect its deformation. The physiological relevance of IVPGs was recognized in catheterized animal models since long time and their alteration was demonstrated in dysfunctional and failing hearts [9, 10]. Since recently, technical advancements in flow imaging method allow the non-invasive evaluation of flow forces, also termed hemodynamic forces, which are the IVPGs averaged over the LV volume thus opening the possibility to test directly the usefulness of flow force assessments in clinical scenarios.

First echocardiographic flow analyses were done using intravenous microbubbles contrast agents, whose rheology is the same of blood particles, that can be easily detected by ultrasound imaging and then tracked by means of image analysis methods (Echo-PIV) [11]. Particular relevance was gained by recent Echo-PIV studies aimed to verify the association of flow imbalance with the risk of LV remodeling. This research line was grounded on the observations that, under normal conditions, flow forces are aligned along the base-apex direction, in compliance with the emptying-filling cyclic path. This natural dynamic flow alignment is invariably altered in any pathological condition connoted by anomalies of the spatial and/or temporal course of the segmental dynamics of the cardiac walls. For this reason, it was hypothesized that the occurrence of non-physiological transversal components of flow forces can represent an

important sign of abnormal cardiac function and even predict the triggering of adaptive mechanisms. To test this conjecture, a population of volumetric responders to cardiac resynchronization therapy (CRT) was studied; they represent a unique physio-pathological model thanks to the possibility of estimating intra-individual variations of the intracavitary PG pattern associated with the interruption/activation of the resynchronizing stimulation [12]. Results demonstrated that flow forces are properly aligned with the LV axis under pacing therapy, while they are altered as soon as pacing is interrupted. Conversely, all patients who do not respond to CRT show preeminent transversal course of PG either during pacing or in basal conditions demonstrating that the response to therapy is always associated with improvement/ /normalization of LV flow dynamics. These observation also support the hypothesis that alteration of a flow alignment can be causally related to LV remodeling [13].

These preliminary studies were soon followed by three-dimensional phase-contrast MRI (often referred as 4D flow MRI), which confirmed that flow forces are consistently aligned with the LV axis in normal subjects while they are noticeably altered in dilated and dysfunctional hearts [14, 15]. 4D Flow MRI also confirmed previous Echo-PIV results that conduction abnormality in heart failure patients with left bundle branch block (LBBB) correlates with deviation of flow forces, and suggest that the latter may be predictive for the response to CRT [16].

Consensus is growing about the relevance of blood motion to the heart physiology and as a potential predictor of LV remodeling after an acute event or a therapeutic procedure [8, 13]. However, advances on clinical applications based on LV fluid dynamics are limited by the complexity or limited accuracy of cardiac flow imaging methods [17–19]. Early results, although promising, still lack of conclusive clinical proofs providing evidence for end-points addressed by fluid dynamics.

Speckle tracking and deformation imaging

Recent years have rather experienced the advent of speckle tracking (ST) technology and the following development of cardiac deformation imaging. ST echocardiography led to a novel conception about LV function, described not only in terms of volume change but also of pattern of deformation characterized by longitudinal and circumferential shortening [20]. Based on LV strain measurements, novel pathophysiological classification of heart failure were proposed as those associated with predominant longitudinal dysfunction, with transmural dysfunction affecting longitudinal and circumferential strain, and with predominant circumferential dysfunction [21, 22]. The technological characteristics of ST technology suggest that global longitudinal and circumferential strain (GLS, GCS) are the most reproducible and appropriate parameters for clinical applications [23]. In this respect, ST technology was demonstrated to be mature for clinical applications. Although ejection fraction (EF) remains the primary measure for assessing the presence of systolic LV dysfunction, in numerous clinical conditions strain measurements were considered complementary, sometime more effective, in detecting alteration in LV function [24].

Speckle tracking and flow imaging

Deformation imaging is progressively entering in the clinical arena for classifying the cardiac function with increased accuracy [20, 25]. Differently, flow imaging provides new physiological insights and promises to be able to detect functional alterations before tissues have undergone to evident, sometime irreversible, modifications. Therefore, flow assessments could become complementary to strain, through the promise of a potentially predictive tool of cardiac outcome after acute events or therapeutic procedures.

However, flow and deformation are intimately connected: cardiac function is about creating and sustaining blood motion, which is achieved through a proper sequence of myocardial contraction and relaxation. Thus, flow forms represent a different aspect of tissue motion whose even microscopic changes may alter the distribution of intracardiac flow forces. The two aspects are so intimately linked that from an appropriate knowledge of tissue motion it is possible to estimate the flow forces, or the IVPGs, that develop inside the cardiac chambers [26]. A validation study compared flow forces computed by 4D Flow MRI with the same obtained from a mathematical model that uses endocardial motion on three apical projections and the size of the aortic and mitral orifice demonstrating the accuracy of the model. Therefore, the knowledge of the LV endocardial motion from ST echocardiography, as it is commonly used to evaluate myocardial strain, also allow estimations of flow forces [27].

Perspectives

Flow imaging technology is primarily represented by 4D Flow MRI. Echocardiography, either Echo-PIV or solutions based on Color-Doppler, is a second option at a lower level in terms of accuracy and reliability [19]; however, novel technological ultrasound solutions could be on their way [28]. Flow imaging methods allow exploring the potential of quantifications based on fluid dynamics.

Flow forces appear currently a promising quantity relating blood motion to cardiac function; it has a rigorous physical significance and appears clinical relevant. Flow forces can be estimated by ST thus their extensive clinical validation becomes relatively easy.

The knowledge of endocardial borders has a long history for the evaluations of volumetric measures and EF. Since the advent of ST technology, the same endocardial borders can be used to evaluate strain. Volumes and EF provide a primary measure of cardiac function; strains represent a second level of information integrative to volumetric measures. Evaluation of flow forces from ST provides a further level of knowledge that is incremental to volumes and strain. These three levels of information are shown in Fig. 1 for a normal subject.

The time profiles of strain curves are somehow comparable to the volume curve and it was natural to use end-systolic strain values as clinical parameters. The time profile of the flow forces brings largely new information and the definition of most appropriate clinical parameters in the different clinical situations is still under development. Two applications are reported below as illustrative examples of the 3-level evaluations based on volumes, strain, and flow forces.

Exemplary clinical cases

The previous literature review eventually highlighted that blood flow and tissue deformation represent two faces of cardiac function and therefore they are deeply interrelated. However, flow and strain are found in literature as separated topics only. We introduce here preliminary results of an integrated analysis where both aspects are evaluated at the same time. This approach is presented in two clinical populations: patients with cardiomyopathy and few subjects who underwent cardiac resynchronization therapy (CRT), with the objective of showing the application of the above concepts into real clinical scenarios. Discussing the clinical relevance of the finding is beyond the scope of this manuscript; these analyses are shown by way of example with the aim of displaying means of integrating measurement based on flow and strain for reaching a deeper understanding of cardiac mechanics at the individual clinical level.

Methods

First, we retrospectively analyzed a population of 33 subjects composed of 13 healthy volunteers (Controls), 9 patients with dilated cardiomyopathy (DCM), and 11 patients with obstructive hypertrophic cardiomyopathy (OHCM), consecutively enrolled in Trieste Heart Muscle Disease Registry [29, 30] between 2008 and 2015. Briefly, diagnosis of DCM and OHCM was defined according to current criteria [31, 32] and all patients underwent extensive clinical and laboratory characterization. Patients underwent a complete echocardiographic evaluation at baseline and periodically during follow up. The average volumetric and strain parameters are reported in Table 1.

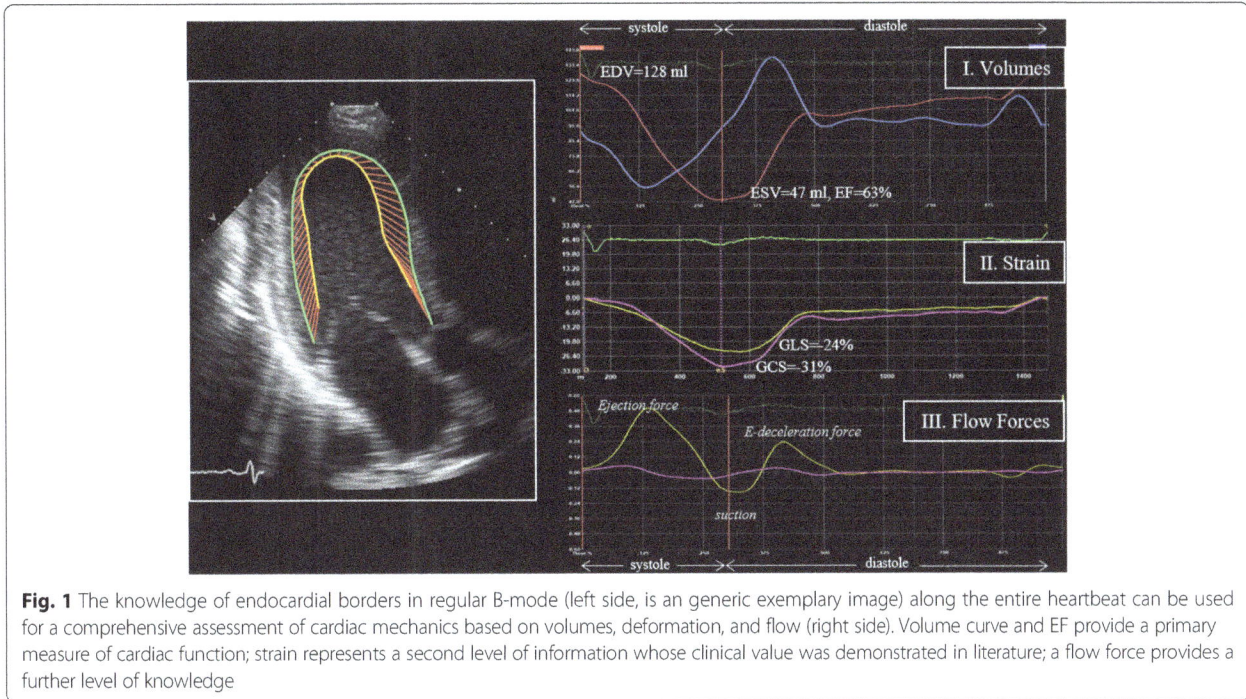

Fig. 1 The knowledge of endocardial borders in regular B-mode (left side, is an generic exemplary image) along the entire heartbeat can be used for a comprehensive assessment of cardiac mechanics based on volumes, deformation, and flow (right side). Volume curve and EF provide a primary measure of cardiac function; strain represents a second level of information whose clinical value was demonstrated in literature; a flow force provides a further level of knowledge

For a second test, 3 patients fulfilling criteria of responders or super-responders to cardiac resynchronization therapy (CRT) [13], were randomly extracted from the CRT registry of our Institution and compared to 3 patients non-responders to CRT [33]. Patients underwent a complete echocardiographic study before implantation (PRE) and few months after the procedure (POST). Table 2 reports the volumetric measures. All patients were then followed-up for a mean period of 3 ± 1 year to assess the long-term effects of resynchronization.

The entire study was performed in accordance with the Helsinki declaration; all subjects provided written informed consent (N.O 43/2009, prot 2161).

During the echocardiographic evaluations, the three echocardiographic apical long axis views (4-ch, 3-ch, and 2-ch) were recorded for offline analysis. Image analysis was performed by a commercially available tool (2D-CPA v.1.3; TomTec Imaging Systems Gmbh, Unterschleissheim, Germany). This ST tool requires drawing the end-systolic (ES) endocardial borders and estimates the border over the entire heartbeat; it then allows

correcting the end-diastolic (ED) one and propagates the correction accordingly over the entire cycle without affecting the previously drawn ES border. Therefore, it gives full control of ES and ED borders from which the EF and GLS are computed as by guidelines [34]. From the same endocardial borders, the LV diameters from base to apex are evaluated and their reduction from ED to ES, averaged of the LV length, gives the GCS. The apical approach to GCS could be less accurate because the entire circumference is not visible from the apical views; this criticality is minimized by using a triplane evaluation thus applying the same approach and the same approximation commonly used in the evaluation of LV volumes. This approach to circumferential strain is more similar to that used in 3D echocardiography because the border follows the tissue during its longitudinal motion and reduce artifacts in deformation such as those that may result from through-plane displacements of 3D geometry that sometime affect the short axis transversal

Table 1 Mean volumetric and deformation parameters of first population

	Controls	DCM	OHCM
EDV [ml]	105 ± 24	233 ± 69	131 ± 47
ESV [ml]	45 ± 12	179 ± 48	44 ± 16
EF [%]	57 ± 6	22 ± 8	65 ± 5
GLS [%]	-20 ± 3	-7 ± 2	-18 ± 3
GCS [%]	-27 ± 5	-8 ± 4	-34 ± 5

Table 2 Volumetric parameters of CRT population

		EDV [ml]			ESV [ml]			EF [%]	
		PRE	POST	Δ%	PRE	POST	Δ%	PRE	POST
1	Resp	210	108	−48%	175	70	−60%	17%	35%
2	Resp	146	69	−53%	103	38	−63%	29%	45%
3	Resp	263	201	−23%	174	98	−43%	34%	51%
4	NR	125	152	+22%	96	113	+18%	23%	26%
5	NR	230	219	−5%	194	185	−5%	16%	16%
6	NR	162	124	−23%	128	87	−32%	21%	30%

projections [23, 35]. All evaluations are performed combining the three apical views. Through this approach the EF and the two global strain, GLS and GCS, are evaluated in a consistent way from the same endocardial border calculations.

Longitudinal and radial displacements, which are described by GLS and GCS, respectively, jointly contribute to the volumetric reduction and to ejection fraction (EF). A relationship to estimate the value of EF from those of myocardial strain was presented in [36] where a further dependence on the average LV diameters and thickness was present. That approach can be recast in simpler terms for endocardial strain values proving the explicit relationship

$$\text{EF} = 1 - (\text{GLS} + 1)(\text{GCS} + 1)^2. \tag{1}$$

This relationship will be used in the analysis of results for demonstrating how longitudinal and circumferential functions combine to volumetric reduction in the different clinical conditions.

The same ST data are then used to evaluate the hemodynamic forces associated with blood flow. A previous study [27] demonstrated that flow forces (which is a synonymous for "hemodynamic forces", "flow momentum" or "average IVPGs" also used in literature) can be estimated from the knowledge of the LV geometry and endocardial velocities, obtained by ST, plus the area of the aortic and mitral orifices. The complete mathematical details of the method for transforming endocardial dynamics into flow forces are reported elsewhere [27] and the concept is only quickly summarized here. The total hemodynamic force, $F(t)$, exchanged between blood and tissues can be computed by the balance of momentum inside the volume $V(t)$ of the LV

$$F(t) = \rho \int_{V(t)} \frac{\partial v}{\partial t} dV + \rho \int_{S(t)} v v_n dS, \tag{2}$$

where $S(t)$ is the surface bounding the volume and v is the velocity vector where the subscript n indicates the outward normal component. The second term in the right-hand-side of the previous formula represents the flux of momentum across the instantaneous LV volume boundary. It can be computed from the velocity at the LV endocardium and at the base, which are known from ST, plus the mean velocity across the mitral and aortic valve, during diastole and systole, respectively, which are the volume rate divided by the valve area. The first term is blood inertia and can be rewritten through the rate of change of the average velocity inside the LV. The longitudinal component of the average velocity can be estimated from mass conservation given the variation of LV shape, known from ST. The main transversal (inferolateral-anteroseptal) components is some more complicated but can also be

estimated from ST data accounting for the transit from inflow to outflow; the other transversal component is mainly due to the orientations of the mitral jet and is not considered here. This approach will be used in the analysis of result to integrate to the volumetric and deformation information with those related to cardiac fluid dynamics.

Results

Strain properties for the first population (Control, DCM, OHCM) are summarized in Fig. 2 in the plane GLS-GCS. From the relationship of formula (1), the curves at constant EF can be drawn on this plane showing regions with same EF value obtained with a different combination of longitudinal and circumferential strain. As expected, the DCM patient, that have reduced EF, also present a reduction of contraction in both strain and are displaced toward the origin with respect to Controls. OHCM patients, that have preserved EF, present a tendency to displace toward the right along the curves with constant EF; this corresponds to a reduction of GLS

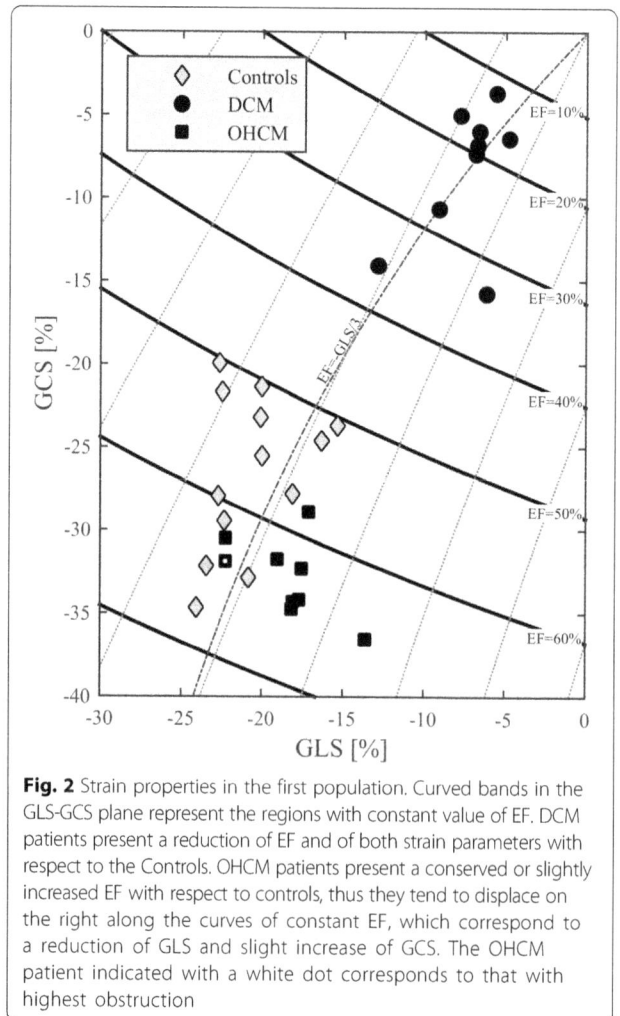

Fig. 2 Strain properties in the first population. Curved bands in the GLS-GCS plane represent the regions with constant value of EF. DCM patients present a reduction of EF and of both strain parameters with respect to the Controls. OHCM patients present a conserved or slightly increased EF with respect to controls, thus they tend to displace on the right along the curves of constant EF, which correspond to a reduction of GLS and slight increase of GCS. The OHCM patient indicated with a white dot corresponds to that with highest obstruction

accompanied by a small increase of GCS to ensure preservation of EF.

The complete time profiles of the longitudinal (base-apex) component of the flow forces in dimensionless form (normalized with volume and expressed in percentage of gravity acceleration or, equivalently, of the weight of the LV blood volume) are reported in Fig. 3 for the three groups. Time scale is adjusted individually, with a common heartbeat frequency and a common ES instant, just improve visual comparability in the graphic representation. All Controls present a consistent pattern of flow forces, DCM patients confirm a depressed function in terms of flow forces as well, OHCM patients present a significant variability where most patients have approximately normal amplitude and a few patients display higher systolic fluctuations. Transversal forces (not shown here) are comparable in the three groups. A synthesis of the overall fluid dynamics differences is given in Fig. 4 where the mean systolic force (or flow impulse [37]) is reported versus EF. In this set, the higher impulse in OHCM patients correspond to higher septal thickness and higher pressure gradients in the outflow tract. The patient with highest impulse, four times higher than in Controls, was reviewed retrospectively to

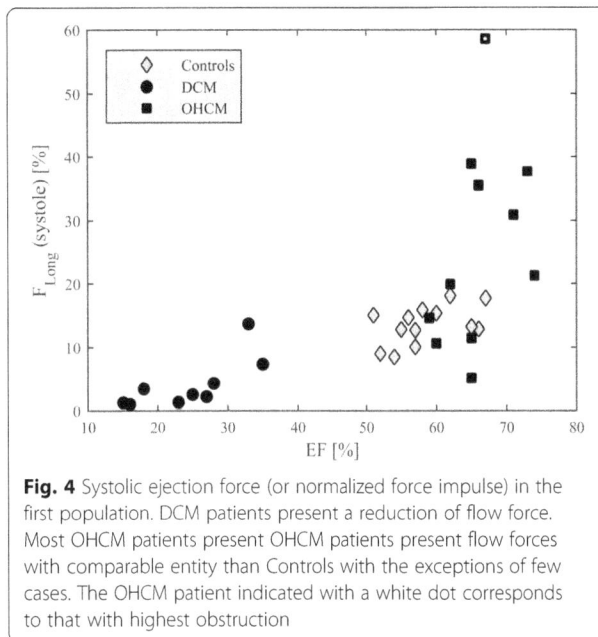

Fig. 4 Systolic ejection force (or normalized force impulse) in the first population. DCM patients present a reduction of flow force. Most OHCM patients present OHCM patients present flow forces with comparable entity than Controls with the exceptions of few cases. The OHCM patient indicated with a white dot corresponds to that with highest obstruction

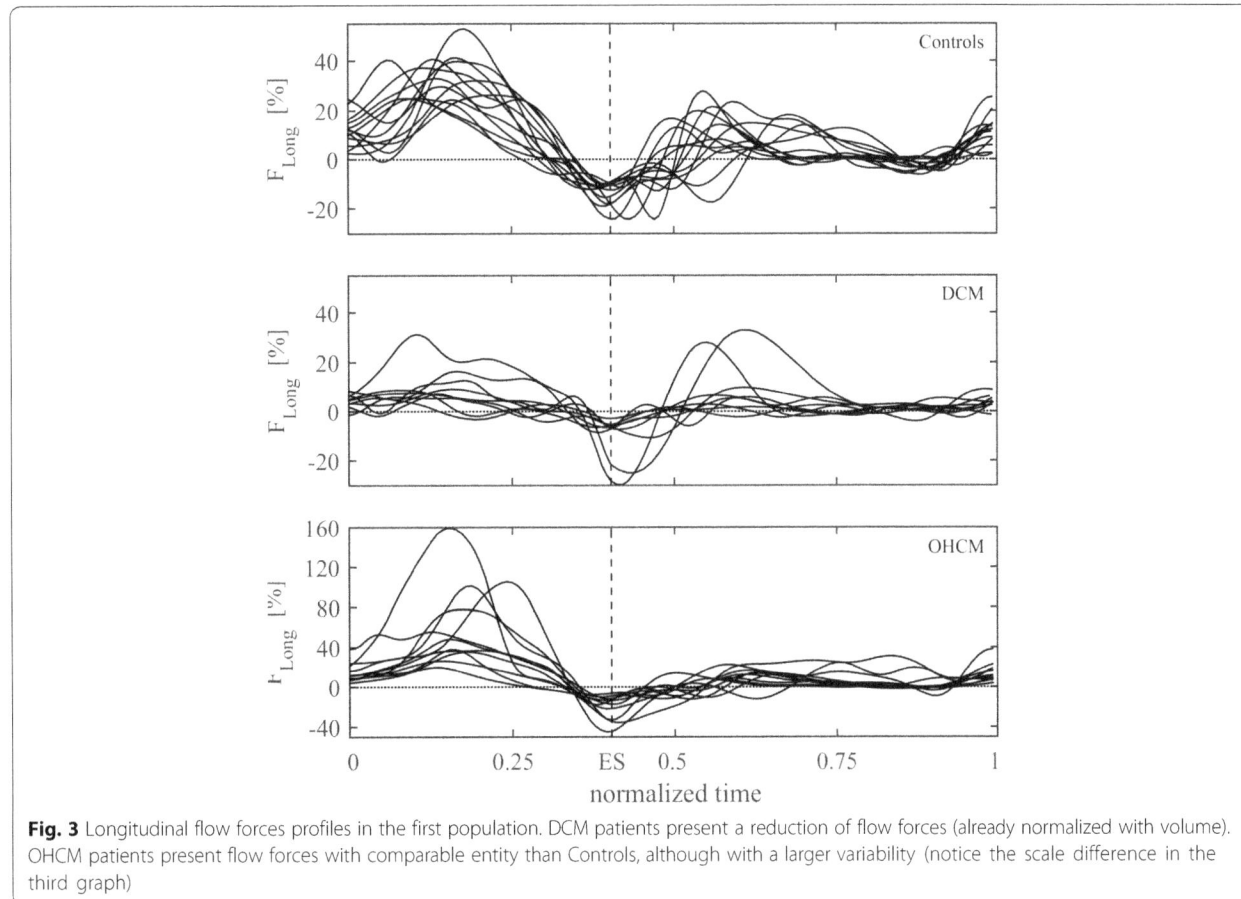

Fig. 3 Longitudinal flow forces profiles in the first population. DCM patients present a reduction of flow forces (already normalized with volume). OHCM patients present flow forces with comparable entity than Controls, although with a larger variability (notice the scale difference in the third graph)

check whether this could correspond to a clinical peculiarity. This patient indeed presented the highest septal thickness (40 mm) in the OHCM group, was asymptomatic, and the only one carrying a mutation of the gene MYH7.

The CRT population was analyzed similarly. Figure 5 shows the data in the same GLS-GCS plane, improvement in EF and strain is found in patients who better responded to therapy (1–3). Non-responders (4–6) present different individual behavior with no or limited improvements. Flow forces clearly witness the differences in clinical outcome. Figure 6 shows the polar distribution of flow forces in two patients: the patient who responded to therapy (#1) presents a clear improvement in the alignment of flow forces; the non-responder patient (#4) exhibits a worsening of such a dynamic alignment, which could support the observed slight reduction of strain. Figure 7 summarizes the individual therapeutic outcome in terms of flow forces, confirming and integrating the observations in terms of volumes and strain.

Discussion

Fluid dynamics provide an alternative viewpoint when looking at cardiac mechanics. Flow forces, or IVPGs, correspond to the ultimate result of LV contraction-relaxation rhythm and, like deformations, play a central role in the description of cardiac function.

The analysis of literature demonstrated a common awareness of the potential relevance of fluid dynamics for clinical assessments; nevertheless, clinical application remained limited. Non-invasive measurements of IVPGs were previously proposed in echocardiography by post-processing of M-mode color Doppler [38–41] or by Echo-PIV [12, 13]; these method present several technical limitations and, also for the unavailability of widespread quantification tools, could not undergo to extensive clinical evaluations. Recently, research in 4D Flow MRI was applied to measuring blood velocities and hemodynamic forces in the heart [14, 15]. Overall, the non-invasive evaluation of hemodynamic force (or IVPGs) appears the most promising clinical application of cardiac fluid dynamics in the short time.

Here we applied a new, previously validated technology that allows quantification of hemodynamic forces using the same ST information used for deformation imaging. This approach, within ST own limitations [23], can highly support diffusion of hemodynamic force measurements by echocardiography. The preliminary clinical applications shown here just by way of example brought evidence that flow force measurements corroborate the findings in terms of volumetric changes and deformations and bring novel incremental information.

Deformation imaging and strain measurements provided an additional level of knowledge of cardiac mechanics with respect to previous evaluations based on volumetric measurement only and parameters like GLS are progressively and firmly entering in the daily clinical practice. Similarly, flow force quantifications is a new field of research promising a further level of knowledge to gain a deeper understanding of cardiac function.

The importance of fluid dynamics, however, may in perspective move beyond the description of cardiac function and extend to the prediction of cardiac outcome. Initial literature results suggest the existence of the intimate relationship between the quality of intraventricular fluid dynamics and longer term geometrical adaptation of the myocardial structure. It was previously suggested [8] that, in LV, endothelial cells are able to sense the loading conditions via shear changes (mechano-sensing), transforming any abnormal condition into adaptive responses (mechano-transduction) [42, 43]. This relationship was previously demonstrated during morphogenesis in embryonic hearts [44, 45]. It was demonstrated that myocardial stretch rapidly activates a plethora of intracellular signaling pathways which decrease the initial load [46]. While extremely efficient, in short time, as a physiological

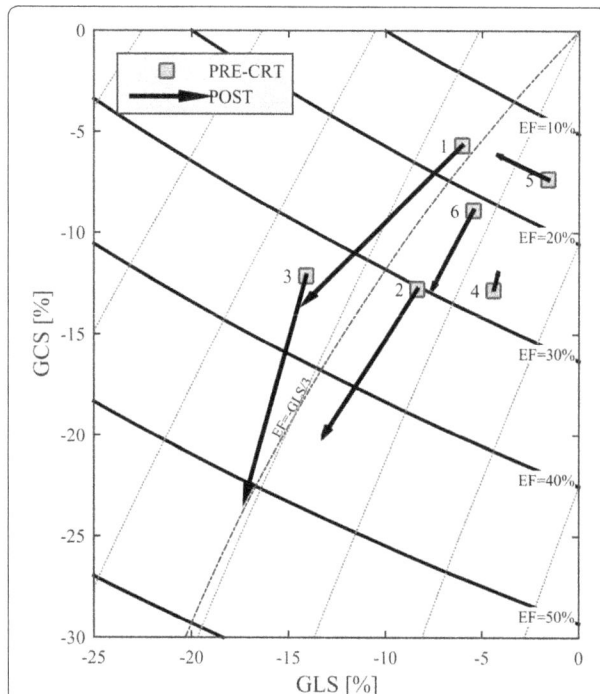

Fig. 5 Strain properties in the CRT patients. Curved bands in the GLS-GCS plane represent the regions with constant value of EF. Responder patients (1–3) present an evident improvement in EF and strain values increases accordingly. Non-responder patients (4–6) display minor improvement in EF and strain

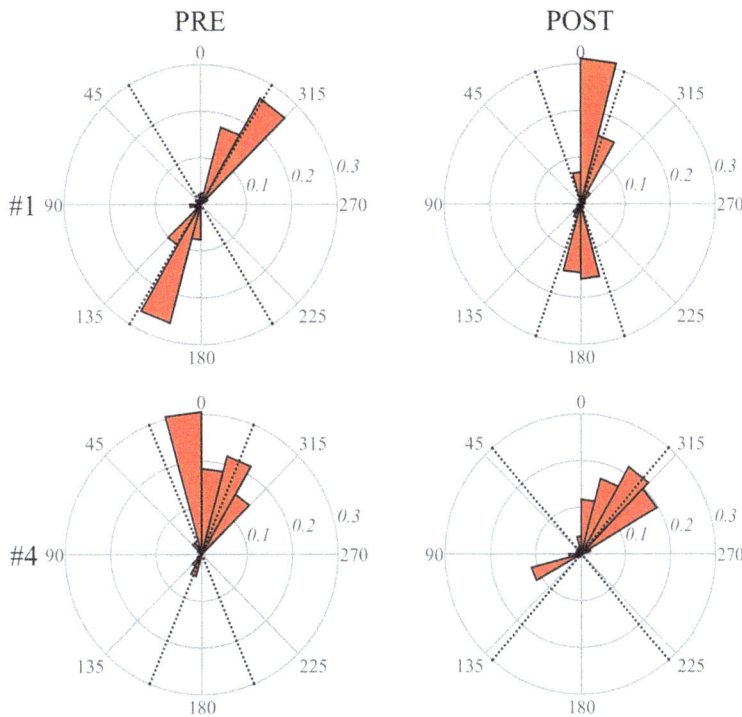

Fig. 6 Polar histogram of the distribution of flow forces during systole. Results are reported PRE- and POST-CRT for a responder patient (#1) and a non-responder (#4), the transversal scale is magnified (2×) to improve visual readability. This representation displays that the therapeutic improvement in alignment of flow force is found in the responder patient only

adaption mechanism, under prolonged overstimulation, this process becomes maladaptive, leading to the development of left ventricular hypertrophy and ultimately to heart failure [47]. In this context, flow forces can provide informative content when creating predictive models that can forecast progression or reversal of LV remodeling following therapeutic interventions.

Conclusion

Fluid dynamics is a promising field of clinical research that can be integrated to volumetric and deformation assessments to provide a further level of knowledge of cardiac mechanics and, possibly, indications of therapeutic outcome. Flow imaging methods like 4D Flow MRI can help to advance research in the field, while novel methods based on ST technology permit an easier access for widespread clinical applications.

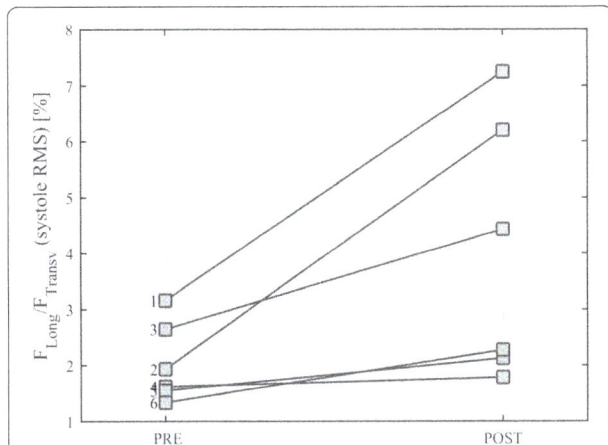

Fig. 7 Changes from PRE- and POST-CRT or the ratio between systolic flow force components during systole, measure by root mean square (RMS). Responder patients (1–3) present an evident improvement of force alignment with therapy as indicated by the increase longitudinal-to-transversal ratio. Non-responder patients (4–6) display no or minor improvement in force alignment

Acknowledgements
Not applicable.

Funding
Author did not receive funding for this study except from salary from the respective institutions.

Authors' contributions
Manuscript design and plan: MDF, DS, GP. Data recording, data processing, quantification and analysis: MDF, DS VDP, PL, RK, DC, GS. Discussion and synthesis of results: GP, MDF, DS, GT, GS. Manuscript writing: GP, MDF, DS, GT. All authors read and approved the final version of the manuscript.

Competing interests
GP and GT receive indirect support from TomTec Gmbh. All other authors declare no competing interest, financial or otherwise.

Author details
[1]Cardiovascular Department, Azienda Ospedaliera Universitaria Integrata of Trieste, Trieste, Italy. [2]Department of Engineering and Architecture, University of Trieste, P.le Europa 1, 34127 Trieste, Italy. [3]Cardiology Division, 'G. D'Annunzio' University, Chieti, Italy.

References
1. Kilner PJ, Yang GZ, Wilkes AJ, Mohiaddin RH, Firmin DN, Yacoub MH. Asymmetric redirection of flow through the heart. Nature. 2000;404:759–61.
2. Pedrizzetti G, Domenichini F. Nature optimizes the swirling flow in the human left ventricle. Phys Rev Lett. 2005;95:1–4.
3. Mangual JO, Kraigher-Krainer E, De Luca A, Toncelli L, Shah A, Solomon S, et al. Comparative numerical study on left ventricular fluid dynamics after dilated cardiomyopathy. J Biomech. 2013;46:1611–7.
4. Carlhäll CJ, Bolger A. Passing strange flow in the failing ventricle. Circ Hear Fail. 2010;3:326–31.
5. Son J-W, Park W-J, Choi J-H, Houle H, Vannan MA, Hong G-R, et al. Abnormal left ventricular vortex flow patterns in association with left ventricular apical thrombus formation in patients with anterior myocardial infarction. Circ J. 2012;76:2640–6.
6. Gharib M, Rambod E, Kheradvar A, Sahn DJ, Dabiri JO. Optimal vortex formation as an index of cardiac health. Proc Natl Acad Sci. 2006;103:6305–8.
7. Abe H, Caracciolo G, Kheradvar A, Pedrizzetti G, Khandheria BK, Narula J, et al. Contrast echocardiography for assessing left ventricular vortex strength in heart failure: a prospective cohort study. Eur Heart J Cardiovasc Imaging. 2013;14:1049–60.
8. Pedrizzetti G, La Canna G, Alfieri O, Tonti G. The vortex—an early predictor of cardiovascular outcome? Nat Rev Cardiol. 2014;11:545–53.
9. Guerra M, Brás-Silva C, Amorim MJ, Moura C, Bastos P, Leite-Moreira AF. Intraventricular pressure gradients in heart failure. Physiol Res. 2013;62:479–87.
10. Courtois M, Kovács SJ, Ludbrook PA. Transmitral pressure-flow velocity relation. Importance of regional pressure gradients in the left ventricle during diastole. Circulation. 1988;78:661–71.
11. Hong G-R, Pedrizzetti G, Tonti G, Li P, Wei Z, Kim JK, et al. Characterization and quantification of vortex flow in the human left ventricle by contrast echocardiography using vector particle image Velocimetry. JACC Cardiovasc Imaging. 2008;1:705–17.
12. Pedrizzetti G, Martiniello AR, Bianchi V, D'Onofrio A, Caso P, Tonti G. Cardiac fluid dynamics anticipates heart adaptation. J Biomech. 2015;48:388–91.
13. Pedrizzetti G, Martiniello AR, Bianchi V, D'Onofrio A, Caso P, Tonti G. Changes in electrical activation modify the orientation of left ventricular flow momentum: novel observations using echocardiographic particle image velocimetry. Eur Heart J Cardiovasc Imaging. 2016;17:203–9.
14. Arvidsson PM, Töger J, Carlsson M, Steding-Ehrenborg K, Pedrizzetti G, Heiberg E, et al. Left and right ventricular hemodynamic forces in healthy volunteers and elite athletes assessed with 4D flow magnetic resonance imaging. Am J Physiol Heart Circ Physiol. 2016;312:H314–28.
15. Eriksson J, Bolger AF, Ebbers T, Carlhäll C-J. Assessment of left ventricular hemodynamic forces in healthy subjects and patients with dilated cardiomyopathy using 4D flow MRI. Physiol Rep. 2016;4:741–7.
16. Eriksson J, Zajac J, Alehagen U, Bolger AF, Ebbers T, Carlhäll C-J. Left ventricular hemodynamic forces as a marker of mechanical dyssynchrony in heart failure patients with left bundle branch block. Sci Rep. 2017;7:2971.
17. Markl M, Kilner PJ, Ebbers T. Comprehensive 4D velocity mapping of the heart and great vessels by cardiovascular magnetic resonance. J Cardiovasc Magn Reson. 2011;13:7.
18. Muñoz DR, Markl M, Mur JLM, Barker A, Fernández-Golfín C, Lancellotti P, et al. Intracardiac flow visualization: current status and future directions. Eur Heart J Cardiovasc Imaging. 2013;14:1029–38.
19. Sengupta PP, Pedrizzetti G, Kilner PJ, Kheradvar A, Ebbers T, Tonti G, et al. Emerging trends in CV flow visualization. JACC Cardiovasc Imaging. 2012;5:305–16.
20. Claus P, Omar AMS, Pedrizzetti G, Sengupta PP, Nagel E. Tissue tracking Technology for Assessing Cardiac MechanicsPrinciples, normal values, and clinical applications. JACC Cardiovasc Imaging. 2015;8:1444–60.

21. Omar AMS, Bansal M, Sengupta PP. Advances in Echocardiographic imaging in heart failure with reduced and preserved ejection fraction. Circ Res. 2016;119:357–74.
22. Sengupta PP, Narula J. Reclassifying heart failure: predominantly Subendocardial, Subepicardial, and Transmural. Heart Fail Clin. 2008;4:379–82.
23. Pedrizzetti G, Claus P, Kilner PJ, Nagel E. Principles of cardiovascular magnetic resonance feature tracking and echocardiographic speckle tracking for informed clinical use. J Cardiovasc Magn Reson. 2016;18:15.
24. Krishnasamy R, Isbel NM, Hawley CM, Pascoe EM, Burrage M, Leano R, et al. Left ventricular global longitudinal strain (GLS) is a superior predictor of all-cause and cardiovascular mortality when compared to ejection fraction in advanced chronic kidney disease. PLoS One. 2015;10:1–15.
25. Schuster A, Stahnke VC, Unterberg-Buchwald C, Kowallick JT, Lamata P, Steinmetz M, et al. Cardiovascular magnetic resonance feature-tracking assessment of myocardial mechanics: Intervendor agreement and considerations regarding reproducibility. Clin Radiol. 2015;70:989–98.
26. Domenichini F, Pedrizzetti G. Hemodynamic forces in a model left ventricle. Phys Rev Fluids. 2016;1:83201.
27. Pedrizzetti G, Arvidsson PM, Töger J, Borgquist R, Domenichini F, Arheden H, et al. On estimating intraventricular hemodynamic forces from endocardial dynamics: a comparative study with 4D flow MRI. J Biomech. 2017;60:203–10.
28. Ekroll IK, Swillens A, Segers P, Dahl T, Torp H, Lovstakken L. Simultaneous quantification of flow and tissue velocities based on multi-angle plane wave imaging. IEEE Trans Ultrason Ferroelectr Freq Control. 2013;60:727–38.
29. Merlo M, Pivetta A, Pinamonti B, Stolfo D, Zecchin M, Barbati G, et al. Long-term prognostic impact of therapeutic strategies in patients with idiopathic dilated cardiomyopathy: changing mortality over the last 30 years. Eur J Heart Fail. 2014;16:317–24.
30. Finocchiaro G, Pinamonti B, Merlo M, Brun F, Barbati G, Sinagra G. Prognostic role of clinical presentation in symptomatic patients with hypertrophic cardiomyopathy. J Cardiovasc Med. 2012;13:810–8.
31. Elliott P, Andersson B, Arbustini E, Bilinska Z, Cecchi F, Charron P, et al. Classification of the cardiomyopathies: a position statement from the european society of cardiology working group on myocardial and pericardial diseases. Eur Heart J. 2008;29:270–6.
32. Elliott PM, Anastasakis A, Borger MA, Borggrefe M, Cecchi F, Charron P, et al. 2014 ESC guidelines on diagnosis and management of hypertrophic cardiomyopathy. Eur Heart J. 2014;35:2733–79.
33. Stolfo D, Tonet E, Merlo M, Barbati G, Gigli M, Pinamonti B, et al. Early right ventricular response to cardiac resynchronization therapy: impact on clinical outcomes. Eur J Heart Fail. 2015;18:205–13.
34. Voigt J-U, Pedrizzetti G, Lysyansky P, Marwick TH, Houle H, Baumann R, et al. Definitions for a common standard for 2D speckle tracking echocardiography: consensus document of the EACVI/ASE/industry task force to standardize deformation imaging. Eur Heart J Cardiovasc Imaging. 2015;16:1–11.
35. Saito K, Okura H, Watanabe N, Hayashida A, Obase K, Imai K, et al. Comprehensive evaluation of left ventricular strain using speckle tracking echocardiography in normal adults: comparison of three-dimensional and two-dimensional approaches. J Am Soc Echocardiogr. 2009;22:1025–30.
36. Stokke TM, Hasselberg NE, Smedsrud MK, Sarvari SI, Haugaa KH, Smiseth OA, et al. Geometry as a confounder when assessing ventricular systolic function: comparison between ejection fraction and strain. J Am Coll Cardiol. 2017;70:942–54.
37. Rushmer RF. Initial ventricular impulse. A potential key to cardiac evaluation. Circulation. 1964;XXIX:268–83.
38. Firstenberg MS, Vandervoort PM, Greenberg NL, Smedira NG, McCarthy PM, Garcia MJ, et al. Noninvasive estimation of transmitral pressure drop across the normal mitral valve in humans: importance of convective and inertial forces during left ventricular filling. J Am Coll Cardiol. 2000;36:1942–9.
39. Greenberg NL, Vandervoort PM, Firstenberg MS, Garcia MJ, Thomas JD. Estimation of diastolic intraventricular pressure gradients by Doppler M-mode echocardiography. Am J Physiol Heart Circ Physiol. 2001;280:H2507–15.
40. Bermejo J, Antoranz JC, Yotti R, Moreno M, García-Fernández MA. Spatio-temporal mapping of intracardiac pressure gradients. A solution to Euler's equation from digital postprocessing of color Doppler M-mode echocardiograms. Ultrasound Med Biol. 2001;27:621–30.
41. Tonti G, Pedrizzetti G, Trambaiolo P, Salustri A. Space and time dependency of inertial and convective contribution to the transmitral pressure drop during ventricular filling. J Am Coll Cardiol. 2001;38:290–1.

23

Prospective assessment of cardiovascular risk parameters in patients with rheumatoid arthritis

Bożena Targońska-Stępniak[1]* ⓘ, Mariusz Piotrowski[1], Robert Zwolak[1], Anna Drelich-Zbroja[2] and Maria Majdan[1]

Abstract

Background: The study presents a prospective follow-up assessment of cardiovascular (CV) risk parameters in patients with rheumatoid arthritis (RA) in comparison with control subjects.

Methods: The study group consisted of 41 RA patients. The following parameters were assessed at subsequent visits [initial (T0), follow-up after 6 years (T6)]: traditional CV risk factors, carotid intima media thickness (cIMT), QTc duration, serum concentration of amino-terminal pro-brain natriuretic peptide (NT-proBNP). A comparative cIMT assessment was performed on 23 healthy controls of comparable age.

Results: The mean (SD) cIMT value in RA patients was significantly higher at T6 than at T0 [0.87 (0.21) vs 0.76 (0.15) mm, $p < 0.001$], the increase in patients with atherosclerotic plaques was noted. Patients with plaques were significantly older, had higher inflammatory parameters. The mean cIMT was significantly higher in RA patients than in controls at both T6, T0 visits. Certain traditional CV risk factors exacerbated during follow up. Unfavorable metabolic parameters and significantly higher cIMT were found in male patients than in female patients at T6. During follow-up, no significant differences in NT-proBNP, QTc were found. There were no significant relationships between cIMT, NT-proBNP, QTc and parameters of disease activity at T6.

Conclusions: During the 6-year course of established RA, significant exacerbation of atherosclerosis was found, revealed by higher cIMT. A careful monitoring should be applied to patients with atherosclerotic plaques and of male gender due to higher burden of CV risk. In long-standing disease, traditional CV risk factors seem to play a key role, beyond the inflammatory activity.

Keywords: Rheumatoid arthritis, Carotid intima media thickness, Cardiovascular disease, Inflammation, Atherosclerosis

Background

Rheumatoid arthritis (RA) is a chronic, progressive, inflammatory joint disease, associated with increased risk of premature atherosclerosis and cardiovascular disease (CVD), to the similar extent as type 2 diabetes [1, 2]. Cardiovascular (CV) death is the leading cause of mortality of patients with RA, responsible for approximately 50% of deaths [3–5]. Traditional risk factors do not fully explain the increased CV risk. Chronic inflammation and high disease activity are reportedly associated with atherosclerotic burden, higher incidence of CVD, chronic heart failure (CHF), and mortality of patients with RA [6, 7].

The increased carotid intima-media thickness (cIMT) and presence of plaques are accepted as strong predictors of generalized atherosclerosis and major CV events in both non-RA and RA subjects [8, 9]. Higher cIMT was reported in RA patients compared with controls [8–11]. Significantly higher N-terminal pro-brain natriuretic peptide (NT-pro-BNP) levels were reported in RA patients, associated with RA duration, disease activity, and inflammatory markers, suggesting a link between inflammation and cardiac stress [11–14]. A relationship was observed between NT-proBNP and cIMT [13]. The

* Correspondence: bozena.stepniak@umlub.pl
[1]Department of Rheumatology and Connective Tissue Diseases, Medical University of Lublin, ul. Jaczewskiego 8, 20-950 Lublin, Poland
Full list of author information is available at the end of the article

increased QTc values were found in RA patients, associated with parameters of disease activity, severity and inflammation [4, 15].

The aim of the study was a prospective assessment of CV risk parameters in patients with established RA, in relation to disease activity and traditional CV risk factors.

Methods

Patients and controls

The study group consisted of RA patients treated at the Department of Rheumatology and Connective Tissue Diseases, Medical University of Lublin. All patients met the American College of Rheumatology (ACR)/European League Against Rheumatism (EULAR) classification criteria for RA [16]. The study was conducted in full compliance with the Helsinki Declaration. The protocol was approved by the Ethics Committee of Medical University of Lublin, with the approval number KE-0254/134/2013. The informed consent for participation in the study was obtained from all participants (patients and controls), after an adequate explanation of the study design.

The study was a part of a research program involving RA patients, to prospectively analyze CV risk factors, both traditional and non-traditional. The assessment presented in the study was performed twice at an average interval of 6 years [73.4 (6.4) months (59–87)], at baseline visit (T0) and current follow-up after 6 years (T6).

RA-related data collection

Demographic and clinical data were obtained through structured interview, review of medical records, self-report questionnaires, and physical examination.

Disease activity was measured using the Disease Activity Score based on evaluation of 28 joints (DAS28), calculated with the number of tender, swollen joints, erythrocyte sedimentation rate (ESR), patient's global disease activity assessment in visual analogue scale (VAS) [17].

The inflammatory burden within the 6-year course of RA was assessed as average of several results of C-reactive protein (CRP). Samples for CRP assessment were taken at consecutive visits, approximately every 6 months.

Erosive form of RA was diagnosed in patients with bone erosions in radiograms of hands and/or feet. Ability to perform daily activities was measured using modified Health Assessment Questionnaire (M-HAQ) [18].

Laboratory tests

Blood was collected after overnight fasting to determine blood cell counts, ESR, serum concentration of CRP, creatinine (Cr), uric acid, glucose, total cholesterol (TC), high-density lipoprotein cholesterol (HDL-C), low-

density lipoprotein cholesterol (LDL-C), triglycerides (TG) at the central laboratory of University Hospital. CRP was measured by immunoturbidimetric assay (upper limit 5 mg/l). Concentrations of TC, HDL-C, TG were measured with standard enzymatic technique (BIOMAXIMA); LDL-C was calculated according to Friedewald formula. Atherogenic index (AI) calculated as ratio TC/HDL-C seems to be more appropriate to assess CV risk in RA than individual cholesterol fractions (normal AI: <4.0 in women and <4.5 in men) [19].

Serum samples were stored at −80° C for further assessment of NT-pro-BNP. Measurement of NT-proBNP concentration was performed using chemiluminescent immunometric assay (IMMULITE 2000 NT-proBNP, Siemens). Reference range according to manufacturer's guidelines is up to 125 pg/ml in patients <75 years and up to 450 pg/ml in older; analytical sensitivity 10 pg/ml. BNP and NT-proBNP levels ≥100 pg/ml are significantly related to cardiac morbidity and mortality [12].

Metabolic and CV biomarkers

Patients were classified as current, ex-smokers or non-smokers. Information about concomitant diseases was taken from medical records. Physical inactivity was defined as lack of regular training. Blood pressure (BP) was assessed in a sitting position. Height and weight were measured barefoot wearing light clothes. Body mass index (BMI) was calculated as the ratio of weight and squared height.

The 10-year risk of fatal CVD using Systemic Coronary Risk Evaluation (SCORE) model was estimated in every patient, with the value ≥5% indicating high or very high risk. According to the EULAR recommendations, the result was multiplied by 1.5 (mSCORE) [20].

Carotid intima-media thickness (cIMT) measurement

Assessment of cIMT was performed at baseline (T0) and follow-up visit (T6) in 41 RA patients and 23 controls. All examinations were performed by the same experienced examiner, with the subject in a supine position, in a quiet, temperature-controlled room; using high-resolution B-mode ultrasound (US) (Logiq 7 GE). IMT was assessed bilaterally in three regions: common carotid artery (CCA), carotid bulb (BULB) and internal carotid artery (ICA). The analyses used the average of maximum IMT from 6 carotid segments (mean cIMT). The cIMT value <0.6 mm is considered as normal, ≥0.9 mm as abnormal. The cIMT value ≥0.6 mm and <0.9 mm is a marker of subclinical atherosclerosis [21]. Plaques were defined as a distinct protrusion >1.5 mm into vessel lumen, with their presence as marker of advanced atherosclerosis [22].

Electrocardiogram assessment

The standard 12-lead transthoracic electrocardiogram (ECG) at 25 mm/s was performed for every patient. Measurement of QTc was performed automatically with normal value 350–430 ms for women and 350–450 ms for men, respectively [23].

Statistics

Variables were tested for normality using the Kolmogorov-Smirnov test. Group differences were tested using Student's t-test and Mann-Whitney U-test for normally and non-normally distributed parameters, respectively. Spearman's or Pearson's correlation test was used to determine association between clinical and laboratory variables. Multivariable analysis (multiple linear regression) was performed according to a forward selection procedure, introducing those variables that showed statistically significant association with certain parameters. For all tests, P values < 0.05 were considered significant.

Results

Demographic, CV risk and RA-related variables in patients

A clinical characteristics of RA patients at T6 has been presented in Table 1.

The study group consisted of 41 patients with long-standing, advanced RA. The disease activity was low (DAS28 $\leq$ 3.2) in over 50% of patients. The value of average CRP (6 years) was slightly above normal range. Most patients had an erosive form of RA and were seropositive (RF-IgM and/or anti-CCP2). Extra-articular manifestations (rheumatoid nodules, sicca syndrome, interstitial lung disease, vasculitis) in the course of the disease were observed in almost 70% of patients (Table 1).

Traditional CV risk factors occurred frequently in RA patients (Table 1).

At T6, disease-modifying antirheumatic drugs (DMARDs) were not used in one patient. Conventional synthetic DMARDs (csDMARDs) used in 39 patients included: methotrexate (MTX) in 33 patients (80.5%), leflunomide 2 (4.9%), antimalarials (hydroxychloroquine or chloroquine) 12 (29.3%), cyclosporine 1 (2.4%). Biological DMARDs (bDMARDs) included: anti-TNF in 12 (29.3%), rituximab 14 (34.1%) and tocilizumab 6 (14.6%).

Characteristics of the healthy volunteers group

The control group consisted of 23 healthy volunteers: 15 women (65.2%) and 8 men (34.8%), with the mean (SD) age of 49.6 (6.2) years (39–62), BMI 25.3 (3.1) kg/m^2 (22.2–31.2). At T6, 10 (43.5%) controls were current/ex-smoker and 6 (26.1%) controls had arterial hypertension.

Table 1 Clinical characteristics of 41 RA patients at follow-up visit (T6)

Variables	Results
Demographic variables:	
Age, years	53.3 (8.7) (28–68)
Gender, F/M	34 (82.9)/ 7 (17)
Cardiovascular risk factors:	
Family history of CVD	20 (48.8)
Current/Ex-smokers	23 (56.1)
Hypertension	17 (41.5)
Diabetes	3 (7.3)
CKD3a (eGFR 45–59 ml/min/1.73 m^2)	2 (4.9)
AI abnormal	11 (26.8)
BMI > 30 kg/m^2	5 (12.2)
Physical inactivity	23 (56.1)
RA related variables	
Disease duration, years	19.2 (9.2) (8–45)
Erosions (X-ray of hands/feet)	35 (85.4)
Extra-articular symptoms	28 (68.3)
Positive RF-IgM	33 (80.5)
Positive anti-CCP2	30 (73.2)
ESR, mm/h	19.2 (16.0) (2–64)
CRP, mg/l	14.35 (37.5) (0.1–228.5)
Average CRP (6 years), mg/l	11.02 (9.9) (0.9–37.3)
Low RA activity (DAS28 $\leq$ 3.2)	23 (56.1)
Current glucocorticoid use	18 (43.9)
Current conventional synthetic DMARD	39 (95.1)
Current biological DMARD	32 (78.1)

Data are presented as mean (SD) (range) or number (%); *AI* atherogenic index, *Anti-CCP2* anti-cyclic citrullinated peptide antibodies, *BMI* body mass index, *CVD* cardiovascular disease, *CKD* chronic kidney disease, *CRP* C-reactive protein; *DAS28* disease activity score in 28 joints, *DMARD* disease modifying antirheumatic drug, *eGFR* estimated glomerular filtration rate, *ESR* erythrocyte sedimentation rate, *RF-IgM* IgM rheumatoid factor

The mean age and BMI did not differ statistically between patients and controls.

Comparison of cIMT between RA patients and controls

The mean value of cIMT was significantly higher in patients than in controls at both visits: current (T6) and baseline (T0) (Table 2).

The significant increase of cIMT value during the 6-year follow-up was noted in both RA patients ($p < 0.001$) and controls ($p < 0.001$). The average increase of cIMT between T0 and T6 (delta IMT) was not significantly different between patients and controls [0.11 (0.18) vs 0.17 (0.09) mm, NS]. Carotid plaques were observed more often in patients than in controls at both T0 and T6 (statistically nonsignificant) (Table 2).

Table 2 Comparison of cIMT and atherosclerotic plaques at T0 and T6 visits in the group of RA patients and controls

Parameters	Group	T0	p	T6	p
Mean cIMT, mm	RA patients	0.76 (0.15) (0.43–1.2)	< 0.001	0.87 (0.21) (0.57–1.77)	0.03
	Controls	0.59 (0.11) (0.4–0.87)		0.76 (0.11) (0.61–1.07)	
Abnormal cIMT (≥0.9 mm)	RA patients	9 (21.9)	0.6	14 (34.1)	0.6
	Controls	1 (4.3)		3 (13.0)	
Atherosclerotic plaques presence	RA patients	6 (14.6)	NS	10 (24.4)	NS
	Controls	1 (4.3)		4 (17.4)	
Bilateral atherosclerotic plaques presence	RA patients	3 (3.7)	NS	7 (17.1)	NS
	Controls	0		1 (4.3)	

Data are presented as mean (SD) (range), *cIMT* carotid intima media thickness

Comparison of clinical and laboratory parameters at T0 and T6 in RA patients

Disease activity assessed with DAS28 diminished significantly between T0 and T6 (Table 3).

Significantly higher cIMT value was found in RA patients at T6 compared with T0 [0.87 (0.21) mm vs 0.76 (0.15), $p < 0.001$] (Table 3).

Most patients had increased cIMT value at both T6 and T0 assessments (Fig. 1). However, during the 6-year follow-up, an increase in the number of patients with defined atherosclerosis (cIMT ≥0,9 mm)

(Fig. 1) and atherosclerotic plaques (Table 3) was observed (statistically nonsignificant). The number of patients with bilateral plaques increased between T0 and T6 (statistically nonsignificant) (Fig. 2).

Serum NT-proBNP concentration and QTc duration did not change significantly between T0 and T6 (Table 3).

Certain traditional CV risk factors (serum uric acid, BMI) and mSCORE exacerbated between T0 and T6 (Table 3). The number of patients with high/very high risk of CV death increased significantly (Table 3).

Table 3 Comparison of clinical and laboratory parameters at T0 and T6 in 41 RA patients

Variables	T0	T6	p
Clinical parameters			
DAS28	4.46 (1.15) (2.58–6.55)	3.33 (1.62) (0.66–6.88)	< 0.001
M-HAQ	1.22 (0.52) (0–2.38)	1.31 (0.52) (0.25–2.38)	NS
SBP, mmHg	123.8 (13.5) (90–160)	128.2 (13.6) (105–160)	NS
BMI, kg/m²	24.8 (3.1) (18.6–29.95)	25.9 (3.4) (17.3–33.2)	0.002
BMI > 30 kg/m²	0	5 (12.2)	0.03
mSCORE, %	0.98 (2.1) (0–12)	2.99 (3.9) (0–18)	< 0.001
High/very high CVD risk	2 (4.9)	10 (24.4)	0.01
QTc, ms	341.9 (60.8) (187–446)	358.8 (59.5) (175–453)	NS
cIMT, mm	0.76 (0.15) (0.43–1.2)	0.87 (0.21) (0.57–1.77)	< 0.001
Carotid plaques presence	6 (14.6)	10 (24.4)	NS
Laboratory parameters			
NT-proBNP, pg/ml	88.9 (78) (12.2–351.2)	126.6 (186.5) (20.1–1175)	NS
Glucose, mg/dl	89.3 (12.9) (54–120)	88.8 (14.5) (67–146)	NS
TC, mg/dl	200.6 (42) (135–325)	206.3 (7.2) (101–318)	NS
HDL-C, mg/dl	59.6 (14.2) (39–87)	60.3 (16.2) (30–102)	NS
LDL-C, mg/dl	119.7 (36.2) (47–232)	120.8 (34.4) (41–190)	NS
Triglycerides, mg/dl	106.5 (45.6) (43–214)	113.0 (53.5) (23–251)	NS
AI (TC/HDL-C)	3.48 (0.81) (2.1–5.5)	3.53 (0.84) (2.0–5.8)	NS
Serum creatinine, mg/dl	0.68 (0.15) (0.4–1.0)	0.66 (0.15) (0.4–1.0)	NS
Serum uric acid, mg/dl	4.0 (0.9) (2.2–5.8)	4.5 (1.1) (2.5–7)	< 0.05

Data are presented as mean (SD) (range) or number (%); *AI* atherogenic index, *BMI* body mass index, *cIMT* carotid intima media thickness, *DAS28* disease activity score in 28 joints, *HDL-C* high-density lipoprotein cholesterol, *LDL-C* low-density lipoprotein cholesterol, *M-HAQ* modified health assessment questionnaire, *NT-proBNP* amino-terminal pro-brain natriuretic peptide, *SBP* systolic blood pressure, *mSCORE* modified Systemic Coronary Risk Evaluation, *TC* total cholesterol

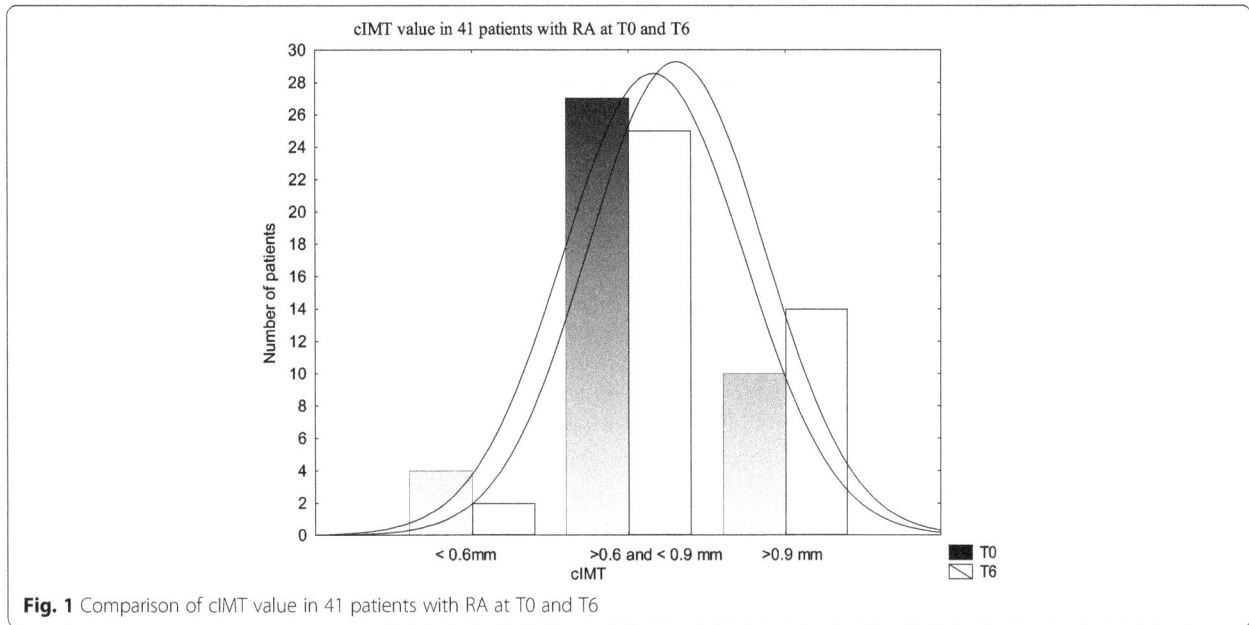

Fig. 1 Comparison of cIMT value in 41 patients with RA at T0 and T6

The other clinical and laboratory parameters did not change significantly (Table 3).

Relationship between CV risk parameters at T0 and T6 in RA patients

There was a strong relationship between the mean cIMT values assessed in RA patients at T6 and T0 ($p < 0.001$). In multiple linear regression analysis, significant association at T0 was confirmed between cIMT and SCORE ($p = 0.001$), NT-proBNP ($p = 0.04$). This relationship was not observed at T6. There were no significant relationships between cIMT, NT-proBNP, OTc and parameters of current disease activity or inflammation as well as average CRP.

Comparison of patients with and without atherosclerotic plaques

Patients with atherosclerotic plaques at T6 were older [59.0 (5.7) vs 51.5 (8.7), $p = 0.02$], had significantly higher CRP concentration [40.6 (72) vs 6.2 (9.5), $p = 0.01$] and white blood cell count (WBC) [7.6 (2.6) vs 5.5 (1.6), $p = 0.006$].

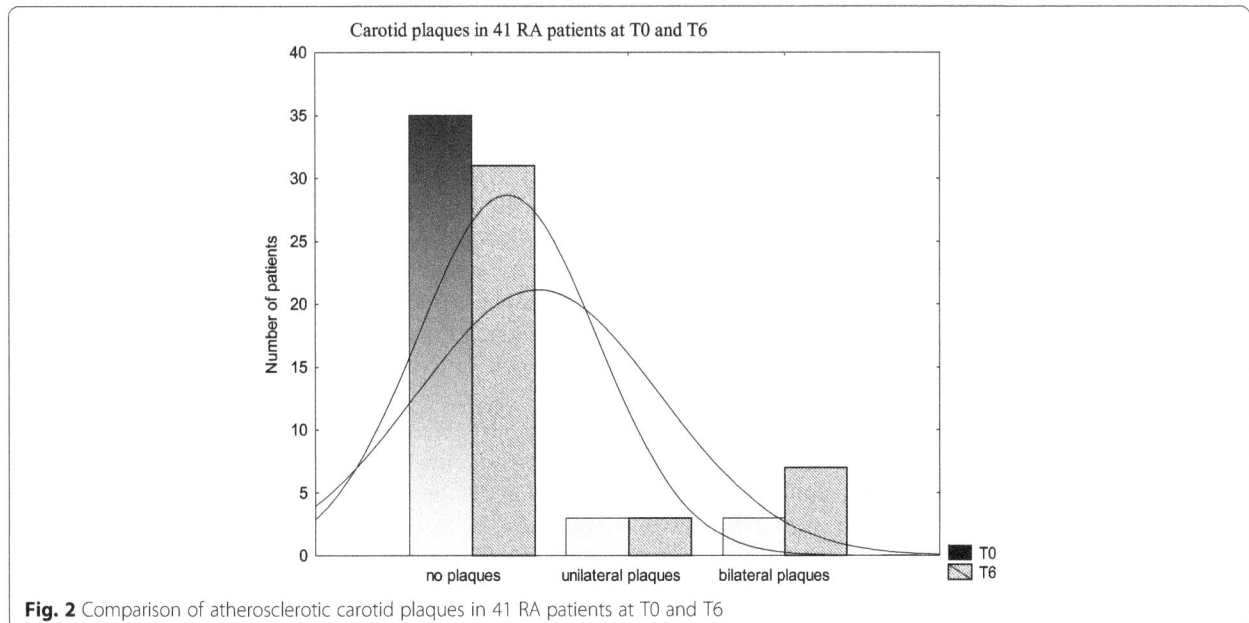

Fig. 2 Comparison of atherosclerotic carotid plaques in 41 RA patients at T0 and T6

Comparison of male and female RA patient

At T0, the mean cIMT value was non-significantly higher in men than in women with RA [0.82 (0.2) vs 0.75 (0.14), NS]. However, at T6, unfavorable CV and metabolic parameters were found in male compared with female patients: significantly higher cIMT [1.1 (0.33) vs 0.82 (0.14), $p < 0.001$], SCORE [6.0 (6.1) vs 2.3 (2.9), $p = 0.04$], uric acid [5.5 (1.0) vs 4.3 (1.0), $p = 0.007$] and lower HDL-C [44.3 (10.7) vs 63.1 (15.4), $p = 0.007$].

In control subjects, the mean cIMT at T6 did not differ significantly between men and women [0.77 (0.13) vs 0.76 (0.1), NS].

Discussion

In this prospective, 6-year follow-up study, exacerbation of atherosclerosis was observed in patients with advanced RA, revealed by a significant increase of cIMT value and an increase in patients with atherosclerotic plaques (non-significant). Patients with atherosclerotic plaques showed significantly higher inflammatory parameters than patients without plaques, suggesting association between inflammatory burden and plaques presence. Especially the presence of bilateral plaques is noteworthy due to significantly higher CV risk and the quadrupled risk of acute myocardial syndrome [24].

Exacerbation of atherosclerosis occurred despite effective control of RA activity. Disease activity according to DAS28 decreased significantly during follow-up, which was associated with active DMARDs treatment. Simultaneously deterioration was found in certain traditional CV risk factors. During follow-up the risk of CV death increased significantly and 25% of patients had high/very high risk of fatal CVD.

The current cIMT was significantly associated only with baseline cIMT assessed 6 years before. No significant relationship was found between current cIMT, NT-proBNP, QTc values and disease activity parameters. The results suggest, that initial state of CV system had a profound effect on further CV risk in the course of RA.

Exacerbation of atherosclerosis, revealed by higher cIMT, was also found in the control group. The cIMT increases were comparable in both groups (patients and controls), which suggests an effect of physiological aging. Similar results were presented in a follow-up study, in which, after 5-year observation, significantly higher cIMT was found in both early RA patients and controls, atherosclerotic plaques were not mentioned [11].

Atherosclerotic plaques were shown to be more predictive of CV events than elevated cIMT, since cIMT value may be associated with arterial wall aging, body size, muscularity [25]. New or progressive carotid plaques were strongly associated with markers of inflammation and disease activity (CRP, swollen joints count) [25]. It seems that in RA, an additional, maladaptive arterial

wall remodeling increases risk of plaque rapture which could explain highly increased CV risk despite a seemingly normal cIMT [26]. According to Semb et al., patients with RA had numerically more atherosclerotic plaques than controls, associated with the presence of RA, but not with the level of RA activity. However, patients in remission and controls had more stable plaques than patients with active disease, pointing to importance of achieving remission [27].

Several hypotheses have been proposed to explain the accelerated atherosclerosis in RA. Thus far, there is no evidence that RA-associated single-nucleotide polymorphisms (SNP) as a group are associated with coronary artery disease [28].

The greater burden of traditional CV risk factors is suggested among RA patients [28, 29]. It seems that classical CV risk factors may be important for generation and progression of stable atherosclerosis, whereas local and systemic high-grade inflammation may contribute to plaque instability and higher rates of acute CV syndromes [30]. Dalbeni et al. found that only age was consistently associated with cIMT and atherosclerotic plaques as major determinant of subclinical atherosclerosis [31]. Male gender is reported to have an impact on cIMT in addition to disease activity parameters [8]. According to data in literature, on average cIMT is higher in men than in women and increases with age [32].

In this study, cIMT value, which was comparable in male and female patients at initial (T0) assessment, became significantly higher in males at the 6-year follow-up. Simultaneously, a higher burden of traditional CV factors and risk of CV death was found in men with RA.

Systemic, immune-mediated inflammation significantly contributes to accelerated atherosclerosis [6]. Effective control of inflammation as a result of DMARDs treatment is associated with CV risk reduction. Significantly lower cIMT was reported in RA patients treated with MTX and correlated with MTX dosage [33]. Significant cIMT reduction was reported in RA patients treated with TNF inhibitors and steadily responsive to therapy [34].

In established RA, NT-proBNP was associated with the disease activity, duration, as well as cIMT [2, 5, 12, 13]. It was suggested that increased NT-proBNP could reflect silent myocardial stress associated with transient ischemia due to atherosclerosis [13]. It was reported that in RA patients without evident CHF, treatment with TNF inhibitor decreased NT-proBNP, suggesting the link between inflammation and cardiac stress [35]. In this study, non-significant increase of NT-proBNP was observed during follow-up, with no clinical symptoms of CHF. The significant association between NT-proBNP and cIMT at T0 was not found at follow-up, which may be considered as a result of active DMARDs treatment.

It seems that traditional CV risk factors in association with high-grade inflammation are responsible for acceleration of atherosclerosis in early course of RA. The results of our study indicate that at follow-up the burden of atherosclerosis is still higher in RA patients than in healthy controls and constantly related to the disease activity. Traditional CV risk factors seem to be important in long-standing advanced RA.

The careful diagnosis and management of CV risk factors should be considered for all RA patients, especially those with atherosclerotic plaques should be treated as high-risk patients.

The main strength of our present study is its prospective design. The same two groups of patients and controls were assessed with a 6-year interval. The detailed characteristics of patients considered all aspects of RA pathology. Another strength is the same specialist who performed all US measurements, thereby eliminating any interpersonal variations.

There are some limitations of the study, including quite small groups of patients and controls. The score used in the study (DAS28) presents only the current disease activity and does not reflect the activity burden over the 6 years. Therefore, further evaluation should be performed on a larger group of patients, considering assessment of the activity burden with other methods.

Conclusions

In this prospective, 6-year follow-up study of patients with established RA, significant exacerbation of atherosclerosis was found, as revealed by higher cIMT and increase in patients with atherosclerotic plaques, despite significant reduction of disease activity. Unfavorable metabolic parameters and significantly higher cIMT in male compared with female patients were noted. The mean cIMT was significantly higher in RA patients than in controls at both assessments. Tight control of inflammation could be an effective method to reduce CV risk. However, in long-standing disease traditional CV risk factors seem to play a key role, beyond inflammatory activity of the disease.

Abbreviations

ACR: American College of Rheumatology; AI: Atherogenic index; bDMARD: biological DMARD; BMI: Body mass index; BP: Blood pressure; BULB: Carotid bulb; CCA: Common carotid artery; CHF: Congestive heart failure; cIMT: carotid intima-media thickness; Cr: Creatinine; CRP: C-reactive protein; csDMARD: conventional synthetic DMARD; CV: Cardiovascular; CVD: Cardiovascular disease; DAS28: Disease Activity Score evaluated in 28 joints; DMARD: Disease-modifying antirheumatic drug; ECG: Electrocardiogram; ESR: Erythrocyte sedimentation rate; EULAR: European League Against Rheumatism; HDL-C: High-density lipoprotein cholesterol; ICA: Internal carotid artery; LDL-C: Low-density lipoprotein cholesterol; M-HAQ: Modified Health Assessment Questionnaire; NT-proBNP: N-terminal pro-brain natriuretic peptide; QTc: Heart rate-corrected QT interval; RA: Rheumatoid arthritis; SCORE: Systemic Coronary Risk Evaluation; TC: Total cholesterol; TG: Triglycerides; TNF: Tumor necrosis factor; US: Ultrasound; VAS: Visual analogue scale

Funding
Medical University of Lublin Grant.

Authors' contributions
BTS contributed to conception and design, contributed to acquisition, analysis and interpretation of data, was a major contributor in writing the manuscript. MP contributed to acquisition, analysis, performed the statistical analyses. RZ contributed to acquisition, analysis and interpretation of data. ADZ performed all the ultrasound examinations, contributed to analysis and interpretation of data. MM contributed to conception and design, contributed to interpretation of data. All authors read and approved the final manuscript.

Competing interests
The authors declare that they have no competing interests.

Author details
[1]Department of Rheumatology and Connective Tissue Diseases, Medical University of Lublin, ul. Jaczewskiego 8, 20-950 Lublin, Poland. [2]Department of Interventional Radiology and Neuroradiology, Medical University of Lublin, ul. Jaczewskiego 8, 20-950 Lublin, Poland.

References

1. Corrales A, Dessein PH, Tsang L, Pina T, Blanco R, Gonzalez-Juanatey C, et al. Carotid artery plaque in women with rheumatoid arthritis and low estimated cardiovascular disease risk: a cross-sectional study. Arthritis Res Ther. 2015;17:55.
2. Provan SA, Angel K, Odegård S, Mowinckel P, Atar D, Kvien TK. The association between disease activity and NT-proBNP in 238 patients with rheumatoid arthritis: a 10-year longitudinal study. Arthritis Res Ther. 2008;10:R70.
3. Pope JE, Nevskaya T, Barra L, Parraga G. Carotid artery atherosclerosis in patients with active rheumatoid arthritis: predictors of plaque occurrence and progression over 24 weeks. Open Rheumatol J. 2016;10:49–59.
4. Lazzerini PE, Capecchi PL, Acampa M, Galeazzi M, Laghi-Pasini F. Arrhythmic risk in rheumatoid arthritis: the driving role of systemic inflammation. Autoimmun Rev. 2014;13:936–44.
5. Provan S, Angel K, Semb AG, Atar D, Kvien TK. NT-proBNP predicts mortality in patients with rheumatoid arthritis: results from 10-year follow-up of the EURIDISS study. Ann Rheum Dis. 2010;69:1946–50.
6. Zhang J, Chen L, Delzell E, Muntner P, Hillegass WB, Safford MM, et al. The association between inflammatory markers, serum lipids and the risk of cardiovascular events in patients with rheumatoid arthritis. Ann Rheum Dis. 2014;73:1301–8.
7. Navarro-Millán I, Yang S, DuVall SL, Chen L, Baddley J, Cannon GW, et al. Association of hyperlipidaemia, inflammation and serological status and coronary heart disease among patients with rheumatoid arthritis: data from the National Veterans Health Administration. Ann Rheum Dis. 2016;75:341–7.
8. Ambrosino P, Lupoli R, Di Minno A, Tasso M, Peluso R, Di Minno MN. Subclinical atherosclerosis in patients with rheumatoid arthritis. A meta-analysis of literature studies. Thromb Haemost. 2015;113:916–30.
9. Wang P, Guan SY, Xu SZ, Li HM, Leng RX, Li XP, et al. Increased carotid intima-media thickness in rheumatoid arthritis: an update meta-analysis. Clin Rheumatol. 2016;35:315–23.
10. Targońska-Stępniak B, Drelich-Zbroja A, Majdan M. The relationship between carotid intima-media thickness and the activity of rheumatoid arthritis. J Clin Rheumatol. 2011;17:249–55.
11. Södergren A, Karp K, Bengtsson C, Möller B, Rantapää-Dahlqvist S, Wållberg-Jonsson S. The extent of subclinical atherosclerosis is partially predicted by the inflammatory load: a prospective study over 5 years in patients with rheumatoid arthritis and matched controls. J Rheumatol. 2015;42:935–42.

12. Mirjafari H, Welsh P, Verstappen SM, Wilson P, Marshall T, Edlin H, et al. N-terminal pro-brain-type natriuretic peptide (NT-pro-BNP) and mortality risk in early inflammatory polyarthritis: results from the Norfolk arthritis registry (NOAR). Ann Rheum Dis. 2014;73:684–90.

13. Targońska-Stępniak B, Majdan M. Amino-terminal pro-brain natriuretic peptide as a prognostic marker in patients with rheumatoid arthritis. Clin Rheumatol. 2011;30:61–9.

14. Avouac J, Meune C, Chenevier-Gobeaux C, Dieudé P, Borderie D, Lefevre G, et al. Inflammation and disease activity are associated with high circulating cardiac markers in rheumatoid arthritis independently of traditional cardiovascular risk factors. J Rheumatol. 2014;41:248–55.

15. Lazzerini PE, Capecchi PL, Laghi-Pasini F. Systemic inflammation and arrhythmic risk: lessons from rheumatoid arthritis. Eur Heart J. 2017;38:1717–27.

16. Aletaha D, Neogi T, Silman AJ, Funovits J, Felson DT, Bingham CO 3rd, et al. 2010 Rheumatoid arthritis classification criteria: an American College of Rheumatology/European League Against Rheumatism collaborative initiative. Arthritis Rheum. 2010;62:2569–81.

17. Prevoo ML, van't Hof MA, Kuper HH, van Leeuwen AN, van de Putte LB, van Riel PL. Modified disease activity scores that include twenty-eight-joint counts: development and validation in a prospective longitudinal study of patients with rheumatoid arthritis. Arthritis Rheum. 1995;38:44–8.

18. Pincus T, Sokka T, Kautiainen H. Further development of a physical function scale on a MDHAQ [corrected] for standard care of patients with rheumatic diseases. J Rheumatol. 2005;32:1432–9.

19. Popa CD, Arts E, Fransen J, van Riel PLCM. Atherogenic Index and high-density lipoprotein cholesterol as cardiovascular risk determinants in Rheumatoid Arthritis: The Impact of Therapy with Biologicals. Mediators Inflamm. 2012;2012:785946.

20. Peters MJL, Symmons DPM, McCarey D, Dijkmans BAC, Nicola P, Kvien TK, et al. EULAR evidence-based recommendations for cardiovascular risk management in patients with rheumatoid arthritis and other forms of inflammatory arthritis. Ann Rheum Dis. 2010;69:325–31.

21. Gonzalez-Gay MA, Gonzalez-Juanatey C, Vazquez-Rodriguez TR, Martin J, Llorca J. Endothelial dysfunction, carotid intima-media thickness and accelerated atherosclerosis in rheumatoid arthritis. Semin Arthritis Rheum. 2008;38:67–70.

22. Gonzalez-Juanatey C, Llorca J, Martin J, Gonzalez-Gay MA. Carotid intima-media thickness predicts the development of cardiovascular events in patients with rheumatoid arthritis. Semin Arthritis Rheum. 2009;38:366–71.

23. Goldenberg I, Moss AJ, Zareba W. QT interval: how to measure it and what is "normal". J Cardiovasc Electrophysiol. 2006;17:333–6.

24. Van Sijl AM, Van Den Hurk K, Peters MJ, Van Halm VP, Nijpels G, Stehouwer CDA, et al. Different type of carotid Arterial Wall remodeling in rheumatoid arthritis compared with healthy subjects: a case-control study. J Rheumatol. 2012;39:2261–6.

25. Giles JT, Post WS, Blumenthal RS, Polak J, Petri M, Gelber AC, et al. Longitudinal predictors of progression of carotid atherosclerosis in rheumatoid arthritis. Arthritis Rheum. 2011;63:3216–25.

26. Evans MR, Escalante A, Battafarano DF, Freeman GL, O'Leary DH, del Rincón I. Carotid atherosclerosis predicts incident acute coronary syndromes in rheumatoid arthritis. Arthritis Rheum. 2011;63:1211–20.

27. Semb AG, Rollefstad S, Provan SA, Kvien TK, Stranden E, Olsen IC, et al. Carotid plaque characteristics and disease activity in rheumatoid arthritis. J Rheumatol. 2013;40:359–68.

28. Jansen H, Willenborg C, Lieb W, Zeng L, Ferrario PG, Loley C, et al. Rheumatoid arthritis and coronary artery disease: genetic analyses do not support a causal relation. J Rheumatol. 2017;44:4–10.

29. Baghdadi LR, Woodman RJ, Shanahan EM, Mangoni AA. The impact of traditional cardiovascular risk factors on cardiovascular outcomes in patients with rheumatoid arthritis: a systematic review and meta-analysis. PLoS One. 2015;10:e0117952.

30. Kitas GD, Gabriel SE. Cardiovascular disease in rheumatoid arthritis: state of the art and future perspectives. Ann Rheum Dis. 2011;70:8–14.

31. Dalbeni A, Giollo A, Tagetti A, Atanasio S, Orsolini G, Cioffi G, et al. Traditional cardiovascular risk factors or inflammation: which factors accelerate atherosclerosis in arthritis patients? Int J Cardiol. 2017;236:488–92.

32. Roman MJ, Naqvi TZ, Gardin JM, et al. American society of echocardiography report. Clinical application of noninvasive vascular ultrasound in cardiovascular risk stratification: a report from the American Society of Echocardiography and the society for vascular medicine and biology. Vasc Med. 2006;11:201–11.

33. Kim HJ, Kim MJ, Lee CK, Hong YH. Effects of methotrexate on carotid intima-media thickness in patients with rheumatoid arthritis. J Korean Med Sci. 2015;30:1589–96.

34. Del Porto F, Laganà B, Lai S, Nofroni I, Tinti F, Vitale M, et al. Response to anti-tumour necrosis factor alpha blockade is associated with reduction of carotid intima-media thickness in patients with active rheumatoid arthritis. Rheumatology (Oxford). 2007;46:1111–5.

35. Peters MJ, Welsh P, McInnes IB, Wolbink G, Dijkmans BA, Sattar N, et al. Tumour necrosis factor {alpha} blockade reduces circulating N-terminal pro-brain natriuretic peptide levels in patients with active rheumatoid arthritis: results from a prospective cohort study. Ann Rheum Dis. 2010;69:1281–5.

24

Are aortic coarctation and rheumatoid arthritis different models of aortic stiffness?Data from an echocardiographic study

Giorgio Faganello[1]* , Giovanni Cioffi[2], Maurizio Rossini[3], Federica Ognibeni[3], Alessandro Giollo[3], Maurizio Fisicaro[1], Giulia Russo[1], Concetta Di Nora[1], Sara Doimo[1], Luigi Tarantini[4], Carmine Mazzone[1], Antonella Cherubini[1], Biancamaria D'Agata Mottolesi[5], Claudio Pandullo[1], Andrea Di Lenarda[1], Gianfranco Sinagra[6] and Ombretta Viapiana[3]

Abstract

Background: Patients who underwent a successful repair of the aortic coarctation (CoA) show high risk for cardiovascular (CV) events. Mechanical and structural abnormalities in the ascending aorta (Ao) might have a role in the prognosis of CoA patients. We analyzed the elastic properties of Ao measured as aortic stiffness index (AoSI) in CoA patients in the long-term period and we compared AoSI with a cohort of 38 patients with rheumatoid arthritis (RA) and 38 non-RA matched controls.

Methods: Data from 19 CoA patients were analyzed 28 ± 13 years after surgery. Abnormally high AoSI was diagnosed if AoSI > 6.07% (95th percentile of the AoSI detected in our reference healthy population). AoSI was assessed at the level of the aortic root by two-dimensional guided M-mode evaluation.

Results: CoA patients showed more than two-fold higher AoSI compared to RA and controls (9.8 ± 12.6 vs $4.8 \pm 2.5\%$ and $3.1 \pm 2.0\%$, respectively; all $p < 0.05$ and in 5 of 19 patients with CoA (26%) AoSI was exceptionally high. The 5 patients with abnormally high AoSI were older with higher BP, LV mass and prevalence of LV diastolic dysfunction. Multiple linear regression analysis revealed that AoSI was independently related to the presence of LV hypertrophy and higher LV relative wall thickness.

Conclusions: CoA patients have higher AoSI levels than RA patients and non-RA matched controls. AoSI levels are abnormally high in a small sub-group of CoA patients who show a very high-risk clinical profile for adverse CV events.

Background

Despite successfully treated, patients with repaired aortic coarctation (CoA) have reduced long-term survival compared with an age and sex matched population [1]. The presence of high systemic blood pressure generally found in these patients together with altered integrity of the aorta due to surgical repair, and/or acquired post-surgery, cause progressive change in the structure and function of arterial vessels [2–4]. Therefore, it is common to find hypertrophy and hyperplasia of smooth muscle cells, together with modification of the matrix protein [5]. The continuous deposition of a variety of proteins,

including collagen, combined with the progressive loss of the elastic matrix leads to a further increase in arterial stiffness and reduction of vascular compliance [6]. Similar features have been found in patients affected by rheumatoid arthritis (RA) which represents a clinical model of acquired extensive arterial disease with abnormal vascular responses [7] to inflammation and/or damaging molecular modulators of immune system. Abnormal aortic elastic properties are associated with older age and higher blood pressure in RA patients [8]. The result of these changes is stiffening of the arteries and consequent increase of aortic stiffness index (AoSI) which is used to evaluate arterial stiffness and it is an independent predictor of cardiovascular morbidity and mortality [9]. AoSI showed a strong correlation with the invasive measurements of arterial stiffness and more popular non-invasive techniques such as pulse wave

* Correspondence: giorgio.faganello@asuits.sanita.fvg.it
[1]Cardiovascular Centre, Department of Cardiology, Azienda Sanitaria Universitaria Integrata di Trieste, via Slataper n°9, 34134 Trieste, Italy
Full list of author information is available at the end of the article

velocity or Tissue Doppler [10–13]. Accordingly, in this study we measured the AoSI of the ascending aorta in patients with successful CoA repair in the long-term period and we compared it with a cohort of RA patients.

Methods
Study population
The study population consisted of 19 non-institutionalized subjects > 18 years of age who consecutively underwent successful repair of CoA during the period from 1964 to 2010 and were subsequently followed-up by the Institute for Maternal and Child Health-IRCCS, Burlo Garofolo and at the Cardiovascular (CV) Center, Maggiore Hospital, Trieste, Italy. Repair of CoA was obtained by: end-to end anastomosis in 9 patients, patch in 4 patients, subclavian flap in 2 patients, subclavian artery flap in 1 patient and percutaneous stent in 3 patients. The mean duration of follow-up was 28 ± 13 years. The patients' inclusion criteria were:

- Residual isthmic gradient by echo-Doppler less than 20 mm Hg;
- Aortic diameter at the site of repair/diaphragmatic aorta ratio more than 0.7 at cardiac MRI
- No associated cardiac abnormalities or moderate/severe valve heart disease;
- No bicuspid aortic valve with moderate/severe regurgitation or stenosis;
- Absence of history of myocardial infarction or prior myocardial revascularization, asymptomatic known LV dysfunction, heart failure, primary cardiomyopathies or myocarditis, atrial fibrillation, chronic kidney disease, obstructive sleep apnea syndrome, RA (all conditions eliciting changes in LV geometry and LV systolic dysfunction). All patients underwent transthoracic echocardiogram, clinical and laboratory evaluation at the CV Center, Maggiore Hospital, Trieste, Italy. Patients expressed their general written consent to the anonymous use of data for their care and research purposes. The study complies with the Declaration of Helsinki as revised in 2000; the locally appointed ethic committee has approved the research protocol.

Rheumatoid arthritis group
A group of 38 patients matched for age, sex, blood pressure, history of hypertension and affected by RA was identified. RA was diagnosed by clinical and laboratory examination according to the American College of Rheumatology criteria [14]. They were selected by a large cohort of patients consecutively recruited from January 2014 to December 2014 in three Italian referral centers (Verona, Trieste, Trento) with fully accessible cardiac units provided in which patients underwent echocardiographic, clinical and laboratory evaluations.

Control group
A control group of 38 subject defined "non-RA patients" matched for age, sex, blood pressure and history of hypertension was identified. RA patients and non-RA controls were studied for the reason to assess the range of values of aortic stiffness in a model of abnormal vascular responses and of acquired chronic arterial disease, respectively. Controls were free of symptoms/signs of cardiac disease and had no history of myocardial illness or valve heart disease, including evidence of more than mild mitral annular calcification at echocardiographic baseline evaluation. These two groups of subjects were statistically comparable with those enrolled into the study for age, sex, blood pressure and hypertension according to the following procedure: a Gower's generalized distance from each of the RA individual and each CoA patient was computed and all patients were ranked in ascending order in the database. The distance was calculated using these variables ordered as follows: age, gender, systolic blood pressure and hypertension. The 38 RA patients and 19 CoA patients were then demarcated and coupled by taking for everyone patient with CoA the two closest controls (selected by a pool of 250 patients). Then, the 19 patients with CoA were compared with a second control group (defined non-RA matched controls), composed of 38 patients, matched for age, sex, blood pressure and prevalence of hypertension by the same statistical procedure described above. The 38 non-RA matched controls were designated by taking for everyone close patient with CoA the two closest control. These subjects were selected by a pool of 180 patients who consecutively performed at our Center a clinical and an echocardiographic evaluation for a CV risk assessment in primary prevention.

Definitions
Arterial hypertension was defined as systolic blood pressure of ≥140 mmHg and/or a diastolic blood pressure of ≥90 mmHg and/or pharmacologically treated high blood pressure. Obesity was diagnosed if patients had body mass index ≥30 kg/m2. Dyslipidemia was defined as levels of total serum cholesterol > 190 mg/dl and or triglycerides > 150 mg/dl or pharmacologically treated high lipid serum levels.

Echocardiography
LV chamber dimensions and wall thicknesses were measured by the American Society of Echocardiography guidelines and LV mass calculated using a necropsy validated formula [15]. LV mass was normalized for height to the 2.7 power and LV hypertrophy was defined as LV mass > 49.2 g/m2.7 for men and > 46.7 for women [16].

Relative wall thickness was calculated as the 2 * end-diastolic ratio posterior wall thickness/LV diameter and indicated concentric LV geometry if > 0.43 (the 97.5 percentile in normal population) [17] LV end-diastolic and end-systolic volumes were measured by the biplane method of disks from 2D apical 4 chamber + 2 chamber views and used to calculate ejection fraction, defined as index of global LV systolic function measured at endocardium. LV ejection fraction < 50% was indicative of LV systolic dysfunction (LVSD). LV systolic function was also assessed by measuring the systolic shortening of the LV minor axis at the midwall level to specifically evaluate the circumferential component of LV systolic function. Midwall shortening was calculated considering the epicardial migration of the midwall during systole caused by the architectural organization of myocardial fibers, as previously described [18]. Midwall end-systolic circumferential stress (sc-MS) was calculated and related to midwall shortening to assess afterload-independent LV systolic function [19]. Thus, sc-MS refers to the ratio observed/predicted midwall shortening for a given end-systolic circumferential stress and corrects for this variable the LV systolic function. sc-MS < 89% (10th percentile of our healthy controls) was indicative of circumferential LVSD. Furthermore, Tissue Doppler study (pulsed wave spectral analysis) was used to measure peak mitral annular systolic velocity (peak S', mean of 4 measurements obtained in septal, lateral, inferior and anterior mitral annular position), as an estimate of longitudinal component of LV systolic function [20]. Peak S' < 8.5 cm/sec (10th percentile of our healthy controls) indicated longitudinal LVSD. Transmitral and pulmonary vein pulsed wave Doppler curves and early diastolic Tissue Doppler velocity of mitral annulus (E') were assessed according to the recommendations of the American Society of Echocardiography [21]. Early diastolic velocity of transmitral flow (E) was divided by E' and used to classify LV diastolic function together with other parameters (E/A ratio of transmitral flow, deceleration time of E and the difference in duration of atrial wave on pulmonary vein flow and atrial wave on transmitral flow) in 4 degrees as proposed by Redfield et al. [22]: normal, mild dysfunction, moderate dysfunction and severe dysfunction. LV end-diastolic pressure was non-invasively estimated by the equation validated by Ommen et al. [23]. Maximal left atrial volume was also computed from 2D apical 4-chamber view using the area - length method and was normalized for body surface area. The residual isthmic gradient was assessed with a standalone, 2.0-MHz, continuous-wave Doppler probe using the modified Bernoulli equation: gradient (mmHg) = $4(V_2^2 - V_1^2)$ m/s, where V_2 was the maximum velocity in the descending aorta and V_1 was the velocity in the descending aorta above the coarctation site when a double shadow could be obtained on Doppler tracing, or

V1 was the velocity in the ascending aorta when a suitable tracing was not obtained [24]. Doppler gradients were considered as the mean of at least 3 consecutive measurements.

Calculation of aortic stiffness

Aortic stiffness was assessed at the level of the aortic root, using a two-dimensional guided M-mode evaluation of systolic (AoS) and diastolic (AoD) aortic diameters, 3 cm above the aortic valve together with blood pressure measured by cuff sphygmomanometer. AoD was obtained at the peak of the R wave at the simultaneously recorded electrocardiogram, while AoS was measured at the maximal anterior motion of the aortic wall [25]. For each diameter five measurements were averaged. The following formula was used for assessing aortic stiffness index (AoSI):

$$(AoSI)\,(\%) \quad = \quad \ln(SBP/DBP)/[(AoS - AoD)/AoD]$$

where ln[systolic blood pressure (SBP)/diastolic blood pressure (DBP)] refers to the natural logarithm of the relative blood pressure (SBP and DBP: systolic and diastolic blood pressure) [26]. Blood pressure was measured at the end of echocardiographic evaluation in supine position. AoD and AoS were evaluated off-line by the principal investigator blinded to the identity of the subject. Reproducibility data on AoSI assessment have been previously reported [27].

Cardiac magnetic resonance

The degree of residual coarctation was determined by spin-echo magnetic resonance imaging of the thoracic aorta. The smallest diameter was measured by hand calipers from internal edge to internal edge of the vascular walls from a combination of 2 views: transverse and sagittal oblique (left anterior oblique equivalent) through the center of the vessel. The smallest diameter was compared with the diameter of the aorta at the diaphragm. Percent narrowing was calculated as: % narrowing = 100 (1 - smallest diameter/diameter at diaphragmatic level).

Statistical analysis

Categorical variables are presented as percentages, while continuous variables are presented as their means and SD. Categorical variables were compared by the chi-square test and continuous variables by the t-test or the Mann–Whitney U-test. The study population was also stratified by status of abnormally high AoSI at baseline. The cut-off value for abnormally high AoSI was a priori identified as 6.07% (the 95th percentile of AoSI calculated in the 113 healthy subjects) as previously reported. Multiple linear regression analysis was computed to assess the variables significantly related to AoSI index in CoA patients.

Variables significantly related to AoSI in univariate tests ($p < 0.01$) were considered in the multivariable model, which included age, body mass index, systolic blood pressure, E/E', LV relative wall thickness and LV hypertrophy. All analyses were performed using statistical package SPSS 19.0 (SPSS Inc. Chicago. Illinois) and statistical significance was identified by two-tailed $p < 0.05$.

Results

Study population

All subjects were free of symptoms and clinical signs of cardiac disease at the time of clinical, laboratory and echocardiographic evaluation. During the 28 ± 13 years of follow-up after surgical intervention, no patient who had undergone successful repair of CoA suffered from an adverse CV event either was hospitalized for any sign or symptoms potentially related to the presence of CV disease. Similarly, RA and non-RA matched controls were analyzed in primary prevention. Clinical and echocardiographic characteristics of the study population compared with

RA patients (mean time from the RA diagnosis 14 ± 10 years) and non-RA matched controls are shown in Tables 1 and 2, respectively. Between all groups, there were no statistical differences in terms of age, sex, body mass index, laboratory data and prevalence of dyslipidemia, type 2 diabetes mellitus and blood hypertension. Despite RA subjects were taking less anti-hypertensive medications compared to CoA patients and controls, blood pressure values were similar between the groups. All groups had LV dimensions within the normal range, however CoA patients showed higher prevalence of LV hypertrophy than controls and RA patients (37% vs 20% vs. 6%, respectively; all $p < 0.05$) associated with a higher end-systolic circumferential stress and lower relative wall thickness, index of concentric LV geometry. Regarding to the parameters of LV systolic function, all three groups showed similar LV ejection fraction and sc-MS (parameter of LV circumferential systolic function), however peak S' (parameter of longitudinal LV systolic function), was significantly lower in CoA subjects than

Table 1 Main clinical characteristics of the 19 study patients with aortic coarctation compared with 38 controls matched for cardiovascular risk factors and 38 patients with rheumatoid arthritis

Variables	Aortic coarctation (19 patients)	Controls (38 patients)	RA (38 patients)
Clinical			
Age (years)	33 ± 12	35 ± 14	37 ± 6
Female gender (%)	37	32	48
Body mass index (Kg/m^2)	23.9 ± 4.0	26.8 ± 4.4	24.2 ± 4.2
Obesity (%)	11	17	9
Hypertension (%)	58	65	41
Dyslipidemia (%)	5	5	15
Active smoker (%)	21	12	28
Diabetes (%)	5	5	3
Systolic blood pressure (mmHg)	127 ± 17	131 ± 19	125 ± 16
Diastolic blood pressure (mmHg)	77 ± 9	83 ± 10	82 ± 10
Heart rate (beats/minute)	68 ± 12	71 ± 14	76 ± 10
Laboratory			
Glycemia (mg/dl)	93 ± 9	98 ± 10	93 ± 9
Hemoglobin (gr/dl)	13.8 ± 1.6	14.6 ± 1.7	14.0 ± 1.2
GFR (ml/min/1.73m^2)	105 ± 26	103 ± 20	108 ± 26
Pharmacological treatment			
Betablockers (%)	32	22	8 [#][§]
ACEi / ARB (%)	32	52	12 [#][§]
Diuretics (%)	16	30	3 [#][§]
Calcium antagonists (%)	11	35	3 [#][§]
Anti-platelets agents (%)	0	1	4
Statins (%)	0	1	1

ACEi Angiotensin-converting enzyme inhibitors, *ARB* Angiotensin T1 receptor blockers, *GFR* Glomerular Filtration Rate, *RA* rheumatoir arthritis
[#] = $p < 0.05$ rheumatoid arthritis (RA) vs coarctation
[§] = $p < 0.05$ RA vs controls

Table 2 Echocardiographic characteristics

Variables	Aortic coarctation (19 patients)	Controls (38 patients)	RA (38 patients)
LV End-diastolic diameter (ml/m^2)	2.9 ± 0.3	2.3 ± 0.4 *	2.6 ± 0.3[#]
LV End-systolic diameter (ml/m^2)	1.9 ± 0.3	1.4 ± 0.4 *	1.7 ± 0.2[#]
LV End-diastolic volume (ml/m^2)	66 ± 19	56 ± 12	51 ± 9 [# §]
LV End-systolic volume (ml/m^2)	27 ± 9	21 ± 6	17 ± 4 [# §]
Relative wall thickness	0.35 ± 0.06	0.40 ± 0.07 *	0.43 ± 0.06 [# §]
Concentric LV geometry (%)	11	45 *	51 [#]
LV mass index (g/m $^{2.7}$)	41 ± 14	38 ± 13	38 ± 7[#]
LV hypertrophy (%)	37	20 *	6 [# §]
Inappropriate LV mass (%)	11	10	36 [# §]
LV stroke volume (ml)	73 ± 25	74 ± 18	59 ± 15 [# §]
Cardiac index (l/min/ m^2)	2.7 ± 0.9	2.4 ± 0.7	2.3 ± 0.6[#]
LV ejection fraction (%)	60 ± 7	63 ± 5	65 ± 5[#]
LV CESS (dynes/cm^2)	166 ± 49	128 ± 48 *	116 ± 28[#]
LV Sc- midwall shortening (%)	101 ± 15	98 ± 10	85 ± 11
Peak S′ (cm/sec)	7.1 ± 1.3	10.5 ± 3.6 *	10.2 ± 1.6[#]
Low peak S′ (%)	84	55 *	27[# §]
Peak E′ (cm/sec)	10.6 ± 3.5	12.3 ± 1.7	13.6 ± 2.2
E wave of transmitral flow (cm/sec)	103 ± 16	86 ± 19 *	75 ± 17[# §]
A wave of transmitral flow (cm/sec)	69 ± 25	64 ± 16	62 ± 15
E / A ratio	1.4 ± 0.36	1.4 ± 0.24	1.3 ± 0.40[#]
E / E′ ratio	10.5 ± 3.6	7.5 ± 2.3 *	5.6 ± 1.1[# §]
LV diastolic dysfunction (%)	11	2 *	3[#]
Maximal left atrial volume (ml/ m^2)	27 ± 11	23 ± 11	18 ± 4
Aortic stiffness index (%)	9.8 ± 12.6	3.1 ± 2.0 *	4.8 ± 2.5[#]
Abnormally high aortic stiffness (% of patients)	26	10	21

CESS circumferential end-systolic stress, *LV* left ventricular; *Peak E′* early diastolic Tissue Doppler velocity of mitral annulus, *Peak S′* peak mitral annular systolic velocity (Tissue Doppler Imaging), *RA* rheumatoid arthritis, *Sc* stress corrected

* = $p < 0.05$ controls vs coarctation;
[#] = $p < 0.05$ rheumatoid arthritis vs coarctation;
[§] = $p < 0.05$ rheumatoid arthritis vs controls

controls and RA patients (7.1 ± 1.3 vs. 10.5 ± 3.6 vs. 10.2 ± 1.6 cm/sec; $p < 0.05$). CoA patients had a greater prevalence of LV diastolic dysfunction as shown by raised E/E' ratio and end-diastolic pressure.

Aortic arterial stiffness

AoSI was significantly higher in the CoA group compared to RA subjects (9.8 ± 12.6% vs. 4.8 ± 2.5%, $p < 0.0001$) and in turn, RA subjects had increased values compared to non-RA matched controls (4.8 ± 2.5% vs. 3.1 ± 2.0, $p = 0.02$) (Fig. 1). The marked increase in AoSI found in CoA patients was essentially due to the presence of 5 subjects showing abnormally high AoSI (mean value 28.9 ± 6.5%) in comparison of the remaining 14 who had AoSI values in the normal range (2.5 ± 1.9%) (Fig. 2). The clinical and echocardiographic characteristics of CoA patients with and without abnormally high AoSI are shown in Table 3. Among CoA group, patients who had abnormally high

AoSI were older, with higher blood pressure values, body mass index, LV mass and worse diastolic function. Four out of five patients were treated with end-to-end anastomosis and only in one case a dacron-patch was used. Multiple linear regression analysis revealed that AoSI was independently related to LV hypertrophy and higher LV relative wall thickness, index of concentric LV geometry (Table 4). Considering the control group, abnormally high AoSI was detected in 4 of 38 (10%) and in 5 of 38 patients with RA (21%). Among the three groups there were no statistically significant differences in the size of the aortic root.

Discussion

In our study, we analyzed AoSI after three decades of follow up in patients who underwent successful CoA repair and we compared it with two different cohorts of patients: the first one, non-RA patients matched for

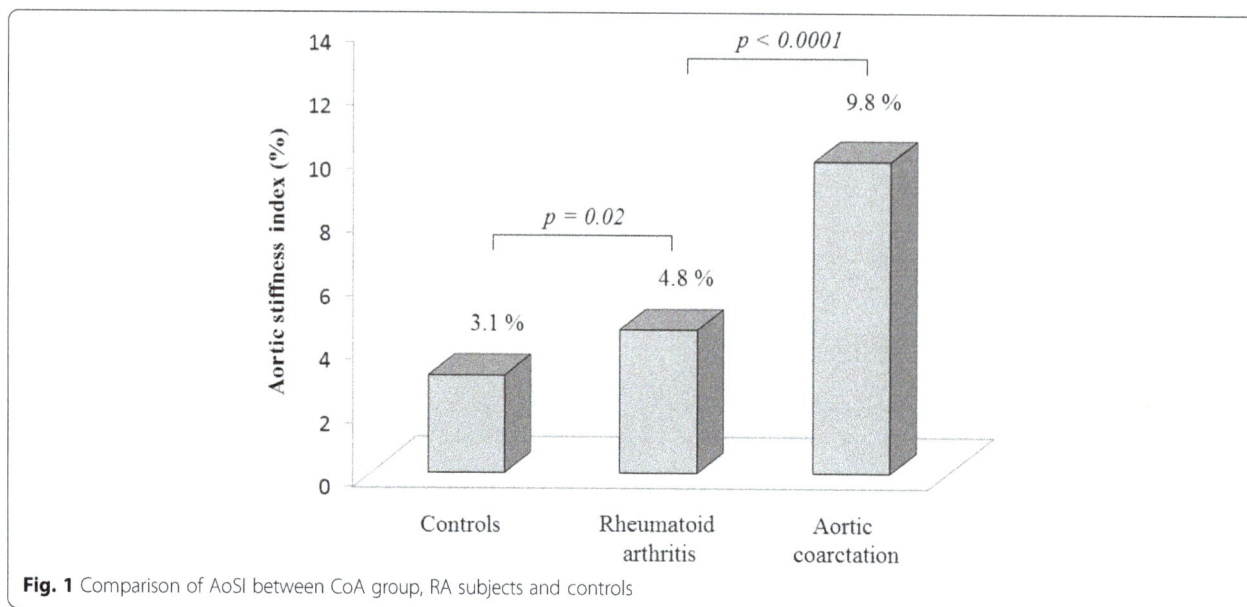

Fig. 1 Comparison of AoSI between CoA group, RA subjects and controls

age, sex, blood pressure and history of hypertension, and the other one, affected by RA. Three main and original findings emerged by our analyses: 1) AoSI was significantly higher in CoA patients than in RA patients or non-RA matched patients; 2) increased AoSI was not homogeneous in CoA patients: two distinct groups, indeed, were identified, the first including near a quarter of subjects who had abnormally high values of AoSI, the second including the remaining three quarter of subjects who had values of AoSI in the normal range; 3) in CoA

patients, AoSI was independently related to LV hypertrophy and concentric LV geometry.

We previously demonstrated persistence of reduced systolic LV long axis and diastolic functions in the long run after successful repair of CoA. In addition, Lam et al. showed that systolic LV long axis dysfunction was associated with increased AoSI in adult patients with corrected CoA, independently from other potential confounders such as hypertension and associated bicuspid aortic valve. More recently, Voges et al. demonstrated a combination

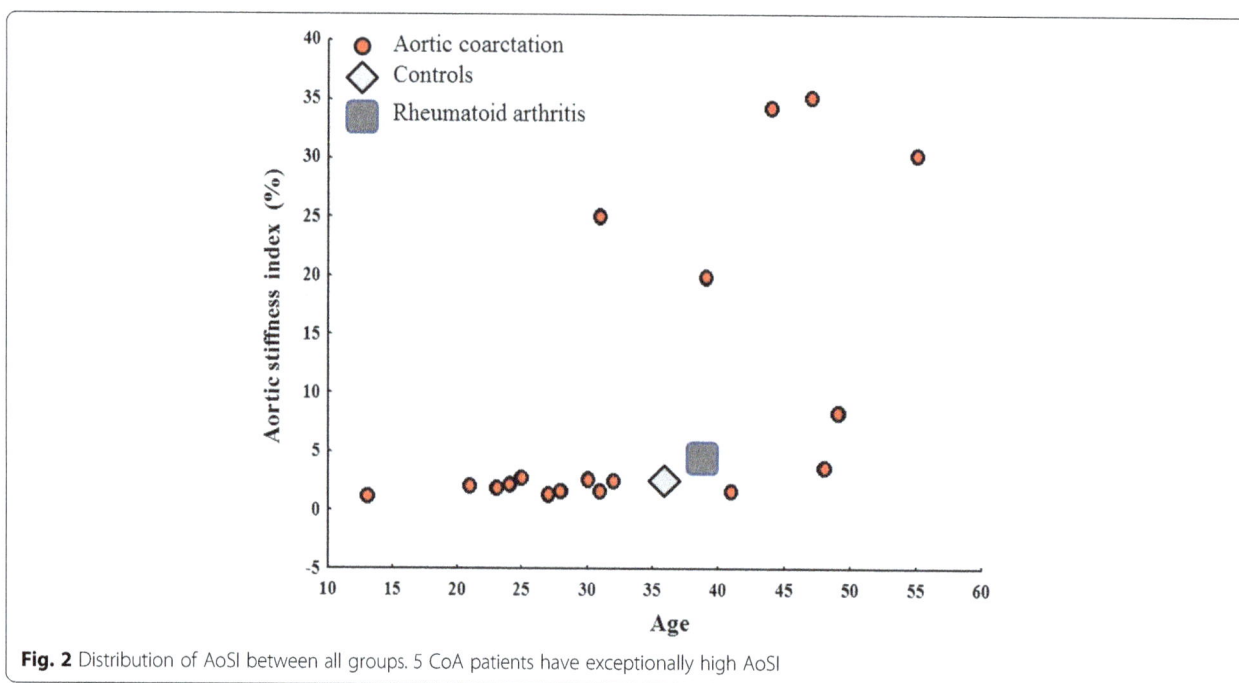

Fig. 2 Distribution of AoSI between all groups. 5 CoA patients have exceptionally high AoSI

Table 3 Variables significantly different between aortic coartaction patients who had abnormally high aortic stiffness and those who had not

Total study population (19 patients)	Abnormally high aortic stiffness NO (14 patients)	Abnormally high aortic stiffness YES (5 patients)	p
Age (years)	30 ± 10	43 ± 9	0.02
Body mass index (Kg/m^2)	22.2 ± 2.7	27.7 ± 4.5	0.004
Systolic blood pressure (mmHg)	120 ± 14	144 ± 14	0.004
Diastolic blood pressure (mmHg)	73 ± 9	83 ± 10	0.04
E / E' ratio	9.5 ± 2.1	13.7 ± 5.1	0.02
LV end-diastolic pressure (mmHg)	14 ± 3	19 ± 6	0.02
Relative wall thickness	0.33 ± 0.04	0.41 ± 0.04	0.002
LV mass index (g/m $^{2.7}$)	36 ± 13	56 ± 5	0.006
LV hypertrophy (%)	15	100	< 0.001
Aortic stiffness index (%)	2.5 ± 1.9	28.9 ± 6.5	< 0.001

E/E' ratio = ratio between peak of early (E) wave of transmitral flow and peak (E') early diastolic Tissue Doppler velocity of mitral annulus

between the impairment of elastic properties in the thoracic aorta with the remodeling of the common carotid artery in young patients nearly fifteen years after CoA repair [28]. Collectively, these findings suggest that CoA might determine aortic wall changes as a systemic vessel disease in humans. Using a clinically representative rabbit model of CoA and correction, Menon et al. [29] quantified mechanical alterations from a 20-mmHg blood pressure gradient in the thoracic aorta and related the expression of key smooth muscle contractile and focal adhesion proteins with aortic remodeling, reduced relaxation and increased stiffness. These structural and functional changes were attributed to a significant increase in non-muscle myosin and reduced smooth muscle myosin heavy chain expression in the proximal arteries of CoA which was not reversed upon blood pressure correction. Furthermore, Gardiner et al. [30] found that, arterial dilation induced by glyceryltrinitrate was significantly impaired in the pre-coarctation vascular bed of young adults who had undergone successful repair of coarctation in childhood. These results may be an important contributor to rest and/or exercise-related hypertension and late morbidity or mortality of these subjects.

Table 4 Variables significantly related to aortic stiffness index (expressed as continuous variable): multiple linear regression analysis

	Standardized coefficients beta	P
Left ventricular hypertrophy	0.62	< 0.001
Left ventricular relative wall thickness	0.34	0.04
Final results multivariate regression model Intercept = − 25.0 Standard error of estimation = 6.9 r ^{2} = 0.74	0.86	< 0.001

Arterial stiffness and AoSI are independent predictors of cardiovascular morbidity and mortality [9]. A number of previous studies confirmed that non-invasive AoSI had a strong correlation with invasive measurements of arterial stiffness, and that the aortic elastic properties deteriorate in patients with coronary artery disease [10, 12]. Vitarelli et al. showed that the measurement of AoSI allows to differentiate hypertensive from healthy adults [11]. In addition, AoSI is increased in women with a previous pregnancy complicated by early onset of pre-eclampsia. Recently, Said et al. demonstrated that AoSI measured by photofletmismography is an independent predictor of cardiovascular events and mortality in a UK large community-based population [9]. From the analysis of our AoSI data, two different phenotypes of repaired CoA patients emerged, corresponding to two distinct pathophysiological models. CoA patients with abnormally high AoSI, indeed, were largely different in comparison with the counterparts with normal AoSI, being older, with higher body mass index, blood pressure, LV mass remodeled in a concentric fashion, and with worse LV diastolic function. In these patients, greater LV hypertrophy and relative wall thickness were possibly due to the persistent LV pressure-overload. So, an older age at the time of intervention seems to promote the development of sky high AoSI more than nearly three decades of follow up with well controlled blood pressure. In our study, we compared LV properties and AoSI in CoA and RA patients. Both diseases are characterized by a lower life expectancy owing to premature CV diseases. RA is a model of acquired extensive arterial disease with abnormal vascular responses due to a number of cytotoxic agents, pro-inflammatory and immuno-modulatory molecules and hyper-functioning neuro-hormonal systems. In line with previous experiences, RA patients had a prevalence of abnormally high AoSI nearly two-fold higher than controls matched for the traditional CV risk factors. Although an increased AoSI is a strong predictor of adverse clinical outcome at mid-term follow-up, our RA subjects were less treated with medications compared to CoA and controls. This data is coherent with that derived by the EPIDAURO registry showing the CV risk stratification missing in daily clinical practice of RA patients [31]. CoA and RA represent different pathophysiological models of aortic disease. The first one is an acquired structural damage primarily caused by hemodynamic factors of longstanding distal obstruction that lead to higher collagen load with a lower elastin and smooth muscle content [32, 33]. The second one is related to non-hemodynamic factors such pro-inflammatory, immunomodulatory, and cytotoxic agents that accelerate vascular atherosclerosis, myocardial fibrosis, and apoptosis by way of direct damage of the myocardial tissue. Despite these different models and magnitude of AoSI, we found several common points. The reduced long-term survival unites CoA and RA patients in the follow up. Persistence or newly developed systemic hypertension and AoSI may cause significant abnormalities in the CV system of both diseases such as LV remodelling and dysfunction, thereby compromising the prognosis.

Study limitations

This study has several limitations. Firstly, it was not adequately powered to determine the effect of other potential confounders (clinical significance of very mild residual narrowing at CoA site, difference between surgical or endovascular treatment approach and usage of antihypertensive medications) on central aortic elastic properties. Secondly, due to the small sample size of the study population, we cannot draw any prognostic inference regarding the detection of abnormally high AoSI condition. Furthermore, the evaluation of AoSI by central pulse pressure as assessed by radial artery tonometry and pulse wave analysis instead of the brachial artery pulse pressure might be more accurate than M-mode-derived aortic recordings and brachial blood pressure we used. Strengths of our study include the very long-term follow-up, the consecutive enrollment of patients, the reliable and appropriate method utilized for the assessment of AoSI, and the comprehensive nature of the dataset.

Conclusions

CoA patients have higher AoSI levels than RA patients and non-RA matched controls. AoSI levels are abnormally high in a small sub-group of CoA patients who show a very high-risk clinical profile for adverse CV events. Although CoA and RA represent two different pathophysiological models of CV disease, they are characterized by common detrimental consequences on LV function and aortic properties. In CoA patients, intervention at an early age before potentially irreversible structural changes

to proximal aorta, might be clinically relevant while in RA patients, appropriate medical treatment to reduce AoSI, might preserve LV geometry and function. These can only be speculative conclusions: nonetheless, the results of this study reinforce the importance of the notion that the measurement of AoSI in CoA and RA patients should conceivably be introduced into routine clinical practice.

Abbreviations
AoD: Diastolic aortic diameter; AoS: Systolic aortic diameter; AoSI: Aortic stiffness index; CoA: Aortic coarctation; CV: cardiovascular; DBP: Diastolic blood pressure; E: Early diastolic velocity of transmitral flow; E′: Early diastolic Tissue Doppler velocity of mitral annulus; LV: Left ventricular; LVSD: LV systolic dysfunction; RA: Rheumatoid arthritis; S′: Mitral annular systolic velocity; SBP: Systolic blood pressure; sc-MS: Midwall end-systolic circumferential stress

Acknowledgements
The authors recognize "Amici del Cuore - Charity" for supporting the publication.

Authors' contributions
GF contributed to the study design, researched data, wrote the manuscript; GC contributed to the study design, performed statistical analysis, researched data, wrote the manuscript; MR, FO, AG, MF, GR, CDN, SD, LT, CM, AC, BDM, and CP researched data, contributed to the discussion and edited manuscript; ADL, GFS and OV contributed to the study design, contributed to the discussion and edited manuscript. All authors read and approved the final manuscript.

Competing interests
The authors declare that they have no competing interests.

Author details
¹Cardiovascular Centre, Department of Cardiology, Azienda Sanitaria Universitaria Integrata di Trieste, via Slataper n°9, 34134 Trieste, Italy. ²Department of Cardiology, Villa Bianca Hospital, Trento, Italy. ³Department of Medicine, Azienda Ospedaliera Universitaria Integrata di Verona, Verona, Italy. ⁴Department of cardiology, Ospedale Civile S. Martino, Belluno, Italy. ⁵Division of Cardiology, Institute for Maternal and Child Health, IRCCS Burlo Garofolo, Trieste, Italy. ⁶Department of Cardiology, Azienda Sanitaria Universitaria Integrata di Trieste, Trieste, Italy.

References
1. Brown ML, Burkhart HM, Connolly HM. Coarctation of the aorta: lifelong surveillance is mandatory following surgical repair. J Am Coll Cardiol. 2013; 62:1020–5.
2. Clarkson PM, Nicholson MR, Barrat-Boyes BG, Neutze JM, Whitlock RM. Results after repair of coarctation of the aorta beyond infancy: 10 to 28 year follow-up with particular reference to late systemic hypertension. Am J Cardiol. 1983;51:1481–8.
3. Faganello G, Fisicaro M, Russo G, Iorio A, Mazzone C, Grande E, Humar F, Cherubini A, Pandullo C, Barbati G, et al. Insights from cardiac mechanics after three decades from successfully repaired aortic Coarctation. Congenit Heart Dis. 2016;11:254–61.
4. Florianczyk T, Werner B. Assessment of left ventricular systolic function using tissue Doppler imaging in children after successful repair of aortic coarctation. Clin Physiol Funct Imaging. 2010;30:1–5.
5. Lam Y-Y, Mullen MJ, Kaya MG, Gatzoulis MA, Li W, Henein MY. Left ventricular long axis dysfunction in adults with "corrected" aortic coarctation is related to an older age at intervention and increased aortic stiffness. Heart. 2009;95:733–9.
6. Mivelaz Y, Leung MT, Zadorsky MT, De Souza AM, Potts JE, Sandor GG. Noninvasive assessment of vascular function in postoperative cardiovascular disease (Coarctation of the aorta, tetralogy of Fallot, and transposition of the great arteries). Am J Cardiol. 2016;118:597–602.

7. Solomon DH, Goodson NJ, Katz JN, Weinblatt ME, Avorn J, Setoguchi S, Canning C, Schneeweiss S. Patterns of cardiovascular risk in rheumatoid arthritis. Ann Rheum Dis. 2006;65(12):1608–12.

8. Cioffi G, Viapiana O, Ognibeni F, Dalbeni A, Orsolini G, Adami S, Gatti D, Fisicaro M, Tarantini L, Rossini M. Clinical profile and outcome of patients with rheumatoid arthritis and abnormally high aortic stiffness. Eur J Prev Cardiol. 2016;23(17):1848–59.

9. Said MA, Eppinga RN, Lipsic E, Verweij N, van der Harst P. Relationship of Arterial Stiffness Index and Pulse Pressure With Cardiovascular Disease and Mortality. J Am Heart Assoc. 2018;7(2).

10. Stefanadis C, Dernellis J, Tsiamis E, Stratos C, Diamantopoulos L, Michaelides A, Toutouzas P. Aortic stiffness as a risk factor for recurrent acute coronary events in patients with ischaemic heart disease. Eur Heart J. 2000;21(5):390–6.

11. Vitarelli A, Giordano M, Germanò G, Pergolini M, Cicconetti P, Tomei F, Sancini A, Battaglia D, Dettori O, Capotosto L, De Cicco V, De Maio M, Vitarelli M, Bruno P. Assessment of ascending aorta wall stiffness in hypertensive patients by tissue Doppler imaging and strain Doppler echocardiography. Heart. 2010;96(18):1469–74.

12. Güngör B, Yılmaz H, Ekmekçi A, Özcan KS, Tijani M, Osmonov D, Karataş B, Taha Alper A, Mutluer FO, Gürkan U, Bolca O. Aortic stiffness is increased in patients with premature coronary artery disease: a tissue Doppler imaging study. J Cardiol. 2014;63(3):223–9.

13. Vitarelli A, Conde Y, Cimino E, D'Angeli I, D'Orazio S, Stellato S, Padella V, Caranci F. Assessment of aortic wall mechanics in Marfan syndrome by transesophageal tissue Doppler echocardiography. Am J Cardiol. 2006;97:571–7.

14. Arnett FC, Edworthy SM, Bloch DA, McShane DJ, Fries JF, Cooper NS, Healey LA, Kaplan SR, Liang MH, Luthra HS, et al. The American rheumatism association 1987 revised criteria for the classification of rheumatoid arthritis. Arthritis Rheum. 1988;31:315–24.

15. Devereux RB, Alonso DR, Lutas EM, Gottlieb GJ, Campo E, Sachs I, Reichek N. Echocardiographic assessment of left ventricular hypertrophy: comparison to necropsy findings. Am J Cardiol. 1986;57:450–8.

16. de Simone G, Devereux RB, Daniels SR, Daniels SR, Koren MJ, Meyer RA, Laragh JH. Effect of growth on variability of left ventricular mass: assessment of allometric signals in adults and children and their capacity to predict cardiovascular risk. J Am Coll Cardiol. 1995;25:1056–62.

17. de Simone G, Daniels SR, Kimball TR, Roman MJ, Romano C, Chinali M, Galderisi M, Devereux RB. Evaluation of concentric left ventricular geometry in humans: evidence for age-related systematic underestimation. Hypertension. 2005;45:64–8.

18. de Simone G, Devereux RB, Koren MJ, Mensah GA, Casale PN, Laragh JH. Midwall left ventricular mechanics: an independent predictor of cardiovascular risk in arterial hypertension. Circulation. 1996;93:259–65.

19. de Simone G, Devereux RB, Roman MJ, Ganau A, Saba PS, Alderman MH, Laragh JH. Assessment of left ventricular function by the midwall fractional shortening/end-systolic stress relation in human hypertension. J Am Coll Cardiol. 1994;23:1444–51.

20. Sohn DW, Chai IH, Lee DJ, Kim HC, Kim HS, Oh BH, Lee MM, Park YB, Choi YS, Seo JD, Lee YW. Assessment of mitral annulus velocity by tissue Doppler imaging in the evaluation of left ventricular diastolic function. J Am Coll Cardiol. 1997;30:474–80.

21. Nagueh SF, Smiseth OA, Appleton CP, Byrd BF 3rd, Dokainish H, Edvardsen T, Flachskampf FA, Gillebert TC, Klein AL, Lancellotti P, et al. Recommendations for the evaluation of left ventricular diastolic function by echocardiography: an update from the American Society of Echocardiography and the European Association of Cardiovascular Imaging. J Am Soc Echocardiogr. 2016;2016(29): 277–314.

22. Redfield MM, Jacobsen SJ, Burnett JC Jr, Mahoney DW, Bailey KR, Rodeheffer RJ. Burden of systolic and diastolic ventricular dysfunction in the community: appreciating the scope of the heart failure epidemic. J Am Med Assoc. 2003; 289:194–202.

23. Ommen SR, Nishimura RA, Appleton CP, Miller FA, Oh JK, Redfield MM, Tajik AJ. Clinical utility of Doppler echocardiography and tissue Doppler imaging in the estimation of left ventricular filling pressures: a comparative simultaneous Doppler-catheterization study. Circulation. 2000;102:1788–94.

24. Aldousany AW, DiSessa TG, Alpert BS, Birnbaum SE, Willey ES. Significance of the Doppler-derived gradient across a residual coarctation. Pediatr Cardiol. 1990;11:8–14.

25. Guenthard J, Zumsteg UWF. Arm-leg pressure gradients on late follow-up after coarctation repair. Possible causes and implications. Eur Heart J. 1996; 17:1572–5.

26. Nistri S, Grande-Allen J, Noale M, Basso C, Siviero P, Maggi S. Aortic elasticity and size in bicuspid aortic valve syndrome. Eur Heart J. 2008;29(4):472–9.

27. Stefanadis C, Stratos C, Boudoulas H, Vlachopoulos C, Kallikazaros I, Toutouzas P. Distensibility of the ascending aorta: comparison of invasive and noninvasive techniques in healthy men and in men with coronary artery disease. Eur Heart J. 1990;11:990–6.

28. Voges I, Kees J, Jerosch-Herold M, Gottschalk H, Trentmann J, Hart C, Gabbert DD, Pardun E. PhamM, Andrade1 AC et al. Aortic stiffening and its impact on left atrial volumes and function in patients after successful coarctation repair: a multiparametric cardiovascular magnetic resonance study J Cardiovasc Magn Reson. 2016;18:56.

29. Menon A, Eddinger TJ, Wang H, Wendell DC, Toth JM, LaDisa JF Jr. Altered hemodynamics, endothelial function, and protein expression occur with aortic coarctation and persist after repair. Am J Physiol Heart Circ Physiol. 2012;303:1304–18.

30. Gardiner HM, Celermajer DS, Sorensen KE, Georgakopoulos D, Robinson J, Thomas O, Deanfield JE. Arterial reactivity is significantly impaired in norm otensive young adults after successful repair of aortic coarctation in childhood. Circulation. 1994;89:1745–50.

31. Faden G, Viapiana O, Fischetti F, Faganello G, Gatti D, Tarantini L, Di Lenarda A, Adami S, Tincani A, Filippini M, et al. Cardiovascular risk stratification and management of patients with rheumatoid arthritis in clinical practice: The "EPIDAURO registry.". Int J Cardiol. 2014;172:534–6.

32. Sehested J, Baandrup U. Different reactivity and structure of the prestenotic and poststenotic aorta in human coarctation. Implications for baroreceptor function. Circulation. 1982;65:1060–5.

33. Cioffi G, Viapiana O, Ognibeni F, Dalbeni A, Giollo A, Gatti D, Mazzone C, Faganello G, Di Lenarda A, Adami S, et al. Combined circumferential and longitudinal left ventricular systolic dysfunction in patients with rheumatoid arthritis without overt cardiac disease. J Am Soc Echocardiogr. 2016;29:689–98.

25

Left atrial strain - an early marker of left ventricular diastolic dysfunction in patients with hypertension and paroxysmal atrial fibrillation

Jonas Jarasunas[*] (iD), Audrius Aidietis and Sigita Aidietiene

Abstract

Background: 2D strain imaging of the left atrium (LA) is a new echocardiographic method which allows us to determine contractile, conduit and reservoir functions separately. This method is particularly useful when changes are subtle and not easily determined by traditional parameters, as it is in arterial hypertension and atrial fibrillation (AF). The aims of our study were: to determine LA contractile, conduit and reservoir function by 2D strain imaging in patients with mild arterial hypertension and paroxysmal AF; to assess LA contractile, conduit and reservoir functions' relation with LV diastolic dysfunction (DD) parameters.

Methods: LA contractile, conduit and reservoir functions together with echocardiographic signs of LV DD were assessed in 63 patients with arterial hypertension and paroxysmal AF. Patients were grouped according to number of signs showing LV DD (annular e' velocity: septal e' < 7 cm/s, lateral e' < 10 cm/s, average E/e' ratio > 14, LA volume index > 34 ml/m^2, peak tricuspid regurgitation velocity > 2.8 m/s) present. Number of patients with 0 signs – 17, 1 sign – 26, 2 signs – 19. Contractile, conduit and reservoir functions were compared between the groups.

Results: Mean contractile, conduit and reservoir strains in all the patients were − 14.14 (± 5.83) %, 15.98 (± 4.85) % and 31.03 (± 7.64) % respectively. Contractile strain did not differ between the groups. Conduit strain was higher in patients with 0 signs compared with other groups ($p = 0.016$ vs 1 sign of LV DD and $p = 0.001$ vs 2 signs of LV DD). Reservoir strain was higher in patients with 0 signs compared with other groups ($p = 0.014$ vs 1 sign of LV DD and $p < 0.001$ vs 2 signs of LV DD).

Conclusions: The patients with paroxysmal AF and primary arterial hypertension have decreased reservoir, conduit and pump LA functions even in the absence of echocardiographic signs of LV DD. With increasing number of parameters showing LV DD, LA conduit and reservoir functions decrease while contractile does not change. LA conduit and reservoir functions decrease earlier than the diagnosis of LV DD can be established according to the guidelines in patients with primary arterial hypertension and AF.

Keywords: Left atrial strain, Diastolic dysfunction, Arterial hypertension, Atrial fibrillation

* Correspondence: jonasjar@gmail.com
Clinic of Cardiac and Vascular Diseases, Institute of Clinical Medicine, Faculty
of Medicine, Vilnius University, Universiteto g. 3, LT-01513 Vilnius, Lithuania

Background

Traditionally the greatest attention during a routine echocardiography is paid to the function of the ventricles and assessment of the atria is limited to measuring the dimensions and volumes of the chambers. Though assessing ventricular function is essential, there is robust data that atrial function is also important and can improve our decision making by determining the risk of cardiovascular events in various conditions [1]. Hypertension is the most common predisposing factor for left ventricular (LV) diastolic dysfunction (DD), which leads to increased left atrial (LA) pressure, its enlargement and fibrosis as well as other proarrhythmic pathological effects on atrial structure and function [2, 3]. These changes cause various cardiac arrhythmias, most commonly atrial fibrillation (AF), an arrhythmia that carries a substantial risk of embolic events. Hypertension and even high-normal blood pressure is a risk factor for developing AF and recent guidelines for the management of arterial hypertension clearly state that AF should be considered a manifestation of hypertensive heart disease [4]. LA function might also be linked to the cardioembolic risk profile in patients with AF and can even provide incremental value for embolism risk stratification over CHA2DS2-VASc score [5, 6]. Recently announced EACVI AFib Echo Europe Registry for assessing relationships of echocardiographic parameters with clinical thrombo-embolic and bleeding risk profile in non-valvular AF aims to determine echocardiographic parameters stratifying prognosis and improving management in categories of AF patients. In this regard LA parameters are among the most promising ones [7].

There are many well established and validated methods to assess left and right ventricular function but the ones for assessing atrial function are lacking. Speckle tracking echocardiography has proven to be useful and applicable not only in the assessment of LV wall motion abnormalities but also in the assessment of LA function. Though the method is more and more studied it is still not widely used in daily clinical practice primarily because there are still some methodological and standardization issues which need to be addressed. The question of normal values is also still valid, though metanalysis by Faraz Pathan et al. was a real step forward in determining normal ranges [8].

One of the most promising areas the method can be used in is hypertension where the LA and LV dysfunctions occuring early in the course of disease can be subtle and not easily determined by traditional echocardiographic parameters [9]. 2D strain parameters of the LA can help to detect increased filling pressures and DD of the LV earlier [10], and, which is very important, antihypertensive treatment can reverse these changes [11].

The aims of our study were: a) to determine LA contractile, conduit and reservoir function by 2D strain imaging in patients with mild arterial hypertension and paroxysmal atrial fibrillation; b) to assess LA contractile, conduit and reservoir functions' relation with LV filling pressure parameters recommended by the American Society of Echocardiography and the European Association of Cardiovascular Imaging [12].

Methods

We assessed 63 patients aged 18–80 with I or II grade primary arterial hypertension and at least one ECG confirmed episode of paroxysmal AF within last year. Only the patients that were in sinus rhythm at the time of investigation were included in the study. Patients with other known causes of AF such as heart failure, coronary heart disease, prior heart surgery, structural heart disease, reduced LV ejection fraction, thyroid dysfunction (assessed by thyroid-stimulating hormone concentration) or renal failure with glomerular filtration rate < 60 ml/min were excluded from the study. Only the ones with hypertension as a possible causative factor for AF were included in the study.

Physical examination, including weight and height was performed. All patients underwent ambulatory blood pressure monitoring, which was carried out according to European Society of Hypertension guidelines [13]. A Meditech card(X)plore monitor and CardioVisions 1.23.0 software were used. The measurements were taken in 20-min intervals during the day and in 40-min intervals during the night. The patients who did not meet the 70% successful measurement criterion were excluded from the analysis.

All the patients had an ECG and sonography of the heart done. Only the ones with acceptable ultrasound image quality were included in the final analysis. A GE Vivid E9 system was used for ultrasound imaging in our study. Routine sonographic examination of the heart was performed as described in the American and European Society of Echocardiography guidelines and their update [14–16] with a cardiac probe M5S-D.

The thicknesses of the interventricular septal and the inferolateral walls as well as LV end-diastolic and end-systolic diameters were obtained from the parasternal short-axis view. LV mass (LVM) was calculated using linear method as recommended in the update Recommendations for cardiac chamber quantification by echocardiography in adults [16]. Cube formula was used:

$$LVM = 0.8 \times 1.04 \left[(LVEDd + PWDd + IVSDd)^3 - LVEDd^3 \right] + 0.6 \, g.$$

where LVEDd is LV end-diastolic internal diameter; PWDd, diastolic posterior wall thickness; and IVSTd, diastolic interventricular septal thickness. To determine

LV hypertrophy LVM was subsequently indexed to body surface area BSA (calculated using DuBois formula). Two waves (E and A) of mitral inflow velocity were recorded using pulsed wave Doppler from the apical 4 chamber view. The velocity waves (e' and a') of mitral annulus septal and lateral regions were recorded using tissue Doppler. When calculating E/e' ratio, an average value of septal and lateral mitral annulus velocities was used.

LV and LA volumes were determined using the biplane disk summation technique from apical 4-chamber and 2-chamber views. LV end systolic and end diastolic volume was recorded, then LV ejection fraction was calculated using these measurements.

Global longitudinal 2D LA strain was analyzed by the speckle tracking technique using GE EchoPAC software. The images were acquired according to the recommendations given by expert consensus statement published in the European Journal of Echocardiography [17]. For analysis we used four-chamber and two chamber apical view images of LA carefully avoiding foreshortening. The focus was set to the level of mid-LA to optimize the image quality. Sector depth and width was adjusted to include as little as possible outside the region of interest. Three consecutive heart cycles were recorded during a single breath hold using a frame rate of > 80 frames/second for offline analysis. The endocardial border of LA was manually traced and a region of interest was manually adjusted to include the entire LA wall thickness. The software selected stable speckles within the LA wall and tracked these speckles frame-by-frame throughout

the cardiac cycle. The entire LA tracking was then divided into 6 segments by the software and tracking quality for each segment was provided. If the tracking was not acceptable, endocardial borders were readjusted until better tracking was achieved. Then, we set the starting point of strain analysis as P-wave onset instead the software preset R-wave peak. The automated software then generated traces depicting the regional longitudinal strain for each segment and calculated global longitudinal strain. Using P wave onset as starting enabled us to define first negative peak, which occurred at maximal LA contraction and represented its contractile function (contractile strain), first positive peak, which occurred at mitral valve opening and represented LA conduit function (conduit strain), and the difference of these peaks, which represented reservoir function (reservoir strain). The values were averaged for all 12 LA segments - 6 in apical four chamber view and 6 in apical two chamber view. LA strain image from four-chamber apical view is shown in Fig. 1. Analogous measurements were performed from apical two-chamber views.

LV diastolic function and filing pressures were evaluated according to the American Society of Echocardiography and the European Association of Cardiovascular Imaging recommendations published in 2016 [12]. The patients were grouped as having none, one, two or three signs of LV DD, according to the guidelines. The variables for identifying LV DD and their cutoffs were annular e' velocity: septal e' < 7 cm/s, lateral e' < 10 cm/s,

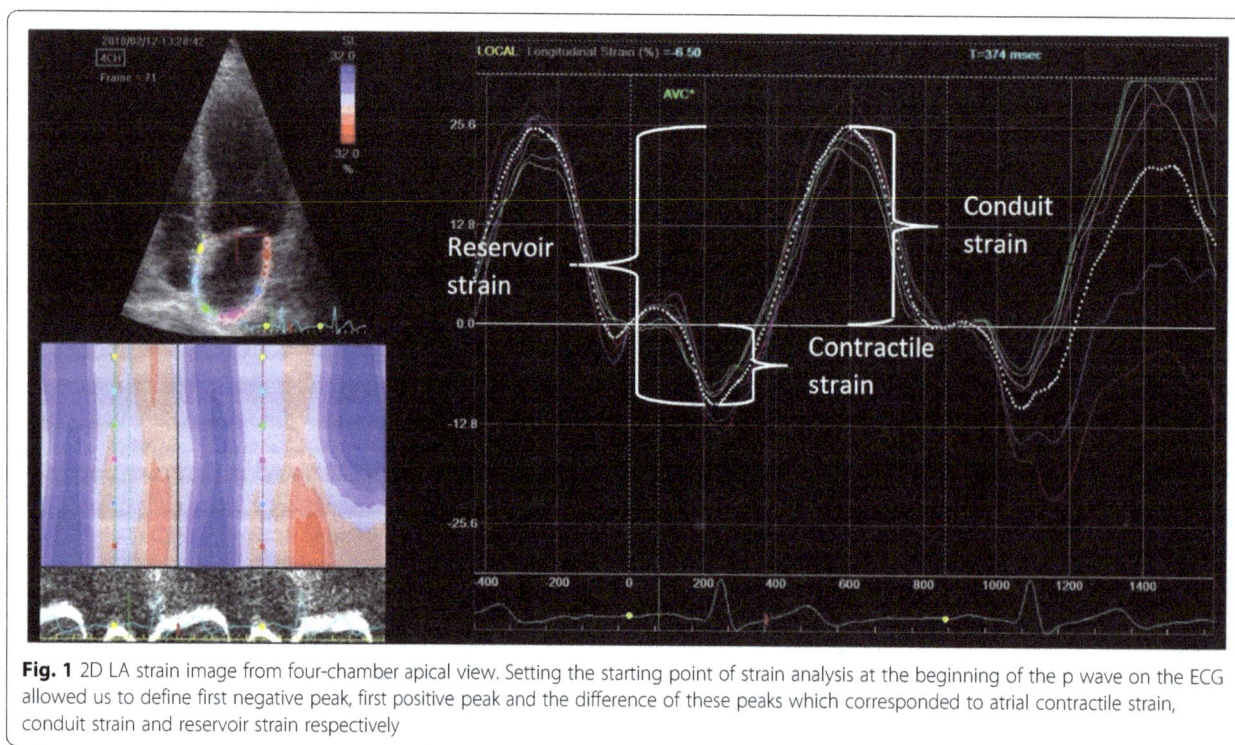

Fig. 1 2D LA strain image from four-chamber apical view. Setting the starting point of strain analysis at the beginning of the p wave on the ECG allowed us to define first negative peak, first positive peak and the difference of these peaks which corresponded to atrial contractile strain, conduit strain and reservoir strain respectively

average E/e' ratio > 14, LA volume index > 34 ml/m², peak tricuspid regurgitation velocity > 2.8 m/s.

The intra- and interobserver variability of contractile, conduit and reservoir LA strains was assessed in 20 randomly selected patients. Intraobserver variability was performed by the same echocardiographer blinded to previous measurements and interobserver variability was performed by a second experienced echocardiographer also blinded to previous measurements. The intraclass correlation coefficient together with the absolute difference divided by the mean of two measurements and given as a percentage were calculated for both intra- and interobserver variability.

For statistical analysis Microsoft Excel and SPSS Statistics 17.0 software was used. The mean values are presented ± standard deviation (SD) or 95% confidence intervals (CI). Shapiro-Wilk test was used to check if the distribution of the data was normal. The means were compared using ANOVA and Fisher's Least Significant Difference test was used for post hoc analysis. Pearson's correlation coefficient was used to test for correlation. *P* value of < 0.05 was considered significant.

Results

Sixty-three patients who met inclusion/exclusion criteria, had acceptable ultrasound picture quality and signed informed consent were included in the final analysis. The patients' demographic, physical examination and blood pressure data is presented in Table 1. Ultrasound of the heart data is presented in Table 2. Intraclass correlation coefficients (95% CI) for intraobserver variability of LA contractile, conduit and reservoir strains were 0.91 (0.79—0.96), 0.92 (0.81—0.97) and 0.94 (0.86—0.98) respectively. The absolute difference divided

Table 1 Demographic, physical examination and blood pressure data of the study population

Variable	Study population (± SD)
Age	63.08 (±11.54)
Male	41%
Height	1.71 (±0.09) m
Weight	86.56 (±15.02) kg
Body mass index (BMI)	29.52 (±4.35) kg/m²
Body surface area (BSA)	1.98 (±0.2) m²
24 h average systolic blood pressure	128.94 (±10.75) mm Hg
24 h average diastolic blood pressure	74.42 (±8.26) mm Hg
Smokers	7.9%
Number of different antihypertensive agents taken daily	1.57 (±1.15)

Table 2 Ultrasound data of the study population

Variable	Study population (± SD)
LV ejection fraction	61.48 (± 5.04) %
LVEDd	5.08 (± 0.5) cm
LV end-diastolic volume	95.16 (± 24.64) ml
IVSDd	1.05 (± 0.12) cm
PWDd	0.91 (± 0.1) cm
Indexed LV mass	92.76 (± 19.7) g/m²
LA diameter	40.86 (± 6.40) mm
LA volume	70.98 (± 20.12) ml
Indexed LA volume (LAVI)	35.80 (± 9.64) ml/m²
E/A ratio	1.11 (± 0.47)
Average septal e'	7.92 (± 0.57) cm/s
Average lateral e'	9.87 (± 2.87) cm/s
E/e' ratio	8.68 (± 2.89)
IVRT	94.31 (± 21.78) ms

by the mean of two measurements for intraobserver variability of LA contractile, conduit and reservoir strains was 5.7%, 5.5% and 4.9% respectively. Intraclass correlation coefficients (95% CI) for interobserver variability of LA contractile, conduit and reservoir strains were 0.89 (0.75—0.96), 0.91 (0.79—0.96) and 0.93 (0.82—0.97) respectively. The absolute difference divided by the mean of two measurements for interobserver variability of LA contractile, conduit and reservoir strains was 8.6%, 6.0% and 5.5% respectively. 2D strain parameters of LA are shown in Table 3. Table 4 shows comparison of contractile, conduit and reservoir strain data of our study population with normal values of healthy individuals according to metanalysis by Faraz Pathan [8].

Seventeen patients had no ultrasound signs of LV DD, 26 patients had one sign, 19 patients had two signs and only 1 patient had 3 ultrasound signs of LV DD, which allowed us to firmly diagnose LV DD according to the guidelines [12]. The single patient who had 3 signs of LV

Table 3 LA strain data of the study population

Variable	Study population (± SD)
Mean contractile strain	−14.14 (± 5.83) %
4CH contractile strain	−13.90 (± 4.51) %
2CH contractile strain	−14.39 (± 9.19) %
Mean conduit strain	15.98 (± 4.85) %
4CH conduit strain	14.99 (± 4.63) %
2CH conduit strain	16.97 (± 5.78) %
Mean reservoir strain	31.03 (± 7.64) %
4CH reservoir strain	28.89 (± 7.30) %
2CH reservoir strain	33.17 (± 9.28) %

Table 4 LA strain data compared with normal values in healthy individuals

Variable	Study population (95% CI)	Normal values according to metanalysis (95% CI) [8]
Mean contractile strain	−14.14 (−15.61--12.67) %	17.4 (16.0–19.0) %
Mean conduit strain	15.98 (14.76–17.20) %	23.0 (20.7–25.2) %
Mean reservoir strain	31.03 (29.11–32.96) %	39.4% (38.0–40.8) %

Contractile, conduit and reservoir strains in patients with mild hypertension and paroxysmal AF are lower compared to normal population

DD was excluded from further analysis, so we had three groups of patients with 0, 1 or 2 signs, showing LV DD. The mean contractile, conduit and reservoir strain values are shown in Table 5. Figures 2, 3 and 4 show graphical comparison of 2D LA strain data between these groups. Contractile strain differences between the groups were not statistically significant, $p = 0.367$. Conduit strain had statistically significant differences between groups. The group without any signs of LV DD had statistically significantly higher conduit strain ($p = 0.016$ vs 1 sign of LV DD and $p = 0.001$ vs 2 signs of LV DD). Reservoir strain also followed the same pattern as conduit strain with the group that had no signs of LV DD having statistically significantly higher reservoir strain values compared with other 2 groups ($p = 0.014$ vs 1 sign of LV DD and $p < 0.001$ vs 2 signs of LV DD). Reservoir strain difference between groups with 1 and 2 signs of LV DD did not meet the cutoff of significance, $p = 0.072$. We also checked for correlation of reservoir strain with average E/e' ratio and found it to be statistically significant ($p < 0.001$) with correlation coefficient – 0.432. Regression analysis and scatter plot are shown in Fig. 5.

Discussion

The method of 2D strain imaging for the evaluation of LA function is being extensively studied and its role in risk determination is constantly increasing. Ability to maintain sinus rhythm after cardioversion or pulmonary vein isolation, reverse atrial remodeling after AF ablation, outcomes in patients with coronary artery disease, exercise capacity in heart failure, development of AF in valvular heart disease, even embolic complications in patients with AF – all these can be predicted by LA strain analysis [6, 18]. Though being so widely used and studied the method suffers from lack of standardization.

One of the main differences in the methodology is the reference point on the ECG. As most of the studies are done using GE software for LV strain analysis, the

default setting is using ventricular cycle and zero reference point by default is set at the apex of R wave. Nevertheless, for the evaluation of atrial function using atrial cycle with zero reference point set at the start of P wave generates negative contractile function strain which is more "physiological" than positive value obtained with R wave reference point. There are more studies done with R being the reference point but most of the experts, including European taskforce members, agree that the onset of the P wave should be used to analyze LA strain in sinus rhythm as we did in our study [19–21].

Of no less importance is the question which parts of LA wall to include in the strain analyses. Expert consensus document of EACVI and EHRA on the role of multi-modality imaging for the evaluation of patients with AF recommends LA strain imaging to be performed only in the lateral wall [19]. This way the influence of nearby structures such as aorta and right atrium can be diminished. Despite that, there have been different approaches in multiple studies from the evaluation of all the segments in 4, 3 and 2 chamber apical views to just 6 segments in 4 chamber apical view. Though methodologically probably the correct approach would be to evaluate all the walls of the LA from 3 apical views [20, 21], the meta-analysis done by Faraz Pathan et al. revealed that the results of the studies using four-chamber view only, four- and two-chamber views, and four-, two-, and three-chamber views were very similar: 38% (95% CI, 35–41%), 41% (95% CI, 39–43%), and 39% (95% CI, 31–47%), respectively, and the difference was not statistically significant ($p = 0.33$) [8].

Our results show that all three LA functions are lower in patients with mild well treated arterial hypertension and paroxysmal AF compared with recently established normal values. These findings suggest that in hypertensive patients changes in the LA myocardium occur very early and support the role of LA strain imaging as an important and a very sensitive marker of hypertensive

Table 5 LA strain values of patients with 0, 1, or 2 signs of LV DD

	Contractile strain mean (± SD)	Conduit strain mean (± SD)	Reservoir strain mean (± SD)
0 signs of LV DD	−15.68 (± 6.73) %	18.87 (± 4.44) %	35.82 (± 6.93) %
1 sign of LV DD	−13.74 (± 5.85) %	15.43 (± 4.57) %	30.48 (± 6.10) %
2 signs of LV DD	−12.96 (± 4.80) %	13.72 (± 4.30) %	26.68 (± 7.68) %

Strain values decrease as there are more signs of LV DD

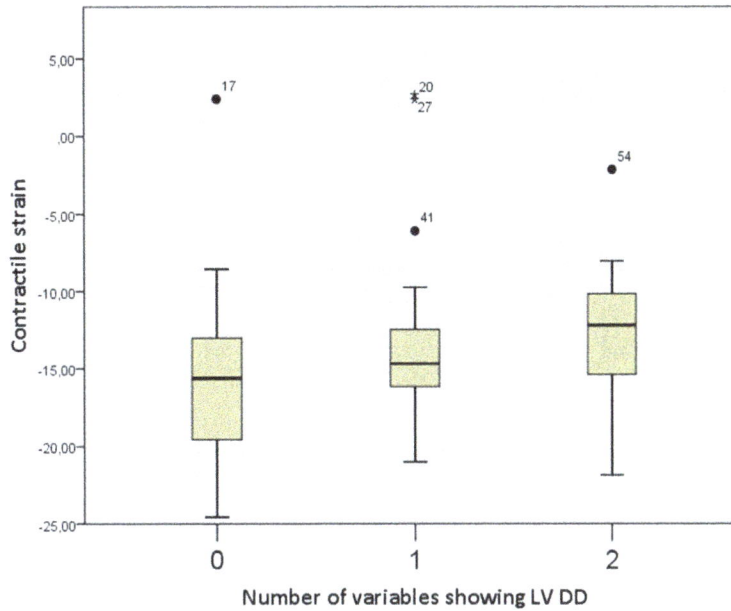

Fig. 2 Contractile strain comparison between groups with different number of LV DD signs. There was no significant difference between the groups, $p = 0.367$

heart disease [22]. Recent data from Melissa Leung that links decreased LA reservoir strain with LA fibrosis, a fundamental component of hypertensive heart disease and AF, makes it even more valid and relevant in these conditions [23].

The second part of our analysis aimed to determine how LA strain parameters change with increasing number of parameters showing LV DD. The relation of LA strain parameters with different LV DD grades has been studied before and it seems that strain parameters follow a distinct pattern with the decreasing LV diastolic function. It has been shown that the most sensitive parameters of LV DD are reservoir and conduit strains, which significantly decrease even in mild LV DD and

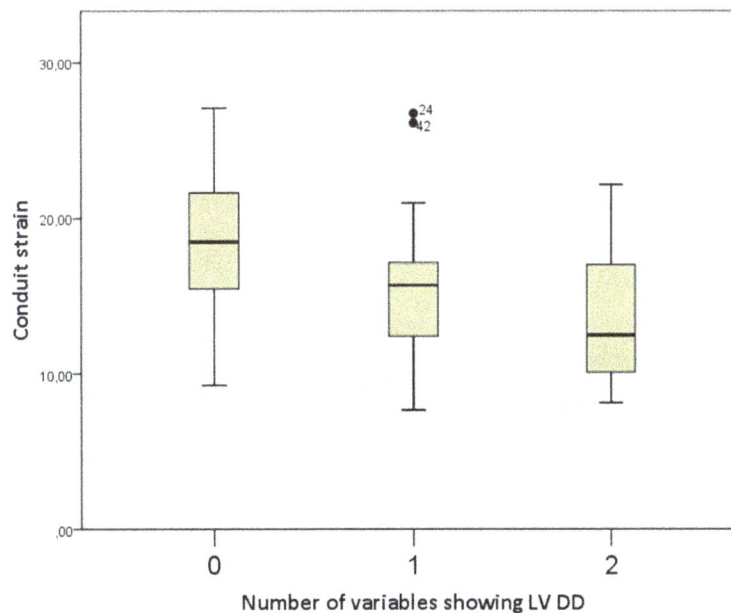

Fig. 3 Conduit strain comparison between groups with different number of LV DD signs. Group with no signs of LV DD had higher conduit strain values ($p = 0.016$ vs 1 sign of LV DD and $p = 0.001$ vs 2 signs of LV DD). Difference between groups with 1 and 2 signs of LV DD were not statistically significant, $p = 0.213$

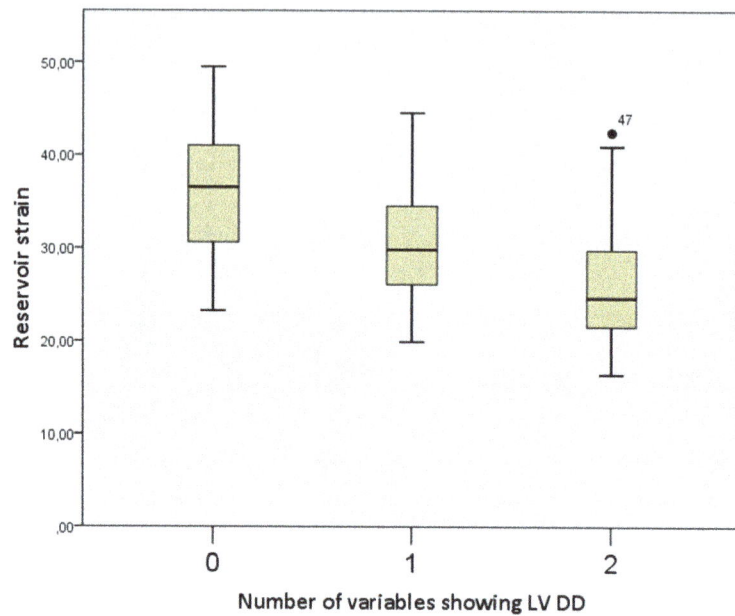

Fig. 4 Reservoir strain comparison between groups with different number of LV DD signs. Group with no signs of LV DD had higher reservoir strain values ($p = 0.014$ vs 1 sign of LV DD and $p < 0.001$ vs 2 signs of LV DD). Difference between groups with 1 and 2 signs of LV DD did not meet the cutoff of significance, $p = 0.072$

continue to decrease as the diastolic function gets worse. ROC curves show that diminished reservoir and conduit strains are superior even to LAVI in diagnosing early-stage LV DD. Meanwhile, contractile strain follows a different pattern. With mild LV DD LA contractility can even increase, dropping only when the DD is obvious [24, 25]. This seems logical and can be explained as reservoir and conduit strains mostly depend on LV longitudinal contraction and LA myocardial compliance whereas contractile strain is mostly influenced by LA myocardial contractility and LV filling pressures [26].

Our results confirm this strain changing pattern with decreasing LV diastolic function with the addition that the LA strain changes precede traditional signs of LV

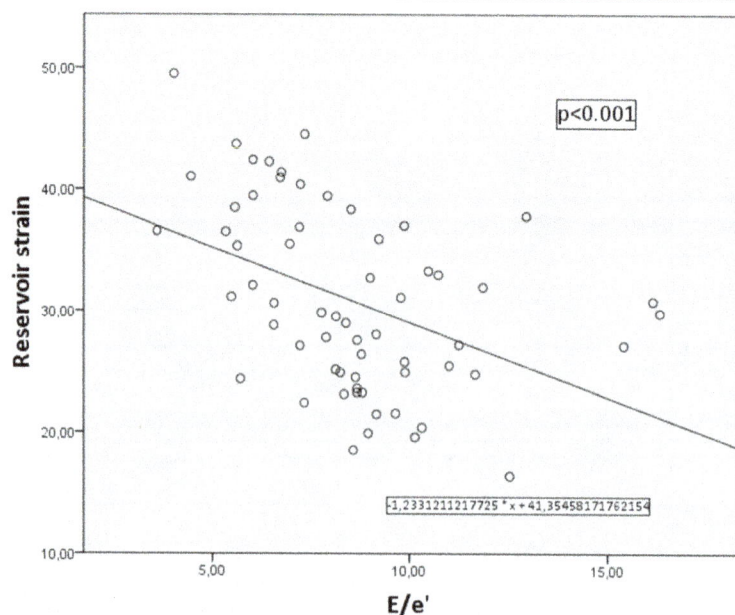

Fig. 5 Scatterplot showing relation between reservoir strain and E/e'. There is significant correlation between marker of LV DD E/e' and reservoir strain

DD. Our patients were early in the course of developing DD as the majority of them had only 1 or 2 signs of LV DD which did not allow us to make an echocardiographic diagnosis of LV DD according to the guidelines [12] but they had already decreased LA strains. With increasing LV filling pressures and decreasing LV diastolic function reservoir and conduit strain values continuously decreased, while contractile strain values did not change or even increased, though it was not statistically significant.

If we followed the recently published guidelines on LV DD [12], only one patient in our study could be firmly diagnosed with LV DD. Significant part with decreased LA strains would fall into the indeterminate LV DD category. Probably this is the area where the LA strain parameters would be most helpful and could allow us to determine the risk of future cardiovascular events better.

Conclusions
The patients with paroxysmal atrial fibrillation and primary arterial hypertension have decreased all 3 – reservoir, conduit and pump – functions assessed by 2D strain imaging even in the absence of echocardiographic signs of increased LV filling pressures. With increasing number of parameters showing high LV filling pressures LA conduit and reservoir functions decrease while contractile does not change or even increase. LA conduit and reservoir functions decrease earlier than the diagnosis of LV DD can be established according to the current guidelines in patients with primary arterial hypertension and AF.

Abbreviations
AF: Atrial fibrillation; CI: Confidence intervals; DD: Diastolic dysfunction; EACVI: European Association of Cardiovascular Imaging; EHRA: European Heart Rhythm Association; LA: Left atrium; LV: Left ventricle; SD: Standard deviation

Acknowledgements
Not applicable.

Funding
Not applicable.

Authors' contributions
JJ contributed to acquisition, analysis and interpretation of the data, was a major contributor in writing the manuscript. AA and SA contributed to conception and design of the paper, analysis and interpretation of the data. All authors read and approved the final manuscript.

Competing interests
The authors declare that they have no competing interest.

References
1. Hoit BD. Left atrial size and function: role in prognosis. J Am Coll Cardiol. 2014;63(6):493–505.
2. Lip GY. Atrial fibrillation in patients with hypertension: trajectories of risk factors in yet another manifestation of hypertensive target organ damage. Hypertension. 2016;68:544–5.
3. Rosenberg MA, Manning WJ. Diastolic dysfunction and risk of atrial fibrillation: a mechanistic appraisal. Circulation. 2012 Nov 6;126(19):2353–62.
4. Williams B, Mancia G, Spiering W, Agabiti Rosei E, Azizi M, Burnier M, Clement DL, Coca A, de Simone G, Dominiczak A, Kahan T, Mahfoud F, Redon J, Ruilope L, Zanchetti A, Kerins M, Kjeldsen SE, Kreutz R, Laurent S, Lip GYH, McManus R, Narkiewicz K, Ruschitzka F, Schmieder RE, Shlyakhto E, Tsioufis C, Aboyans V, Desormais I. 2018 ESC/ESH Guidelines for the management of arterial hypertension. Eur Heart J. 2018;39(33):3021–104.
5. Obokata M, Negishi K, Kurosawa K, Tateno R, Tange S, Arai M, Amano M, Kurabayashi M. Left atrial strain provides incremental value for embolism risk stratification over CHA$_2$DS$_2$-VASc score and indicates prognostic impact in patients with atrial fibrillation. J Am Soc Echocardiogr. 2014;27:709–716.e4.
6. Leung M, van Rosendael PJ, Abou R, Ajmone Marsan N, Leung DY, Delgado V, Bax JJ. Left atrial function to identify patients with atrial fibrillation at high risk of stroke: new insights from a large registry. Eur Heart J. 2018 Apr 21;39(16):1416–25.
7. Galderisi M, Donal E, Magne J, Lo Iudice F, Agricola E, Sade LE, Cameli M, Schwammenthal E, Cardim N, Cosyns B, Hagendorff A, Neskovic AN, Zamorano JL, Lancellotti P, Habib G, Edvardsen T, Popescu BA. Rationale and design of the EACVI AFib Echo Europe registry for assessing relationships of echocardiographic parameters with clinical thromboembolic and bleeding risk profile in non-valvular atrial fibrillation. Eur Heart J Cardiovasc Imaging. 2018 Mar 1;19(3):245–52.
8. Pathan F, D'Elia N, Nolan MT, et al. Normal ranges of left atrial strain by speckle-tracking echocardiography: a systematic review and meta-analysis. J Am Soc Echocardiogr. 2017;30:59–70.e8.
9. Xu TY, Sun JP, Lee AP, Yang XS, Ji L, Zhang Z, et al. Left atrial function as assessed by speckle-tracking echocardiography in hypertension. Medicine (Baltimore). 2015;94:e526.
10. Morris DA, Belyavskiy E, Aravind-Kumar R, Kropf M, Frydas A, Braunauer K, Marquez E, Krisper M, Lindhorst R, Osmanoglou E, Boldt LH, Blaschke F, Haverkamp W, Tschöpe C, Edelmann F, Pieske B, Pieske-Kraigher E. Potential Usefulness and Clinical relevance of adding left atrial strain to left atrial volume index in the detection of diastolic dysfunction diastolic dysfunction. JACC Cardiovasc Imaging. 2018;11(10):1405–15.
11. Degirmenci H, Duman H, Demirelli S, Bakirci EM, Hamur H, Inci S, Simsek Z, Askin L, Arisoy A, Lazoglu Z. Assessment of effect of irbesartan and nebivolol on the left atrium volume and deformation in the patients with mildmoderate hypertension. Eur Rev Med Pharmacol Sci. 2014;18(6):781–9.
12. Nagueh SF, Smiseth OA, Appleton CP, Byrd BF, Dokainish H, Edvardsen T, Flachskampf FA, Gillebert TC, Klein AL, Lancellotti P, Marino P, Oh JK, Popescu BA, Waggoner AD. Recommendations for the evaluation of left ventricular diastolic function by echocardiography: an update from the American Society of Echocardiography and the European Association of Cardiovascular Imaging. Eur Heart J Cardiovasc Imaging. 2016 Dec;17(12):1321–60.
13. O'Brien E, Parati G, Stergiou G, Asmar R, Beilin L, Bilo G, Clement D, de la Sierra A, de Leeuw P, Dolan E, Fagard R, Graves J, Head GA, Imai Y, Kario K, Lurbe E, Mallion JM, Mancia G, Mengden T, Myers M, Ogedegbe G, Ohkubo T, Omboni S, Palatini P, Redon J, Ruilope LM, Shennan A, Staessen JA, vanMontfrans G, Verdecchia P, Waeber B, Wang J, Zanchetti A, Zhang Y. European Society of Hypertension position paper on ambulatory blood pressure monitoring. J Hypertens. 2013;31:1731–68.
14. Lang RM, Bierig M, Devereux RB, Flachskampf FA, Foster E, Pellikka PA, Picard MH, Roman MJ, Seward J, Shanewise J, Solomon S, Spencer KT, St John Sutton M, Stewart W. Recommendations for chamber quantification. Eur J Echocardiogr. 2006 Mar;7(2):79–108.
15. Gottdiener JS, Bednarz J, Devereux R, Gardin J, Klein A, Manning WJ, Morehead A, Kitzman D, Oh J, Quinones M, Schiller NB, Stein JH, Weissman NJ. American Society of Echocardiography recommendations for use of echocardiography in clinical trials. J Am Soc Echocardiogr. 2004 Oct;17(10):1086–119.
16. Lang RM, Badano LP, Mor-Avi V, Afilalo J, Armstrong A, Ernande L, Flachskampf FA, Foster E, Goldstein SA, Kuznetsova T, Lancellotti P, Muraru D, Picard MH, Rietzschel ER, Rudski L, Spencer KT, Tsang W, Voigt JU. Recommendations for cardiac chamber quantification by echocardiography

in adults: an update from the American Society of Echocardiography and the European Association of Cardiovascular Imaging. J Am Soc Echocardiogr 2015;28:1–39.e14.

17. Mor-Avi V, Lang RM, Badano LP, Belohlavek M, Cardim NM, Derumeaux G, Galderisi M, Marwick T, Nagueh SF, Sengupta PP, Sicari R, Smiseth OA, Smulevitz B, Takeuchi M, Thomas JD, Vannan M, Voigt JU, Zamorano JL. Current and evolving echocardiographic techniques for the quantitative evaluation of cardiac mechanics: ASE/EAE consensus statement on methodology and indications endorsed by the Japanese Society of Echocardiography. Eur J Echocardiogr. 2011 Mar;12(3):167–205.

18. Hoit BD. Evaluation of left atrial function: current status. Structural Heart. 2017. https://doi.org/10.1080/24748706.2017.1353718.

19. Donal E, Lip GYH, Galderisi M, Goette A, Shah D, Marwan M, et al. EACVI/EHRA expert consensus document on the role of multi-modality imaging for the evaluation of patients with atrial fibrillation. Eur Heart J Cardiovasc Imaging. 2016;17(4):355–83.

20. Rimbas RC, Dulgheru RE, Vinereanu D. Methodological gaps in left atrial function assessment by 2D speckle tracking echocardiography. Arq Bras Cardiol. 2015 Dec;105(6):625–36.

21. Hayashi S, Yamada H, Bando M, et al. Optimal analysis of left atrial strain by speckle tracking echocardiography: P-wave versus R-wave trigger. Echocardiography. 2015;32:1241–9.

22. De Simone G, Mancusi C, Esposito R, De Luca N, Galderisi M. Echocardiography in arterial hypertension. High Blood Press Cardiovasc Prev. 2018 Jun;25(2):159–66.

23. Leung M, Abou R, van Rosendael PJ, van der Bijl P, van Wijngaarden SE, Regeer MV, Podlesnikar T, Ajmone Marsan N, Leung DY, Delgado V, Bax JJ. Relation of echocardiographic markers of left atrial fibrosis to atrial fibrillation burden. Am J Cardiol. 2018 Aug 15;122(4):584–91.

24. Brecht A, Oertelt-Prigione S, Seeland U, Rucke M, Hattasch R, Wagelohner T, Regitz-Zagrosek V, Baumann G, Knebel F, Stangl V. Left atrial function in preclinical diastolic dysfunction: two-dimensional speckle-tracking echocardiography-derived results from the BEFRI trial. J Am Soc Echocardiogr. 2016 Aug;29(8):750–8.

25. Singh A, Addetia K, Maffessanti F, Mor-Avi V, Lang RM. LA strain for categorization of LV diastolic dysfunction. J Am Coll Cardiol Img. 2017;10:735–43.

26. Donal E, Behagel A, Feneon D. Value of left atrial strain: a highly promising field of investigation. Eur Heart J Cardiovasc Imaging. 2015;16:356–7.

26

How I do it: feasibility of a new ultrasound probe fixator to facilitate high quality stress echocardiography

O. A. E. Salden[1][*] (iD), W. M. van Everdingen[1], R. Spee[2], P. A. Doevendans[1,3] and M. J. Cramer[1]

Abstract

Background: Stress echocardiography (SE) has recently regained momentum as an important diagnostic tool for the assessment of both ischemic and non-ischemic heart disease. Performing SE during physical exercise is challenging due to a suboptimal patient position and vigorous movements of the patient's chest. This hampers a stable ultrasound position and reduces the diagnostic performance of SE. A stable ultrasound probe position would facilitate producing high quality images during continuous measurements. With Probefix (Usono, Eindhoven, The Netherlands), a newly developed tool to fixate the ultrasound probe to the patient's chest, stabilization of the probe during physical exercise is possible.

Implementation and results: The technique of SE with the Probefix and its' feasibility are evaluated in a small pilot study. Probefix fixates the ultrasound probe to the patient's chest, using two chest straps and a fixation device. The ultrasound probe position and angle may be altered with a relative high degree of freedom. We tested the Probefix for continuous echocardiographic imaging in 12 study subjects during supine and upright ergometer stress tests. One patient was unable to perform exercise and in two study subjects good quality images were not achieved. In the other patients (82%) a stable probe position was obtained, with subsequent good quality echocardiographic images during SE.

Conclusion: We have demonstrated the feasibility of the Probefix support during ergometer tests in supine and upright positions and conclude that this external fixator may facilitate continuous monitoring of cardiac function in a group of patients.

Keywords: Stress echocardiography, Ultrasound, Probe, Fixation

Background

Stress echocardiography (SE) is a non-invasive and cost-effective tool to test myocardial function and hemodynamics during exercise [1]. It has most frequently been applied for the assessment of known or suspected ischemic heart disease, and has recently regained momentum as an important diagnostic tool [2]. The indications for the use of SE in non-ischemic heart disease are continuously evolving, as a consequence SE has also become widely implemented to assess various conditions other than ischemic heart disease, such as the assessment of systolic or diastolic heart failure, valvular heart disease, congenital heart disease, athletes' hearts, and the presence of inotropic contractile reverse in patients eligible for cardiac resynchronization therapy (CRT) [1, 3, 4].

SE during physical exercise is closest to normal physiological conditions as it preserves the integrity of the electromechanical response and provides valuable information about the patients' functional status. Pharmacological stress testing, contrastingly, does not replicate the complex hemodynamics and neurohormonal changes that are triggered by exercise [3, 5–7]. SE during physical exercise requires a treadmill or ergometer with dedicated equipment for exercise protocols. Unfortunately, physical exercise hampers a stable ultrasound probe position and echocardiographic image quality [8]. During physical exercise, the thorax moves due

---

* Correspondence: o.a.e.salden@umcutrecht.nl
[1]Department of Cardiology, University Medical Centre Utrecht, P.O. Box 85500, 3508 GA Utrecht, The Netherlands
Full list of author information is available at the end of the article

to vigorous cycling or running and heavy breathing. Both movements hamper a stable ultrasound probe position with manual application of the ultrasound probe. Additionally, due to the patient's position during exercise induced SE, obtaining high quality images is challenging. Yet, image quality is imperative for obtaining an accurate diagnosis, as anomalies can be subtle. Consequently, SE is often performed directly after peak exercise, to reduce the motion artefacts caused by exercise. However, according to previous trials that assessed the diagnostic accuracy of exercise testing, continuous SE during exercise is superior to post-exercise testing as it can detect even small, quickly reversible wall motion abnormalities. Post-exercise testing, on the other hand, can miss important information about the existence, extension, and location of ischemia [5, 6].

SE during physical exercise would be more feasible and easy if a stable ultrasound probe position can be maintained throughout the test, whilst at the same time high quality images are being produced. With Probefix (Usono, Eindhoven, The Netherlands), a newly developed tool to fixate the ultrasound probe to the patient's chest, the probe position is stabilized during echocardiography. Thereby Probefix enables stable and continuous echocardiographic measurements over time. Probefix additionally removes the necessity for sonographers to manually hold the probe during continuous stress testing, thereby enabling hands-free continuous measurements. We therefore believe that this device has the potential to improve the implementation of SE. In the present paper, we report the technique of SE with the Probefix and test its' feasibility.

Implementation
Probefix
Probefix is a non-invasive tool which provides lengthy and stable fixation of an ultrasound probe to the body. The Probefix consists of several parts that together enable fixation of the ultrasound probe to the patient's chest for continuous echocardiographic examination (Fig. 1). The device is attached to the patient's chest with two chest straps (Fig. 2). The horizontal and vertical chest strap may be adjusted to the patients' chest size by the velcro tape. The external holder of the fixator has three rings to attach the flexible chest straps. The external holder has three silicon feet by which it is placed onto the patient's chest. Within the external holder an internal holder fixates the ultrasound probe. Nonetheless, the probe angle can be altered with a relative high freedom of degrees in any direction, thus enabling rotating from, for example, the apical four chamber to two- and three chamber position. The internal holder can also be positioned up- and downward in the external ring, thereby affirming the probe towards the chest. The

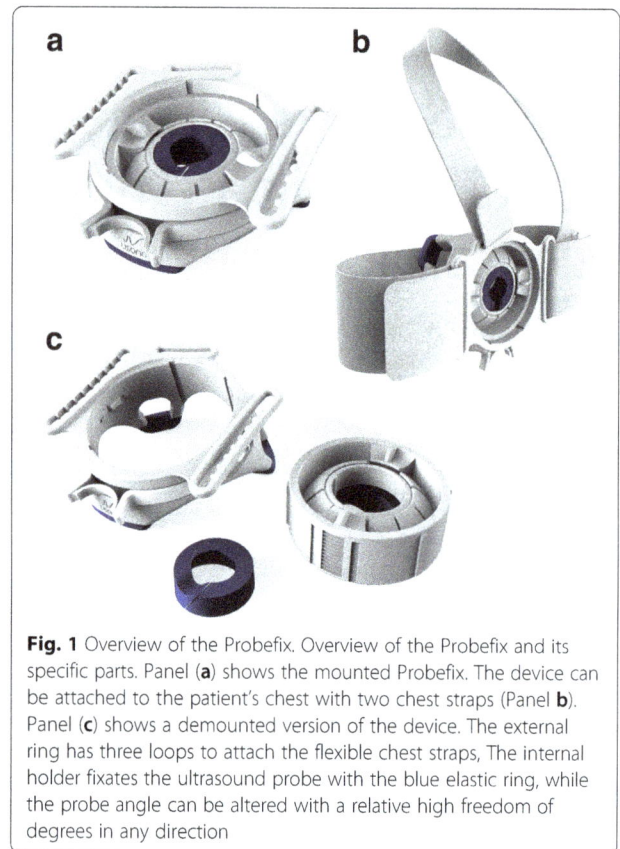

Fig. 1 Overview of the Probefix. Overview of the Probefix and its specific parts. Panel (**a**) shows the mounted Probefix. The device can be attached to the patient's chest with two chest straps (Panel **b**). Panel (**c**) shows a demounted version of the device. The external ring has three loops to attach the flexible chest straps, The internal holder fixates the ultrasound probe with the blue elastic ring, while the probe angle can be altered with a relative high freedom of degrees in any direction

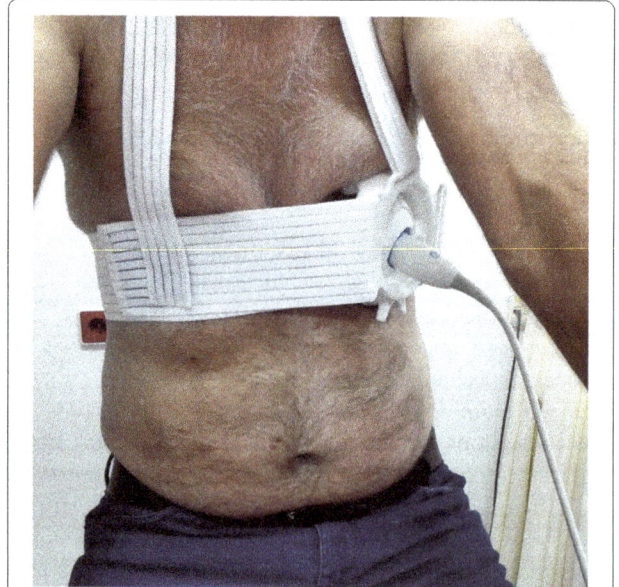

Fig. 2 Apical fixation of the Probefix for echocardiography. The ultrasound probe (M5Sc, GE Healthcare, Milwaukee, USA) is fixated to the patient's chest with the Probefix. The patient is sitting upright on the bicycle ergometer. First the optimal apical four chamber position is searched for without the fixator. Next, the probe is placed in the Probefix, which is then fixated to the patient by attaching the chest straps

probe itself is held in the internal ring by a blue elastic ring, which is moulded to match the shape of the specific ultrasound probe. By using different elastic rings, ultrasound probes of different sizes and manufacturers can be fixated in the universal Probefix.

Set up

Stress echocardiography requires a treadmill or bicycle ergometer with a dedicated system for stress protocols. The ergometer can be either upright or supine, depending on the available equipment (Figs. 3 and 4). During bicycle stress tests, a 12-lead ECG can be recorded simultaneously, combining a standard ergometer test and stress echocardiography (Fig. 3). Alongside the exercise module, an echocardiographic machine is positioned. Connected to the ultrasound machine is a conventional 2D or 3D brightness mode (B-mode) ultrasound probe.

Before positioning the ultrasound probe at the ideal acoustic window, the probe is loosely connected to the Probefix, without fixating the device to the patient's body. This set up, allows for accurate, manual

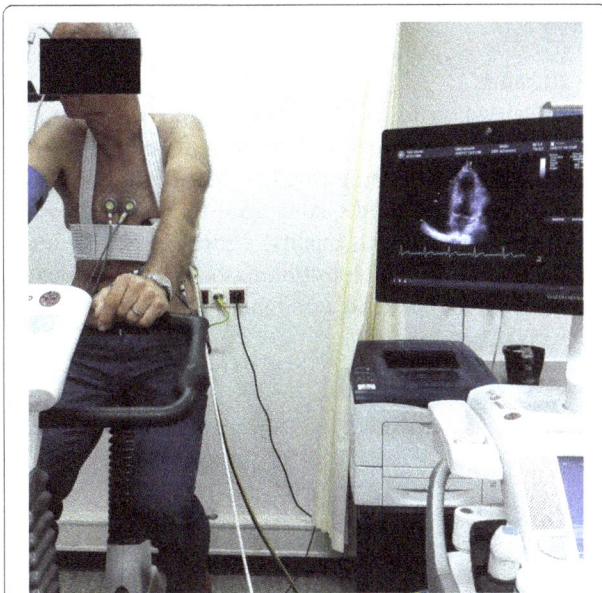

Fig. 4 Supine bicycle ergometer test with stress echocardiography. Example of stress echocardiography with a patient lying on a supine bicycle ergometer. The table is tilted towards the left, to optimize the image quality of the apical four chamber view. The probe (X5-1, Philips Medical Systems, Best, The Netherlands) is fixated with Probefix and angulated in the optimal position. See the online movie for an overview of the supine bicycle test with echocardiography using the Probefix (Additional file 2)

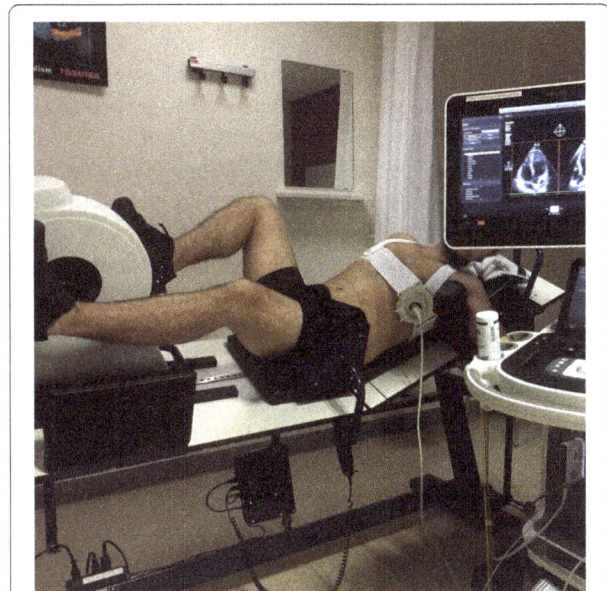

Fig. 3 Upright bicycle ergometer test with stress echocardiography. Stress echocardiography during upright bicycle ergometer test with Probefix. The CASE ergometer machine (GE Healthcare, Milwaukee, US) is connected to the Ergoline bicycle (Ergoline GmbH, Bitz, German). The GE Vivid9 ultrasound machine is positioned on the left side of the patient to facilitate apical positioning of the ultrasound probe (M5Sc, GE Healthcare, Milwaukee, USA). With the ultrasound probe fixated in the apical position, continuous monitoring of the apical four chamber view is displayed on the echocardiographic monitor (Vivid9, GE Healthcare, Milwaukee, USA). Simultaneous electrocardiographic (ECG) monitoring is performed during an exercise protocol. See the online movie for an overview and results of the upright bicycle test with echocardiography using the Probefix (Additional file 1)

positioning of the ultrasound probe at the optimal position. When the desired acoustic window is identified, the Probefix can be fixated to the patient's chest with the two Velcro straps. The horizontal chest strap is positioned first and the vertical chest strap is fixated next. Both should be firmly attached to the patient's chest. The internal holder of the Probefix can then be pushed towards the chest to achieve a firm position, while rotating the ultrasound probe is still feasible.

Measurements

During stress echocardiography, 2D or 3D B-mode images of the left ventricle may be obtained during various stages of physical exercise. Alternatively, pulsed wave or continuous wave Doppler recordings may be obtained over the cardiac valves. The ultrasound probe can be rotated and angulated to acquire all desired imaging planes (e.g. the apical two chamber, apical three chamber or apical four chamber view). Several parameters can be assessed, such as, ventricular function, valvular and subvalvular gradients and regurgitant flows. Implementation of a 3D ultrasound probe is even more convenient, as multiple 2D imaging planes can be recorded without rotating the probe.

Pilot study set up

We performed SE with the Probefix in healthy volunteers and in patients from our outpatient clinic. Exclusion criteria were pharmacological stress testing and the necessity to perform imaging in both apical and parasternal view, because during stress test it is very challenging to relocate the Probefix. All patients that received exercise induced SE, for the assessment of valvular disease or CRT device optimization in January and February 2018 were asked for participation ($n = 6$). In addition we asked six healthy volunteers (colleagues) to undergo SE with Probefix. All volunteers signed informed consent prior to stress testing. Stress tests were performed at supine or upright bicycle ergometer and stress protocol were adjusted to the subjects physical fitness (Figs. 3 and 4). Study subject were tested until maximal exercise levels were achieved. In the healthy volunteers we performed imaging in either short axis view or apical view (depending on the best image quality) and we assessed whether during SE the image quality was sufficient for wall motion analysis. In patients from our outpatient clinic we used local imaging protocols according to the objectives of the diagnostic test.

Stress tests were performed on an Ergoline bicycle (Ergoline GmbH, Bitz, German) ergometer. For echocardiographic examination GE Vivid7 or Philips iE33 ultrasound machines were used, with 2D echo probes (M5Sc, GE Healthcare, Milwaukee, USA and X5-1, Philips Medical Systems, Best, The Netherlands). The study complied with the Declaration of Helsinki and the protocol was issued by the local Medical Research Ethics Committees (MREC/METC) as non-WMO (Medical Research Involving Human Subjects Act) research.

Results

We performed SE in six heathy subjects and six patients of which a detailed description is given in Table 1. One patient was not able to perform exercise and was therefore excluded from further analysis. Subjects that were included in the feasibility study were 55% male, had a mean age of 42 ± 21 year, and a mean body mass index of 25 ± 5. Most outpatient subjects were tested for the evaluation of valvular disease (Fig. 5), while in one patient SE was performed for echocardiography-guided CRT device optimization. In two study subject, the image quality at baseline was insufficient to test Probefix. In all other subjects, the acoustic windows remained of good quality during increased load, and the echo probe remained stable at the fixated position. There was no repositioning necessary. The application of Probefix therefore was feasible in 9 out of 11 subjects (82%).

Fixating Probefix to the patient at the best echocardiographic window took less than 5 min in all patients. Both supine and upright testing resulted in good quality echocardiographic images during exercise as is visualized in the two additional movie files (see Additional files 1 and 2).

Discussion

We have demonstrated the feasibility of the Probefix in the field of SE for performing continuous, hands-free echocardiographic monitoring over time. In 82% of subjects, we acquired good quality acoustic windows, which remained of sufficient quality during increased load, without the need for repositioning the probe. Attaching the device to the patients was rapidly performed.

Table 1 Patients overview

Subject	Age	Gender	BMI	Indication	Stress test	Echo view	Quality baseline	Quality mid exercise	Quality max exercise	Probefix feasible
Patient 1	76	male	29.3	gradient MV	supine	AP4CH	good	good	good	yes
Patient 2	80	male	26.7	gradient MV	supine	AP4CH	good	good	n/a	n/a
Patient 3	34	female	21.3	device optimization in CRT patient	Supine	AP4CH	moderate	moderate	moderate	yes
Patient 4	82	female	33.2	gradient AoV	Supine	AP5CH	good	good	good	yes
Patient 5	19	female	22.2	gradient AoV	Supine	AP5CH, AP3CH	poor	n/a	n/a	no
Patient 6	43	female	35.2	gradient MV	Supine	AP4CH	good	good	good	yes
Volunteer 1	58	male		quality check	Upright	AP4CH	good	good	n/a	yes
Volunteer 2	35	male	23.1	quality check	Supine	AP4CH	good	good	good	yes
Volunteer 3	28	male	20.5	quality check	Supine	PSAX/AP4CH	poor	n/a	n/a	no
Volunteer 4	27	male	23.5	quality check	Supine	AP4Ch	moderate	moderate	moderate	yes
Volunteer 5	28	male	24.9	quality check	Supine	AP4CH	good	good	good	yes
Volunteer 6	27	female	21.1	quality check	Supine	AP4CH	good	good	good	yes

An overview of patients and volunteers that participated in the pilot study. Age, gender, body mass index (*BMI*), indication for stress test and feasibility of the Probefix is displayed. *MV* mitral valve, *AoV* aortic valve, *AP3CH* apical three chamber, *AP4CH* apical four chamber, *AP5CH* apical five chamber, *PSAX* parasternal short axis

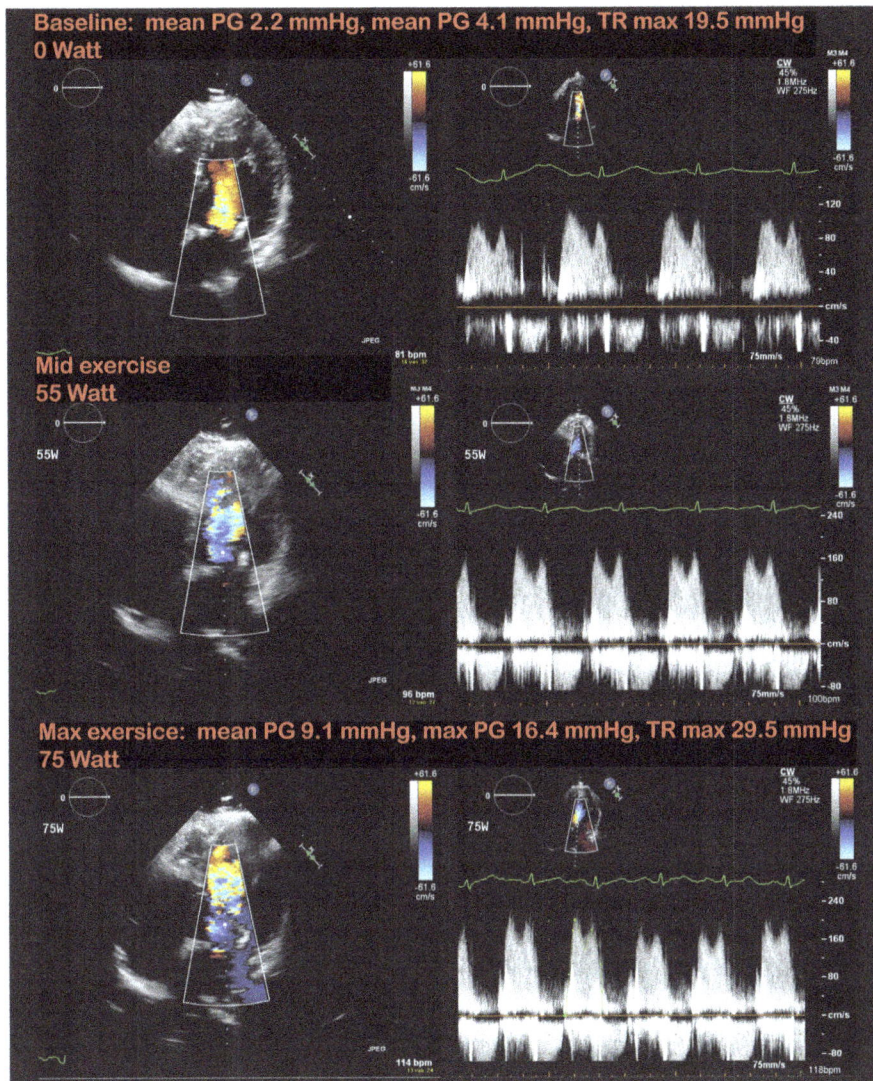

Fig. 5 Stress echocardiography of mitral valve. SE performed with the Probefix in patient six. The patient had a history of mitral valve plasty due to P2 leaflet prolapse. Patient experienced progressive dyspnoea, fatigue and weight gain after surgery. SE was performed to assess the mitral valve pressure gradient during exercise, which was not elevated. At baseline and at peak exercise, right ventricular filling pressures were also assessed with continuous wave Doppler of the tricuspid valve

Strengths and limitations

The inherent limitations associated with a small, pilot study should be acknowledged. Nevertheless, this study is the first to describe a new technique for facilitating continuous ultrasound measurements. The superiority of continuous echocardiographic measurements during exercise over post-exercise testing has previously been demonstrated by the studies of Dagianti et al. and Badruddin et al. [5, 6].

We demonstrate the feasibility of Probefix in five out of six healthy volunteers and four out of five patients from our outpatient clinic. There are however also limitations to its' implementation. Firstly, due to the fixation of the echo probe, it is challenging to change from e.g.

the parasternal view to the apical view during exercise testing. Fixating two Probefix devices to the patients' chest could be a solution to this problem, however this is not possible in all patients due to lack of space on the patients' thorax. Secondly, due to poor baseline echocardiographic windows, SE with Probefix will not be achievable in all patients. As a result of these limitations we believe that the primary application of the Probefix are echocardiographic imaging protocols in which only one view (either apical or parasternal) is required. Consequently, patients with valvular disease and patients whom undergo diastolic function testing are especially suitable for SE with the Probefix. In this patient group we strongly believe that Probefix facilitates continuous monitoring of cardiac function during SE. Because Probefix removes the necessity for sonographers to manually hold the probe during continuous stress testing, this could also reduce the risk of repetitive strain injuries. However more research is needed to test this hypothesis. As Probefix is a new device scientific proof of its added value is of importance. This article explores the possibilities of Probefix in the field of (stress) echocardiography. A trial on the efficacy of this device must be executed.

Clinical implications

We demonstrated the feasibility of Probefix in the field of SE. In addition to achieving high quality, stable, hands-free continuous echocardiographic monitoring during exercise, the Probefix has far reaching potential. Continuous monitoring of cardiac function with Probefix could be implemented for the assessment of contractile reserve for response prediction to CRT or for monitoring of myocardial function and hemodynamics under certain physiological or pharmacological conditions [3, 9]. Another application for Probefix could be continuous monitoring of cardiac output at the intensive care department or during cardiac and non-cardiac surgery. A recent case report by our hospital demonstrated for the first time the successful treatment of severe mitral regurgitation through transthoracic echocardiography-guided MitraClip placement [10]. Transcatheter MitraClip placement is traditionally performed using transesophageal echocardiography. However, a history of esophagectomy left the patient involved unfit for transesophageal echocardiography. In special cases like this, the Probefix could facilitate continuous transthoracic echocardiographic measurements. At the same time, the exposure to ionizing radiation of the cardiologist is reduced. As a safe distance to the radiation beam can be secured during measurements.

Conclusion

In this pilot study, the feasibly of Probefix is demonstrated for stress echocardiography during ergometer tests in supine and upright positions. Although SE with Probefix will not be achievable in all patients due to extensive SE imaging protocols or poor image quality, we believe that the Probefix enables good quality continuous echocardiographic monitoring. Therefore Probefix is able to improve the implementation of an existing diagnostic tool. Validation and scientific proof of the efficacy of this device must be further studied in a larger patient cohort.

Abbreviations
B-mode: Brightness mode; CRT: Cardiac resynchronization therapy; SE: Stress echocardiography

Acknowledgements
The authors acknowledge Benjamin Tchang from Usono for supplying the Probefix during the stress tests.

Funding
Not applicable.

Authors' contributions
OS, WE and RS performed the stress echocardiography tests. OS and WE were a major contributor in writing the manuscript. All authors read and approved the final manuscript.

Competing interests
The authors declare that they have no competing interests.

Author details
[1]Department of Cardiology, University Medical Centre Utrecht, P.O. Box 85500, 3508 GA Utrecht, The Netherlands. [2]Department of Cardiology, Maxima Medisch Centrum, Veldhoven, The Netherlands. [3]Netherlands Heart Institute, Central Military Hospital, Utrecht, The Netherlands.

References
1. Sicari R, Nihoyannopoulos P, Evangelista A, Kasprzak J, Lancellotti P, Poldermans D, et al. Stress echocardiography expert consensus statement—executive summary: European Association of Echocardiography (EAE) (a registered branch of the ESC). Eur Heart J. 2009;30:278–89.
2. Vrints CJ, Senior R, Crea F, Sechtem U. Assessing suspected angina: requiem for coronary computed tomography angiography or exercise electrocardiogram? Eur Heart J. 2017;38(23):1792–800.
3. Lancellotti P, Pellikka PA, Budts W, Chaudhry FA, Donal E, Dulgheru R, et al. The clinical use of stress echocardiography in non-ischaemic heart disease: recommendations from the European Association of Cardiovascular Imaging and the American Society of Echocardiography. J Am Soc Echocardiogr. 2017;30:101–38.
4. Obokata M, Kane GC, Reddy YNV, Olson TP, Melenovsky V, Borlaug BA. Role of diastolic stress testing in the evaluation for heart failure with preserved ejection fraction: a simultaneous invasive-echocardiographic study. Circulation. 2017;135:825–38.
5. Dagianti A, Penco M, Bandiera A, Sgorbini L, Fedele F. Clinical application of exercise stress echocardiography: supine bicycle or treadmill? Am J Cardiol. 1998;81(98):62G–7G.
6. Badruddin SM, Ahmad A, Mickelson J, Abukhalil J, Winters WL, Nagueh SF, et al. Supine bicycle versus post-treadmill exercise echocardiography in the detection of myocardial ischemia: a randomized single-blind crossover trial. J Am Coll Cardiol. 1999;33(6):1485–90.
7. Armstrong WF, Zoghbi WA. Stress echocardiography: current methodology and clinical applications. J Am Coll Cardiol. 2005;45:1739–47.
8. Peteiro J, Bouzas-Mosquera A, Estevez R, Pazos P, Pineiro M, Castro-Beiras A. Head-to-head comparison of peak supine bicycle exercise echocardiography and treadmill exercise echocardiography at peak and at post-exercise for the detection of coronary artery disease. J Am Soc Echocardiogr. 2012;25:319–26.
9. Ciampi Q, Carpeggiani C, Michelassi C, Villari B, Picano E. Left ventricular contractile reserve by stress echocardiography as a predictor of response to cardiac resynchronization therapy in heart failure: a systematic review and meta-analysis. BMC Cardiovasc Disord. 2017;17:223.
10. Hart EA, Teske AJ, Voskuil M, Stella PR, Chamuleau SAJ, Kraaijeveld AO. Transthoracic echocardiography guided MitraClip placement under conscious sedation. JACC Cardiovasc Interv. 2017;10(3):e27–9.

27

Realization of fully automated quantification of left ventricular volumes and systolic function using transthoracic 3D echocardiography

Lina Sun, Haiyan Feng, Lujia Ni, Hui Wang and Dongmei Gao[*]

Abstract

Background: Study on automated three-dimensional (3D) quantification of left heart parameters by using Heartmodel software is still in the early stage and fully automatic analysis was not clearly achieved. The aim of our study was to evaluate the performance of this new technology in measuring left ventricular (LV) volume and ejection fraction (EF) in patients with a variety of heart diseases on the basis of rationally determining the default endocardial border values.

Methods: Subjects with a variety of heart diseases were included prospectively. High quality Heartmodel images were selected to determine the end-diastolic and end-systolic default values of endocardial border. The accuracy and reproducibility of automated three-dimensional echocardiography (3DE) for measuring LV end-diastolic volume (EDV), end-systolic volume (ESV) and EF were evaluated with the traditional manual 3DE as the relative standard.

Results: Ninety seven subjects were enrolled in the study. The default endocardial border values were determined as 66% and 40% for end-diastole (ED) and end-systole (ES), respectively. Most of the subjects (84/97) were automatically analyzed by Heartmodel software without manual adjustment, revealing a close correlation of automated 3DE with manual 3DE in measuring EDV, ESV and EF (r-values: EDV: 0.96, ESV: 0.97, EF: 0.96). The EDV and ESV values obtained by automated 3DE were higher than those measured by manual 3DE (biases: EDV: 16 ± 18 ml, ESV: 11 ± 12 ml). The intra- and inter-observer reproducibility of automated 3DE was better than that of manual 3DE. Automated 3DE with manual adjustment showed good consistency with manual 3DE in assessing the impairment degree of systolic function in patients with wall motion abnormalities ($n = 58$), (Kappa = 0.74, $P = 0.00$).

Conclusion: Fully automated 3DE quantification of LV volume and EF could be achieved in most patients. Since automated 3DE was accurate and more reproducible, it could replace the existing manual 3DE technology and be routinely used in clinical practice.

Keywords: 3D echocardiography, Cardiac chamber quantification, Fully automated analysis

Background

Accurate measurement of left ventricular (LV) volume and ejection fraction (EF) is essential to determine the prognosis in patients with various heart disease, and consequently helps in establishing treatment decisions as eligibility criteria in many clinical trials [1, 2]. Cardiac magnetic resonance (CMR) is now considered the gold standard for measuring LV volume and EF. However, it

is very expensive and cannot be used by bedside patients or patients with implanted devices. Currently, transthoracic echocardiography (TTE) remains to be the technique of choice for imaging. The biplane method of disks summation (modified Simpson's rule) is the most commonly used technology for measuring LV volume and EF. However, due to technical shortcomings of apex foreshortening and geometrical assumptions, the results are not very satisfactory. Transthoracic three-dimensional echocardiography (3DE) overcomes the above shortcomings. Although volumes tended to be underestimated on 3DE, the accuracy of

---

* Correspondence: sunlina@jlu.edu.cn
Department of Ultrasound, China-Japan Union Hospital of Jilin University,
126 Xiantai Street, Changchun, Jilin 130033, China

3DE was comparable with that of CMR when measuring LV volume and EF [3]. But 3DE, especially traditional manual 3DE, is not widely used in clinical practice due to its time-consuming measurements [4].

In order to apply 3DE technology for routine clinical examination, the newly developed Heartmodel software (HeartModel[A.I.]; Philips Healthcare, Andover, MA, USA) that realizes the rapid and automated three-dimensional (3D) quantitative analysis of LV volume and EF can be used. But the study on automated 3DE technology is still in its early stages due to the following reasons: Firstly, the Heartmodel software detects more robustly the inner and outer extents of the myocardial tissue – those being at the interface of the blood-tissue and the compacted myocardium, whereas the LV endocardial border between them needs to be subjectively defined by the operator himself. It is well known that the correct endocardial border setting is essential for the accurate measurement of LV volume and EF, which is also the basis for comparing this novel measurement technology with the traditional ones. However, there are still no optimal rationally-determined default endocardial border values that can be routinely used at clinic so far. Secondly, previous studies have reported a great deal of manual editing needed in a large proportion of enrolled subjects following the automated analyses [5–11], which Obviously did not fulfill the function of complete automated measurement for LV volume and EF, hence still has the disadvantage of time consumption. Since one of the reasons might be the lack of reasonable default border values they could refer to, the default endocardial border values should be first determined properly before the evaluation of this new technique, which consequently reduced the manual editing after automated contouring and in turn helped to realize the objective and complete automated quantitative analysis of LV volume and EF. Hence, the purpose of this study was to evaluate the accuracy and reproducibility of automated 3DE technology in measuring LV volume and EF in patients with a variety of heart diseases on the basis of rationally determining the default endocardial border values.

Methods
Study design
Patients with a variety of heart diseases were included prospectively. A full-volume image used for manual 3D measurements and two Heartmodel images acquired over a 5 min period were collected in each patient by an experienced physician (DM.G.). Image quality was determined by using a five point scale in which 1, clear display of all 17 segments, well visualization of endocardial trabeculae and clear differentiation from the myocardium in at least 12 segments; 2, visualization of all wall segments and clear differentiation of endocardial

trabeculae from the myocardium in 6–12 segments; 3, visualization of all wall segments and clear differentiation of endocardial trabeculae from the myocardium in less than 6 segments; 4, dropout of less than or equal to three segments but visualization of adjacent segments within the same territory; 5, dropout of more than 3 segments. Images in scale 5 were considered poor image quality and excluded from the study. After completing the image acquisition for all subjects, the high quality Heartmodel images in scale 1 were selected for determining the default endocardial border values. Then all Heartmodel images were automated analyzed with the determined default endocardial border values. The time interval for the analysis of two Heartmodel images in each subject should be at least one week and it was applied in a random order. If the automated contouring of endocardial border was not satisfactory, manual editing can be performed. Similarly, each full volume image was analyzed twice by manual 3DE using blinded method. The time required to obtain LV volume and EF with the two methods was recorded. The averaged values of two automated 3D measurements were compared to those from two manual 3D measurements to determine the consistency and differences between the two methods in measuring LV volume and EF. The intra-observer reproducibility of the two methods was also evaluated. Besides, to assess the inter-observer reproducibility of the two methods, 15 subjects were randomly selected and a second dataset was retained by another physician (LN.S.) using the same device in the same place, and the images were analyzed by the same physician (LN.S.). The EF values of patients with wall motion abnormalities was further divided into normal range (male $\geq$ 52%, female $\geq$ 54%), mildly abnormal (41–51% for male, 41–53% for female), moderately abnormal (30–40% for both male and female) and severely abnormal (<30% for both male and female) according to the American society of echocardiography and the European association of cardiovascular imaging [12]. Results were compared to evaluate the consistency between automated 3DE and manual 3DE in assessing the degree of impaired systolic function.

Patients
Between February 2017 and August 2017, 103 patients undergoing TTE in our ultrasound room were prospectively included when there was adequate time for the examination. This study has been approved by the institutional review board and all enrolled subjects have signed the informed consent form. Patients with severe heart malformation or with atrial fibrillation were excluded.

Automated 3DE
Automated 3DE was performed using the EPIQ system (Philips Medical Systems, Andover, MA, USA) and an

X5–1 phased-array transducer with the patient placed in the left lateral decubitus position. After connecting the electrocardiogram, the apical 4-chamber view was displayed with the LV in the center along the volume axis. The X-plane button on the screen was clicked, and the clear imaging of the LV was confirmed on the biplane display. Then the HM ACQ button on the screen was clicked to collect the Heartmodel image. Before acquisition of each image, the images were optimized for endocardial visualization by modifying the gain, compress, and time gain compensation controls. The posture of the patient was adjusted to reduce the shielding of pulmonary gas. Focus was set on the mitral valve -papillary muscle level. The HVR full volume and the Auto SCAN were activated under the HM ACQ mode. Then the stored heartmodel image was called out for automated analysis of LVEDV, LVESV and EF using Heartmodel software.

The mechanism of automated 3DE involves detection of LV endocardial surfaces throughout the cardiac cycle using Heartmodel software, which utilized an adaptive analytics algorithm that consists of knowledge-based identification of initial global shape and orientation followed by patient specific adaptation. As opposed to the detection of single endocardial border, the Heartmodel software detects more robustly the inner and outer extents of the myocardial tissue, i.e., the interface of the blood-tissue and the compacted myocardium. The recognized tissue was divided into 100 slides (0%–100%), where the blood-tissue interface was presented as 0% and the interface of compacted myocardium as 100%. The LV endocardial border between them was subjectively defined by the operator. Taking the measurement of LV volume using CMR as a reference, we included the trabecular muscle in the LV cavity volume [13]. Therefore the endocardial border was defined as the interface between the trabecular muscle and the LV myocardium (Fig. 1). After completing the image acquisition for all subjects, the high quality Heartmodel images were selected for determining the default endocardial border values. With the prerequisite of blinding method on LV volume and EF, the following operations were performed to calculate the default endocardial border values: Firstly, both the ED and ES default endocardial border values were set to 0%; secondly, an experienced physician (DM.G.) adjusted the global ED and ES slides to the closest desired border and recorded the numbers separately. The above operations were repeated on all high quality images, and the ED and ES numbers were added and then the averages were calculated, which were considered as the default endocardial border values and subsequently were applied to all Heartmodel images. If the operator was not satisfied with the automated contouring, manual adjustment was needed, including global and regional editing.

Manual 3DE

The full-volume images for manual 3D analysis were obtained using the same machine and probe. The images were also obtained from apical 4-chamber view. Full-volume image was required from 4 wedge-shaped subvolumes, which were stitched over 4 consecutive cardiac cycles in a single breath-hold. When capturing the images, the image should be adjusted as in automated 3D to produce the best endocardial visibility. Prototype software QLAB (QLAB 10.5, 3DQ-Advanced, Philips Medical Systems, Bothell, Washington) was adopted for analyzing the full volume images. The 3D volume data were displayed and modified in 3 different cross-sections, which included conventional 2D 4- and 2-chamber views and a short-axis view. The following steps were performed on the end-diastolic and end-systolic frames. First, the users aligned the multiplanar view to maximize the LV cavity long- and short-axes in the 2- and 4-chamber views. Four mitral annular and 1 apical points were then placed on the left ventricle as landmarks in each view. Then, the initial endocardial surface was manually adjusted in multiple apical planes, while including the papillary muscle and endocardial trabeculae in the LV cavity, and its position was corrected as necessary in multiple arbitrary cut planes until the best match was visually verified and the final LVEDV, LVESV, and LVEF values were then recorded.

Statistics

The correlation between the LV parameters measured by automated 3DE and the ones by manual 3DE was tested using Spearman coefficient. Bland-Altman analysis was used to assess the bias and limits of agreement. Wilcoxon matched paired test was used to verify the significance of the biases. Intra- and inter-observer variability was calculated as the absolute difference of the corresponding pair of repeated measurements as a percentage of their mean in each patient and then averaged over the study group. Kappa test was used to analyze the consistency of categorical data. $P < 0.05$ was considered as statistically significant. Continuous variables are presented as mean $\pm$ standard deviation, if normally distributed, or median and interquartile range (IQR) if non-normally distributed; number and percentages are presented for categorical variables.

Results

Of the 103 subjects included in this study, the image quality of them was classified as scale 1 ($n = 32$ vs $n = 36$), scale 2 ($n = 13$ vs $n = 17$), scale 3 ($n = 16$ vs $n = 11$), scale 4 ($n = 36$ vs $n = 35$) and scale 5 ($n = 6$ vs $n = 4$) with automated 3DE and manual 3DE, respectively. 6 patients were excluded because of poor image quality including 2 patients had poor Heartmodel image quality and 4 patients had poor image quality for both Heartmodel

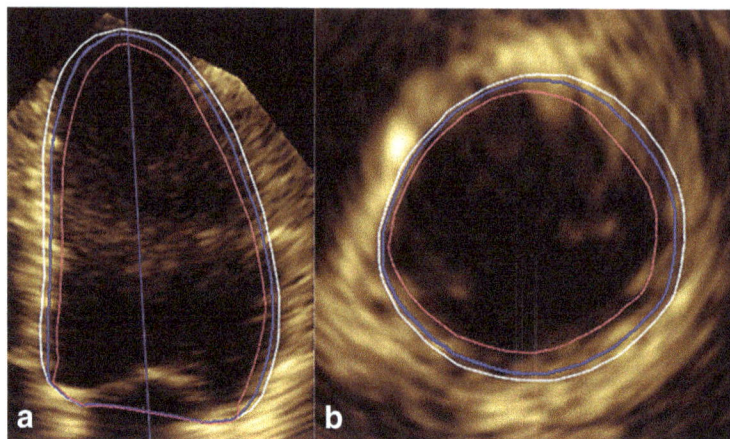

Fig. 1 (a) LV apical 4-chamber view and (**b**) basal short-axis view in ED showed that the Heartmodel software detected the inner and outer extents of the myocardial tissue, i.e., the blood-tissue interface (red line) and the interface of compacted myocardium (white line), which were assigned to slides of 0% and 100%, respectively. The LV endocardial border (blue line) between them was subjectively defined by the operator, and in this case, it was at the slide of 68%

and full-volume. Finally, the study group consisted of 97 subjects, and the 32 subjects who showed high Heartmodel image quality on scale 1 were used to determine the default endocardial border values. The default values of the endocardial border were set at the slides of 66% (66.38 ± 4.56%, range 57%–75%) and 40% (39.78 ± 3.72%, range 33%–47%) for ED and ES, respectively. The baseline demographic and clinical characteristics of all the enrolled subjects and 32 subjects who were used to obtain the default values were shown in Table 1.

With the above default border values, 13 subjects required manual adjustment after automated contouring, including 8 cases with apical wall motion abnormalities (Fig. 2), 3 patients with hypertrophic cardiomyopathy and 2 patients with LV wall thickening up to or more than 15 mm due to hypertensive heart disease ($n = 1$) or aortic valve stenosis ($n = 1$). The time required for the LV volume and EF measurements by automated 3DE was 1.12 ± 0.31 min and 3.74 ± 1.62 min for those who did not require manual adjustment and the 13 subjects who needed manual adjustment after automated contouring, respectively, whilst it was 4.93 ± 2.38 min using manual 3DE.

A strong correlation was noted between the automated and the manual 3D measurements of LVEDV, LVESV and LVEF. However, a statistically significant difference was observed between the two methods. Compared with manual 3DE, EDV and ESV obtained by automated 3DE were higher (Table 2, Fig. 3, Fig. 4).

The automated 3DE showed better correlation with manual 3DE for classifying the impairment degree of systolic function in patients with wall motion abnormalities ($n = 58$) with manual adjustment (Kappa = 0.74, $P = 0.00$) than without adjustment (Kappa = 0.63, $P = 0.00$).

Although there were 10 patients who were assigned to different impairment classification between manual 3DE and automated 3DE with manual adjustment, the EF difference was within 5% in 6 patients. (Table 3).

The results of intra- and inter-observer variability were shown in Table 4. Intra- and inter-observer reproducibility of automated 3DE were better than those of manual 3DE.

Table 1 Baseline demographic and clinical characteristics of study subjects

Variables	All subjects ($n = 97$)	Subjects used to determine the default endocardial border values ($n = 32$)
age(y)	52 ± 14	55 ± 13
men	60(62%)	18(56%)
Systolic blood pressure (mmHg)	140 ± 22	140 ± 22
Diastolic blood pressure (mmHg)	87 ± 12	86 ± 12
Heart rate (beats/min)	76 ± 13	72 ± 14
Primary diagnosis		
Coronary heart disease	38(39%)	12(38%)
Valvular heart disease	12(12%)	5(16%)
Hypertensive heart disease	14(15%)	4(12%)
Dilated cardiomyopathy	8(8%)	4(12%)
Hypertrophic cardiomyopathy	3(3%)	0(0%)
Congenital heart disease	4(4%)	0(0%)
No specific heart disease	18(19%)	7(22%)
Frame rate (Hz)		
Automated 3DE datasets	19 ± 3	19 ± 3
Manual 3DE datasets	21 ± 5	23 ± 6

Data are expressed as mean ± SD or as number (percentage)

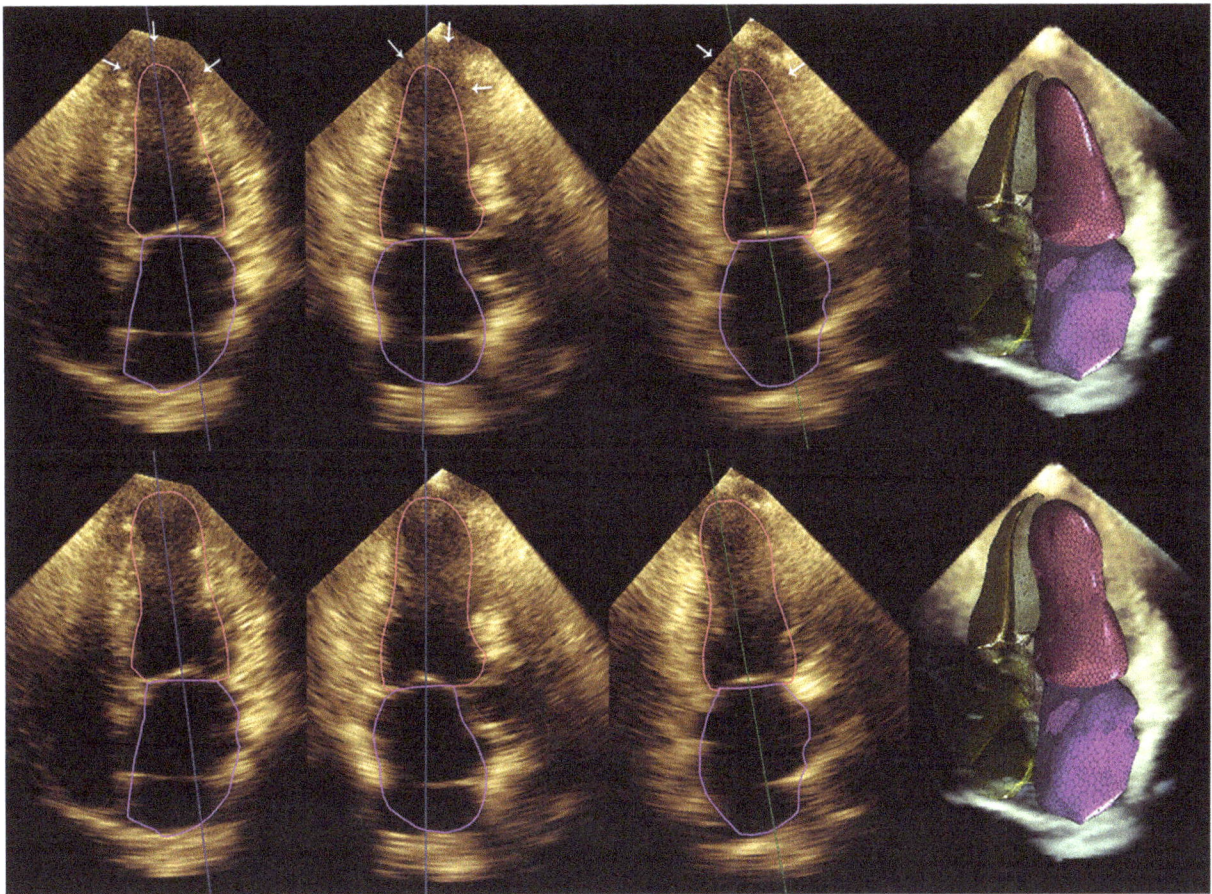

Fig. 2 The top line showed the apical segments with regional wall motion abnormality were not correctly recognized (arrow), then manual adjustment was needed (the bottom line)

Discussion

This study showed that the automated 3DE measurement, assisted with few manually adjusted Heartmodel images (13/97), was highly accurate in measuring LV volume and EF in patients with a variety of heart diseases. In addition, it was more timesaving and reproducible than the manual 3DE. The LVEDV and LVESV values obtained by automated 3DE were higher compared to manual 3DE, and there was a good consistency in assessing the impairment degree of systolic function in patients with wall motion abnormalities with these two technologies.

The Heartmodel software was designed to automatically measure LV volume and EF in order to reduce subjective factors, increase reproducibility and save time. However, previous studies on automated 3DE demonstrated a large amount of manual editing following after the automated contouring [5–11]. The purpose of fully automated measurement was therefore not clearly

Table 2 Comparison of LV volume and EF measured by automated 3DE and manual 3DE

	Automated 3DE measurements	Manual 3DE measurements as relative standard	Correlation (r value)	P value	Bias
LVEDV with manual adjustment, ml	143 (108 to 214)	133 (103 to 200)	0.964	0.00	16 ± 18
LVEDV without manual adjustment, ml	148 (109 to 214)	133 (103 to 200)	0.961	0.00	17 ± 18
LVESV with manual adjustment, ml	75 (42 to 152)	66 (36 to 130)	0.972	0.00	11 ± 12
LVESV without manual adjustment, ml	74 (43 to 150)	66 (36 to 130)	0.968	0.00	11 ± 12
LVEF with manual adjustment, %	49 (35 to 61)	51 (34 to 63)	0.964	0.00	−1 ± 3
LVEF without manual adjustment, %	52 (35 to 61)	51 (34 to 63)	0.956	0.00	−1 ± 4

3 DE 3-dimensional echocardiography, *Bias* measurement of automated 3DE - measurement of manual 3DE, *LVEDV* left ventricular end-diastolic volume, *LVESV* left ventricular end-systolic volume, *LVEF* left ventricular ejection fraction
Data were expressed as mean ± SD or as median (interquartile range)

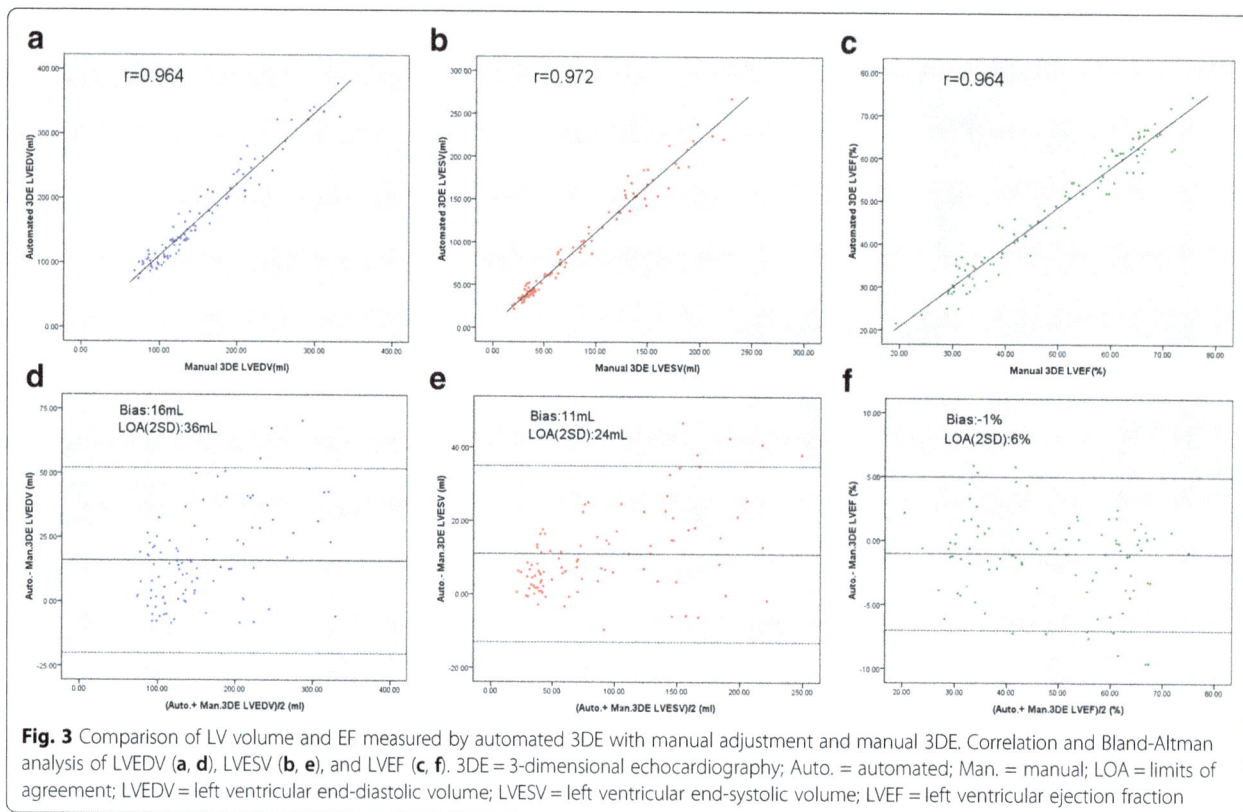

Fig. 3 Comparison of LV volume and EF measured by automated 3DE with manual adjustment and manual 3DE. Correlation and Bland-Altman analysis of LVEDV (**a**, **d**), LVESV (**b**, **e**), and LVEF (**c**, **f**). 3DE = 3-dimensional echocardiography; Auto. = automated; Man. = manual; LOA = limits of agreement; LVEDV = left ventricular end-diastolic volume; LVESV = left ventricular end-systolic volume; LVEF = left ventricular ejection fraction

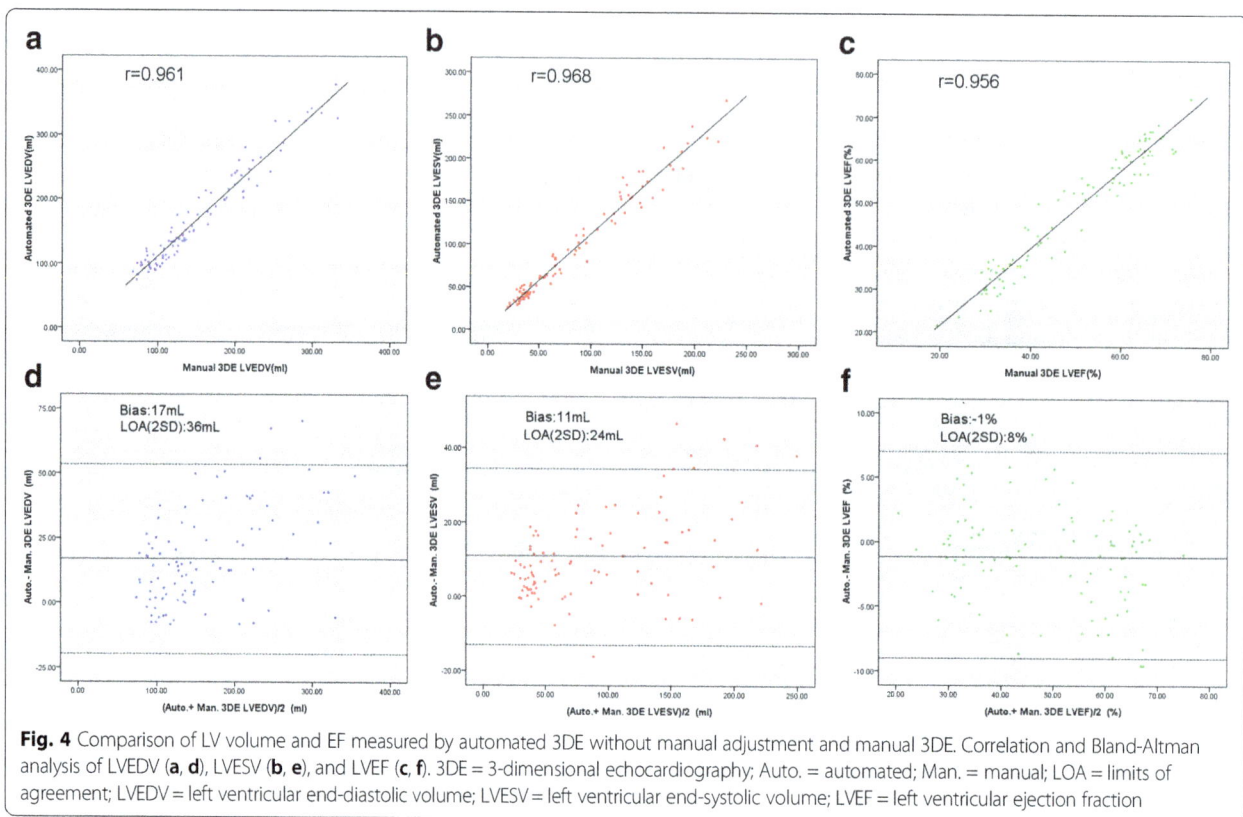

Fig. 4 Comparison of LV volume and EF measured by automated 3DE without manual adjustment and manual 3DE. Correlation and Bland-Altman analysis of LVEDV (**a**, **d**), LVESV (**b**, **e**), and LVEF (**c**, **f**). 3DE = 3-dimensional echocardiography; Auto. = automated; Man. = manual; LOA = limits of agreement; LVEDV = left ventricular end-diastolic volume; LVESV = left ventricular end-systolic volume; LVEF = left ventricular ejection fraction

Table 3 Classification of the impairment degree of systolic function in patients with wall motion abnormalities

Automated 3DE	Manual adjustment							
Manual 3DE	A		B		C		D	
	Yes	No	Yes	No	Yes	No	Yes	No
A	5	6	2	1	0	0	0	0
B	1	3	13	10	1	2	0	0
C	0	0	2	2	24	24	4	4
D	0	0	0	0	0	2	6	4

3DE 3-dimensional echocardiography
A = normal range (male ≥ 52%, female ≥ 54%); B = mildly abnormal (male 41–51%, female 41–53%); C = moderately abnormal (30–40% for both male and female); D = severely abnormal (<30% for both male and female)

achieved, and the advantages of the new technology were not presented totally. Our study tended to realize the automated measurement to the greatest extent by rationally setting the default endocardial border values. Among the 97 enrolled patients, only 13 images required manual editing. Special attention should be paid to the fact that all the 8 patients with apical wall motion abnormalities were incorrectly automated contoured (Fig. 2). The reason may be that the apical myocardium located in the near field of ultrasound was not clear in apical 4-chamber view because of reverberation artifact and focus location which was set at the mitral valve-papillary muscle level. This in turn affected the recognition and tracking of the endocardium in the apex region by Heartmodel software. We suppose that the wall motion of apical segments was approximately estimated on the basis of basal and midventricular segment wall motion. Our conjecture was supported by the following phenomena: for patients with global wall motion abnormalities or without wall motion abnormalities, the software can correctly outline the apical endocardium because the amplitude of LV wall motion in these cases was essentially the same in all segments, whilst for patients with regional wall motion abnormalities in the apical segments, the Heartmodel software seemed to outline the apical endocardium according to the basal and midventricular segment wall motion instead of tracing the true position of apical endocardium. Therefore, when apical wall motion was inconsistent with the basal and midventricular segment motion, attention should be paid whether manual adjustment was needed in apical segments. The other 5 patients who needed manual

adjustment consisted of 3 patients with hypertrophic cardiomyopathy and 2 patients with prominent LV wall thickening due to hypertensive heart disease or aortic valve stenosis. Uneven wall thickening and hypoechoic myocardium close to the endocardium accounted for the inaccurate automated contouring. According to our study, fully automated quantification of LV volumes and systolic function using Heartmodel software could be achieved in most patients and manual adjustment was needed merely in the minority of the patients.

In this study, the default endocardial border values were set as 66% and 40% for ED and ES, respectively. EDV and ESV obtained by automated 3DE were higher compared to manual 3DE, and the bias for EDV and ESV were 16 ± 18 ml and 11 ± 12 ml, respectively. The different methods of determining the endocardial border with the automated and manual 3DE accounted for the biases: On automated 3DE, although the endocardial border cannot be clearly explored in most patients, the more robustly recognized inner and outer extents of the myocardial tissue, i.e., the interface of the blood-tissue and the compacted myocardium can be easily detected by Heartmodel software. In our study we obtained the default endocardial border values from high quality heartmodel images, which represented the relative position of the endocardial border between the inner and outer extents of the myocardial tissue with varying heart shapes and sizes. Then all the subsequent Heartmodel images were automated analyzed with the determined default border values. So technically we could count trabeculae muscle in the LV volume on automated 3DE regardless of the image quality. On the contrary, on manual 3DE, although the trabeculae was planned to be counted in LV volume, the spatial resolution in most patients was insufficient to clearly define the endocardial trabeculae, which was, as a result, lumped together with the myocardium rather than being included in the LV cavity. This was the most significant potential source of volume underestimation by 3DE [14]. Most previous studies but two [6, 11] supported that the LV volumes obtained by automated 3DE were higher than those by manual 3DE [5, 8–10]. In addition, automated 3DE and CMR were compared in three studies, and results showed that the LV volumes were still underestimated by automated 3DE [7, 8, 11]. A meta-analysis of 34 studies reported that the overall pooled biases of manual

Table 4 Intra- and inter-observer variability comparison

Variability (%)	Manual 3DE			Automated 3DE with manual adjustment			Automated 3DE without manual adjustment		
	EDV	ESV	EF	EDV	ESV	EF	EDV	ESV	EF
Intra-observer	6 ± 4	9 ± 7	8 ± 5	5 ± 4	6 ± 5	6 ± 5	5 ± 4	6 ± 4	6 ± 5
Inter-observer	8 ± 5	10 ± 7	7 ± 3	5 ± 4	8 ± 5	7 ± 4	5 ± 4	8 ± 5	7 ± 4

3DE 3-dimensional echocardiography, *EDV* end-diastolic volume, *ESV* end-systolic volume, *EF* ejection fraction

3DE were −19.1 ± 17.1 ml and −10.1 ± 14.9 ml for EDV and ESV compared with CMR [3]. According to our results, the measured values using automated 3DE might be very close to that of CMR values. A multicentric study also came up with the result that the automated 3DE measurements were closer to that of CMR than manual 3DE [15].

Practically, EF is the most important index in assessing the cardiac function for clinicians. Previous studies have reported that automated 3DE and manual 3DE were highly consistent in measuring EF. While some studies suggested no significant difference between the two methods [5, 6, 11], two studies found that the EF measured by automated 3DE was slightly lower than that measured by manual 3DE [8, 10]. Our study arrived at similar result with the bias −1%, which might be explained by the fact that the frame rate of full volume image was slightly higher than that of Heartmodel images. The impairment degree of EF in patients with wall motion abnormalities was further classified in the present study and the results showed that the automated 3DE with manual adjustment showed better correlation with manual 3DE than that without adjustment. Without manual adjustment, automated 3DE tended to overestimate the EF measurement in patients with regional kinetic abnormalities of the apex and underestimate it in patients with prominent LV wall thickening.

Manual 3DE has been considered the most reproducible ultrasonic technology for measuring LV volume and EF so far [16]. According to our results, the reproducibility among inter- and intra-observer using automated 3DE was better than those using manual 3DE in measuring EDV, ESV and EF. This was consistent with a multicentric validation study describing both inter- and intra-observer variability were lower for the automated measurements than conventional manual technology for all parameters [6]. The lower variability of the automated method might be explained by the fact that the automated 3DE measurement did not require much experience to operate and automated analytic method was more objective.

This study has some limitations. Firstly, CMR was currently recognized as the gold standard for measuring LV volume and EF; however, manual 3DE rather than CMR was used as a reference standard in our study. Although the volume tended to be underestimated, the accuracy of manual 3DE was proved to be comparable with that of CMR [3]. In order to warrant the accuracy as standard, all of full-volume images for manual 3DE were analyzed by an experienced physician. Secondly, our sample size was not large enough to include all kinds of heart diseases, and further research is still needed to improve the results.

Conclusion

Automated 3DE could measure LV volume and EF accurately and fully automated quantification could be achieved in most patients. Since it was timesaving and more reproducible, automated 3DE could replace the existing manual 3D technology and be routinely used in clinical practice.

Abbreviations
3-D: Three-dimensional; 3DE: Three-dimensional echocardiography; CMR: Cardiac magnetic resonance; ED: End-diastole; EDV: End-diastolic volume; EF: Ejection fraction; ES: End-systole; ESV: End-systolic volume; IQR: Interquartile range; LV: Left ventricular; TTE: Transthoracic echocardiography

Acknowledgements
Not applicable

Funding
Not applicable

Authors' contributions
DG contributed to study design, images acquisition and data analysis. LS contributed to images acquisition, data analysis and had a major contribution in writing. HF helped in the literature search, data analysis and manuscript writing. LN helped in data analysis and manuscript revise. HW helped in the literature search, data analysis and manuscript revise. All authors read and approved the final manuscript.

Competing interests
The authors declare that they have no competing interests.

References
1. MossAJ ZW, Hall WJ, Klein H, Wilber DJ, Cannom DS, Daubert JP, Higgins SL, Brown MW, Andrews ML. Prophylactic implantation of a defibrillator in patients with myocardial infarction and reduced ejection fraction. N Engl J Med. 2002;346:877–83. [PubMed]
2. Packer M, Fowler MB, Roecker EB, Coats AJ, Katus HA, Krum H, Mohacsi P, Rouleau JL, Tendera M, Staiger C, et al. Effect of carvedilol on the morbidity of patients with severe chronic heart failure: results of the carvedilol prospective randomized cumulative survival (COPERNICUS) study. Circulation. 2002;106:2194–9. [PubMed]
3. Dorosz JL, Lezotte DC, Weitzenkamp DA, Allen LA, Salcedo EE. Performance of 3-dimensional echocardiography in measuring left ventricular volumes and ejection fraction: a systematic review and meta-analysis. J Am Coll Cardiol. 2012;59:1799–808. [PubMed]
4. Jenkins C, Chan J, Hanekom L, Marwick TH. Accuracy and feasibility of online 3-dimensional echocardiography for measurement of left ventricular parameters. J Am Soc Echocardiogr. 2006;19:1119–28. [PubMed]
5. Spitzer E, Ren B, Soliman OI, Zijlstra F, Van Mieghem NM, Geleijnse ML. Accuracy of an automated transthoracic echocardiographic tool for 3D assessment of left heart chamber volumes. Echocardiography. 2017;34:199–209. [PubMed]
6. Medvedofsky D, Mor-Avi V, Amzulescu M, Fernández-Golfín C, Hinojar R, Monaghan MJ, Otani K, Reiken J, Takeuchi M, Tsang W, et al. Three-dimensional echocardiographic quantification of the left-heart chambers using an automated adaptive analytics algorithm: multicentre validation study. Eur Heart J Cardiovasc Imaging 2017; doi: https://doi.org/10.1093/ehjci/jew328. [PubMed]
7. Levy F, Schouver ED, Lacuzio L, Civaia F, Rusek S, Dommerc C, Marechaux S, Dor V, Tribouilloy C, Dreyfus G. Performance of new automated transthoracic three-dimensional echocardiographic software for left ventricular volumes and function assessment in routine clinical practice: Comparison with 3 Tesla cardiac magnetic resonance. Arch Cardiovasc Dis 2017; doi:https://doi.org/10.1016/j.acvd.2016.12.015. [PubMed].

8. Tsang W, Salgo IS, Medvedofsky D, Takeuchi M, Prater D, Weinert L, Yamat M, Mor-Avi V, Patel AR, Lang RM. Transthoracic 3D Echocardiographic left heart chamber quantification using an automated adaptive analytics algorithm. JACC Cardiovasc Imaging. 2016;9:769–82. [PubMed]

9. Otani K, Nakazono A, Salgo IS, Lang RM, Takeuchi M. Three-dimensional Echocardiographic assessment of left heart chamber size and function with fully automated quantification software in patients with Atrial fibrillation. J Am Soc Echocardiogr. 2016;29:955–65. [PubMed]

10. Feng C, Chen L, Li J, Wang J, Dong F, Xu J. Three-dimensional echocardiographic measurements using automated quantification software for big data processing. J Xray Sci Technol. 2017;25:313–21. [PubMed]

11. Yang LT, Nagata Y, Otani K, Kado Y, Otsuji Y, Takeuchi M. Feasibility of one-beat real-time full-volume three-dimensional echocardiography for assessing left ventricular volumes and deformation parameters. J Am Soc Echocardiogr. 2016;29:853–60. [PubMed]

12. Lang RM, Badano LP, Mor-Avi V, Afilalo J, Armstrong A, Ernande L, Flachskampf FA, Foster E, Goldstein SA, Kuznetsova T, et al. Recommendations for cardiac chamber quantification by echocardiography in adults: an update from the American Society of Echocardiography and the European Association of Cardiovascular Imaging. J Am Soc Echocardiogr. 2015;28:1–39. [PubMed]

13. Thavendiranathan P, Liu S, Verhaert D, Calleja A, Nitinunu A, Van Houten T, De Michelis N, Simonetti O, Rajagopalan S, Ryan T, et al. Feasibility, accuracy, and reproducibility of real-time full-volume 3D transthoracic echocardiography to measure LV volumes and systolic function: a fully automated endocardial contouring algorithm in sinus rhythm and atrial fibrillation. JACC Cardiovasc Imaging. 2012;5:239–51. [PubMed]

14. Mor-Avi V, Jenkins C, Kühl HP, Nesser HJ, Marwick T, Franke A, Ebner C, Freed BH, Steringer-Mascherbauer R, Pollard H, et al. Real-time 3-dimensional echocardiographic quantification of left ventricular volumes: multicenter study for validation with magnetic resonance imaging and investigation of sources of error. JACC Cardiovasc Imaging. 2008;1:413–23. [PubMed]

15. Medvedofsky D, Mor-Avi V, Byku I, Singh A, Weinert L, Yamat M, Kruse E, Ciszek B, Nelson A, Otani K, et al. Three-dimensional Echocardiographic automated quantification of left heart chamber volumes using an adaptive analytics algorithm: feasibility and impact of image quality in nonselected patients. J Am Soc Echocardiogr. 2017;30:879–85. [PubMed]

16. Thavendiranathan P, Grant AD, Negishi T, Plana JC, Popović ZB, Marwick TH. Reproducibility of echocardiographic techniques for sequential assessment of left ventricular ejection fraction and volumes: application to patients undergoing cancer chemotherapy. J Am CollCardiol. 2013;61:77–84. [PubMed]

Permissions

The contributors of this book come from diverse backgrounds, making this book a truly international effort. This book will bring forth new frontiers with its revolutionizing research information and detailed analysis of the nascent developments around the world.

We would like to thank all the contributing authors for lending their expertise to make the book truly unique. They have played a crucial role in the development of this book. Without their invaluable contributions this book wouldn't have been possible. They have made vital efforts to compile up to date information on the varied aspects of this subject to make this book a valuable addition to the collection of many professionals and students.

This book was conceptualized with the vision of imparting up-to-date information and advanced data in this field. To ensure the same, a matchless editorial board was set up. Every individual on the board went through rigorous rounds of assessment to prove their worth. After which they invested a large part of their time researching and compiling the most relevant data for our readers.

The editorial board has been involved in producing this book since its inception. They have spent rigorous hours researching and exploring the diverse topics which have resulted in the successful publishing of this book. They have passed on their knowledge of decades through this book. To expedite this challenging task, the publisher supported the team at every step. A small team of assistant editors was also appointed to further simplify the editing procedure and attain best results for the readers.

Apart from the editorial board, the designing team has also invested a significant amount of their time in understanding the subject and creating the most relevant covers. They scrutinized every image to scout for the most suitable representation of the subject and create an appropriate cover for the book.

The publishing team has been an ardent support to the editorial, designing and production team. Their endless efforts to recruit the best for this project, has resulted in the accomplishment of this book. They are a veteran in the field of academics and their pool of knowledge is as vast as their experience in printing. Their expertise and guidance has proved useful at every step. Their uncompromising quality standards have made this book an exceptional effort. Their encouragement from time to time has been an inspiration for everyone.

The publisher and the editorial board hope that this book will prove to be a valuable piece of knowledge for researchers, students, practitioners and scholars across the globe.

Contributors

Jiaqi Shen, Qiao Zhou, Yue Liu, Runlan Luo, Bijun Tan and Guangsen Li
Department of Ultrasound, The Second Affiliated Hospital of Dalian Medical University, Dalian 116027, China

Martijn F.H. Maessen, Ayla Grotens and Maria T.E. Hopman
Department of Physiology, Radboud university medical center, Nijmegen, The Netherlands

Thijs M.H. Eijsvogels and Dick H.J. Thijssen
Department of Physiology, Radboud university medical center, Nijmegen, The Netherlands
Research Institute for Sports and Exercise Sciences, Liverpool John Moores University, Liverpool, UK

Hendrik H.G. Hansen
Department of Radiology and Nuclear Medicine, Radboud university medical center, Medical UltraSound Imaging Center (MUSIC), 6500, HB, Nijmegen, The Netherlands

Marco Paterni, Clara Carpeggiani, Eugenio Picano, Lorenza Pratali, Luna Gargani and Maria Grazia Andreassi
Institute of Clinical Physiology, National Research Council, Pisa, Italy

Quirino Ciampi
Cardiology Division, Fatebenefratelli Hospital, Benevento, Italy

Rodolfo Citro, Eduardo Bossone and Francesco Ferrara
Heart Department, University Hospital "San Giovanni di Dio e Ruggi d'Aragona", Salerno, Italy

Antonello D'Andrea and Giuseppe Pacileo
Division of Cardiology, Monaldi Hospital, Second University of Naples, Naples, Italy

Maria Chiara Scali
Cardiology Department, Pisa University and Nottola (Siena) Hospital, Pisa, Italy

Lauro Cortigiani
Cardiology Department, San Luca Hospital, Lucca, Italy

Iacopo Olivotto and Fabio Mori
Cardiology Department, Careggi Hospital, Florence, Italy

Maurizio Galderisi
Department of Advanced Biomedical Sciences, Federico II University Hospital, Naples, Italy

Marco Fabio Costantino
Cardiology Department, San Carlo Hospital, Potenza, Italy

Giovanni Di Salvo
Pediatric Cardiology Department, Brompton Hospital, London, UK.

Fausto Rigo
Division of Cardiology, Ospedale dell'Angelo Mestre-Venice, Mestre, Italy

Nicola Gaibazzi
Cardiology Department, Parma University Hospital, Parma, Italy

Giuseppe Limongelli
Pediatric Cardiology Department, Monaldi Hospital Clinics, Naples, Italy

Bruno Pinamonti and Laura Massa
Cardiology Department, University Hospital "Ospedale Riuniti", Trieste, Italy

Marco A. R. Torres
Hospital de Clinicas de Porto Alegre, Universidade Federal do Rio Grande do Sul, Porto Alegre, Brazil

Marcelo H. Miglioranza
Cardiology Institute of Rio Grande do Sul, Porto Alegre, Brazil

Clarissa Borguezan Daros
Cardiology Division, Hospital San José, Criciuma, Brazil

José Luis de Castro e Silva Pretto
Hospital Sao Vicente de Paulo, Hospital de Cidade, Passo Fundo, Brazil

Ana Djordjevic-Dikicand Branko Beleslin
Cardiology Clinic, Clinical Center of Serbia, Medical School, University of Belgrade, Belgrade, Serbia

Albert Varga and Gergely Agoston
Institute of Family Medicine, University of Szeged, Szeged, Hungary

Attila Palinkas
Department of Internal Medicine, Elisabeth Hospital, Hodmezovasarhely, Hungary

Dario Gregori
Department of Biostatistics, University of Padua, Padua, Italy

Paolo Trambaiolo
Department of Cardiology, Sandro Pertini Hospital, Rome, Italy

Sergio Severino
Cardiology Department, Monaldi Hospital, Naples, Italy

Ayana Arystan
RSE, Medical Centre Hospital of the President's Affairs Administration of the Republic of Kazakhstan, Astana, Kazakhstan

Paolo Colonna
Cardiology Hospital, Policlinico of Bari, Bari, Italy

Micael Waldenborg
School of Medical Sciences, Faculty of Medicine and Health, Örebro University, 70182 Örebro, Sweden
Department of Clinical Physiology, Faculty of Medicine and Health, Örebro University, 70182 Örebro, Sweden

Mats Lidén
School of Medical Sciences, Faculty of Medicine and Health, Örebro University, 70182 Örebro, Sweden
Department of Radiology, Faculty of Medicine and Health, Örebro University, 70182 Örebro, Sweden

Per Thunberg
School of Medical Sciences, Faculty of Medicine and Health, Örebro University, 70182 Örebro, Sweden
Department of Medical Physics, Faculty of Medicine and Health, Örebro University, 70182 Örebro, Sweden

Stina Jorstig
School of Medical Sciences, Faculty of Medicine and Health, Örebro University, 70182 Örebro, Sweden
Biomedical Engineering, Örebro University Hospital, 70185 Örebro, Sweden

Rosa Sicari
CNR, Institute of Clinical Physiology, Via G. Moruzzi, 1, 56124 Pisa, Italy

Lauro Cortigiani
Department of Cardiology, San Luca Hospital, Lucca, Italy

Marcel L. Geleijnse, Wim B.Vletter, Ben Ren, Tjebbe W. Galema, Nicolas M.Van Mieghem and Peter P. T.de Jaegere
From the department of Cardiology, Thoraxcenter, Erasmus University Medical Center, Thoraxcenter, Ba304, 's-Gravendijkwal 230, 3015, CE, Rotterdam, The Netherlands

Osama I.I.Soliman
From the department of Cardiology, Thoraxcenter, Erasmus University Medical Center, Thoraxcenter, Ba304, 's-Gravendijkwal 230, 3015, CE, Rotterdam, The Netherlands

From the Cardialysis Cardiovascular Core Laboratory, Rotterdam, The Netherlands

Luigi F. M. Di Martino
From the department of Cardiology, Ospedali Riuniti, Università degli Studi di Foggia, Foggia, Italy

Huimei Huang, Qinyun Ruan, Meiyan Lin, Lei Yan, Chunyan Huang and Liyun Fu
Department of Ultrasound, the First Affiliated Hospital of Fujian Medical University, Fuzhou 350005, China

Steinbuch and APG Hoeks
Biomedical Engineering, Cardiovascular Research Institute Maastricht, Maastricht University, Maastricht, The Netherlands

A van der Lugt
Radiology, Erasmus Medical Center, Rotterdam, The Netherlands

AC van Dijk
Radiology, Erasmus Medical Center, Rotterdam, The Netherlands
Neurology, Erasmus Medical Center, Rotterdam, The Netherlands.

E Hermeling
Radiology, Maastricht University Medical Center, Maastricht, The Netherlands

FHBM Schreuder and MTB Truijman
Radiology, Maastricht University Medical Center, Maastricht, The Netherlands
Clinical Neurophysiology, Maastricht University Medical Center, Maastricht, AZ, TheNetherlands
Neurology, Maastricht University Medical Center, Maastricht, The Netherlands

WH Mess
Clinical Neurophysiology, Maastricht University Medical Center, PO Box 58006202 Maastricht, AZ, TheNetherlands

J Hendrikse
Radiology, University Medical Center Utrecht, Utrecht, The Netherlands

PJ Nederkoorn
Neurology, Academic Medical Center, Amsterdam, The Netherlands

Maxime Fournet, Elena Galli, Raphael Martins, Philippe Mabo, J. Claude Daubert and Christophe Leclercq
Cardiologie et CIC-IT 1414, Centre Hospitalier Universitaire de Rennes, F-35000 Rennes, France
LTSI, Université Rennes 1, INSERM, F-35000 Rennes, France

Alfredo Hernandez
LTSI, Université Rennes 1, INSERM, F-35000 Rennes, France

Erwan Donal
Cardiologie et CIC-IT 1414, Centre Hospitalier Universitaire de Rennes, F-35000 Rennes, France
LTSI, Université Rennes 1, INSERM, F-35000 Rennes, France
Service de Cardiologie, Hôpital Pontchaillou, CHU Rennes, F-35033 Rennes, France

Anne Bernard
LTSI, Université Rennes 1, INSERM, F-35000 Rennes, France
Service de Cardiologie, CHU Tours, F-37000 Tours, France

Sylvestre Marechaux
Service de Cardiologie, Saint Philibert Catholic University Hospital, Lille, France

Miikka Tarkia1, Matti Haavisto1, Virva Saunavaara1, Tuula Tolvanen1, Mika Teräs1 and Juhani Knuuti
Turku PET Centre, University of Turku and Turku University Hospital, Kiinamyllynkatu 4-8, Turku 20520, Finland

Haitham Ballo
Turku PET Centre, University of Turku and Turku University Hospital, Kiinamyllynkatu 4-8, Turku 20520, Finland
Heart Center, Turku University Hospital and University of Turku, Turku, Finland

Antti Saraste
Turku PET Centre, University of Turku and Turku University Hospital, Kiinamyllynkatu 4-8, Turku 20520, Finland
Heart Center, Turku University Hospital and University of Turku, Turku, Finland
Institute of Clinical Medicine, University of Turku, Turku, Finland

Anne Roivainen
Turku PET Centre, University of Turku and Turku University Hospital, Kiinamyllynkatu 4-8, Turku 20520, Finland
Turku Center for Disease Modeling, University of Turku, Turku, Finland.
6Institute of Clinical Medicine, University of Turku, Turku, Finland

Marjatta Strandberg
Heart Center, Turku University Hospital and University of Turku, Turku, Finland

Christoffer Stark and Tommi Vähäsilta
Heart Center, Turku University Hospital and University of Turku, Turku, Finland
Research Centre of Applied and Preventive Cardiovascular Medicine, University of Turku, Turku, Finland

Timo Savunen
Research Centre of Applied and Preventive Cardiovascular Medicine, University of Turku, Turku, Finland

Ville-Veikko Hynninen
Department of Anesthesiology, Intensive Care, Emergency Care and Pain Medicine, Turku University Hospital, Turku, Finland

Boris Brodkin, Vladimir Khalameizer, Amos Katz and Avishag Laish-Farkash
Department of Cardiology, Barzilai Medical Center, Ben-Gurion University of the Negev, Ashkelon, Israel

Chaim Yosefy
Department of Cardiology, Barzilai Medical Center, Ben-Gurion University of the Negev, Ashkelon, Israel
Noninvasive Cardiology Unit, Barzilai Medical Center, Ashkelon 78306, Israel

Yulia Azhibekov
Department of Imaging, Barzilai Medical Center, Ben-Gurion University of the Negev, Ashkelon, Israel

Nicola Gaibazzi, Guido Pastorini, Andrea Biagi, Francesco Tafuni, Claudia Buffa, Silvia Garibaldi, Francesca Boffetti and Giorgio Benatti
Department of Cardiology, Parma University Hospital, Via Gramsci 14, 43123 Parma, Italy

Roberta Esposito, Federica Ilardi, Vincenzo Schiano Lomoriello, Regina Sorrentino, Vincenzo Sellitto, Giuseppe Giugliano, Giovanni Esposito and Bruno Trimarco
Department of Advanced Biomedical Sciences, Division of Cardiology, Federico II University Hospital, Naples, Italy

Maurizio Galderisi
Department of Advanced Biomedical Sciences, Division of Cardiology, Federico II University Hospital, Naples, Italy
Interdepartimental Laboratory of Cardiac Imaging, Federico II University Hospital, Via S. Pansini 5, bld 1, 80131 Naples, Italy

Yasunobu Hayabuchi, Akemi Ono, Yukako Homma and Shoji Kagami
Department of Pediatrics, Tokushima University, Kuramoto-cho-3, Tokushima 770-8305, Japan

Jelena Čelutkienė, Gitana Zuozienė, Irena Butkuvienė, Birutė Petrauskienė, and Pranas Šerpytis
Clinic of Cardiac and Vascular Diseases, Faculty of Medicine, Vilnius University, Vilnius, Lithuania

Centre of Cardiology and Angiology, Vilnius University Hospital Santariskiu Klinikos, Vilnius, Lithuania

Greta Burneikaitė
Clinic of Cardiac and Vascular Diseases, Faculty of Medicine, Vilnius University, Vilnius, Lithuania
Centre of Cardiology and Angiology, Vilnius University Hospital Santariskiu Klinikos, Vilnius, Lithuania
Room No A311, Santariskiu str. 2, 08661 Vilnius, Lithuania

Aleksandras Laucevičius
Clinic of Cardiac and Vascular Diseases, Faculty of Medicine, Vilnius University, Vilnius, Lithuania
Centre of Innovative Medicine, Vilnius, Lithuania

Evgeny Shkolnik
Moscow State University of Medicine and Dentistry, Moscow, Russia
Yale- New Haven Health Bridgeport Hospital, Connecticut, United States of America

Amir Lerman
Division of Cardiovascular Diseases, Mayo Clinic, Rochester, Minnesota, United States of America

Jureerat Khongkaew, Tharrittawadha Potat and Phatchara Thammawirat
Queen Sirikit Heart Center of the Northeast, Faculty of Medicine, Khon Kaen University, Khon Kaen, Thailand

Dujdao Sahasthas
Division of Cardiology, Department of Medicine, Khon Kaen University, Khon Kaen, Thailand

Christine Prieschenk, Franziska Eckert, Christoph Birner and Lars S. Maier
Department of Internal Medicine II, University Hospital Regensburg, Franz-Josef-Strauss Allee 11, D-93053 Regensburg, Germany

Alexander Dietl
Department of Internal Medicine II, University Hospital Regensburg, Franz-Josef-Strauss Allee 11, D-93053 Regensburg, Germany
Comprehensive Heart Failure Center Würzburg, University Hospital and University of Würzburg, Würzburg, Germany

Andreas Luchner
Department of Internal Medicine II, University Hospital Regensburg, Franz-Josef-Strauss Allee 11, D-93053 Regensburg, Germany
Department of Internal Medicine I, Klinikum St. Marien, Amberg, Germany

Stefan Buchner
Department of Internal Medicine II, University Hospital Regensburg, Franz-Josef-Strauss Allee 11, D-93053 Regensburg, Germany
Department of Internal Medicine II, Sana Kliniken Cham, Cham, Germany

Hongmin Zhang, Xiaoting Wang, Qing Zhang and Dawei Liu
Department of Critical Care Medicine, Peking Union Medical College Hospital, Chinese Academy of Medical Sciences, 1# Shuai Fu Yuan, Dong Cheng District, Beijing 100730, China

Xiukai Chen
Pittsburgh Heart, Lung, Blood and Vascular Medicine Institute, University of Pittsburgh, Pittsburg, PA 15261, USA

Min-Kyung Kang
Division of Cardiology, Kangnam Sacred Heart Hospital, Hallym University Medical Center, Seoul, South Korea

Boyoung Joung, Chi Young Shim, In Jeong Cho, Yangsoo Jang, Namsik Chung, Byung-Chul Chang and Jong-Won Ha
Division of Cardiology and Cardiovascular Surgery, Severance Cardiovascular Hospital, Yonsei University College of Medicine, 134 Shinchon-dong, Seodaemun-gu, Seoul 120-752, Republic of Korea

Woo-In Yang
Division of Cardiology, CHA Bundang Medical Center, CHA University, Seongnam, South Korea

Jeonggeun Moon
Division of Cardiology and Cardiovascular Surgery, Department of Internal Medicine, Gachon University of Medicine and Science, Incheon, South Korea

Lingyun Kong and Xiuzhang Lv
Echocardiography Department of Heart Center, Beijing Chao-Yang Hospital, Capital Medical University, 8 Gongren Tiyuchang Nanlu, Chaoyang District, Beijing 100020, China

Ziwang Li
Department of Cardiology, Jiang Xi Yichun Hospital of Traditional Chinese Medicine, Jiang Xi, China

Jingrui Wang
Department of Cardiology, Beijing Daxing District people's Hospital, Beijing, China

Annelie Blumrich, Sarah Brix, Anna Foryst-Ludwig and Ulrich Kintscher
Institute of Pharmacology, Center for Cardiovascular Research, Charité-Universitaetsmedizin Berlin, Hessische Str. 3-4, 10115 Berlin, Germany

Jana Grune
Institute of Pharmacology, Center for Cardiovascular Research, Charité-Universitaetsmedizin Berlin, Hessische Str. 3-4, 10115 Berlin, Germany
German Center for Cardiovascular Research (DZHK), partner site Berlin, 10117 Berlin, Germany
Institute of Physiology, Charité University Medicine Berlin, Charitéplatz 1, 10117 Berlin, Germany

Cathleen Drescher and Christiane Ott
German Center for Cardiovascular Research (DZHK), partner site Berlin, 10117 Berlin, Germany

Department of Molecular Toxicology, German Institute of Human Nutrition Potsdam-Rehbruecke (DIfE), 14558 Nuthetal, Germany

Tilman Grune
German Center for Cardiovascular Research (DZHK), partner site Berlin, 10117 Berlin, Germany
Department of Molecular Toxicology, German Institute of Human Nutrition Potsdam-Rehbruecke (DIfE), 14558 Nuthetal, Germany
German Center for Diabetes Research (DZD), 85764 Muenchen-Neuherberg, Germany

Sarah Jeuthe and Daniel Messroghli
German Center for Cardiovascular Research (DZHK), partner site Berlin, 10117 Berlin, Germany
Internal Medicine/Cardiology, Deutsches Herzzentrum Berlin, Augustenburger Platz 1, 13353 Berlin, Germany
Department of Cardiology, Charité University Medicine Berlin, Augustenburger Platz 1, 13353 Berlin, Germany

Wolfgang M. Kuebler
German Center for Cardiovascular Research (DZHK), partner site Berlin, 10117 Berlin, Germany
Institute of Physiology, Charité University Medicine Berlin, Charitéplatz 1, 10117 Berlin, Germany

Matteo Dal Ferro, Davide Stolfo, Valerio De Paris, Pierluigi Lesizza, Renata Korcova, and Gianfranco Sinagra
Cardiovascular Department, Azienda Ospedaliera Universitaria Integrata of Trieste, Trieste, Italy

Dario Collia and Gianni Pedrizzetti
Department of Engineering and Architecture, University of Trieste, P.le Europa 1, 34127 Trieste, Italy

Giovanni Tonti
Cardiology Division, 'G.D'Annunzio' University, Chieti, Italy

Bożena Targońska-Stępniak, Mariusz Piotrowski, Robert Zwolak, and Maria Majdan
Department of Rheumatology and Connective Tissue Diseases, Medical University of Lublin, ul. Jaczewskiego 8, 20-950 Lublin, Poland

Anna Drelich-Zbroja
Department of Interventional Radiology and Neuroradiology, Medical University of Lublin, ul. Jaczewskiego 8, 20-950 Lublin, Poland

Giorgio Faganello, Maurizio Fisicaro, Giulia Russo, Concetta Di Nora, Sara Doimo, Carmine Mazzone, Antonella Cherubini, Claudio Pandullo and Andrea Di Lenarda
Cardiovascular Centre, Department of Cardiology, Azienda Sanitaria Universitaria Integrata di Trieste, via Slataper n°9, 34134 Trieste, Italy.

Giovanni Cioffi
Department of Cardiology, Villa Bianca Hospital, Trento, Italy

Maurizio Rossini, Federica Ognibeni, Alessandro Giollo and Ombretta Viapiana
Department of Medicine, Azienda Ospedaliera Universitaria Integrata di Verona, Verona, Italy

Luigi Tarantini
Department of cardiology, Ospedale Civile S. Martino, Belluno, Italy

Biancamaria D'Agata Mottolesi
Division of Cardiology, Institute for Maternal and Child Health, IRCCS Burlo Garofolo, Trieste, Italy

Gianfranco Sinagra
Department of Cardiology, Azienda Sanitaria Universitaria Integrata di Trieste, Trieste, Italy

Jonas Jarasunas, Audrius Aidietis and Sigita Aidietiene
Clinic of Cardiac and Vascular Diseases, Institute of Clinical Medicine, Faculty of Medicine, Vilnius University, Universiteto g. 3, LT-01513 Vilnius, Lithuania

O. A. E. Salden, W. M. van Everdingen and M. J.Cramer
Department of Cardiology, University Medical Centre Utrecht, 3508 GA Utrecht, The Netherlands

P. A. Doevendans
Department of Cardiology, University Medical Centre Utrecht, 3508 GA Utrecht, The Netherlands
Netherlands Heart Institute, Central Military Hospital, Utrecht, The Netherlands

R. Spee
Department of Cardiology, Maxima Medisch Centrum, Veldhoven, The Netherlands

Lina Sun, Haiyan Feng, Lujia Ni, Hui Wang and Dongmei Gao
Department of Ultrasound, China-Japan Union Hospital of Jilin University, 126 Xiantai Street, Changchun, Jilin 130033, China

Index